THE MULTICONTEXT APPROACH TO COGNITIVE REHABILITATION

A METACOGNITIVE STRATEGY INTERVENTION TO OPTIMIZE FUNCTIONAL COGNITION

THE MULTICONTEXT APPROACH TO COGNITIVE REHABILITATION

A METACOGNITIVE STRATEGY INTERVENTION TO OPTIMIZE FUNCTIONAL COGNITION

JOAN TOGLIA AND ERIN R. FOSTER

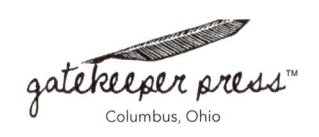

gatekeeper press
Columbus, Ohio

The Multicontext Approach to Cognitive Rehabilitation: A Metacognitive Strategy Intervention to Optimize Functional Cognition

Published by Gatekeeper Press
2167 Stringtown Rd, Suite 109
Columbus, OH 43123-2989
www.GatekeeperPress.com

Copyright © 2021 by Joan Toglia

All rights reserved

Except as indicated below, no parts of this book may be reproduced, translated, transmitted, in any form, or by any means, electronic or mechanical, including photocopying, recording, information storage or retrieval without written permission from the authors.

ISBN (paperback): 9781662903113
eISBN: 9781662903120

Library of Congress Control Number: 2020944570

These materials are intended for use only by qualified professionals

Limited Photocopy License for Appendices: The authors grant non-assignable limited permission to individual purchasers of this book to reproduce all materials in the Appendices for personal use or clinical use with individual clients. This license does not grant the right to reproduce these materials for resale or redistribution, or in other publications, websites, file-sharing sites, internet, handouts or slides for lectures, workshops or webinars. Permission to reproduce these materials for these purposes must be obtained in writing from the authors. Duplication of this material for commercial purposes is prohibited.

Contents

About The Authors vii
List of Figures, Tables, Exhibits ix
Foreword xiii
Introduction xv

Part I.	**Foundational Knowledge and Skills** 1
Chapter 1.	**Cognition, Occupational Performance, and Participation** 3
	• The Central Role of Cognition in Everyday Life 3
	• Functional Cognition and the Role of Occupational Therapy 4
	• Cognition and Daily Function 4
	• Factors Affecting Cognitive Health 9
Chapter 2.	**Functional Cognition: Understanding How Executive Function and Memory Impairments are Expressed in Everyday Life** 12
	• Executive Function 12
	• Memory 28
Chapter 3.	**Self-Awareness, Metacognition, and Self-Efficacy** 37
	• The Impact of Self-Awareness Limitations 37
	• The Dynamic Comprehensive Model of Awareness 38
	• Implications of the Dynamic Comprehensive Model of Awareness for Assessment 43
	• Implications of the Dynamic Comprehensive Model of Awareness for Treatment 44
	• Defensive Denial 46
Chapter 4.	**The Dynamic Interactional Model of Cognition: Activity and Environmental Demands** 50
	• Overview of the Dynamic Interactional Model of Cognition 50
	• Analyzing and Manipulating Activity and Environment Demands 54
Chapter 5.	**Assessing Functional Cognitive Performance** 64
	• Methods of Performance-Based Assessment 64
	• Performance Analysis based on the Dynamic Interactional Model of Cognition 65
	• Dynamic Interaction Model and Treatment Planning 75
Part II.	**Cognitive Rehabilitation Intervention: The Multicontext Approach** 77
Chapter 6.	**Introduction to the Multicontext Approach** 79
	• Overview of the Multicontext Approach 79
	• Background of the Multicontext Approach 83
	• For Whom is the Multicontext Approach Most Appropriate? 87
	• Knowledge and Skills Needed to Implement the Multicontext Approach 88
Chapter 7.	**Cognitive Strategies** 90
	• What are Strategies? 90
	• Strategy Use in the Multicontext Approach 100

Chapter 8.	**Structuring Treatment Activities to Promote Awareness and Strategy Transfer**	108
	• Overview of Generalization and Transfer	108
	• Promoting Generalization and Transfer	109
	• Sideways Learning: The Horizontal Activity Transfer Continuum	111
Chapter 9.	**Introduction to Metacognitive Strategy Interventions and Guided Learning**	121
	• Metacognitive Strategy Intervention	121
	• Instructional Approaches in Metacognitive Strategy Interventions	122
Chapter 10.	**The Metacognitive Framework: Guidelines for Mediated Learning within Multicontext Treatment Sessions**	131
	• Pre-Activity Discussion	132
	• During-Activity Mediation	139
	• Post-Activity Discussion	146
	• End of Session: Methods to Enhance Connections to Everyday Life	150
Chapter 11.	**The Multicontext Approach: Assessing Treatment Delivery and Client Response**	154
	• The Multicontext Approach and Treatment Fidelity	154
	• Client Response to Treatment Sessions: Observing, Tracking, and Documenting Progress	157
Chapter 12.	**Goal Setting and Measuring Functional Outcomes**	163
	• Goal Setting and Adjustment for People with Cognitive Impairment	164
	• Documenting Functional Goals and Progress	169
	• Assessing Outcomes	172
	• Distal Outcome Measures	175
Chapter 13.	**The Multicontext Approach: Putting It All Together**	176
	• Steps of the Multicontext Approach	177
	• Learning and Gaining Proficiency in the Multicontext Approach	177
	• What does a Multicontext Treatment Session Look Like?	182
	• Challenges in Implementing the Multicontext Approach	187
	• Typical Frequently Asked Questions	188
Part III.	**Clinical Applications of the Multicontext Approach**	193
Chapter 14.	**Applying the Multicontext Approach Across Different Clinical Problems or Contexts**	195
	• Client-related Factors	195
	• Treatment Setting	204
Chapter 15.	**Case Examples of the Multicontext Approach**	210
	• Case 1: Inpatient Setting, Stroke	210
	• Case 2: Outpatient Day Program, Traumatic Brain Injury	216
	• Case 3: In-Home Treatment, Parkinson's Disease	222
Resources		229
References		231
Part IV.	**Tools, Resources, and Supplementary Material**	247
	• Appendix A: Learning Activities for Therapists	249
	• Appendix B: Assessment and Observational Tools	285
	• Appendix C: Treatment Forms	313
	• Appendix D: Supplementary Material	359

About The Authors

Joan Toglia, PhD, OTR/L, FAOTA is internationally recognized as a leader in cognitive rehabilitation and occupational therapy. She is an Adjunct Clinical Professor of Cognitive Science in Rehabilitation Medicine at Weill Cornell Medical College, NY; Professor of Occupational Therapy, and Dean of the School of Health and Natural Sciences at Mercy College, NY. Dr. Toglia has over 30 years of experience in Occupational Therapy, with a specialization in neurorehabilitation and cognitive impairments following acquired brain injury. Her advanced graduate and doctoral work in Educational Psychology includes specializations in cognition and learning as well as measurement and evaluation.

Dr. Toglia has contributed extensively to the field of cognitive-perceptual rehabilitation as a clinician, author, educator, and researcher. She has presented over 300 workshops and lectures on cognitive rehabilitation to clinicians throughout the United States and around the world including Hong Kong, South Africa, Israel, Europe, Canada, and South America. Her work has focused on theory, assessment methods, and intervention strategies to support and optimize cognitive function across different populations. Dr. Toglia's publications include a co-edited book, assessment tools, and over 75 journal articles and book chapters. Motivated by a clinical need to address challenges in self-awareness and learning observed in people with brain injury, she is one of the first clinicians and authors to apply metacognitive strategy principles to Cognitive Rehabilitation and hence developed the Multicontext Approach. Dr. Toglia has been recognized for her leadership and contributions to Cognitive Rehabilitation Theory and Practice by the American Occupational Therapy Association through an Achievement Award and appointment to the Roster of Fellows of the American Occupational Therapy Association.

ORCID ID: https://orcid.org/0000-0002-6902-6853
Website: www.multicontext.net

Erin R. Foster, PhD, OTD, OTR/L is an Assistant Professor in Occupational Therapy, Neurology, and Psychiatry at Washington University School of Medicine in St. Louis, MO. Dr. Foster has over 15 years of experience in occupational therapy and cognitive rehabilitation research, with a specialization in aging, neurorehabilitation, functional cognition, and intervention development and testing. Her doctoral work in Rehabilitation and Participation Science and post-doctoral work in clinical investigation and clinical neuroscience involved advanced training in rehabilitation research, neurodegenerative disease, cognitive neuroscience, behavioral intervention development and testing, self-management, functional cognition, and research design and methods.

Dr. Foster directs the Cognitive and Occupational Performance Laboratory, which generates knowledge to guide the development of more effective and comprehensive rehabilitation programs for individuals with neurological disorders and cognitive dysfunction. She is recognized nationally and internationally for her work in functional cognition and Parkinson's disease. She has received federal and foundation funding for her research, which includes studies on cognitive strategy-based interventions and, specifically, the Multicontext Approach. She has numerous peer-reviewed publications and national and international presentations on these topics. In addition, she teaches occupational therapy students in a variety of related subjects and has trained occupational therapy practitioners in the use of the Multicontext Approach.

ORCID ID: https://orcid.org/0000-0003-1625-2125

List of Figures, Tables, Exhibits

FIGURES

Figure 1.1	Cycle of Cognitive Decline	10
Figure 2.1	Executive Functions	13
Figure 2.2	Initiation Deficits on a Continuum from Severe to Mild	16
Figure 2.3	A Functional Example Illustrating the Supervisory Attentional System (SAS) Model	19
Figure 2.4	Two Aspects of Long-Term Memory	31
Figure 2.5	Two Memory Systems with Different Learning Methods	33
Figure 3.1	General vs. Online Awareness	39
Figure 3.2	Different Levels of Self-Awareness	42
Figure 3.3	Activity Experiences Promote Changes in Self-Awareness	45
Figure 3.4	Factors that Influence the Expression of Impaired Awareness and Denial	47
Figure 4.1	Dynamic Interactional Model of Cognition (1992, 1998, 2005, 2011)	51
Figure 4.2	Influence of External and Internal Factors on Functional Cognition	53
Figure 4.3	Dynamic Interactional Model and Performance Errors	54
Figure 4.4	Executive Function Skills of Person versus Activity or Context Demands	55
Figure 6.1	Multicontext Treatment Approach	80
Figure 6.2	Multicontext Treatment Phases	83
Figure 7.1	Conceptualizing and Defining Strategies	91
Figure 8.1	Increasing Transfer Distance: The Appearance of Activities is Gradually Changed	112
Figure 8.2	Sideways Learning	118
Figure 8.3	Limited Awareness and the Continuum of Client-Centered Practice	119
Figure 9.1	Different Ways to Promote Strategy Use	122
Figure 10.1	Metacognitive Framework	132
Figure 10.2	Decision Tree for Pre-Activity Phase	139
Figure 10.3	Summary of Mediation During an Activity and Indications for Use	145
Figure 12.1	Sub-goal Ladder	166
Figure 12.2	Goal Mapping: Breaking Down a Larger Goal into Subcomponents	166

TABLES

Table 2.1	Terminology: Attention and Executive Function	14
Table 2.2	Problem-Solving Stages (IDEAL) and Examples of Dysfunction	25
Table 2.3	Organizational Skills: Function and Dysfunction	27
Table 4.1	Activity Characteristics: Effect on Executive Function Performance	56
Table 4.2	Examples of Functional Tasks: Variations in Activity Demands	57
Table 4.3	Manipulating Task Components to Increase or Decrease Demands on Executive Function	58
Table 4.4	Varying Cognitive Demands of Motor Activities by Changing Directions	59
Table 4.5	Physical and Social Environmental Characteristics that Increase Demands on Executive Function Skills	61
Table 5.1	Performance-Based Testing Methods	65
Table 6.1	The Multicontext Approach: Key Treatment Components	82
Table 6.2	Comparison of Core Multicontext Treatment Components Over Time	85
Table 7.1	Strategy Attributes	92
Table 7.2	Strategy Attribute Worksheet Example	93
Table 7.3	Types of Strategy-Based Intervention	102
Table 7.4	Obstacles to Strategy Use	103
Table 7.5	Characteristics that Affect the Quality of Strategy Use	105
Table 9.1	Hierarchical Cues From Least to Most Assistance	123
Table 9.2	Comparison of Therapist-Directed versus Guided Learning Methods	124
Table 9.3	General Mediation Guidelines	125
Table 9.4	Differences in Type and Content of Guided Questions	128
Table 10.1	Task-Specific Assessment for Making Cookies	147
Table 11.1	Side-by-Side Comparison of Routine and Multicontext Treatment	155
Table 11.2	Tracking Progress Across Treatment Activities	160

Table 12.1	Conventional 5-point Goal Attainment Scale (Turner-Stokes, 2009)	171
Table 12.2	Modified 3-point Goal Attainment Scale for Self-Ratings	171
Table 12.3	Example Goal Rating Scale for the Functional Goal of "Cooking Dinner 1x/Week"	172
Table 12.4	Joe's Goal Rating Scale for the Goal of Decreasing Reliance on Others	173
Table 12.5	Goal Rating Across Treatment	173

EXHIBITS

Exhibit 1.1	Cognitive Instrumental Activities of Daily Living and Variations in Complexity	5
Exhibit 1.2	Negative Behaviors	6
Exhibit 1.3	Social Communication Skills	8
Exhibit 2.1	Behaviors Associated with Working Memory Dysfunction	15
Exhibit 2.2	Behaviors Associated with Initiation Dysfunction	17
Exhibit 2.3	Behaviors Associated with Disinhibition	20
Exhibit 2.4	Examples of Tasks or Situations that Place Increased Demands on Cognitive Flexibility	22
Exhibit 2.5	Behaviors Associated with Reduced Cognitive Flexibility	23
Exhibit 2.6	Summary of Key Executive Function Components	28
Exhibit 2.7	Encoding Strategies	29
Exhibit 2.8	Type of Memory?	30
Exhibit 2.9	Clinical Signs of Primary Amnestic Disorder	31
Exhibit 2.10	Analyzing Memory Complaints	35
Exhibit 3.1	Different Objects of General Awareness	41
Exhibit 3.2	Subskills: Online Awareness of Performance	42
Exhibit 3.3	Key Components of the Dynamic Comprehensive Model of Awareness	43
Exhibit 3.4	Techniques to Increase Self-Efficacy	45
Exhibit 3.5	Key Guidelines to Promote Self-Awareness	46
Exhibit 3.6	Strategies for Managing Denial	48
Exhibit 4.1	Sample Patterns of Cognitive Behaviors	52
Exhibit 4.2	Sample Cognitive Performance Errors	53
Exhibit 4.3	Schedule Module: Same Activity Places Different Demands on Executive Function by Changing Directions	60
Exhibit 4.4	Environmental Modifications that Facilitate Cognitive Performance	62
Exhibit 5.1	Sample Cognitive Performance Observation Tool Activity: Gathering items for a new recipe	70
Exhibit 5.2	Pizza Phone Delivery Task: Analysis of Task Errors (NO cues or assistance provided)	71
Exhibit 5.3	Sample of Multi-step Activity Error Analysis	72
Exhibit 5.4	Sample Dynamic Interactional Model (DIM): Treatment Planning	75
Exhibit 6.1	Goals of the Multicontext Approach	81
Exhibit 6.2	Who is Best Suited for the Multicontext Approach?	87
Exhibit 7.1	Examples of Types of Lists	94
Exhibit 7.2	Self-Verbalization or Self-Talk Strategies	95
Exhibit 7.3	Mental Imagery or Mental Practice Strategies	96
Exhibit 7.4	Examples of Strategies with Acronyms	97
Exhibit 7.5	Activity Management Strategies	98
Exhibit 7.6	Examples of Negative Beliefs and Thinking	99
Exhibit 7.7	Action Plan to Manage Frustration and Anger	100
Exhibit 7.8	Emotional Regulation Strategies	100
Exhibit 7.9	Strategies and Difficulty Level	104
Exhibit 8.1	Explicitly Addressing Transfer during Treatment: Guidelines for Therapists	110
Exhibit 8.2	Treatment Methods to Promote Positive Transfer	110
Exhibit 8.3	Sample Activity Theme: Search and Locate	113
Exhibit 8.4	Multicontext Treatment Activity Planning Worksheet: Increasing Transfer Distance	114
Exhibit 8.5	Sample Multicontext Horizontal Activity Structure Across Treatment Sessions: Basic (search and locate)	116
Exhibit 8.6	Sample Multicontext Horizontal Activity Structure Across Treatment Sessions: Complex Activity	116
Exhibit 9.1	Evidence for Metacognitive Strategy Intervention	122
Exhibit 9.2	General Therapeutic Methods	129
Exhibit 10.1	Components of the Pre-Activity Discussion	132
Exhibit 10.2	Pre-Activity Discussion: Examples of General Questions	133
Exhibit 10.3	Pre-Activity Discussion: Indications for Use	134
Exhibit 10.4	Pre-Activity Questions to Prompt Connections to Previous Activities (Optional)	134
Exhibit 10.5	Pre-Activity General Questions for Identification of Challenges	135
Exhibit 10.6	Pre-Activity General Questions for Strategy Generation	136
Exhibit 10.7	During Activity Mediation: Observe the Process of Activity Performance	140
Exhibit 10.8	During Activity Mediation: When is it Used?	141

Exhibit 10.9	During Activity: Examples of General Mediation Questions	142
Exhibit 10.10	During Activity: General Mediation Questions for Error Recognition (poor awareness)	142
Exhibit 10.11	During Activity: General Mediation Questions for Error Recognition (Partial Awareness)	143
Exhibit 10.12	During Activity: General Reflection on Performance Observations	143
Exhibit 10.13	During Activity: General Mediation Questions that Focus on Strategy Execution and Effectiveness	144
Exhibit 10.14	Components of the Post-Activity Phase	146
Exhibit 10.15	Post-Activity Questions: Examples of General Questions	147
Exhibit 10.16	Post-Activity Questions: General Questions for Awareness of Strategy Use	148
Exhibit 10.17	Post-Activity Questions: General Questions for Identification of Challenges	149
Exhibit 10.18	Post-Activity: General Questions for Strategy Generation	149
Exhibit 10.19	End of Session: Strategy Bridging Methods	150
Exhibit 10.20	End of Session: General Strategy Bridging Questions	151
Exhibit 10.21	Clinician Guide: Multicontext Metacognitive Framework Summary	152
Exhibit 11.1	Common Therapist Errors in Implementing Multicontext Treatment Treatment approach	157
Exhibit 11.2	Key Multicontext Treatment Session Targets	158
Exhibit 12.1	Sample Short-term Goals Consistent with the Multicontext Approach	170
Exhibit 13.1	Steps of the Multicontext Approach	177
Exhibit 13.2	Gaining Foundational Knowledge and Skills: Advice for the Therapist	178
Exhibit 13.3	Assessment and Synthesis of Results: Advice for the Therapist	179
Exhibit 13.4	Observing and Analyzing Strategy Use: Advice for the Therapist	180
Exhibit 13.5	Creating a Horizontal Treatment Activity Continuum: Advice for the Therapist	181
Exhibit 13.6	Practicing Mediated Learning Methods: Advice for the Therapist	182
Exhibit 13.7	Assessing and Documenting Treatment Delivery, Client Progress and Outcomes: Advice for the Therapist	183
Exhibit 13.8	Sample Outline of Multicontext Treatment Sessions	184
Exhibit 14.1	Examples of Focused Goals	197
Exhibit 14.2	Pre-Discussion Example: Goal of staying focused on task for 10 minutes	197
Exhibit 14.3	Sample Cognitive Log	200
Exhibit 14.4	Activity Challenge Log and Plan	201
Exhibit 14.5	Strategies for Spatial Neglect	202
Exhibit 14.6	Example of How to Use the Multicontext Approach Within an Interprofessional Team	206
Exhibit 14.7	Care Partner Log of Everyday Functional Cognitive Challenges	207
Exhibit 14.8	Multicontext Approach: Consistent Group Format	208

Foreword

The goal of rehabilitation is to enable and facilitate human participation in everyday activities that are meaningful to life. It involves helping people acquire key skills and practices which empower them to care for themselves and others, as well as perform tasks and roles of significance to their lives.

The advent of this new publication is both highly timely and long overdue. The Multicontext (MC) approach, initially introduced in 1991, represents a metacognitive strategy-based intervention approach to cognitive rehabilitation, designed to promote and enhance strategy use, self-awareness, and self-monitoring skills over a range of functional activities. This rich approach incorporates numerous functional assessment tools based upon the principles of dynamic assessment, self-awareness, executive functions, and use of strategy; all these tools notably evidence high ecological validity.

At the outset, the approach was designated for people with acquired brain injury; however, over the years, it has been successfully implemented with additional populations with neurological conditions, neurodevelopmental disabilities, severe mental illness, and autism spectrum disorders.

This new book provides in-depth coverage of both the underlying theoretical concepts and key treatment elements of the MC approach and includes many case studies to highlight implementation principles in clinic settings. Importantly, the text provides documentation of ongoing research enterprises that have accompanied the use of the MC approach, thus serving to support and validate the MC approach.

Both authors of this book are involved clinicians, professors, and scientists who have dedicated their careers to treating clients, promoting the MC approach worldwide, and stimulating the conduct of rigorous research on multiple facets of the MC approach with varied populations.

I look forward eagerly to use this important resource book in my personal toolbox, encouraging my students in their first steps as clinicians, and stimulating the research pursuits of my graduate students. Thank you to Joan Toglia and Erin Foster for contributing this valuable book and thereby promoting our profession.

—Naomi Josman, Ph.D. OT (I)
Faculty Associate Dean for Research
Department of Occupational Therapy
Faculty of Social Welfare & Health Sciences
University of Haifa,
Israel.

Introduction

The purpose of this book is to provide practical information, tools, and guidelines for implementation of the Multicontext (MC) approach. The MC approach is a metacognitive strategy-based intervention approach to cognitive rehabilitation that was designed to promote and enhance strategy use, self-awareness, and self-monitoring skills across functional activities. Metacognitive strategy interventions are evidence-based and have been demonstrated to be more effective compared to conventional rehabilitation for people with executive dysfunction (Goverover, et al 2007; Cicerone et al., 2019). In this text, in-depth coverage of the theoretical concepts and key treatment elements of the MC approach provides readers with a comprehensive view of this approach and its application.

The MC approach is a complex, multi-component intervention. A unique focus of the MC approach from its inception has been the integration of learning principles to promote transfer and generalization into intervention design, methods, and techniques. Treatment is purposely structured to maximize the application of cognitive strategies across activities and everyday functioning. Additionally, mediated learning techniques and a metacognitive framework are structured around functional activity experiences to promote self-awareness, strategy use, and self-monitoring skills during activity performance. The focus is on methods used to obtain a successful outcome rather than cognitive deficits, and the instructional techniques are designed to empower the person to figure out performance problems and generate solutions themselves. These are features essential to promoting a sense of control and self-efficacy. This text specifies and operationalizes the key components of the MC approach and provides tools and specific guidelines for its application in clinical practice and research.

The MC approach was initially developed in 1991 for individuals with cognitive impairments resulting from acquired brain injury. As such, most of the examples in this manual are of adults with stroke, acquired brain injury, or other neurological conditions. However, the intervention principles and techniques are broad and have been used with other populations with cognitive or learning difficulties including children and adolescents (Cermak, 2018; Waldman-Levi & Steinmann Obermeyer, 2018) as well as those with mental health conditions (Josman & Regev, 2018). Thus, although much of the content in this manual focuses on adults with neurological conditions, the MC approach can be applied across a variety of populations and contexts.

The book consists of 15 chapters that are divided into 4 parts. Each chapter begins with an outline of the contents and concludes with a summary and key points. Extensive appendices (A-D) supplement the information in the chapters and provide learning activities, worksheets, tools, and other resources that can be used to support the implementation of the MC approach.

PART I. FOUNDATIONAL KNOWLEDGE AND SKILLS

The first section of this book (Chapters 1-5) provides critical background knowledge on functional cognition, self-awareness, the Dynamic Interactional Model (DIM) of cognition, performance analysis, and tools for assessment. Chapters 1 and 2 focus on understanding functional cognition and interpreting functional cognitive performance. A solid understanding of the underlying components of cognition is necessary to identify and analyze cognitive performance errors within functional activities as well as to help clients learn strategies to control cognitive performance errors. The components of executive functioning and memory are reviewed to provide an understanding of cognitive functional difficulties as a foundation for intervention. Information is provided on how executive function and memory deficits can manifest or be observed in everyday activities, behavior, social interactions, and life situations. Clinical examples of functional cognitive difficulties are integrated throughout these chapters.

An in-depth view of the multidimensional nature of self-awareness is provided in Chapter 3. The distinction between online awareness of performance within the context of an activity and general awareness that is outside the context of an activity or specific situation is emphasized. This distinction is important because the MC approach focuses on online awareness of performance. This chapter, therefore, provides important background for observing and interpreting performance as well as for developing an MC intervention plan.

Chapter 4 introduces the Dynamic Interactional Model (DIM) of cognition and highlights how cognitive performance can vary with changes in characteristics of the environment or activity. A framework for analysis and manipulation of cognitive activity demands is reviewed as a foundation for interpreting functional cognitive performance. Chapter 5 builds upon this information and presents different methods for observing, analyzing, and interpreting functional cognitive performance. Examples of practical clinical assessment tools that are based on the Dynamic Interactional Model are described in the chapter and included within appendices.

PART II. COGNITIVE REHABILITATION INTERVENTION: THE MULTICONTEXT APPROACH

The second section of this book (Chapters 6-13) specifies the key components of the MC approach, focuses on treatment methods, and provides detailed information on implementation of the MC approach. An overview of the MC approach is presented in Chapter 6, including its treatment components, evolution, and evidence. Chapters 7-10 provide knowledge and practical guidelines for implementation of each of the three key treatment ingredients (strategies, transfer and generalization, metacognition). Strategies are discussed in Chapter 7 including examples of strategies for various cognitive performance problems. Methods for observing and analyzing strategy use are reviewed. Chapter 8 introduces specific methods for structuring treatment activities along a horizontal continuum that represents increasing transfer distance to promote generalization of self-monitoring skills and strategy use across functional activities. Detailed guidelines for using mediated learning techniques and a structured metacognitive framework within treatment sessions accompanied by sample scripts, examples, and worksheets are provided in Chapters 9 and 10.

Methods for assessing adherence and quality of MC treatment delivery and summarizing client responses within and across individual treatment sessions is reviewed in Chapters 11. A therapist fidelity tool is presented and examples of ways to track, document, and summarize clients' progress within treatment are described. Chapter 12 integrates best practice goal-setting principles with MC approach principles and focuses on measuring and documenting intervention outcomes (i.e., pre- to post-treatment change). Implementation of the MC approach requires a shift in thinking and practice and an investment of time and effort to learn, practice, and apply the methods described. Suggestions and guidelines for the therapist to learn, implement, and gain proficiency in this approach are provided in Chapter 13.

PART III. CLINICAL APPLICATIONS OF THE MULTICONTEXT APPROACH

The third section of this book (Chapters 14-15) illustrates varied clinical applications of the MC approach across different client populations and contexts. Chapters 14 and 15 use clinical scenarios and case descriptions to illustrate how the MC approach can be tailored to meet the needs of a wide range of clinical problems or settings and can be used within interprofessional teams and with family collaboration.

PART IV. TOOLS, RESOURCES, AND SUPPLEMENTARY MATERIAL

The final section of the book consists of four appendices with resources, tools, worksheets, supplementary information, and additional summaries of key concepts, that can be used to implement the MC approach. The appendices are also available in a separate digital file available for download and easy printing (see Part IV, page 249 for website and passcode).

The appendices are organized into four themes: (A) Learning Activities for Therapists, (B) Assessment and Observational Tools, (C) Treatment Forms, and (D) Supplementary Material. These are each described below:

Appendix A – Learning Activities for Therapists: This includes reflective exercises to increase knowledge and skills in the area of executive functioning, interpretation of functional cognitive scenarios, and mediated learning techniques. Sample answers or analysis of selected questions are included.

Appendix B – Assessment and Observational Tools: This includes worksheets for systematically observing, analyzing, interpreting, and summarizing functional cognitive performance.

Appendix C – Treatment Forms: This includes treatment planning worksheets that can be used by therapists, worksheets that can be used with clients (including a sample treatment session), a treatment fidelity tool, and forms for documenting treatment observations.

Appendix D – Supplementary Material: This includes expanded information on concepts from the chapters, guidelines, summaries, and completed examples of selected worksheets.

This book provides in-depth and comprehensive coverage of the MC approach. By presenting foundational knowledge underlying its core concepts, clearly specifying its key components, and providing practical information, guidelines, and tools for treatment delivery, it is hoped that this book will promote wide and skilled implementation of the MC approach in clinical practice and research to optimize the occupational performance and participation of individuals with cognitive impairment.

PART I

FOUNDATIONAL KNOWLEDGE AND SKILLS

CHAPTER 1

Cognition, Occupational Performance, and Participation

In this chapter, we describe the critical role that cognition has in all aspects of daily life and define the concept of *functional cognition*. The cognitive dimensions of key areas of daily life are reviewed and the broad impact that cognitive changes can have on participation in meaningful activities and life roles is highlighted. Additional factors that can affect cognitive health are also reviewed.

CONTENTS OF CHAPTER 1

The Central Role of Cognition in Everyday Life
Functional Cognition and The Role of Occupational Therapy
Cognition and Daily Function
    Instrumental Activities of Daily Living
    Leisure
    Work
    Behavior and Personality
    Social Function
    Emotional Regulation
    Self-Identity and Self-Efficacy
    Coping and Resilience
Factors Affecting Cognitive Health
Summary and Key Points

THE CENTRAL ROLE OF COGNITION IN EVERYDAY LIFE

Adaptive and independent functioning requires the integration and synthesis of cognitive skills. Cognition refers to mental processes involved in gaining knowledge, understanding, and reasoning. It encompasses a broad range of areas, including attention, thinking, learning, memory, visuospatial skills, and executive functions. Cognition allows us to process and assimilate all parts of an activity or situation, as well as learn new information. Therefore, changes in cognition can affect all aspects of daily life and participation. A variety of medical, mental health, and neurological conditions are associated with cognitive deficits that negatively impact daily function such as schizophrenia, acquired brain injury (ABI), multiple sclerosis, Parkinson's disease (PD), lupus, congestive heart failure, critical illness, and cancer (Toglia & Katz, 2018). Even mild cognitive impairments that are not easily discerned by others can affect participation in complex occupational or social activities (Foster & Hershey, 2011).

Executive functioning (EF) has taken a prominent role in contemporary literature on cognition and this manual reflects that emphasis. EF is described broadly as a set of inter-related cognitive abilities that coordinate, regulate and control thinking processes and are associated with the ability to engage in goal-directed and independent behavior (Miyake & Friedman, 2012). This conceptualization of EF includes a wide range of cognitive skills that overlap with attention and memory, including the ability to inhibit distractions, keep track of information, shift focus of attention between task components, adjust to changing demands, prioritize, select strategies, monitor performance and use feedback to adjust responses and actions.

EF plays an essential role in functional performance, wellness, and participation. For example, EF consistently relates to instrumental activities of daily living (IADL), employment, functional outcome, and people's ability to engage in and benefit from rehabilitation (Laakso et al., 2019; Royall et al., 2007; Shea-Shumsky, et al., 2019; Skidmore et al., 2010). Decreased EF has also been identified as a predictor of falls, future stroke risk, and functional decline in the elderly (Liu-Ambrose, et al., 2007). Further, among the elderly, decreased EF increases the risk for institutionalization (Laakso et al., 2019) and predicts difficulty in medication management as well as hospital readmission (Anderson & Birge, 2016; Buslovich & Kennedy, 2012).

FUNCTIONAL COGNITION AND THE ROLE OF OCCUPATIONAL THERAPY

Optimization of cognition is essential for engagement in meaningful occupations and well-being. However, the role of the occupational therapist (OT) is not to isolate, diagnose and treat specific cognitive impairments but rather to use background knowledge of cognition to analyze and promote functional cognitive performance (Giles et al., 2020). The concept of *functional cognition* integrates underlying cognitive skills and everyday task performance (Skidmore, 2017; Wesson & Giles, 2019). It has been defined as how an individual "uses and integrates his or her thinking and performance skills to accomplish complex everyday activities" (Giles et al., 2017, p.1). Functional cognition, therefore, incorporates EF, metacognition, and other cognitive skills within the context of the demands of the activity and environment (Giles et al., 2020). This is further clarified in the following definition of functional cognition, as "the observable performance of everyday activities resulting from the dynamic interaction between motor abilities, activity demands, and the task environment, which is guided by cognitive abilities" (Wesson, et al., 2016, p. 336). This definition specifically accounts for motor performance and the performance context. In essence, functional cognition describes how cognition is applied in daily life across the spectrum of activity complexity to influence occupational performance and participation.

While other team members such as a neuropsychologist provide comprehensive information on the type and extent of cognitive impairments compared to the norm, OTs can provide information on functional cognition. To do this, OTs analyze actual performance across a wide range of cognitively demanding everyday activities and conditions. Functional cognitive performance, which reflects the integration of cognitive skills, is different from performance on structured tests designed to isolate specific cognitive skills. This is supported by studies that have found moderate relationships, ranging from 0.27 to 0.60 at best, between standardized tests of cognition and performance-based functional cognitive measures (Chaytor et al., 2006). The large amount of unexplained variance highlights the unique information provided by direct observation of functional cognition. Information on functional cognition complements that of neuropsychological assessment and provides the multi-disciplinary team with valuable insight into the person's ability to manage expected daily activities, routines, and roles. This is important in planning intervention or post-discharge care (Giles et al., 2020).

OT plays a key role in promoting functional cognitive performance and participation across all of life's occupations by providing skilled evaluation and intervention. This involves analyzing the supports needed to successfully manage expected activities, roles, or responsibilities as well as modification of routines, the environment, and lifestyle. It also includes helping a person cope with and manage cognitive performance problems by enhancing self-efficacy, self-awareness, and strategy use, which is the focus of intervention in this manual.

COGNITION AND DAILY FUNCTION

Instrumental Activities of Daily Living

Cognition, particularly EF, consistently relates to IADL (Mansbach & Mace, 2018; Royall et al., 2007; Vaughan & Giovanello, 2010). Basic activities of daily living (ADL) such as personal hygiene, dressing, and eating are performed routinely or automatically and rely heavily on physical abilities and procedural memory (Mlinac & Feng, 2016). Procedural memory involves memory for skills, procedures, or "how-to" information and is acquired with repetition and practice (Mlinac and Feng, 2016). Because procedural memory is typically accessed and used without conscious awareness, basic ADL is relatively resistant to the effects of impairments in attention, declarative memory, or EF except in severe cases. Therefore, an individual with cognitive dysfunction can be completely independent in basic ADL yet have significant difficulty in IADL such as maintaining a household, shopping, and moving within the community.

Compared to basic ADL, IADL has greater cognitive demands, including sequencing multiple steps or actions for goal completion, multitasking, and the integration of cognitive processes. Indeed, a study of basic ADL and IADL in people with Parkinson's disease found selective relationships with motor and EF such that motor, but not executive function was associated with basic ADL, whereas executive, but not motor function was associated with IADL (Cahn et al., 1998). Numerous studies across a range of clinical populations demonstrate the association between EF and IADL performance (Lipskaya-Velikovsky et al., 2019; Mansbach & Mace, 2018; Royall et al., 2007).

Instrumental activities of daily living (IADL) can be divided into activities that have higher physical demands such as vacuuming, taking out the garbage, sweeping, mowing the lawn, or walking a dog and activities that have higher cognitive demands such as managing money, preparing meals, and planning social events (termed cognitive IADL, C-IADL). Exhibit 1.1 below illustrates how C-IADL can further range in cognitive complexity. Simple C-IADL tasks are more familiar, contain fewer steps, and require less planning or problem solving. Complex C-IADL tasks are more novel, less predictable, and place greater demands on multitasking, planning, decision-making, and problem-solving capacities. Also, complex C-IADL tends to be less structured and may have more than one possible solution. Lifestyle factors and personal experiences affect the extent to which an activity presents cognitive challenges. For example, a cooking task that may be considered complex for some people may be perceived as relatively easy by someone who previously worked as a chef in a restaurant.

Executive function (EF) has been described as a major determinant of health management and maintenance (Allan et al., 2016). The ability to avoid health risk behaviors and maintain a healthy lifestyle directly involves higher-level cognitive skills such as initiating, planning, and decision-making and the ability to learn

Exhibit 1.1 Cognitive Instrumental Activities of Daily Living and Variations in Complexity

Simple C-IADL	Complex C-IADL
• Make coffee, tea, or hot chocolate	• Organize and manage medications
• Heat an item in microwave	• Plan and choose a menu based on a budget and create a shopping list
• Make a simple or routine breakfast, lunch, or dinner	• Multistep cooking task; new recipe with a large number of ingredients
• Determine correct amount of money for a purchase less than $10.00	• Carry out a series of errands at different times
• Address an envelope for mailing	• Search internet and find least expensive plane fare
• Laundry or fold clothes	• Set table for 8-10 people
• Set table for 2 people	• Create and organize a schedule for an outside visitor based on a list of criteria
• Put away groceries	
• Empty dishwasher	• Keep papers and financial records organized
• Place 1 or 2 appointments on a calendar	
• Make a phone call to a family member or friend	• Complete and file forms (taxes, insurance)
	• Create a budget and/or analyze expenses over the past 3 months
• Pack a bag for an overnight stay	
• Send an e-mail or text message to a family member or friend	• Use information from bus schedules and maps to get to a new location, figure out cost to get to a specific location, etc.
• Pay 1 bill	• Reading a map and figuring out directions in an unfamiliar location
• Compare 2 prices and determine the more expensive item	
• Look up 1 item on the internet	• Plan a birthday party
	• Composing a letter or report

new routines or information. For example, adopting a new exercise or fitness routine or new dietary restrictions (e.g., no-salt diet) require modification of existing habits and the ability to maintain, keep track of and monitor progress toward a goal. Compliance with medical or health recommendations also involves understanding cause and effect or the consequences of not following through with health practitioner recommendations (Toglia & Katz, 2018). Indeed, cognition is associated with medication adherence across a variety of populations, and problems in medication adherence, in turn, are associated with poorer clinical outcomes, reduced quality of life, and higher long-term health costs, including hospitalizations (Zogg et al., 2012).

Leisure

Participation in leisure activities, particularly those that entail active engagement with novel information, can be mentally challenging and cognitively complex (Toglia & Golisz, 2017). Leisure exploration and participation necessitate cognitive skills such as initiation, planning, organization, flexibility, and learning new information. This is demonstrated by studies showing decreased leisure skills in people with cognitive impairments. For example, people with ABI experience reduced leisure participation that can persist for years post-injury and is predicted, in part, by executive dysfunction (Fleming et al., 2011). Persisting limitations in meaningful activities contribute to restricted participation in one's community, poorer psychosocial functioning, reduced overall life satisfaction, and quality of life (Toglia & Golisz, 2017).

Work

Work requires many complex cognitive operations such as decision-making, problem solving, remembering tasks and procedures, planning, scheduling, recognizing and correcting performance errors, and communicating with others. It has been argued that work is becoming more mental than physical in nature, posing primarily cognitive, emotional, and social demands (Kompier, 2006). Maintaining or returning to employment, which is a key contributor to life satisfaction and quality of life, is often a problem for people with neurological conditions and cognitive impairment (Gustafsson et al., 2015; Kavaliunas et al., 2017; Murphy et al., 2013; van der Kemp et al., 2019). EF, in particular, has been significantly related to return to work (Fride et al., 2015), productivity (Ownsworth & Shum, 2008), vocational outcome (Wong et al., 2019), and work performance (O'Brien & Wolf, 2010) following ABI across many different studies. Even mild cognitive deficits can have a significant impact on the ability to satisfactorily complete work tasks. For example, Wolf, et al. (2009) found that among people returning to work following a mild stroke (indicating no significant aphasia, spatial neglect, or motor impairment), 52% reported difficulty concentrating, 46% reporting working slower, 31% reported difficulty keeping organized, and 42% reported not being able to do the job as well.

Behavior and Personality

Changes in cognition can cause changes in personality and behavior (Ylvisaker et al., 2005). For example, a person previously described as a "go-getter" and "outgoing" may appear passive, rarely starting activities or conversations with others. Conversely, a person previously viewed as reserved or quiet may now constantly interrupt others, blurt out inappropriate remarks in social situations, and talk to strangers. These two different personality changes reflect deficits in different aspects of EF (initiation and inhibition, respectively). Review the list of negative behaviors in Exhibit 1.2. As you read the following sections and Chapter 2, think about underlying cognitive problems that could explain each of these behaviors and complete the worksheet in Appendix A.1.

Even mild cognitive deficits can contribute to negative behavioral characteristics that may be misinterpreted by others. A person who was previously very conscientious and dependable may now be perceived as unreliable due to a failure to carry out plans or tasks. Subtle cognitive difficulties can be reflected in reduced empathy or reduced ability to put oneself in another person's shoes. The person may appear rigid or self-centered, as they are unable to think beyond the here and now or adopt another person's

---

Exhibit 1.2 Negative Behaviors

- Careless, lack of effort, lazy, unmotivated
- Repeatedly makes the same mistakes, does not learn from experiences
- Does not follow directions
- Lack of follow-through, leaves tasks unfinished
- Lack of concern about others, self-centered
- Rude, interrupts others
- Resistant, stubborn, argumentative
- Inconsistent work, unpredictable
- Irresponsible, not trustworthy, unreliable
- Low frustration tolerance, angry reactions, emotional outbursts that are out of proportion to the situation

perspective. They may be thinking about what they want to do without the capacity to look beyond themselves to the potential consequences of their actions or how they might affect others (Toglia & Golisz, 2017). This is illustrated in Clinical Example 1.1.

> **Clinical Example 1.1 Personality Change**
>
> John went into the room where his two children were watching their favorite TV show and suddenly changed the channel without saying a word. The children started crying. His wife came in and told him to change the channel back, but he refused, became very angry, and started yelling.

In Clinical Example 1.1, John was overfocused on his needs. He was unable to simultaneously attend to the larger context of the situation or recognize why his actions were upsetting to others. He was only able to view the situation in one way. John's wife described this situation as a dramatic change in behavior and indicated he would have never done something like this before the injury.

Family members, friends, or co-workers readily recognize that something is wrong or different but may not understand what the problem is. They may attribute observed behaviors to lack of motivation, interest, incompetence, or psychological issues. Inconsistent or fluctuating performance, that can result from cumulative activities, fatigue, stress, environmental distractions, and small changes in task directions or structure can further compound these misinterpretations. The person may have no difficulty with tasks or act normally on one day and the next day be unable to complete similar tasks or behave inappropriately. Friends may not know how to respond and may gradually stop calling or visiting. Personality changes can create tensions in relationships. Additional support and strategies for significant others are needed to help them understand, cope, and manage these changes.

Therefore, information on perceived behavioral and personality changes is important to obtain, as it can indicate underlying subtle cognitive difficulties that may place a person at risk for functional performance problems, reduced social participation, interpersonal conflicts, and social isolation. Appendix B.1 - B.2 has an informal checklist that can be completed by the client and a significant other to detect perceived changes as a result of brain injury (Toglia & Golisz, 2017).

Social Function

Participation in social situations or activities involves integration of cognitive skills such as attending to and remembering verbal and non-verbal information, organizing thoughts, inferring meaning, making decisions, and processing and interpreting conversations or interactions with people in our social world. Social communication itself involves a complex interaction of cognitive abilities, self-monitoring of speech and language, awareness of social rules and boundaries, and emotional control (Dahlberg et al., 2007; McDonald et al., 2014). Personality, emotions, past experiences, and other factors interact with cognitive processes in social situations (Ybarra & Winkielman, 2012). The term "social cognition" refers to the wide range of cognitive capacities that enable a person to communicate with others, interpret the social context, and engage in the appropriate social behaviors (Njomboro, 2017). This includes the capacity to understand others' perspectives, beliefs, intentions, and feelings, or emotional state. The term *theory of mind* has been used to specifically refer to social-cognitive skills that enable us to interpret social cues and infer other people's (and our own) mental state (McDonald, 2013). Review the list of social communication and skills in Exhibit 1.3. As you read the following sections, think about the cognitive skills that could impact these social abilities (Dahlberg, et al., 2007; McDonald, et.al., 2016) and complete the learning activity in Appendix A.2.

Significant associations between cognitive impairment and reduced social functioning have been reported across different ages as well as across mental health and neurological conditions (Njomboro, 2017; Ucok et al., 2006; Yeates et al., 2004). EF impairments decrease perspective-taking and can result in insensitive, impulsive, or childish remarks (McDonald et al., 2014). Decreased awareness or inability to understand the unacceptability of one's behavior further contributes to conflicts with others. Reduced initiation of conversation or questions and difficulty attending to one's conversational partner may be observed and interpreted as disinterest by others. Communication may be overly repetitive, fragmented, disorganized, tangential, or ineffective. Also, memory deficits can result in forgetting people's names, forgetting to call someone back, losing track of social engagements, missing a close friend's birthday, or a lack of follow-through with plans and promises made to others. Friends or significant others may take these lapses personally, think that the person no longer cares for them, or perceive the person as someone that can no longer be relied on (Toglia & Golisz, 2017).

Social cognitive difficulties contribute to a breakdown of communication and social or interpersonal relationships that leads to social isolation and loneliness. For example, conversations with people with TBI have been described by others as less socially rewarding, less interesting, less appropriate, and more effortful (Dahlberg et al., 2007). The impact of social cognitive deficits on life satisfaction, employment, functional outcome, and quality of life

> **Exhibit 1.3 Social Communication Skills**
>
> - Eye contact
> - Keep conversations focused on the topic
> - Keep track of what was already stated
> - Sustain a meaningful conversation
> - Shift with changes in topic, speakers
> - Wait for turn before speaking and self-monitor one's reactions
> - Start conversations and keep the conversation going
> - Recall and maintain continuity between previous conversations and interactions
> - Attend to and recognize others' actions, verbal and nonverbal social cues
> - Simultaneously attend to the content of conversation and context
> - Express thoughts in an organized way
> - Understand different perspectives
> - Make inferences about the intentions, beliefs, or emotional state of others
> - Anticipate and recognize consequences of saying something that might evoke unpleasant reactions from others
> - Show empathy
> - Awareness and monitoring of one's tone of voice, facial expressions, nonverbal cues, and emotions
> - Ability to interpret sarcastic remarks and humor

underscores the importance of addressing this area in treatment (Spikman et al., 2012; Ubukata et al., 2014).

Emotional Regulation

Emotional regulation is the ability to modulate and monitor one's emotional reactions. People with EF difficulties may overreact emotionally to an insignificant or trivial event. They may over-focus on a small part of a situation and have difficulty seeing the broader picture or they may have difficulty inhibiting actions or responses as in Clinical Example 1.2.

> **Clinical Example 1.2 Emotional Regulation**
>
> Richard was walking into a store and a stranger accidentally bumped into him. Richard reacted with anger because he thought the stranger bumped into him on purpose. The stranger immediately apologized, but Richard started yelling at the stranger, in an angry, loud, and threatening tone. He created a scene and security officers were called.

Richard exhibited heighten emotional reactivity. He overreacted to an insignificant event. His angry emotional outburst was out of proportion to the situation. Richard impulsively jumped to an erroneous assumption and was unable to appropriately control or regulate his emotions.

In contrast to emotional reactivity, a person with brain injury might also exhibit dampened emotional responses with reduced drive, flat affect, or minimal emotional reactions to significant events. Changes in emotional regulation can also result in difficulty suppressing emotions. The person might cry easily or excessively, laugh inappropriately, or become overly anxious without an appropriate reason or trigger. These difficulties can further contribute to difficulties in social communication and personal relationships (Salas et al., 2019).

Self-Identity and Self-Efficacy

Changes in cognitive abilities disrupt the continuity of one's life and can lead to a subjective loss of a sense of self and perceived control. Cognitive characteristics are closely associated with one's identity. For example, a person may describe themselves as detail-oriented, decisive, or highly organized. In the context of a neurological condition, these characteristics may no longer apply because the brain processes information differently, and familiar ways of approaching tasks are often no longer effective. Also, as discussed above, changes in cognition can result in personality, social, and behavior changes that effectively produce a "different person." The person may experience a lack of self-coherence, including a loss of a sense of who they are and what their future might be. For example, the following is a quote from a brain injury survivor:

> *I had almost 30 years of being one way and now I don't think the same, I don't learn the same and there are things I am no longer able to do that I took for granted before. I don't know myself anymore . . . . I am not sure who I am. I can't predict the way things will turn out . . . . I never know when lightning is going to strike. I make stupid mistakes all the time. My brain is messed up.*

The above quote reflects feelings of uncertainty, loss of self-identity, low self-esteem, and loss of control over performance (decreased self-efficacy) that have resulted from cognitive changes. Reported changes in self-identity are common following brain injury or traumatic events and can result in psychological and emotional distress (Beadle et al., 2016).

Cognitive self-efficacy refers to "people's beliefs about their capabilities to use memory or other cognitive skills effectively in various situations" (Bandura, 1995). Of note, beliefs about cognitive capabilities are distinctly different from knowledge or awareness of one's cognitive abilities (discussed in Chapter 3). A person may believe that their performance is outside of their control. For example, they may be unsure if a task they previously took for granted will turn out right or if difficulties might be encountered during tasks that they used to complete relatively easily. Negative beliefs such as "there is nothing I can do" or "my brain is messed up" impede information processing and strategy use, thus adversely affecting functional performance and creating a negative cycle (Toglia & Kirk, 2000). The quote below also reflects low self-efficacy:

> *I can't keep anything straight. I know I am not going to be able to remember this. This is what happens when you get old (have Parkinson's disease; have a head injury, etc.).*

Perceived self-efficacy for the management of cognitive symptoms is consistently related to life satisfaction and predicts quality of life in people with brain injury (Cicerone & Azulay, 2007). Low self-efficacy negatively affects activity choices, strategy use, effort, motivation, and willingness to engage in an activity. It can also increase anxiety or depression and reduce self-confidence and psychological adjustment (Brands et al., 2019). Low self-efficacy, therefore can negatively impact treatment engagement and outcome (Bandura, 1997; Gage and Polatajko, 1994). If a person perceives a loss of control over cognitive performance or feels there is little they can do to influence outcomes, then they will tend to withdraw from cognitively challenging activities and situations both during therapy and in everyday life. In therapy, this ultimately may result in poor treatment engagement and less than maximal treatment gains.

A strategy-based intervention approach will not be useful if a person believes there is little that can be done to improve their performance. This can be further complicated by diminished self-awareness and understanding of the changes that have occurred as discussed in Chapter 3. It is therefore important to help people with cognitive limitations rebuild their sense of self-identity and self-efficacy while simultaneously addressing both knowledge and beliefs regarding cognitive functional abilities using a holistic, multi-component, and strategy-based intervention approach (Cicerone & Azulay, 2007; Toglia, 2018).

Coping and Resilience

Coping with adverse situations requires imagining various possibilities or alternatives to one's current situation and adopting a "what if" perspective, generating new strategies or options, and looking at a situation from different perspectives. These abilities require initiation, flexibility, and abstract thought. It is not surprising, therefore, that EF is positively correlated with adaptive coping and resilience (Kegel et al., 2014) and that individuals with ABI have been shown to have restricted coping skills that are limited in variability (Brands et al., 2014). Reduced coping abilities following a brain injury can lead to increased stress, anxiety, or depression (Toglia & Golisz, 2017). This makes it important to have long-term psychological supports in place to help a person deal with life challenges when needed.

FACTORS AFFECTING COGNITIVE HEALTH

Many factors can affect cognition including poor sleep, nutrition, fatigue, chronic pain, medication side effects, depression, anxiety, emotional status, and physical health. Emotional and physical well-being influence cognition in ways that can challenge learning and make it more difficult to remember, pay attention, self-regulate, plan, organize thoughts, make decisions, and reason (Toglia & Katz, 2018).

The effects of stress on cognition are well documented

(Tsai, et al., 2019). All of us need cognitive skills to manage daily life, but stress makes it more difficult to use the skills we have. Stress makes it harder to access knowledge, plan, prioritize, problem solve, monitor behavior, and use good judgment. Toxic stress or prolonged stress has damaging effects on learning, behavior, and health across the lifespan (Blair & Raver, 2016; Cermak & Toglia, 2018). In contrast, when people are feeling healthy, well-rested, and are more relaxed, they are better able to solve problems, make sound decisions, learn and adapt to change (Majd et al., 2017). Stress management methods such as breathing exercises, meditation, mindfulness, and guided imagery should be considered within cognitive rehabilitation programs to optimize function.

Depression, in particular, has been linked with decreased attention, EF, memory, and strategy use (Bortolato et al., 2016; Zebdi et al., 2016). Similarly, anxiety can interfere with information processing and impair the ability to concentrate and remember. Anxiety disorders are consistently associated with deficits in EF such as cognitive flexibility, planning, strategy use, and the organization and monitoring of behavior (Ferreira & Monteiro, 2018). If depression or anxiety is suspected or diagnosed, treating these conditions may improve cognitive performance.

Mental and physical fatigue, which are common symptoms of many health and neurological disorders, including multiple sclerosis, Parkinson's disease, and traumatic brain injury, can impair cognitive task performance as well (Bol et al., 2010). Mental fatigue has been cited as one of the most significant causes of accidents in modern society (Ishii et al., 2014). Mental fatigue is the inability to sustain cognitive performance and mental energy during increased sensory stimulation, mental activity, or when cognitive tasks are performed for extended periods. A disproportionate amount of time is often needed to restore mental energy levels after a period of mental exhaustion (Palm et al., 2017). Mental fatigue is correlated with speed of processing, decreased attention, and working memory tests (Jonasson et al., 2018). It is also associated with sleep problems, mood swings, irritability, and stress intolerance (Johansson & Ronnback, 2014). In persons with brain injury, long-term mental fatigue is associated with unemployment and uniquely contributes to disability, after controlling for injury severity, executive functions, and depression status (Palm et al., 2017).

The functional cognitive problems caused by these factors can further negatively impact activity performance and participation, self-efficacy, coping, emotional state, and health maintenance. This can create a negative cycle as illustrated in Figure 1.1 and suggests that other health, lifestyle, and emotional factors need to be addressed within rehabilitation programs, to optimize functional cognition or prevent functional cognitive decline (Toglia & Katz, 2018).

SUMMARY

This chapter described functional cognition and how changes in cognition can impact the ability to engage in meaningful occupations. The essential role of cognition in all aspects of daily life, including IADL, health maintenance and promotion, leisure, work, behavior, personality, social function, interpersonal relationships, and adaptive functioning cannot be overstated.

The relationships between cognition, occupational

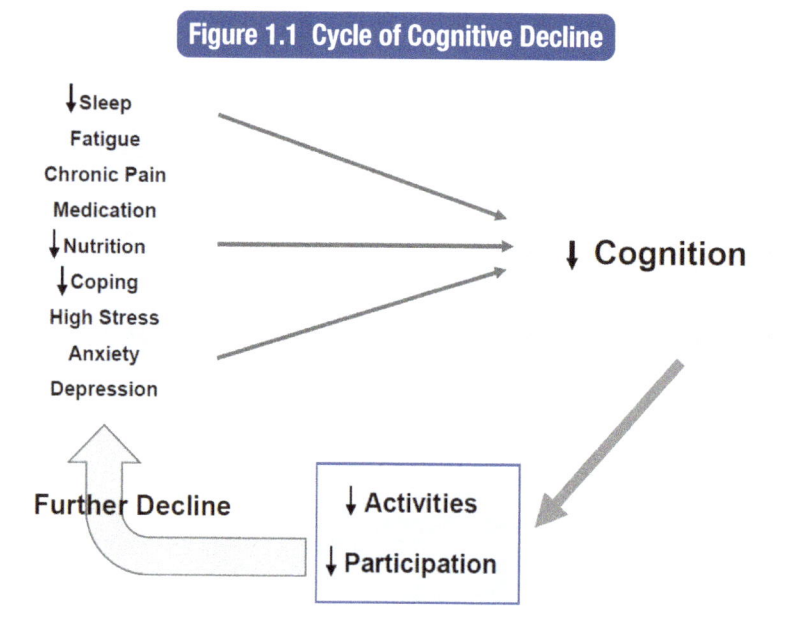

Figure 1.1 Cycle of Cognitive Decline

↓Sleep
Fatigue
Chronic Pain
Medication
↓Nutrition
↓Coping
High Stress
Anxiety
Depression

→ ↓ Cognition

→ ↓ Activities / ↓ Participation

→ Further Decline

performance, and participation are bidirectional and problems in any can result in a downward spiral that leads to further decline. In addition to directly impacting a person's ability to engage in their occupations, changes in cognitive abilities can manifest as negative behaviors or personality characteristics, and this can disrupt interpersonal relationships and communication, decrease social support, and lead to social isolation. Cognitive dysfunction can also have a profound impact on one's self-efficacy and self-identity as well as diminish their coping and resilience skills. These changes, along with other factors that affect cognitive health such as poor sleep, stress, pain, or depression, can create a negative cycle that exacerbates cognitive decline and negative functional outcomes.

Given the critical importance of cognition and its influence across all areas of life, a multidisciplinary team approach is required for successful outcomes. Intervention programs for people with cognitive challenges need to adopt a broad and holistic perspective, considering all areas of functioning and factors that may affect cognitive health. In addition to addressing meaningful activities, this includes addressing psychological, behavioral, and social difficulties. The contribution of OT, with its focus on functional cognition, was discussed in this chapter. However, each team member, including physicians, neuropsychologists, speech-language pathologists, physical therapists, social workers, and family members additionally bring unique expertise and perspectives that together provide a comprehensive approach to treatment.

While this chapter presented a broad view of the impact of cognitive dysfunction on everyday life, the next chapter (2) focuses more narrowly on discrete components of executive function and memory and their influence on everyday tasks or situations.

KEY POINTS

- Executive function (EF) has a prominent role in contemporary literature on cognition because it consistently relates to life activities, social and interpersonal functioning, health, and well-being.

- Functional cognition reflects the integration of cognitive skills within the context of the demands of the activity and environment. OTs have a unique role in assessing and promoting performance in functional cognitive activities.

- Basic, routine ADL have low cognitive demands and are relatively resistant to the effects of EF impairments.

- Executive function is consistently related to IADL. IADL are not all or none but vary in cognitive complexity and are influenced by previous experiences and familiarity. This implies that IADL assessment needs to consider a wide range of IADL tasks.

- Cognitive impairments can be manifested in behaviors and personality changes that are misunderstood and misinterpreted by others (e.g., disinterest, self-centered, lazy, rude, or stubborn). Breakdown of social communication skills and emotional regulation can further contribute to problems in interpersonal relationships and social participation.

- Changes in cognitive abilities can disrupt one's sense of who they are, leading to a loss of self-identity and diminished self-confidence and self-efficacy.

- Lower EF abilities increase risk for negative behaviors, poor coping skills, and diminished activity engagement, which in turn negatively impact emotions, health, and well-being; thereby creating a cycle of cognitive decline.

- Given the impact of cognition and EF on all areas of daily life, participation, and overall health, intervention programs need to adopt a broad, multidisciplinary, and holistic perspective.

Chapter 2

Functional Cognition: Understanding How Executive Function and Memory Impairments are Expressed in Everyday Life

A solid understanding of the underlying components of cognition is necessary to identify and analyze cognitive performance errors within functional activities as well as to help clients learn strategies to control cognitive performance errors. This chapter provides an overview of the main components of executive function (EF) and memory, common clinical signs and complaints associated with deficits in these functions, and examples of how deficits can manifest in the performance of daily activities.

> **CONTENTS OF CHAPTER 2**
>
> **Executive Function**
> Basic Components of Executive Function and the Impact on Daily Life
> - Working Memory
> - Initiation
> - Inhibition
> - Cognitive Flexibility
> - Metacognition
>
> Integration of Executive Function Components and Higher-Level Cognitive Skills
> - Problem solving
> - Organization
> - Multitasking
> - Executive Function Summary
>
> **Memory**
> Memory Processes: Registering, Retaining, Retrieval
> - Clinical Scenarios Illustrating Problems with Different Memory Processes
>
> Types of Memory and the Impact on Daily Life
> - Declarative Memory
> - Procedural Memory
> - Prospective Memory
>
> Memory Summary
>
> **Summary and Key Points**

EXECUTIVE FUNCTION

Given the critical importance of EF skills in daily functioning, participation, and treatment outcome as described in Chapter 1, it is important to look more closely at the underlying dimensions of EF and understand how EF deficits manifest in everyday activities. Executive functions underlie the ability to cope with a cognitively demanding activity. One way to better understand EF is to try activities that are cognitively challenging and require the integration of cognitive skills. Appendix A.3-A.4 has four different EF activities to try with an accompanying reflection worksheet (Appendix A.5).

Executive function is an umbrella term that encompasses the cognitive processes required for adaptive responses to novel, unfamiliar, unpredictable, or unstructured situations (skill acquisition, task challenges). It involves an interrelated set of abilities that allow us to translate intentions into coordinated actions, override automatic behaviors, control impulses, mentally hold and manipulate information, stay goal-focused, shift between ideas or task steps, and manage changing priorities. EF is essential for learning, adapting to new situations, meeting unanticipated challenges, multitasking, and breaking out of routines or habits (Miyake & Friedman, 2012; Toglia & Katz, 2018).

A person with EF deficits may be completely independent in routine activities and situations but may have difficulty performing these tasks in new environments or coping with unfamiliar activities. Repetitive practice of a task increases automaticity and decreases requirements for EF skills so that as a new activity is practiced and becomes routine, the need for executive function skills diminishes. However, if there is a new environment or something unexpected occurs while performing a routine task, EF skills are needed to manage and cope with the situation (Toglia et al., 2018).

Multitasking requirements or unstructured activities that involve initiation of a goal and plan can increase the probability of observing EF deficits (Toglia & Katz, 2018). Multitasking requires coordination and shifting between different subtasks or task components and keeping track of information that may be constantly changing. Unstructured or ambiguous situations also place demands on EF skills because they require asking questions, seeking information, or initiating and generating alternative plans.

EF consists of unitary global functions as well as diverse and separate dimensions that may function independently. For example, executive control has been described as a global EF function that is analogous to the CEO of the brain and helps to select strategies and coordinate and regulate mental activities (Miyake & Friedman, 2012). At the same time, EF includes separate skills that develop according to separate trajectories. There is a lack of consensus on the specific subskills that comprise EF, but the core components of EF that have been most consistently described in contemporary developmental literature include working memory, inhibition, and flexibility (Best et al., 2009; Karr et al., 2018). Initiation is also often included as a core EF component, particularly in literature on stroke and brain injury (Laakso et al., 2019). These core skills are thought to provide the substrate for higher-level skills such as organization, planning, reasoning, and problem solving (Diamond, 2013; Miyake & Friedman, 2012).

Figure 2.1 shows how the basic core components of EF work together in an integrated manner to provide a foundation for higher-level thinking skills and all aspects of life activities. For the most part, the description of EF in this manual follows this contemporary conceptualization.

Of note, traditional conceptualizations of EF described higher-level thinking skills such as planning, problem

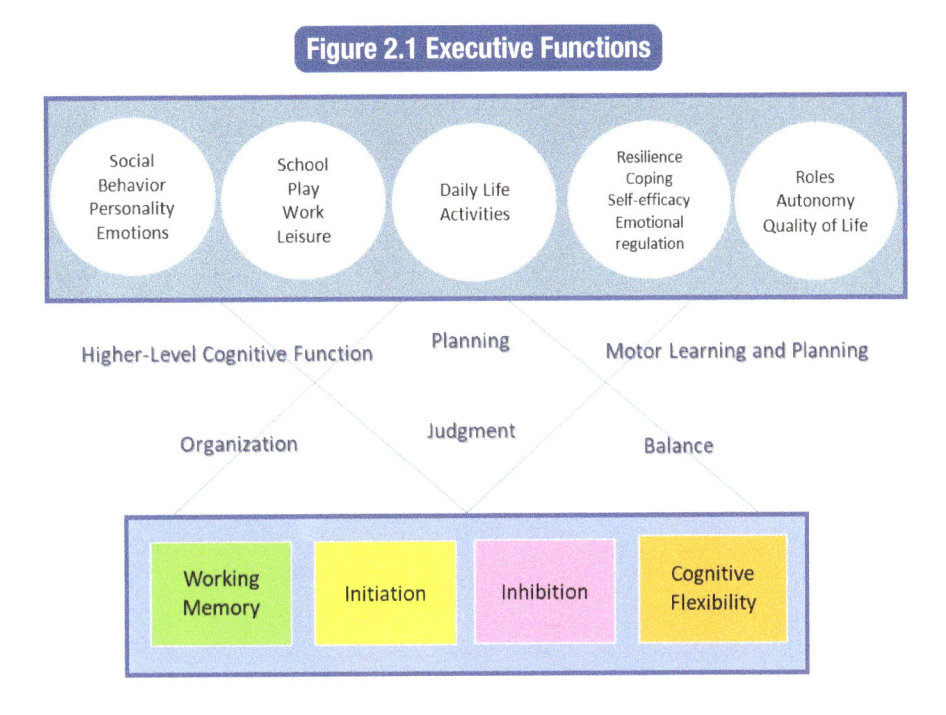

Figure 2.1 Executive Functions

- Social Behavior Personality Emotions
- School Play Work Leisure
- Daily Life Activities
- Resilience Coping Self-efficacy Emotional regulation
- Roles Autonomy Quality of Life

Higher-Level Cognitive Function   Planning   Motor Learning and Planning

Organization   Judgment   Balance

| Working Memory | Initiation | Inhibition | Cognitive Flexibility |

Basic Executive Functioning Components

Table 2.1 Terminology: Attention and Executive Function

Attention Terms	Description	Executive Function Terms
Selective Attention	Focusing on relevant information and ignoring or inhibiting irrelevant information	Inhibition
Sustained Attention	Maintaining mental energy over time or sustained performance and persistence over time	Mental energy
Mental Tracking	Keeping track of information within immediate awareness	Working memory
Shifting or Alternating Attention	Mentally shifting attention, ideas, thoughts, or actions as a result of either external conditions or self-initiated decisions	Flexibility
Divided Attention	Simultaneously attending to more than one task	Dual tasking or Multitasking

solving, organization, decision-making, and reasoning as part of the core EF components that supervise lower-level abilities (Cramm et al., 2015). In these previous views, EF was thought to emerge in late childhood or early adolescence and be localized to the prefrontal cortex. In contrast, and as mentioned above, contemporary conceptualizations of EF consider higher-level thinking skills as a product of EF, resulting from core EF components such as working memory, inhibition, and flexibility (Cermak & Toglia, 2018; Suchy, 2016).

It is now recognized that aspects of EF emerge in infancy and continue to develop into the third decade of life (Zelazo & Carlson, 2012). In addition, EF is mediated by widely distributed and interconnected neural networks that include prefrontal areas as well as other cortical and subcortical structures such as the basal ganglia and cerebellum (Blair et al., 2016). Newer conceptualizations of EF now also encompass what were previously categorized as attentional skills (Diamond, 2013). Table 2.1 lists previous constructs in the area of attention that have been re-conceptualized within the concept of EF. Self-monitoring, or metacognition, is sometimes included within the umbrella of EF (Bjorklund & Causey, 2017; Kennedy & Coelho, 2005); however, others have discussed metacognition as a related but separate ability (Spiess et al., 2016).

BASIC COMPONENTS OF EXECUTIVE FUNCTION AND THE IMPACT ON DAILY LIFE

This section reviews basic EF skills including working memory, initiation, inhibition, and cognitive flexibility. Definitions, descriptions, behaviors associated with dysfunction, and functional examples are presented for each EF component.

Working Memory

Working memory (WM) keeps information "online" or active in one's mind during an activity so that it stays accessible or remains within immediate awareness. Mental information within WM is held temporarily for < 1 minute unless it is actively rehearsed or transferred to long-term storage for later retrieval. WM is limited in capacity. This limitation is defined as 7 +/- 2 bits or "chunks" of information, indicating that a greater amount of information can be held in WM at one time if information is associated or grouped together (Baddeley et al., 2015). Familiarity, therefore, influences WM capacity because it is easier to recognize patterns and associate or group information under familiar conditions. Some models of WM propose that WM capacity depends on executive control functions that make use of stored information in long-term memory (Chai et al., 2018).

WM has been described as a mental "sketchpad" because it allows us to temporarily store information for immediate use and then update or erase it as needed (Baddeley et al., 2015). However, WM is not just temporary storage. It provides the ability to mentally track and manipulate information in one's mind so that comparisons can be made. This is highlighted by the multicomponent model of WM that describes the role of the central executive system in WM, including attentional control and manipulation of information (Baddeley & Hitch, 1974; Baddeley, 2012).

Working memory is thought to underlie a wide range

of cognitive processes including planning, sequencing, organization, problem solving, reasoning, and comprehension. WM deficits are common in a range of conditions across diagnostic categories and ages including attentional deficit disorder, learning disabilities, schizophrenia, stroke, traumatic brain injury, and Parkinson's disease (Duval et al., 2008). WM is also affected by aging. Significant differences have been observed between younger and older adults in WM skills (Chai et al., 2018).

WM includes the following skills:

1. *Short-term storage of information* – Immediate recall of information just presented or maintaining information for less than a minute. This includes keeping information active in one's mind during an activity (Baddeley et al., 2015).

2. *Updating information* – As new information is received, old information is discarded, suppressed, revised, or replaced with the new information from moment to moment. For example, when listening to a phone recording, "press 1 for sales, press 2 for orders," etc., one needs to discard information that is not needed and update or replace it with new information (Diamond & Ling, 2016).

3. *Manipulation of information* – This goes beyond holding on to information and includes selecting, comparing, or manipulating information. An example is searching online to compare prices for an airline ticket: after obtaining a price from one airline, you hold the information in your mind as you search and compare the price to another airline. Another example is mental math: adding the cost of several items to purchase or determining the tip amount and new bill total in your mind (Duval et al., 2008).

4. *Dual tasking* – Keeping track of two or more things simultaneously. An example is listening to the radio or news while making a salad or cooking an item on the stove.

Limitations in WM reduce the amount of information that a person can keep in mind or attend to at once. In a multistep task, this makes it difficult to know where you are in a sequence such as what you have just done and what you need to do next. Similarly, the ability to plan, organize, problem solve, make sound decisions or learn new information will be compromised if a person cannot keep track of all of the variables or all parts of a task or situation (Diamond & Ling, 2016).

Limitations in WM may also make it difficult to keep a goal or goals in mind during completion of an activity. Goals impose structure on behavior and actions. If goals are not maintained in working memory during a task, actions become disorganized or random and activities may be left unfinished or incomplete. This has also been described as *goal neglect* (Chan et al., 2008; Levine et al., 2011). Exhibit 2.1 presents common WM complaints.

Working memory is particularly influenced by fatigue, anxiety, stress, depression, pain, or other internal factors (Johansson et al., 2009; Salazar-Villanea et al., 2015). For example, if one is using WM mental resources to attend to other concerns, worries or emotions, performance will likely suffer. Therefore, it is important to recognize other factors that might influence WM performance.

Functional clinical examples and client quotes are presented to illustrate how WM deficits can impact performance of everyday tasks. After each of the following examples, an analysis of the functional situation is presented. Specific strategies that can be used to help a person manage difficulties in WM and other EF components are included in Chapter 7 and Appendix D.1.

> **Exhibit 2.1 Behaviors Associated with Working Memory Dysfunction**
>
> - I can't keep my mind on what I'm doing.
> - I forget what I came into a room for.
> - I can't do more than one thing at a time.
> - I lose track of what I'm trying to say.
> - I lose track of what I just did.
> - I forget what I am supposed to do next.
> - I constantly have to ask people to repeat things.
> - I have to re-read what I just read.
> - I lose track of information in the middle of a task.

Functional Cognitive Examples of Working Memory Dysfunction

> **Clinical Example 2.1 Working Memory: Work Task**
>
> "I have always used Excel at work, and I am good with numbers but as I went from one screen to the next, I found myself losing mental track of the information. I kept having to go back to the previous screen multiple times. I couldn't hold on to the information or the steps that I had just completed. It took me more than twice as long to complete a simple work task."

This higher-level client indicates that although she can complete work tasks, everything takes her twice as long because she has to constantly review previous steps and information (due to an inability to hold information in mind).

> **Clinical Example 2.2 Working Memory: Cooking**
>
> Carol put pasta in boiling water and then proceeded to make a salad. As she was making the salad, she received a phone call and walked into another room to take the call. After she hung up the call, she went onto her computer to check e-mails, unaware that she had left pasta cooking on the stove.

Carol lost track of what she had been doing after an interruption. Once she left the kitchen to take a phone call, she no longer had a visual cue to remind her of her goal. She became engaged in a different activity. She completely forgot that she left pasta cooking on the stove. Her WM limitations resulted in a failure to maintain or keep track of her initial goal and created a safety hazard (leaving pot on stove). This type of behavior is an example of goal neglect.

> **Clinical Example 2.3 Working Memory: Self-Care**
>
> Kevin was asked to put his comb, toothbrush, toothpaste, razor, and shaving cream into a basket and bring them to the bathroom. He only brought his shaving cream into the bathroom.

Kevin was given a list of directions, but he could not hold all of the information in his mind at the same time. The amount of information presented exceeded his WM capacity. He only remembered the last item that was stated.

INITIATION

Initiation includes the ability to begin tasks and actions as well as the ability to generate mental ideas, thoughts, and plans. Deficits in initiation can result in a reduction in goal-directed behavior and sustained activity (Lane-Brown & Tate, 2010). Apathy or "adynamia" may be present with a flat affect, inertia, passivity, a loss of spontaneity, and diminished interest, drive, or motivation to engage in previous activities. Decreased initiation following brain injury is different from depression because it is not accompanied by the typical signs of depression such as hopelessness, despair, decreased appetite, or sleep (Lane-Brown & Tate, 2011).

A person can have intact cognitive skills in other areas but may fail to initiate and follow through with intentions, plans, or goals. If a task is started, the person may have difficulty maintaining performance. Tasks may be stopped right after they begin. There is often a dissociation between what one says they will do and what they actually do. The person may verbally state that they need to pay a bill and be able to recite the steps but then neglect to fully carry out their intentions unless prompted by others to do so (Oddy et al., 2009).

Figure 2.2 illustrates how initiation deficits can range in severity and affect activities across the spectrum of complexity. At the more severe end of the continuum, difficulty "getting started" may be observed in routine tasks such as getting ready in the morning. If someone reminds the person to get washed or dressed, he or she has no difficulty, but they do not initiate these activities themselves. Or, once activities are started, the person may end prematurely or fail to initiate the next step, thereby requiring cues throughout an activity to "keep going" (Toglia & Golisz, 2017).

Mild difficulties in initiation may only be observed under novel or unstructured situations that require seeking information, asking questions, generating goals, ideas, or plans, or investigating something new. For example, vague or ambiguous directions such as "make reservations for a restaurant for two guests" requires active seeking of information. The person needs to determine day and time, type of meal (lunch or dinner), location, and food preferences.

Figure 2.2 Initiation Deficits on a Continuum from Severe to Mild

Difficulty initiating rote, routine activities	Begins routine activities but stops activity prematurely (needs cues to go from step to step)	Difficulty getting started and persisting in less familiar or less structured activities May not recognize need for action	Difficulty generating and initiating plans, thoughts or ideas in unstructured or complex situations

People with decreased initiation can demonstrate a large discrepancy between performance in structured versus unstructured conditions or between routine versus unfamiliar situations. Although the person may have knowledge and skills to perform an activity, they will exhibit greater difficulties if the activity format or directions are presented in an open-ended or less structured manner. This is important to consider because many assessments and treatment activities are highly structured, making it difficult to observe subtle initiation deficits, particularly within a clinic or hospital setting (Toglia & Golisz, 2017). Exhibit 2.2 includes clinical observations and behaviors indicative of initiation deficits.

Difficulty Formulating versus Carrying Out Intentions

It is important to understand if the observed problems in initiation are related to difficulty generating an intention or formulating goals and ideas or if they represent difficulty translating an intention or goal into action. A person who has difficulty forming intentions or goals themselves may still be able to carry out a plan formulated by others. Initiation deficits, however, can also be related to an inability to carry out intentions once they are formed or provided (Oddy et al., 2009). A person might be able to generate and/or state the goal and all of the steps of a task but still fail to carry out the task. If a person is observed to have difficulty beginning an activity, the following questions should be considered to determine the source of the problem:

- Can the person repeat what needs to be done?
- Can he/she formulate or understand the goal?
- Does he/she know the steps of the task or have a plan?
- Can he/she generate ideas for the plan?
- Does he or she want to do the activity?

An inability to repeat what needs to be done could indicate difficulty in working memory. The person may have not started the task because they forgot what they were supposed to do. An answer of "no" to the questions above, except for the last question, suggests that the person has difficulty formulating goals, plans, or ideas for action. If the person is given a plan or the activity is structured with clearly identified steps, they will likely be able to carry it out, as long as it is something that they want to do.

An answer of "yes" to all of the questions above suggests that the person may have difficulty translating intentions into action. In this situation, providing the person with a plan or additional structure may not help. There is a disassociation between what a person says he is going to do or one's plans and what the person actually does. Stronger cues within the environment such as video prompts, demonstrations, tactile cues, or very specific plans with small and detailed steps may be needed to increase the ability to execute actions. It is also important to differentiate between the person that does not initiate because they do not have motivation or interest to do the activity versus someone who wants to do activities but cannot get themselves started (Oddy et al., 2009).

Functional Cognitive Examples of Initiation Dysfunction

> **Clinical Example 2.4 Initiation: Generating Ideas**
>
> Sue was asked what she could make for dinner and she said hamburgers, but she couldn't think of anything else. Her mind was blank. When given prompts, she could think of additional ideas, but she needed someone to prompt her to keep the ideas flowing.

Sue had trouble generating ideas or brainstorming and experienced a "mind blank." She was unable to access or

> **Exhibit 2.2 Behaviors Associated with Initiation Dysfunction**
>
> - "Just sits there."
> - Slow in getting started or needs help to get started.
> - Appears passive, disinterested, unmotivated.
> - Starts but stops prematurely.
> - Needs cues to move from step to step or to "keep going."
> - Not sure where or how to begin.
> - Decreased idea generation.
> - Decrease in spontaneous behavior and communication.
> - May not recognize the need for action.
> - Lack of spontaneous conversation. Does not initiate asking questions of others.
> - Requires prompts to engage in activities.
> - Has difficulty responding to open-ended questions and often says "I can't think of anything."
> - Has difficulty elaborating on answers to questions or yes/no responses.

retrieve information from episodic memory even though she had the knowledge (as demonstrated when prompted). Sue needed external prompts to think of additional items and did not initiate scanning her environment or asking herself questions (e.g. other meat dinners? fish or pasta meals? side dishes?) to prompt ideas. The ability to generate ideas or brainstorm requires self-questions, self-cues, or mental searching.

> **Clinical Example 2.5 Initiation: Structured vs. Unstructured Directions**
>
> Frank was asked to copy an e-mail. He did so without difficulty but when he was asked to compose an e-mail to a friend he just sat there and stared at the screen. Three minutes went by and he had not done anything.

Clinical Example 2.5 illustrates the discrepancy between structured and unstructured tasks in the context of decreased idea generation. Frank had no trouble copying information that was provided and following directions in a structured task, but he was unable to initiate, plan, or organize his thoughts with open-ended directions. A small change in directions or provision of information can significantly influence performance.

> **Clinical Example 2.6 Initiation: Adynamia**
>
> Kathy scored within normal limits on a neuropsychological assessment; however, there is a marked discrepancy between Kathy's scores on standardized tests and her everyday function. Kathy's husband describes her as someone who has always been vibrant, energetic and involved in many activities. He states that she has changed. She no longer has initiative and appears lazy and disinterested. For example, he indicates that unless prompted, she does not make lunch or dinner. If they are planning to go grocery shopping, she no longer initiates looking in the refrigerator to see what is needed. She does not have the desire to be involved in previous interests or activities. For example, Kathy used to enjoy playing the piano and swimming but now no longer initiates doing so. If prompted, she engages in activities; however, without prompts from another person, she would spend the entire day doing nothing. She takes a long time to get up and get ready in the morning and often sits and watches the same channel on TV for hours. She has little sense of time (date or time of day) and hours can pass without her realizing it. Kathy has no difficulty sleeping and there have been no changes in appetite.

Clinical Example 2.6 illustrates the signs of apathy and the impact of problems in initiation on personality and everyday life. Kathy does not have clinical signs of depression. She appears to be content doing nothing; however, when prompted she engages in an activity. She seems to be unable to spontaneously "get started" with activities on her own. A person with apathy can be perceived by others as lazy, depressed, or unmotivated. For someone who was previously described as vibrant and energetic, this can represent a dramatic personality change. Support for family members to understand and manage these behaviors is needed.

INHIBITION

Inhibitory control is a fundamental component of goal-focused behavior, self-regulation, and self-control (Cermak & Toglia, 2018). Inhibition is commonly described as the ability to suppress or override automatic responses to familiar situations or the environment; however, inhibition also includes other aspects such as controlling interference, attention, motor responses, emotions, or behaviors (Best et al., 2009). This top-down control allows a person to control impulses, ignore distractions to remain goal-focused, plan, troubleshoot, or adapt to unexpected circumstances and changes (Burgess et al., 2006; Chan et al., 2008).

Inhibitory control can therefore be subdivided into the following:

1. *Attentional inhibition* or *interference control* or involves the ability to ignore irrelevant information or distractions and stay goal-focused or "on task."
2. *Cognitive inhibition* involves the ability to resist or suppress extraneous thoughts.
3. *Self-control over actions* involves premeditation or the ability to think and reflect on consequences before acting, as well as controlling behaviors such as the ability to resist temptations.
4. *Self-control over emotions and emotional responses* involves modulating or managing one's emotional state.
5. *Delay of gratification* involves the ability to defer an immediate pleasure for a greater reward at a later time (Diamond, 2013).

Attentional inhibition or the ability to suppress unimportant or competing stimuli allows thought and action to be focused on goal-relevant information. Suppression of distracting information depends on previous experience with the distractors as well as top-down control. Inhibition of irrelevant processing has been described as an important function of selective attention (Miyake & Friedman 2012). If all information presented is perceived to have equal importance, one is unable to focus, set priorities, make decisions, or solve problems. This can result in a tendency to become easily overwhelmed. Environments or tasks with an increased number of stimuli place greater demands on attentional inhibition or the ability to manage distractions. Inhibitory control of attention is critically important to selectively focus on goals and complete everyday tasks (van Moorselaar & Slagter, 2020).

Several theoretical models can be used to explain disinhibition. The Supervisory Attentional System (SAS) model (Shallice & Burgess, 1991) explains it as a problem with top-down executive control in the following way: Behavior in novel or unpredictable situations and routine situations require different levels of attentional resources or executive control. Routine and familiar situations require little executive control and instead are driven in a "bottom-up" manner by the immediate environment and external stimuli. In contrast, in non-routine situations, the SAS is responsible for exerting top-down executive control to override automatic, habitual, or reflexive responses to external stimuli and response in a flexible manner. This top-down control allows a person to inhibit impulses, plan, troubleshoot, or adapt to unexpected circumstances and changes. Prefrontal cortical regions are thought to support this controlled processing. Impairments of the SAS reduce top-down executive control and result in the expression of lower level, habitual responses. Behaviors are more immediate, automatic, and dependent on environmental influence (stimulus-bound, environmental dependency).

Individuals with a lack of top-down control can easily become sidetracked, fail to "stay on task," and stray away from the goal (e.g., goal neglect). Figure 2.3 illustrates the functional application of the SAS model. In Figure 2.3, the person has a goal to enter the store to buy milk. As the person enters the store, attention is automatically captured by salient, but irrelevant items in the environment (bright signs for bakery items, announcement of items on sale). The person wanders over to the bakery section and purchases several items but returns home without the milk. In this situation, inability to inhibit irrelevant stimuli resulted in goal neglect or failure to maintain actions toward the goal. Top-down control helps the person inhibit distractions and remain goal focused (buying milk). If top-down control is inactivated or impaired, behavior is triggered automatically by environmental stimuli (bright signs) and the person is unable to inhibit distractions or automatic actions.

Other models explain this lack of goal-focused behavior as a limitation in processing resources, such as WM (Chan et al., 2008; Levine et al., 2011). The person is unable to simultaneously maintain the goal in WM while performing the activity. As the initial goal and plan fade, actions become disorganized and the person strays away from the goal (Chan et al., 2008; Levine et al., 2011). Goal neglect, therefore, can be related to limitations in working memory, disinhibition, or a combination of both.

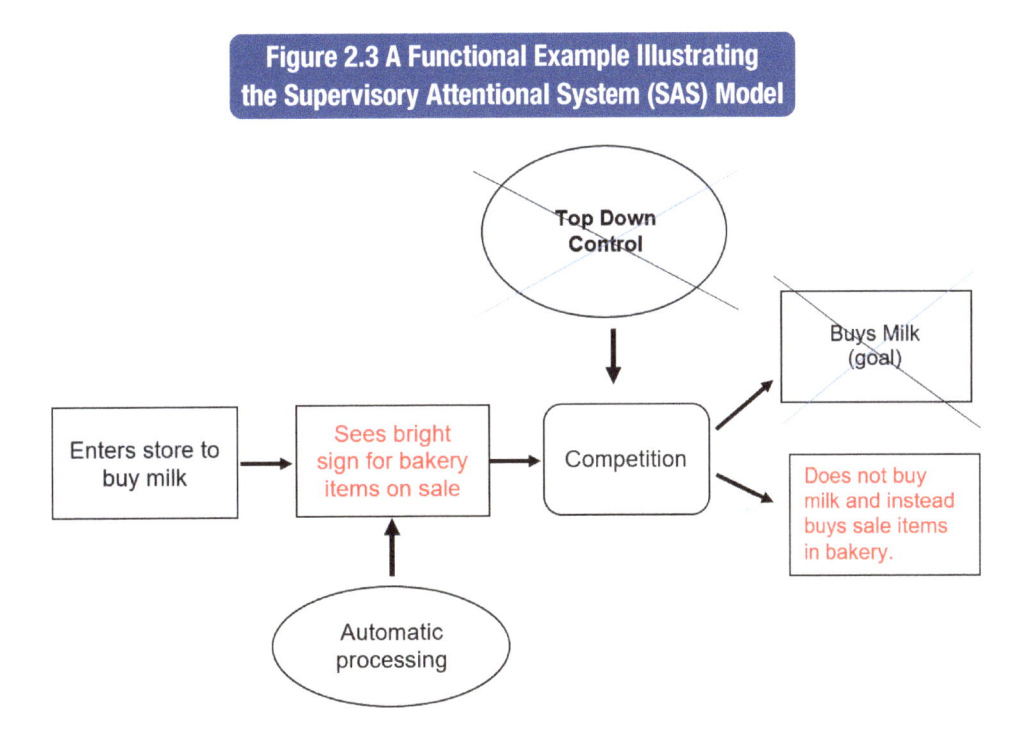

Figure 2.3 A Functional Example Illustrating the Supervisory Attentional System (SAS) Model

The ability to resist impulsive responses and distractions, to stop a behavior at the appropriate time, and to regulate emotional responses contributes to goal-directed behavior. Disinhibition can be observed as difficulty withholding responses or stopping ongoing activity, failure to pace speed of actions, failure to analyze situations before acting or speaking, difficulty ignoring irrelevant or competing information, limited perseverance, and an inability to delay gratification. Exhibit 2.3 lists behaviors that are indicative of disinhibition.

Individuals with decreased inhibitory control tend to exhibit actions that are triggered automatically by external stimuli (e.g., social or physical environment) rather than executed in a controlled and deliberate manner according to internal stimuli (e.g., goals). Similar to problems in initiation, inhibition deficits can be observed on a continuum ranging from severe deficits in impulsivity and distractibility that overshadow performance on nearly all daily tasks to those that are only observed in unfamiliar, challenging, or novel situations.

As an extreme example, the sight of an object may cause the person to grab it and start using it at an inappropriate time. This has been termed as *utilization behavior* or *environmental dependency* (Besnard et al., 2011). Actions are triggered automatically by environmental stimuli, rather than by top-down, internal executive control.

Disinhibition is also linked to behavioral disturbances and difficulty in self-regulation, or emotional regulation (Diamond, 2013). Impulsive behaviors can result in increased irritability, loss of temper, emotional outbursts, decreased frustration tolerance, impatience, and poor decision-making or judgment abilities (Rochat et al., 2010).

Functional Cognitive Examples of Disinhibition

Clinical Example 2.7 Disinhibition: Organizing Medications

Martha was asked to put pills in a medication organizer according to a medication schedule. She immediately began putting pills into the organizer, even though she had not yet been given the medication schedule. As a result, the majority of pills in the organizer did not correspond to the schedule.

Martha saw the familiar medication organizer, and this triggered an automatic response of filling the organizer with pills. Her behavior was driven by the stimulus (medication organizer) rather than adhering to the medication schedule through top-down control. Normally, EF skills override automatic actions or habits and allow a person to adhere to task requirements.

Clinical Example 2.8 Disinhibition: Incomplete Tasks

In an interview, Sarah stated, "I have become more and more scattered when I do things at home. For example, I may start to make something for lunch; then while doing that, I come across an item that needs to be in the bathroom. While in the bathroom, I find a book that I was reading and put it in the bedroom, where I start hanging clothes in the closet which is all disorganized, so I start taking everything from the closet shelves and start to rearrange them. Then . . . I remember that I was making lunch. . . . It's not harder; it just takes much longer."

Sarah is unable to complete tasks. She moves randomly from one task to another and becomes easily sidetracked by extraneous items that capture her attention. Behavior is driven by salient stimuli in the environment and Sarah easily strays from the goal. She is unable to suppress irrelevant information or distractions in her environment (attentional inhibition) and, as a result, behavior lacks focus and goal direction. Sarah may eventually complete her tasks, but overall performance appears to be haphazard, inefficient and requires increased time.

Exhibit 2.3 Behaviors Associated with Disinhibition

- Impulsive – does not think before acting or talking
- Makes careless mistakes
- Does or says embarrassing things when in the company of others
- Interrupts others
- Jumps into tasks without planning ahead or thinking of consequences
- Begins a task before reading or listening to all of the directions or determining if they have the needed materials
- Distracted by irrelevant information
- Gets sidetracked or easily goes "off-task"
- Exhibits lack of perseverance or persistence (jumps from one thing to the next)
- Displays excessive emotions or overreactions to situations
- Easily overwhelmed – cannot inhibit irrelevant or extraneous information
- Makes quick decisions without stopping to think things through
- Appears to disregard boundaries or rules

> **Clinical Example 2.9 Disinhibition: Making a Sandwich**
>
> Jayden was asked to make lunch and chose a ham and cheese sandwich. He immediately started the task and went to the refrigerator before directions were completed. He ate the cheese and some of the ham before he brought it to the table. Jayden removed items from the refrigerator very quickly. In the process, he mistook salad dressing for mustard and took out English muffins instead of bread. He had to make numerous trips back and forth to the refrigerator to return incorrect items and to retrieve items needed.

Jayden has difficulty inhibiting actions. He jumped into the task without preplanning or carefully gathering needed items. He exhibited a lack of self-control or an inability to delay gratification by eating items for the sandwich as soon as he saw them. He also selected multiple irrelevant items, suggesting an automatic response to salient stimuli or impulsive actions that resulted in a lack of attention to detail.

COGNITIVE FLEXIBILITY

Two dimensions of cognitive flexibility have been described: reactive flexibility and spontaneous flexibility (Eslinger & Grattan, 1993). Reactive flexibility involves task switching or shifting behaviors, actions, attentional focus, or plans according to task demands or the context of a situation. Spontaneous flexibility is the ability to generate a variety of ideas or shift perspectives as a result of self-initiated decisions. Both types of flexibility are needed for higher-level thinking, reasoning, and problem solving (Rende, 2000; Whiting et al., 2015).

Task switching, a key aspect of reactive flexibility, refers to the ability to shift between task steps, rules, activities, or situations. Successful task switching involves inhibition of previous responses or activated mental sets (Best et al., 2009). Inflexibility in task switching is observed as perseveration. Perseveration is defined as repetition or continuation of a previous activity or response without the appropriate stimulus. The person is unable to terminate their current responses or activity and instead may repeat the same actions, errors, ideas, or thoughts multiple times (Sandson & Albert, 1984). Four forms of perseveration are distinguished in the literature (Hotz & Helm-Estabrooks, 1995; Sandson & Albert, 1984):

1. *Perseveration of activities* or *stuck-in-set perseveration* involves inappropriate maintenance of a current mental set, concept, or activity so that the person is unable to adapt to a new situation. For example, a person may be unable to shift from addition of numbers to subtraction or multiplication.

2. *Recurrent perseveration* involves unintentional repetition of a specific response after an intervening stimulus or response. For example, a person who is asked what he had for lunch indicates *grilled cheese,* salad, Jell-o, milk, and *grilled cheese.*

3. *Continuous perseveration* involves inappropriate repetition of a current action within a task, without interruption. For example, a person writing the word "gym" wrote the word as "gymmmmm."

4. *Ideational perseveration* involves the inappropriate repetition of an idea or thought. For example, the person brings up the same topic multiple times during a conversation.

Tasks that are presented quickly (one after another) or that involve shifting back and forth between two or more different tasks, moving from one step to another, or that have changing rules and circumstances present particular challenges for a person with decreased flexibility. Also, changes that are unpredictable or occur without warning present a higher level of challenge compared to tasks that have a predictable, alternating pattern of expected responses.

Similarities and differences between tasks also appear to influence task switching. For example, it is easier to shift between very different tasks such as bouncing a ball and combing hair. It is more difficult to shift between similar tasks or steps, such as moving from one related topic to the next in a conversation or shifting between steps when making dinner (preparing salad, checking on and basting a roast in the oven, checking vegetables cooking on the stove). Similarly, a person with moderate or severe inflexibility will likely have difficulty switching between using a knife for spreading butter and cutting. Exhibit 2.4 provides examples of situations or tasks that may pose difficulties for a person with cognitive flexibility impairment.

Modification of actions, behaviors, plans, or activities based on changing circumstances is important in adjusting or adapting to new, unexpected, or challenging daily life situations. Similarly, modification of the environment to make tasks or emotions more manageable or change the course of a situation is also a key aspect of flexibility and adaptation (Salas et al., 2019).

Milder deficits in cognitive flexibility are not always readily observable. A person may tend to exhibit a "stickiness of thinking": they have difficulty shifting mindsets, letting go of a thought or idea, and coping with unanticipated changes or events. For example,

> **Exhibit 2.4 Examples of Tasks or Situations that Place Increased Demands on Cognitive Flexibility**
>
> - Shifting with topic shifts in a conversation or discussion
> - Changes in rules or directions on the same page or within the same activity
> - Moving from one activity to another within a session
> - Difficulty with sorting tasks that require shifting back and forth to different groups or categories
> - Emptying dishwasher and placing glasses in one cabinet and cups in a different cabinet
> - Shifting between numerical operations (e.g., adding, subtracting)
> - Following a multi-step activity (shifting from step to step)
> - Shifting between different tasks (multitasking)
> - Shifts in story plot or characters when watching TV or reading a story
> - Tasks that require a trial and error approach
> - Coming up with alternative activity plans (e.g., if it starts raining on the way to the pool; if the restaurant has run out of the dish you wanted to order)
> - Brainstorming ideas or alternative solutions to problems

if plans to go to a movie have changed, the person may have difficulty adapting to the new plans. Transitions or changes to regular routines, environments, or activities can be particularly challenging. The person may also exhibit changes in personality or behavior and appear self-centered, close-minded, argumentative, and stubborn because they are only able to view situations in one way. In addition to cognitive flexibility, the person may have difficulty modifying their emotional reactions in response to environmental changes. This has been also termed as *affective shifting* (Salas et al., 2019).

Cognitive flexibility allows us to view situations from different perspectives, produce a variety of ideas, generate alternative responses, and adjust responses based on feedback or circumstances. Decreased flexibility can result in a rigid, ineffective approach to problem solving. The person may overfocus on one aspect of a task or situation, view a situation in just one way, or be unable to alter responses when faced with obstacles. The same solution or methods are tried repeatedly, even though it is clear that they are not working. There is an inability to think about the problem in different ways or generate alternate methods or solutions (Rende, 2000). Similarly, the ability to cope with a disability involves having a repertoire of flexible strategies so that options or alternatives to one's situation can be considered as described in Chapter 1.

The ability to brainstorm ideas, "think outside the box", represent the same information in different ways, mentally consider different connections and possibilities, imagine "what if?" or think abstractly all require spontaneous and reactive cognitive flexibility and are key components of learning, higher-level thinking, creativity, and generalization (Diamond, 2013). Exhibit 2.5 lists clinical signs and symptoms associated with reduced cognitive flexibility. Functional Cognitive examples are presented below.

Functional Cognitive Examples of Reduced Cognitive Flexibility

> **Clinical Example 2.10 Inflexibility: Wearing the Same Clothes**
>
> Tom wears the same shirt and pants every day, even though he acknowledges they are dirty and need to be washed. He also brings up the same topic for discussion (getting a new apartment) multiple times during a treatment session. When asked if he already brought up the topic, he acknowledges that he did, but proceeds to talk about the same issues again.

Tom has difficulty with changes in routines. He knows that his shirt should be washed and that the same topic had been brought up before in conversations, but he continues with the same clothes and topics. He has difficulty "letting go" and adapting to change.

> **Clinical Example 2.11 Inflexibility: Alternate Solutions**
>
> One day, Jim unintentionally arrived two hours early for his physical therapy appointment because he had written down the wrong time. When confronted with two free hours, Jim decided to sit in his car. He later told his therapist that he wanted to do something productive with his time but could not think of a different activity to fill the hours. Instead, he sat in his car waiting for the two hours to pass.

Jim knew there was a problem. He came up with one solution (sit in car) and could not generate other alternative solutions (reduced spontaneous flexibility). This is similar to idea generation discussed under initiation. It might be that Jim could not initiate mental searching or self-cues to

> **Exhibit 2.5 Behaviors Associated with Reduced Cognitive Flexibility**
>
> - Rigid, fixated on ideas, actions, or thoughts
> - Repeats the same actions, errors, or verbal statements (perseveration)
> - Brings up the same argument multiple times (can't let it go)
> - Brings up the same topic of conversation multiple times
> - Finds it hard to stop repeating, saying or doing things once started
> - Lack of variability in response
> - Difficulty with movements or actions requiring rapid shifts in directions
> - Slowness in serial tasks
> - Unable to adjust responses or behavior with feedback
> - Irritation or confusion with any sudden changes in the environment, situation, or routine
> - May appear rigid, stubborn, inflexible, unwilling to compromise
> - Intolerance to change in routine, schedules, or plans
> - Unable to adjust approach or deal with unexpected obstacles or situations
> - Difficulty making transitions between activities
> - Difficulty thinking of alternate solutions to problems or brainstorming

generate ideas, but it could also be that Jim perseverated on just one solution or idea and could not let it go. Inability to generate ideas may be related to initiation, reduced flexibility, or a combination of both.

> **Clinical Example 2.12 Inflexibility: Adjusting Methods**
>
> Bill is putting together a new toy that he ordered for his daughter. Two of the parts are not fitting together because he has them lined up incorrectly. Instead of reading the instructions or rotating the pieces, he continues to try to force them together and eventually ends up breaking one of them. He gets very angry and calls customer service to complain that the toy was either not made properly, or they sent him the wrong parts.

Bill persisted in using the same incorrect method of fitting the toy parts together, even though it was apparent it was not working. He was unable to change or adjust his approach. He could not recognize that there may have been an alternate solution and instead blamed it on the toy manufacturer.

METACOGNITION

Metacognition is central to the Multicontext (MC) approach and is covered in depth in Chapters 3, 9 and 10. It is briefly mentioned here since it is often included as a component of EF. Metacognition is a broad term that involves knowledge, thinking, and reflection about one's cognition and how one goes about learning (Bjorklund & Causey, 2017). Flavell et al. (2002) described metacognition as including two main aspects:

1. *Self-knowledge of oneself, task, and strategies* – This includes knowledge of one's cognitive strengths and limitations and their interactions with task demands as well as knowledge about when, why, and how to use strategies.

2. *Self-monitoring and self-regulation* – This involves planning, self-questioning, checking work to detect or recognize errors, correcting errors, monitoring progress toward goals, using strategies when needed, and reflecting on and assessing one's own performance.

The Dynamic Comprehensive Model of Awareness (DCMA) (Toglia & Kirk, 2000) discussed in Chapter 3 integrates literature on self-awareness, self-efficacy, and metacognition as a foundation for assessment and treatment.

INTEGRATION OF EXECUTIVE FUNCTION COMPONENTS AND HIGHER-LEVEL COGNITIVE SKILLS

As described previously, EF can be thought of as including both distinct and separate components (i.e., WM, initiation, inhibition, and cognitive flexibility) and unitary global functions (e.g., cognitive control) that work together in an integrated manner to coordinate and control other cognitive operations (Miyake & Friedman, 2012). According to most current conceptual models, these EF capacities provide the foundation for higher-level cognitive skills including planning, sequencing, multitasking, problem solving, organization, reasoning, abstraction, decision-making, and self-regulation. These skills have also been described as "executive cognitive function skills" or ECFs and differentiated from more basic executive functions or EF (Suchy, 2016). From this perspective, higher-level cognitive skills or ECFs are a product of the integration of EF components and control functions. In this way, people can exhibit difficulty in higher-level cognitive skills for many different reasons (Toglia & Katz, 2018).

For example, a person can have difficulty sequencing an activity due to difficulty keeping track of the steps (WM), inability moving to the next step (initiation and/or flexibility), tendency to become sidetracked (inhibition and/or WM), repeat previous steps (flexibility or WM), or a failure to self-check and monitor performance (metacognition).

Similarly, abstraction requires the ability to simultaneously hold in mind all qualities of an object, experience, or situation (WM), whereas a concrete way of dealing with situations is to overfocus or react to only one aspect. Abstraction also requires focusing on the most relevant qualities while looking beyond the immediate experience or stimulus (inhibition), viewing different perspectives to formulate hypotheses or "what ifs," and using imagination/creativity (initiation and flexibility). This integration of EF skills allows us to think symbolically or use analogies, reflect on previous experiences, formulate perspectives for the future, and plan goals. In contrast, *concreteness* is characterized by an inability to disassociate oneself from one's immediate surroundings (Goldstein, 1990). Stimuli are responded to as if they existed only in the setting that they are presented (environmental dependency). The person is "stuck in the moment" and has difficulty thinking beyond their current thoughts, perspective, or situation and seeing the broader picture. It should be noted that concrete thinking has also been described as an attitude or mode of functioning that influences one's interpretation of experiences (Salas et al., 2013).

Below we use the examples of problem solving, organization, and multitasking to further illustrate how higher-level cognitive skills involve the combination and coordination of core EF components as well as other cognitive processes and how dysfunction in these skills can arise from many sources.

PROBLEM SOLVING

Here, we use the Bransford and Stein (1993) IDEAL model of problem solving (Table 2.2) to show how poor problem solving can result from a variety of cognitive behaviors, which themselves may be caused by impairment in a number of component cognitive processes.

It is helpful to keep the IDEAL problem-solving stages in mind as well as the wide variety of behaviors that could contribute to performance breakdown as a person attempts to manage problems or obstacles during performance.

Functional Cognitive Example of Problem Solving

The below scenario presents a problem and four deficient methods for solving the problem. Each flawed solution reflects different aspects of EF dysfunction.

John parked his car in a large parking garage at a mall two hours away from his house. He could not find the car when he returned to the garage.

Sample of deficient problem solving that might be observed with EF deficits:

1a. John immediately assumed the car was stolen and called the police to report the car as stolen without looking further or considering that he forgot where he had parked it.

   Analysis: Impulsively jumps to a conclusion without considering other possibilities and does not define the problem accurately.

1b. Later, he found the car but did not call the police back to explain he had found it.

   Analysis: Focuses on the "here and now" and does not think ahead to consider possible consequences of not calling the police back to let them know the car was found (does not identify problem).

2. John walks around the same floor or area repeatedly looking for his car and becomes increasingly frustrated. He does not remember where he parked it and does not know what else to do.

   Analysis: John is unable to generate alternative solutions and is stuck on using the same method of searching (difficulty initiating or exploring other strategies).

3. John realizes he forgot where he parked his car and is overwhelmed because the garage is so big. He decides to call a friend, but his friend is not answering the phone. He walks randomly to different floors and areas without a systematic search plan. He walks outside and sees a hotel across the street. He checks in and stays there overnight without a plan.

   Analysis: John generates random and inefficient methods solutions without a clear plan (difficulty in exploring strategies)

4. John thinks of a systematic plan to search each floor, but as he is walking around, he is text messaging his friends, stopping at vending machines, talking to strangers, answering phone calls and he loses

track of which floor he is on and which floors were already searched.

Analysis: John thinks of a plan but is unable to carry out the plan effectively (difficulty in the execution of the plan due to difficulty with inhibiting distractions and keeping track of information).

ORGANIZATION

Similar to problem solving, the concept of organization is also very broad. Different types of organizational skills are identified in Table 2.3. These different types of organizational skills are not necessarily related. For example, a person may have difficulty organizing time

Table 2.2 Problem-Solving Stages (IDEAL) and Examples of Dysfunction

Problem-solving Stage	Dysfunctional Cognitive Behavior
I = Identify the problem *Involves preliminary exploration, attention and awareness of the environment, ability to understand cause and effect.*	• Person does not recognize that a problem or obstacle exists. • Person is unable to predict the consequences of an obstacle or action.
D = Define the problem precisely *Analyzing conditions of the problem and constructing a meaningful internal representation of the problem.*	Incomplete analysis of the problem due to: • Omitting details or steps • Over attention on one aspect of the problem at the exclusion of another relevant aspect • Encoding unnecessary dimensions of the problem • Not seeking out or searching for additional information (to help define the problem) • Poor allocation of resources - Does not take adequate time to study the conditions of the problem • Inability to simultaneously keep track of all the relevant conditions of the problem • Concrete thinking - Interprets the issues literally and fails to see the whole picture
E = Explore possible strategies *Formulating a plan, trying alternate strategies, and testing hypotheses.*	• Tends to approach problems in a haphazard, trial and error manner • Difficulty deciding how to approach the problem • Difficulty predicting future events • Decreased planning • Chooses inefficient strategies • Has difficulty using organizational strategies to group or classify information • Has difficulty shifting to alternate strategies when needed • Difficulty producing different hypotheses (poor hypothesis formation) • Difficulty letting go of a hypothesis once it has been proven wrong (maintaining hypothesis)
A = Act *Carrying out or executing the strategy or plan.*	• Difficulty initiating the plan of action • Difficulty remembering and following the plan • Becomes sidetracked - Loses track of the original goal • Difficulty persisting with the task. Tends to withdraw when the task becomes too difficult. • Decreased ability to monitor speed - Impulsivity or excessively slow • Loses track of time
L = Look at the effects *Comparing final solution with original conditions of the problem.*	• Difficulty recognizing errors • Difficulty correcting errors once they are identified

but have no difficulty organizing space and materials or thoughts and ideas.

A wide array of cognitive impairments can underlie different types of organizational difficulties. For example, disorganization in time, materials and space, communication, or task steps may be related to an impulsive, unsystematic approach, lack of attention to details, inability to keep track of items or materials simultaneously, inability to recognize patterns, difficulty making connections or associations between similar thoughts, ideas or objects, inability to think ahead, difficulty keeping the goal in mind, or poor awareness of the level of structure needed to support task performance. This suggests that careful analysis across different types of organizational tasks is needed to characterize strengths and weaknesses and to understand the problems contributing to a breakdown in performance.

Functional Cognitive Example of Organization

> **Clinical Example 2.13 Organization of a Work Task**
>
> Karen was asked to organize and plan two meetings at work. This included e-mailing participants; setting a time and day that people would be available; planning a time that the meetings would not overlap or interfere with other events; reserving a room; sending a calendar invite to all participants and sending the agenda to participants. Karen accurately planned the meetings so that they did not overlap with each other or other events. She wrote concise and well-organized e-mails to participants; however, the following errors were observed.
>
> - Sent out e-mails but used the wrong list (mixed it up with another list).
> - Planned the meeting time but did not check conference room availability first and will need to change the meeting due to room unavailability.
> - Included the time and location but not the day on the e-mail invite.
> - Mixed up the two meetings and attached the wrong agenda to the e-mails.
> - Failed to send the e-mail to two people who were on the invite list for one meeting.
> - Used the wrong invite list for the second meeting.

Although Karen was able to organize time of the meetings and communicate appropriately in e-mails, she had difficulty with organization of task steps (sequencing, keeping track of all information) and materials (agenda, meeting lists). This could reflect limitations in a combination of basic EF components (failure to keep track of what she just did or what needs to be done next, inability to shift attention, inhibit distractions, or initiate and seek information).

MULTITASKING

Multitasking involves the ability to carry out and interleave multiple steps or subtasks of complex activities in a coordinated manner. Although multitasking can be described as doing several things at once, there are different views of multitasking. Some authors describe multitasking as performing concurrent tasks or two or more tasks at the same time (Just & Buchweitz, 2016), while others distinguish between *concurrent* or *serial* multitasking. Serial involves interleaving several tasks that overlap in time because one subtask is not finished, while another must start. Each task or subtask is done one at a time but requires switching back and forth, rather than concurrent performance. It has been proposed that different brain mechanisms may underlie these two forms of multitasking. It is also not clear if multitasking describes features of an activity or situation that the individual has to manage or if it represents a distinct EF ability (e.g., similar to WM) (Burgess, 2015).

Multitasking involves all of the EF components described in this chapter, including switching between two or more subtasks, organization of time and materials, estimating time, as well as managing challenges or problems as they occur. In multitasking, EF components are simultaneously working together in an interwoven fashion. An example is making a meal. Substeps need to be carried out at the right time or in a synchronized way within a task rather than one at a time. The person needs to switch back and forth between a pot on the stove and a dish in the oven while preparing a salad and setting the table. The person may have difficulty multitasking due to failure to keep track of all the steps or subtasks simultaneously (WM); inability to switch tasks or let go of a subtask and switch to another (flexibility); difficulty keeping track of time or remembering a subtask that needs to be completed at a certain time (prospective memory); or tendency to get sidetracked by irrelevant tasks such as reading other recipes in a cookbook (inhibition). Alternatively, each EF component or subtask might be intact in isolation, but performance of complex tasks in multitasking situations may be inefficient and disorganized due to the lack of synchronization between subtasks or subgoals (Suchy, 2016). The observation that individual EF or task components can be intact yet performance can disintegrate when individual tasks need to be interleaved or performed concurrently has led to

Table 2.3 Organizational Skills: Function and Dysfunction

Type of Organization	Disorganization: Signs and Symptoms
Organization of Materials and Personal Space *Arrange and maintain materials, objects, personal belongings, and information (e.g., computer files, notes) for tasks in a manner that facilitates easy identification or location and efficiency in performance.*	Unsystematic and haphazard approach, frequently loses things, is unprepared, appears irresponsible, work is messy and may appear to lack effort, forgets or omits information, needed items, or parts of tasks.
Organization of Thoughts and Ideas in Written and Verbal Communication *Communicate ideas or thoughts in a manner that easily conveys the main points or ideas.*	Tangential, moves randomly from one idea or thought to the next, difficult to understand the main point, includes irrelevant and extraneous information or details.
Organization of Information or Task Steps *Group or associate related items, consolidate or reduce the amount of information, break up a large task into smaller parts, generate a table, chart or other system to structure separate pieces of information.*	Tries to tackle a large task at once without breaking down the information, easily becomes overwhelmed by the amount of information or number of task steps, unable to detect similarities or patterns of similarities so that information can be grouped together more efficiently. Randomly jumps from one part of a task to another.
Organization of Time *Estimate, allocate, plan and budget appropriate time for projects, activities and daily schedules.*	Difficulty planning, prioritizing, and coordinating different parts of an activity or day; runs out of time and fails to complete planned activities, allocates too much time for some activities and not enough time for other activities, does not consider all aspects (location, day, time, people involved) in arranging schedules, fails to anticipate potential conflicts or obstacles in schedule.

the emerging view of multitasking as a separate ability (Burgess, 2015; Just & Buchweitz, 2016).

Functional Cognitive Example of Multitasking

Clinical Example 2.14 presents a high-functioning person who scores within normal limits on standardized neuropsychological tests but demonstrates functional cognitive difficulties.

> **Clinical Example 2.14 Multitasking During Cooking**
>
> Susan performed well on tests of neuropsychological tests including working memory, flexibility, initiation, and inhibition. Susan was asked to make breakfast for three people including a cheese omelet, coffee, tea, and toast so that everything would be ready at the same time. Susan put the toast in the toaster, started the coffee, and then began the omelet last. She stopped to get the toast out of the toaster and forgot to put the cheese in the omelet. As she was pouring coffee into the cups, she realized she had forgotten to make tea. Once she was finished preparing breakfast, she started to set the table. By the time everything was served, it was cold.

Susan did not demonstrate problems with individual components of EF. She also did not have difficulty with performing tasks such as making coffee or making an omelet in isolation. However, her performance fell apart in a multitask situation that involved the coordination and interleaving of multiple tasks.

EXECUTIVE FUNCTION SUMMARY

Executive functions (EF) are a set of cognitive processes that subserve the ability to execute and control goal-directed behavior, particularly in non-routine, non-automatic situations. EF dysfunction is characterized by a disassociation between knowledge and action. A person with EF dysfunction may be able to accurately verbalize plans and "say the right things" but fail to carry out plans or self-monitor performance effectively. EF symptoms vary with structure, familiarity, predictability, and activity or environmental features. Since EF demands are reduced in habitual or automatic activities, EF symptoms are least apparent in routine situations. People with EF dysfunction have the most difficulty with unstructured activities, ambiguous directions, novel tasks, unexpected events, unfamiliar environments, and unpredictable or multitasking situations. The effect of activity and environmental demands on performance is discussed further in Chapter 4.

Deficits in EF are prevalent across many neurological and mental health conditions and can affect daily performance and participation in a variety of ways. Two people with executive dysfunction can exhibit very different clinical presentations and experience distinct difficulties in everyday tasks as illustrated throughout this chapter through a variety of functional cognitive examples (see learning activity in Appendix A.6). This is because executive dysfunction is not a unitary disorder. It represents a cluster of deficiencies. There are several theories, frameworks, and conceptualizations of EF. In this chapter, EF components were described as a foundation for higher-level thinking skills and are summarized in Exhibit 2.6.

In addition, metacognition, or the awareness and appraisal of one's abilities and performance, is often considered an EF (described in detail in Chapter 3). Higher-level cognitive skills such as problem solving, organization, reasoning, and self-regulation require the coordination and integration of EF components with metacognition and other cognitive skills (e.g., memory). Individual EF components may be intact; however, the person may have difficulty in functional cognitive activities that require the integration, interleaving, or synchronization of subtasks or steps.

Similarly, social communication, behaviors, and interactions with others also reflect the integration of executive function skills as discussed in Chapter 1. Appendix A.1 and A.2 ask the reader to identify how behavioral characteristics and social skills can be reflective of underlying EF components.

MEMORY

Memory is the retention of information over time. It provides us with continuity from day to day and frees us from dependency on here-and-now situations. It gives us the ability to reflect upon experiences, learn, and use information to influence future actions. Memory is not a unitary or isolated skill. It is a multi-step process that interacts and overlaps with executive function and other cognitive skills (Baddeley et al., 2015; Toglia, 1993b; Wilson, 2013). The following section describes the general memory process as well as different types of memory and provides clinical descriptions and examples of functional memory problems.

MEMORY PROCESSES: REGISTERING, RETAINING, RETRIEVAL

The process of memory can be described in a simplified way as the three R's:

1. *Registering* – Taking in information.
2. *Retaining* – Storing or holding on to information over time.
3. *Retrieval* – Searching for, finding, and pulling out previously stored information.

Registration includes the process of *encoding*. Encoding refers to mental operations that the person does at the time of study or input to process information. For example, in studying information that will need to be recalled later, a person may use multiple skills and strategies to take in information efficiently (Toglia, 1993a). Examples of such encoding strategies are presented in Exhibit 2.7.

As you review the list of strategies, you can see that good encoding involves many different cognitive skills including attention and components of EF. Craik and Lockhart's (1972) levels of processing theory explains how greater depth of processing during encoding leads to better retention and retrieval. The more one thinks about new information, elaborates upon it, or associates it with previous experience or meaning during encoding, the more likely it is to be remembered. If information is not well attended to or is simply repeated without connecting

---

Exhibit 2.6 Summary of Key Executive Function Components

- **Working Memory**: Holding information in mind to complete a task; updating and manipulating information; keeping track.
- **Initiation**: Beginning an activity; seeking information; generating ideas, plans, or strategies; persisting or completing all parts of activity.
- **Inhibition**: Controlling impulses and automatic tendencies; stopping behavior; thinking before acting; pacing actions; following or selecting according to rules or criteria; ignoring or managing distractions or irrelevant information; delaying responses.
- **Flexibility**: Shifting between ideas, thoughts, and tasks; moving freely from one step, activity, or situation to another; going back and forth between stimuli or rules; viewing situations from different perspectives; revising plans; adapting to changing circumstances.

> **Exhibit 2.7 Encoding Strategies**
>
> - Actively scans the material to be remembered and looks at all aspects
> - Identifies the most important information or details to be remembered
> - Identifies context or theme
> - Spontaneously shifts focus of attention to different stimuli to be remembered
> - Categorizes or chunks related items together
> - Tests self during study time
> - Verbally repeats or rehearses information to self
> - Maintains concentration on material to be remembered
> - Asks self-questions about the to-be-remembered material
> - Link a series of items or events into a story
> - Creates mental images of the to-be-remembered items
> - Associates new info with familiar experiences or information

information to one's experiences or somehow infusing it with meaning, it is likely that it will be processed superficially and will not be retained or accessible for retrieval.

Deep or strategic encoding involves using the EF components discussed above. There are many ways that cognitive impairments in these processes can limit encoding operations and, therefore, memory performance. For example, individuals with difficulties in initiation may not initiate use of encoding strategies such as association, elaboration, or verbal rehearsal. Those with difficulty in inhibition may fail to attend to relevant information or may impulsively move on to the next piece of information after only a quick glance. Those with problems in cognitive flexibility may over attend or become stuck on certain aspects, failing to process all information, or may only think about the information in one way. These are just a few ways in which other cognitive processes can interfere with the encoding of information necessary for retention and retrieval (Toglia 1993a).

Retention involves holding on to information over time or storing information for later use. Registration and retention in short-term memory overlap with WM in that they involve taking in information and holding it temporarily in one's mind during a task. Immediate recall, the ability to recall information within 60 seconds, is thought to be related to the encoding of information and WM. If information in working or short-term memory needs to be used later, it is transferred to long-term memory for storage over prolonged time (Baddeley et al., 2015). Once information is in storage, practice or testing over expanded time intervals (e.g., 5 minutes, 15 minutes, 30 minutes, one hour) can help increase retention of information over time. This has also been referred to as expanded rehearsal or spaced retrieval (Wilson, 2013). If information can be recalled as needed, learning has taken place.

Retrieval involves searching for, finding, and pulling previously-stored information out of memory when it is needed. Delayed recall or recall of information after several minutes to hours after presentation requires the ability to retrieve information from longer-term memory storage. Similar to encoding, or the process of getting information in, retrieval also involves the use of strategies and multiple cognitive skills to get information out (Toglia, 1993b).

For example, when trying to remember where you put something, you might try to mentally visualize and retrace your steps backwards in the order in which you completed tasks on that day. Similarly, when trying to recall an event or information, you might think back to the input situation and ask yourself a series of questions (e.g., Where was I? What time was it? Who was I with?) or try to think of the overall context first before thinking about specifics. This self-questioning process involves cognitive skills such as initiation, sustained attention, information seeking, association, and the ability to generate relevant questions and search in an organized manner (Toglia, 1993a).

Retrieval demands can differ depending on the level of cues present:

1. *Free Recall (most demanding)* – The person is asked to recall information or an event without cues. This requires self-initiation of an effective and organized search strategy.

- *Cued Recall* – The person is asked to recall information or an event after being provided with cues that facilitate retrieval. Cues may consist of items associated with the to-be-remembered information or a category in which the information belongs.

- *Recognition (least demanding)* – The person is asked to identify target stimuli from multiple choices, an array of stimuli, or through continuous presentation of stimuli.

If the person is not able to freely recall information but can retrieve information with cues or through recognition, it implies that information was stored in memory but could not be easily accessed. If the person does not recall information with cues or through recognition, it implies that there was difficulty with the consolidation or storage of information over time (Wilson, 2013). However, this explanation is somewhat of an oversimplification because the stages of memory are interdependent. If information is not encoded well to begin with, it is more difficult to consolidate it in storage and retrieve it. As you read the two clinical examples (2.15 and 2.16), identify similarities and differences, and think about how these examples reflect different types of memory problems.

Clinical Scenarios Illustrating Problems with Different Memory Processes

Clinical Example 2.15 Reading and Retention #1

Nicolas was asked to read an article in a magazine and remember the key points. As he was reading the article, he became distracted by an ad in the magazine and skipped over parts of the article. He read quickly without thinking about the meaning of the article or associating it with previous experiences. After reading the article, he only recalled 3 out of 15 facts. After 20 minutes, he still recalled the same three facts from the article.

Clinical Example 2.16 Reading and Retention #2

Ian was asked to also read an article in a magazine and remember the key points. Ian read carefully, underlined keywords, and wrote notes in the margin. He recalled 14 out of 15 facts immediately after reading the article, but after 20 minutes, he could only recall three facts. He was provided with cues; however, they did not help him retrieve additional material.

In both clinical examples, the delayed recall score is the same (3), but there is a difference in immediate recall. In Clinical Example 2.15, Nicolas demonstrates ineffective encoding of information, and this impairs his immediate recall. Other cognitive impairments, such as disinhibition, appear to be limiting Nicolas's ability to efficiently process and take in information. Although he registers a limited amount of information, this information is maintained over time and can be retrieved. Decreased immediate recall with minimal loss of information between immediate and delayed recall is a common clinical scenario and implies that the observed memory deficit is secondary to other cognitive impairments. This suggests that improving attention and EF skills, including the use of good encoding strategies, will improve memory performance as a by-product (Toglia, 1993a).

In contrast, in Clinical Example 2.16, Ian can take in information adequately as demonstrated by intact immediate recall. He used effective strategies during reading and attended to the material. The information, however, was quickly forgotten over time so that there was a large discrepancy between immediate and delayed recall even when support for retrieval was provided (cues). Ian appeared to be unable to hold or store new information in memory. In this situation, treatment strategies might include helping Ian use external devices such as a digital notebook, video clips, or pictures of daily events to compensate for decreased ability to retain or store information over time.

TYPES OF MEMORY AND THE IMPACT ON DAILY LIFE

In addition to the general processes of memory, there are different types of memory that are important for everyday function. Short-term and WM, both involved in temporarily holding information for recall and processing, are described above. Long-term memory, which is for lasting retention (i.e., anything over a few minutes) of information or skills, is often divided according to the type of information being stored. Long-term memory can be broadly divided into declarative and procedural memory, with declarative memory being further subdivided into episodic and semantic memory (Levy, 2018). Figure 2.4 illustrates the different components of long-term memory. Long-term memory can also be classified according to the temporal direction of the memories into retrospective and prospective memory.

Exhibit 2.8 presents questions that reflect different types of long-term memory. After you read this section, see if you can identify the type of memory to which each question corresponds.

Declarative Memory

Declarative memory, or "knowing that/what," is memory of facts and events. It involves conscious, deliberate, and explicit processing of information and experiences (Baddeley et al., 2015). Semantic and episodic memory are types of declarative memory.

Exhibit 2.8 Type of Memory?

1. When did you last ride a bicycle?
2. What is a bicycle?
3. How do you ride a bicycle?
4. Meet me at 3:00 to ride a bicycle.

Answers at end of chapter

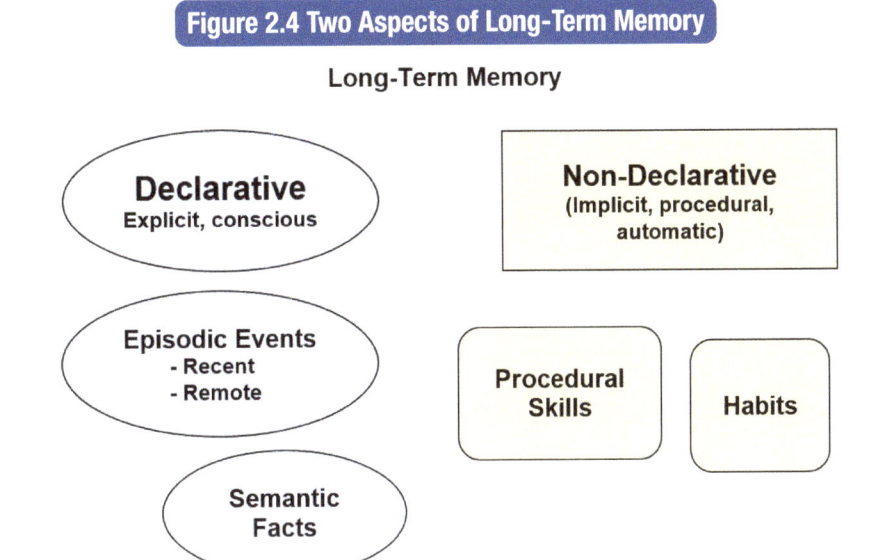

Figure 2.4 Two Aspects of Long-Term Memory

Long-Term Memory

- **Declarative** — Explicit, conscious
  - Episodic Events
    - Recent
    - Remote
  - Semantic Facts
- **Non-Declarative** (Implicit, procedural, automatic)
  - Procedural Skills
  - Habits

Semantic Memory

Semantic memory involves general knowledge of the world, including knowledge about objects, people, facts, definitions, concepts, and words. Unlike episodic memory, it is context-independent. It has been speculated that "semantic memories" result from an accumulation of similar episodic memories and that they become "knowledge" when we are no longer able to retrieve individual learning episodes (Baddeley et al., 2015). Examples of semantic memories include knowing that an orange is a fruit, knowing who the first president of the United States was, or knowing the capital city of England. Semantic memory is typically preserved following brain injury, Alzheimer's disease, most other neurological conditions, and with normal aging. As an exception, semantic dementia is a neurodegenerative disorder characterized by a progressive loss of semantic memory. Individuals demonstrate decreased ability to link names of objects to their concepts and lose the meaning of words (Budson & Price, 2005b). This can significantly impact activities of daily living. For example, the person may be unable to follow a shopping list in the grocery store or order from a menu because they do not remember what certain food names such as quiche or potatoes mean. Recipes may be difficult to follow as words such as ½ cup or ½ tablespoon may not be understood. The person may use words incorrectly such as saying "water" instead of "milk," use vague terms and have difficulty understanding what other people are saying (Bier & Macoir, 2010).

Episodic Memory

Episodic memory is memory for information from specific personally experienced events or moments in time. It allows us to draw on our past experiences and provides continuity of information and experiences from day to day (Baddeley et al., 2015). Episodic memory may be recent or remote. Recall of a conversation that occurred earlier in the day or remembering what one ate for dinner the night before are examples of recent episodic memories, as are the clinical scenarios presented earlier in this section (Clinical Examples 2.15 and 2.16). Memory of a wedding that occurred five years earlier or of a significant event from childhood are examples of remote episodic memories.

Episodic remembering is a complex process involving several brain regions. As such, episodic memory impairments are seen in a variety of neurological conditions. In Alzheimer's disease, episodic memory is among the first and most severely affected cognitive domains (Budson & Price, 2005a). Episodic memory impairments are characterized by rapid forgetting with poor delayed recall or recognition and difficulty learning and remembering new information. Isolated impairments in episodic memory have been described as primary or anterograde amnestic disorder (clinical signs outlined in Exhibit 2.9).

It is rare to observe severe memory deficits without impairments in other cognitive skills in everyday clinical

Exhibit 2.9 Clinical Signs of Primary Amnestic Disorder

- Rapid forgetting (poor episodic memory)
- Normal immediate recall
- Other cognitive skills relatively intact
- Preserved procedural learning

practice; however, primary amnestic disorders can occur, particularly with hippocampal damage.

Autobiographical Memory

Autobiographical memory is a type of personal memory that represents a combination of episodic and semantic memory. In autobiographical memory, information and events from one's own life are recalled from one's specific point of view. This helps to anchor one's sense of self and provides continuity over time. Autobiographical memory includes both memories of specific events such as memory of the first meeting with one's spouse or a past vacation, as well as recall of general information from a time period such as the name of famous people or important historical dates (Baddeley et al., 2015).

Functional Cognitive Examples of Declarative Memory Dysfunction

> **Clinical Example 2.17 Episodic Memory: Recall of Recent Events**
>
> Sophia can recall events from her childhood, but she cannot recall food that she ate, people she was with, conversations, events, or activities that she engaged in yesterday or within the last week.

Clinical Example 2.17 illustrates an impairment in recent episodic memory, but intact remote or long-term episodic memory. This pattern of forgetting is often seen in people with early Alzheimer's disease or anterograde amnesia from, for example, a brain injury. Repeated viewing of pictures or video clips of past events has been shown to stimulate episodic memory (Selwood et al., 2020) and could be used with someone like Sophia.

> **Clinical Example 2.18 Episodic Memory: Recall of Therapy Session**
>
> When the occupational therapist (OT) asked Liz to recall what she did in therapy yesterday, she did not remember. The OT gave Liz hints, but she still could not recall. The OT showed Liz two activities and asked her to choose the activity that she had done yesterday. Liz was able to choose the correct activity.

Similar to example 2.17, example 2.18 illustrates an impairment in recent episodic memory. It also shows how someone can have impaired free recall of information but can recognize the information correctly when it is presented. This implies intact encoding and storage of information but impaired retrieval or ability to access information. In this situation, treatment might focus on helping a person create or learn to search for retrieval cues to prompt memory.

> **Clinical Example 2.19 Semantic Memory**
>
> Jason went to the grocery store with a shopping list prepared by his wife. When he got to the store, he realized that he had forgotten what several items on the list looked like. For example, he wasn't sure what lettuce was and needed to ask for assistance. Similarly, he was not sure what apples were and mistakenly selected plums.

Jason has impaired semantic memory that is interfering with IADL such as following a shopping list in the grocery store. The use of a smartphone to retrieve semantic information from visual online dictionaries or the internet could be used to compensate for semantic memory difficulties (Bier et al., 2015).

Procedural Memory

Procedural memory, or "knowing how," is memory for how to execute skills, routines, and procedures, particularly the use of objects and body movements. It involves automatic, unconscious, and implicit processing during the performance of tasks or activities. Examples are knowing how to ride a bicycle, how to operate a microwave oven, or how set an alarm on a watch. Procedural memory is acquired by "doing" and repetitive practice. A person may remember how to transfer out of a wheelchair (procedural memory), but they might not remember who taught it to them or where they learned it (declarative memory). A person may be able to drive a manual transmission car (procedural memory), but they may not be able to verbalize to someone how they do it (declarative memory). Procedural memory can be preserved despite significant deficits in episodic memory. For example, in Alzheimer's disease, procedural memory is often spared until late in the disease (Budson & Price, 2005a). Repetitive practice of a functional task using errorless learning methods capitalizes on procedural memory. Errors are avoided because they can contaminate memory for the procedure and remain within procedural memory (Tailby & Haslam, 2003).

Figure 2.5 illustrates how learning methods differ for declarative and procedural memory. Declarative memory is learned through trial and error, effort, and strategies while procedural memory is learned by doing, practice, and repetition. A key distinction is that procedural memory does not require conscious recollection (Wilson, 2013).

Functional Cognitive Examples of Procedural Memory Dysfunction

> **Clinical Example 2.20 Procedural Memory: Remembering Procedures**
>
> Larry has Parkinson's disease. He remembered what he did yesterday and recalled a conversation he had with his daughter without difficulty, but he forgot how to make coffee. As he began to make coffee, he realized had forgotten how to operate the coffee machine and did not know what to do first. He had to stop and think carefully about each step and was unsure that he was doing it correctly even though he had made coffee every morning for years.

Larry has intact episodic memory but has lost memory for "how to" make coffee. He was unable to carry out a procedure of task steps that had been automatic. Larry previously did not have to think about what he was doing when he made coffee – he just did it. His procedural memory for making coffee has disintegrated. Procedural memory disorders are most commonly observed in Parkinson's disease (Budson & Price, 2005a).

> **Clinical Example 2.21 Procedural Memory: Skill Acquisition**
>
> Janice has early Parkinson's disease, and she and her husband have joined a tai-chi class. Although she eventually learns the movements and positions, it takes her a lot longer than her husband. She finds she still has to think about them, whereas they seem to be more automatic for him.

As illustrated in Clinical Example 2.21, procedural memory dysfunction can also manifest as the inability to learn new motor skills or slower skill acquisition. Skills are eventually acquired, but it may take longer or require more practice. Pictures or video clips of task sequences or exercises can be used repeatedly to facilitate procedural learning or to support performance and then gradually faded.

Prospective Memory

The discussion of memory thus far has focused on *retrospective memory* or memory of past episodes. In contrast, *prospective memory* involves remembering to do something in the future. Prospective memory is a multi-faceted cognitive construct encompassing the ability to remember to execute delayed intentions at the appropriate moment in the future (McDaniel & Einstein, 2007). Prospective memory plays a central role in daily occupational performance and participation, as it serves to bind together goal-directed actions and enables people to carry out their plans and wishes meaningfully and appropriately (Burgess et al., 2001; Morris & Gruneberg, 1992). For some prospective memory tasks, called event-based tasks, the appropriate moment to execute an intention is signaled by an external support or cue. Examples of everyday event-based prospective memory tasks include mailing a letter when you pass the mailbox, taking the dish out of the oven when the timer rings, and giving someone a message when you see them. In activity-based tasks, which are a subtype of event-based tasks, the trigger for action is one's own preceding behavior; for example, taking medication after breakfast or turning your cell phone to vibrate when you enter a meeting. In time-based prospective memory tasks, the appropriate moment to execute an intention is a certain time or the passage of a specified amount of time (Raskin et al., 2018; Umanath et al., 2016). Examples of everyday time-based prospective memory include remembering to attend a meeting at 3:00 p.m. or refill the parking meter in two hours. Some

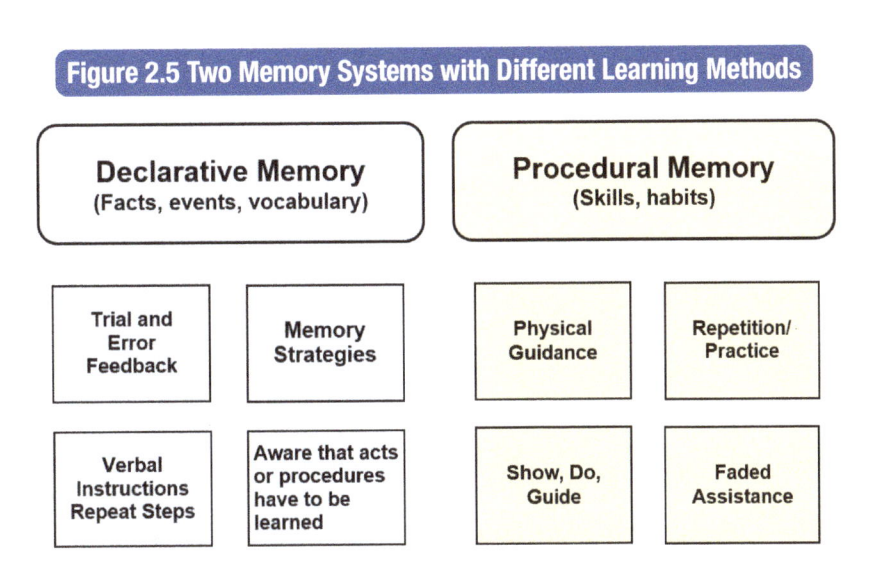

Figure 2.5 Two Memory Systems with Different Learning Methods

- **Declarative Memory** (Facts, events, vocabulary)
  - Trial and Error Feedback
  - Memory Strategies
  - Verbal Instructions Repeat Steps
  - Aware that acts or procedures have to be learned
- **Procedural Memory** (Skills, habits)
  - Physical Guidance
  - Repetition/Practice
  - Show, Do, Guide
  - Faded Assistance

time-based tasks are recurring, such as remembering to check the pot on the stove every few minutes until it starts to boil. Time-based prospective memory tasks are more cognitively demanding than other types of prospective memory tasks because they depend on self-initiated processes and are not prompted by external cues (Palermo et al., 2018).

Prospective memory performance can be described as a process consisting of four phases (Rummel & McDaniel, 2019):

1. *Intention formation* – The intention to execute an action at a particular moment in the future is formed and encoded.
2. *Intention retention* – The intention is retained in long-term memory over a delay period while performing other unrelated tasks (i.e., ongoing activity).
3. *Intention retrieval* – The appropriate moment (i.e., cue) occurs and the intended action is retrieved from memory and initiated.
4. *Intention execution* – The intention is successfully carried out.

This process involves the integration of episodic memory and EF skills. It requires the episodic memory processes of encoding, retaining, and retrieving the contents of the intention (i.e., what to do) and when to do it. It also requires EF skills such as maintaining an intention in mind while completing other unrelated activities (WM), self-initiated intention retrieval and execution (initiation), and stopping or interrupting an ongoing activity to switch to the intention (inhibition, flexibility). The extent of demand on EF processes can depend on features of the specific prospective memory task. For example, tasks with obvious external cues (e.g., an alarm) can be retrieved relatively automatically, whereas time-based tasks or event-based tasks without obvious cues require attentional monitoring to detect the appropriate moment for action. Tasks with numerous or complex intentions may require more strategic or deep encoding to be recalled, and tasks that must occur amid many competing activities (e.g., a busy day or week) may require detailed planning (Anderson et al., 2017).

Prospective memory is akin to the higher-level cognitive skills described above (e.g., problem solving, organization). It involves multiple steps and can take different forms, all of which differentially involve the coordination of various cognitive processes. In this way, prospective memory failures (i.e., forgetting to do something) can arise from a number of sources, so a detailed performance analysis should be conducted to pinpoint what task and person-related features may be impacting performance.

Functional Cognitive Examples of Prospective Memory Dysfunction

Clinical Example 2.22 Prospective Memory: Remembering to Take Medication

Carlos remembers to take his medication when his son sets alarm reminders for him. As soon as Carlos hears the alarm, he knows it means that he needs to take his medication. Without an alarm, he is unreliable in taking his medication.

Clinical Example 2.23 Prospective Memory: Remembering to Make a Phone Call

When Esther heard the phone ring, she realized she had forgotten to call her daughter as promised at 3:00 p.m.

Clinical Examples 2.22 and 2.23 illustrate how prospective memory can be impaired while retrospective memory is intact. In both situations, the person can remember on their own what it is they are/were supposed to do (i.e., take medication, call daughter); however, they do/did not remember to carry out the intended task at the appropriate moment until cued. In these two examples, time-based prospective memory is impaired, but event-based prospective memory (triggered by cues) is intact.

MEMORY SUMMARY

In summary, memory is a process that involves taking in, storing, and retrieving information. There are distinctive types of memory related to the different types of information being processed as well as to temporal components (short- vs. long-term; past vs. future). Inability to recall information from one day to the next results in dependency on others for information, limits the ability to learn from experiences, and disrupts the sense of continuity in one's life. It can also interfere with therapy, as it can result in limited carryover from one treatment session to the next and from treatment to everyday life.

Functional problems can vary considerably depending on the extent, process, and type of memory involved. Therefore, it is important to understand the source of memory impairment in a client. Clinically, when a person complains of memory problems, the nature of the complaint should be analyzed to determine the type(s) of memory that could be affected (Exhibit 2.10).

Impairments in WM, prospective memory, and recent episodic memory are most frequently observed in clinical

> **Exhibit 2.10 Analyzing Memory Complaints**
>
> *Do memory complaints relate to*
>
> - Recent past events (earlier that day, day before, or week before)? *(episodic memory - recent)*
> - Keeping track of information during a task? *(working memory)*
> - Holding information for very short time periods (minutes)? *(short-term memory)*
> - Remembering to carry out future intentions? *(prospective memory)*
> - Remembering how to do something? *(procedural memory)*
> - Remembering facts and meanings of words? *(semantic memory)*
> - Remembering events from the past? *(episodic memory - remote)*

practice. Different types of memory problems have different implications for treatment. For example, WM difficulties require strategies to help the person keep track of all aspects of a task, whereas prospective memory difficulties may require strategies to keep track of time or retrieve future intentions.

In addition, the extent that memory difficulties are related to decreased ability to encode or retrieve information as a result of other cognitive problems versus an inability to consolidate new memories or hold onto information over time (storage) also has treatment implications. Strategies such as rehearsal, association, or simplifying the to-be-remembered items by condensing information into key words or images help enhance encoding of information, whereas repeated viewing of pictures or video clips of past events may facilitate retention of episodic memories. Chapter 7 and Appendix D.1 include specific strategies for memory dysfunction.

SUMMARY

This section reviewed the definitions and clinical signs of impairments in EF and memory and provided examples of the impact of said impairments on functional cognitive performance. Learning activities are provided in Appendix A to help the reader integrate the information presented and to provide the opportunity to self-assess functional cognitive skills. For example, Appendices A.1-A.5 requires analysis of behavior and social skills from an EF perspective as well as identification of EF skills within simulated activities or exercises. Appendix A.6 presents a variety of brief, everyday functional cognitive scenarios to provide the opportunity to practice analysis and interpretation of cognitive performance errors.

Executive function and memory are multi-faceted cognitive constructs. As such, identifying a person as having deficits in EF or memory is too general to be useful for treatment because the clinical picture and intervention approach can be so varied. Even when impairments in the specific components of EF or memory are identified, a range of functional cognitive difficulties can arise. Functional cognitive performance is complex, as it requires an intricate interplay of cognitive skills with activity and environmental demands and other non-cognitive personal factors (e.g., experience, fatigue, medication). Also, the expression of similar cognitive impairments in the performance of functional tasks may be highly varied both across and within individuals.

A thorough understanding of EF, memory, and how cognitive impairments can be expressed in the context of functional activities can help facilitate communication between OTs and other team members. It is also necessary background information for using the MC approach, as it helps therapists analyze, manipulate, and grade cognitive functional activities, interpret performance observations, and identify cognitive performance errors. This process is described in Chapters 4 and 5 and forms the foundation for helping a person understand and manage cognitive performance errors within the context of everyday life.

KEY POINTS

- The key dimensions of EF include WM, initiation, inhibition, and flexibility. These core components work together in an integrated manner to provide a foundation for higher-level cognitive skills such as problem solving, organization, abstract thinking, or multitasking.
- Memory is a multi-component process, which includes the registering, retaining, and retrieving of information.
- Other cognitive skills are used during the encoding and retrieval of information.
- Different types of memory tasks, such as recall of facts (semantic), recall of how to do something (procedural), recall of a personal event (episodic), or remembering to carry out a future intention (prospective) involve different types of memory that reflect different neural processes.

- Executive function and memory are complex and interrelated skills. A wide range of functional cognitive difficulties can be observed with EF and memory limitations.
- Intact EF or memory component skills in isolation do not necessarily result in intact functional performance. Cognitive functional performance requires the integration and synchronization of cognitive skills and is influenced by the environment, activity demands, and personal experience.

Answers to Exhibit 2.8: (1) episodic memory, (2) semantic memory, (3) procedural memory (4) prospective memory (time-based)

Chapter 3

Self-Awareness, Metacognition, and Self-Efficacy

A comprehensive understanding of the multidimensional components of self-awareness is needed as a foundation for interpreting assessment, as well as planning and implementing cognitive rehabilitation interventions. This chapter provides an overview of a theoretical model of awareness, including its relationship to self-efficacy and metacognition, types of self-awareness deficits, and clinical manifestations and implications for assessment and treatment. Factors that contribute to the expression of awareness limitations and defensive denial are also reviewed.

CONTENTS OF CHAPTER 3
The Impact of Self-Awareness Limitations
The Dynamic Comprehensive Model of Awareness
    Relationship between Self-Awareness, Metacognition, and Self-Efficacy
    The Distinction between General (Offline) Awareness and Online Awareness
    Variations in Awareness across Domains and the Object of Awareness
    Online Awareness of Performance
    Depth of Awareness

Implications for Assessment
    Assessing General Awareness
    Assessing Online Awareness
Implications for Treatment
    Building Self-Efficacy
    A Focus on Online Awareness
Defensive Denial
    Interaction of Denial Reactions and Impaired Self-Awareness
    Denial and Treatment Implications
Summary and Key Points

THE IMPACT OF SELF-AWARENESS LIMITATIONS

A significant proportion of individuals with acquired brain injury do not recognize that their cognitive-perceptual abilities or daily functioning have changed. A large discrepancy between one's subjective view and actual performance can present a major challenge in rehabilitation. An individual who does not have concerns about their functioning will not be actively engaged in treatment. In addition, a failure to recognize limitations in performance will result in a tendency to try activities that are beyond their capacity, thus compromising safety. It is not surprising, therefore, that self-awareness is strongly associated with function, safety, compliance, realistic goal setting, independence, caregiver burden, and functional outcome across different ages and diagnostic categories (Gould et al., 2015; Hurst et al., 2018; Ownsworth & Clare, 2006; Ownsworth, Desbois, et al., 2006; Robertson & Schmitter-Edgecombe, 2015; Toglia & Maeir, 2018; Villalobos et al., 2019). The consistent relationship between awareness, function, and outcomes highlights the importance of understanding the complex nature of awareness and addressing awareness in treatment.

THE DYNAMIC COMPREHENSIVE MODEL OF AWARENESS

The Dynamic Comprehensive Model of Awareness (DCMA) proposed by Toglia and Kirk (2000) further elaborates on the construct of self-awareness described in the Dynamic Interactional Model of cognition (Chapter 4) and provides an important foundation for the metacognitive framework used within the Multicontext (MC) approach. The DCMA builds upon the Pyramid model of awareness described by Barco et al. (1991) to provide an understanding of the complex nature of self-awareness. The Pyramid model identified three interdependent awareness levels that are hierarchical: 1) *Intellectual Awareness,* or knowing that one has limitations, 2) *Emergent Awareness,* or recognizing problems as they are occurring, and 3) *Anticipatory awareness,* or the ability to recognize that a problem is likely to occur as a result of an impairment. The Pyramid model was the first clinical model of self-awareness to highlight the multi-dimensional nature of awareness and incorporate metacognitive concepts within the description of self-awareness deficits. The DCMA re-conceptualizes these different aspects of self-awareness and proposes a multi-component model that broadens and further explains the different aspects of self-awareness as well as the factors that influence the expression of awareness deficits.

The DCMA focuses on the associations between metacognition, self-efficacy, and self-awareness. It proposes a dynamic relationship between knowledge, beliefs, task demands, self-monitoring skills, and the context of an activity or situation. Self-awareness is not static. Consistent with the Dynamic Interactional Model of cognition (Chapter 4), it varies depending on characteristics of the activity or environment such as complexity, meaningfulness, value, or familiarity. It also varies with personal factors such as personality, emotional factors, beliefs, culture, and life experiences. Differences in self-awareness can be observed across tasks or contexts as well as across stages of recovery. The following sections describe the different aspects of the DCMA.

Relationship between Self-Awareness, Metacognition, and Self-Efficacy

The terms self-awareness, metacognition, and self-efficacy are derived from different bodies of literature; however, the constructs overlap. Metacognition overlaps with the concept of self-awareness, but both concepts also have distinct or unique aspects. In the broad sense, *self-awareness* encompasses sense of individuality, self-identity, autobiographical experiences, and one's personal narrative (Morin, 2009). It goes beyond the understanding of one's strengths and weaknesses and includes level of consciousness, recognizing one's thoughts and actions as one's own (sense of agency), knowing that one is distinct from the environment, and the capacity for self-reflection (Kircher & David, 2003). Impaired self-awareness following a neurological illness or injury has been described as a failure to gain conscious or explicit access to information regarding one's state of perceptual, cognitive, or motor function (McGlynn & Schacter, 1989).

Metacognition includes self-knowledge of cognitive abilities, task characteristics, and strategies, but it does not include the broader aspects of self-awareness such as sense of agency and consciousness. Metacognition also includes monitoring and regulation of one's cognition. This includes use of metacognitive skills such as anticipating the difficulty level of a task, planning the way to approach a task, monitoring comprehension, analyzing thinking, sustaining effort over time, and evaluating progress towards task completion (Flavell et al., 2002).

Metacognitive skills help us determine which task components will be easy and which will be challenging so we can anticipate performance challenges and plan our course of action to avoid or lessen them. They also help us recognize, in the moment, if activity performance is going well or not and what does or does not work to support performance (Toglia & Kirk, 2000). People with highly developed metacognitive skills are often good problem solvers because they recognize flaws or gaps in their own thinking and can explain their thought processes. As a result, people with good metacognition are more strategic and are better learners than those with poor metacognition. People with low levels of metacognition have difficulty in accurately judging their level of skill or knowledge in a specific area. They typically over-estimate their abilities and do not anticipate challenges. As a result, effort and persistence are limited, performance is poorer, and errors may come as a surprise, causing frustration (Gutierrez & Price, 2017). Studies have shown that those who are low achieving academically tend to overestimate performance compared to those who are high achievers (Job & Klassen, 2012). Similarly, a study found that those with schizophrenia who overestimated functioning had lower scores on an index of rehabilitation potential, compared to those who were accurate or underestimated their functioning (Harris & Rempfer, 2020).

There is a close inter-relationship between self-awareness of one's cognitive processes and beliefs about one's own cognitive capabilities, or *cognitive self-efficacy*. Cognitive self-efficacy is an individual's perceived confidence and belief in their capabilities to manage cognitive symptoms or performance problems and succeed in cognitively challenging activities (Toglia & Kirk, 2000; West et al., 2008).

Social cognitive psychologists view self-knowledge as a constructive process that cannot be separated from one's beliefs and subjective interpretations. Self-perceptions and beliefs about abilities affect the activities in which one chooses to engage, the speed and intensity of performance, and the allocation of effort, resources, and strategy use (Toglia & Kirk, 2000). For example, successful use of strategies requires an understanding of one's abilities and limitations as well as self-efficacy. If a person inaccurately perceives a task as easy (low self-awareness, metacognition), they are not likely to initiate strategies, modify task methods, request assistance, or closely attend to and monitor performance because they may not think it is needed. On the other hand, a person who is aware of task challenges but has low self-efficacy might fail to initiate strategies because they do not believe that there is anything that can be done to help their performance.

Decreased self-awareness can also lower self-efficacy. Failure to accurately appraise the level of task challenge can lead to unexpected task outcomes (i.e., poorer performance than expected). If the individual has beliefs about themselves that are incongruent with their abilities, they will likely fail to meet their goals or expectations. As a result, perceived sense of control or self-efficacy may be significantly altered. This further decreases motivation, effort, and engagement in activities, resulting in a negative performance cycle.

The Distinction between General (Offline) Awareness and Online Awareness

The DCMA emphasizes the distinction between awareness of one's abilities that exist outside the context of a task (*general or offline awareness*) and that which is activated during task performance (*online awareness*). This distinction shares similarities with Flavell's initial description of metacognition, which includes both knowledge and monitoring components (Flavell et al., 2002), but it is expanded, modified, and reframed within the context of the awareness literature. This distinction also shares similarities with the description of intellectual awareness versus emergent or anticipatory awareness in the Pyramid model (Barco et al., 1991). Unlike the Pyramid model of awareness, however, the DCMA views these constructs within a non-hierarchical and dynamic relationship. The differences between general and online awareness are summarized in Figure 3.1.

General awareness and online awareness can be described as awareness outside and inside the context of

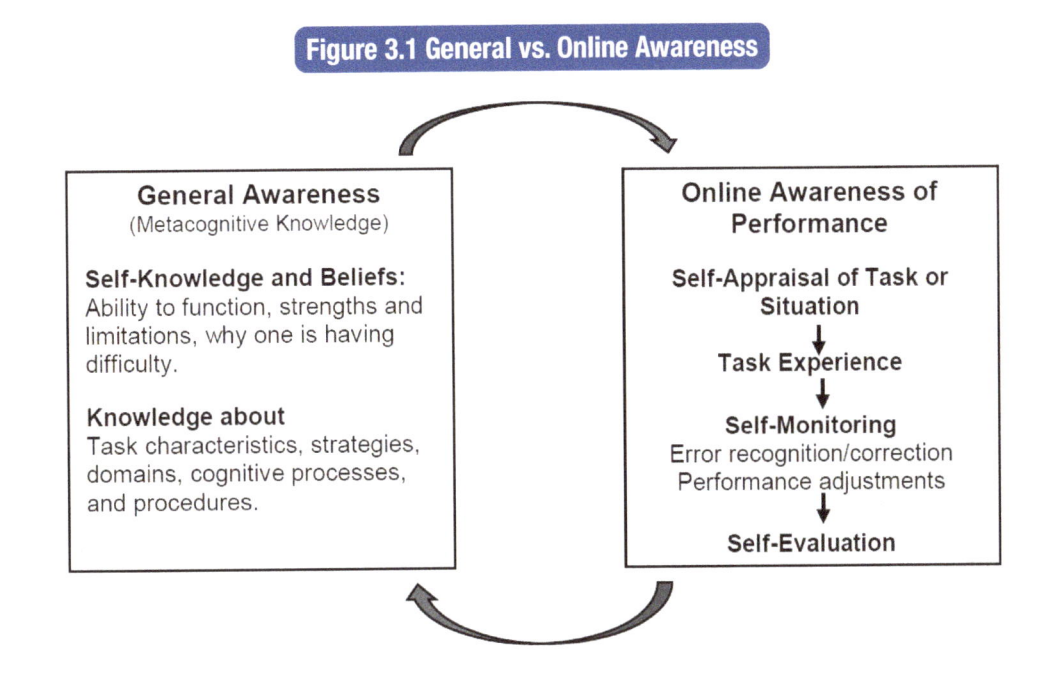

Figure 3.1 General vs. Online Awareness

General Awareness
(Metacognitive Knowledge)

Self-Knowledge and Beliefs:
Ability to function, strengths and limitations, why one is having difficulty.

Knowledge about
Task characteristics, strategies, domains, cognitive processes, and procedures.

Online Awareness of Performance

Self-Appraisal of Task or Situation
↓
Task Experience
↓
Self-Monitoring
Error recognition/correction
Performance adjustments
↓
Self-Evaluation

activity performance, although this is somewhat of an oversimplification. *General awareness* includes beliefs and subjective perceptions of one's functioning, performance, and cognitive abilities that are offline or unrelated to a task. It includes beliefs or thoughts about general factors that may be contributing to difficulties in function and ability to perform future tasks. It also includes metacognitive knowledge of cognitive processes, task demands, and how, when, or why strategies are used. The term general awareness is similar to but broader than, intellectual awareness, which is typically described as knowledge of one's abilities and limitations (Toglia & Kirk, 2000). Most of the literature on self-awareness of cognitive limitations has focused on general awareness, as it is assessed through an interview outside of the context of performance.

In contrast, *online awareness* of performance is activated within the context of a specific task or situation. In the DCMA, online awareness (also described as *awareness of performance*) includes metacognitive skills such as appraisal of task difficulty, self-monitoring (e.g., error detection or correction), self-evaluation, and awareness of effectiveness of task methods (Toglia & Maeir, 2018). The terms *online error monitoring* or *error self-regulation* more specifically describe error detection and correction while a person is performing an activity or at the moment (Doig, Fleming, & Lin, 2017; O'Keeffe et al., 2007). The term online awareness (instead of online monitoring) has also been used to describe awareness at the moment (Doig, Fleming, Ownsworth, et al., 2017). It is important to note that we and the DCMA use the term online awareness more broadly as that which occurs within a task context and includes awareness immediately preceding, during, and following task performance.

The distinction between general and online awareness suggests that knowledge of a problem (general awareness) does not necessarily mean that the person can recognize the problem when it occurs (online awareness). This is illustrated in Clinical Examples 3.1 and 3.2.

Clinical Example 3.1 General Knowledge versus Online Awareness

Interview: I have difficulties staying focused on the task.

Later: During bill-paying activity, client turns off radio, removes extraneous materials and distractions from table, asks others not to interrupt, and turns off the phone ringer.

Clinical Example 3.2 General Knowledge versus Online Awareness

Interview: I have difficulties staying focused on the task.

Later: During bill-paying activity, client gets sidetracked by a story on the news, becomes distracted by a phone call and a magazine on the table and forgets about the bill-paying task.

Both clients in Clinical Examples 3.1 and 3.2 express the same cognitive concern during an interview, but they differ in online awareness. The first client (Clinical Example 3.1) acknowledges difficulty in staying focused and recognizes the need to remove distractions and extraneous information during an activity. The second client (Clinical Example 3.2) also acknowledges difficulties in staying focused but is unable to use this knowledge during an activity to monitor performance and effectively manage distractions. As a result, there are significant differences in function.

The DCMA suggests that online awareness is dynamic and changes within and across activities, whereas general awareness is relatively stable and changes slowly with repeated experiences. Pre-existing knowledge of abilities, strategies, or task experiences that are stored in long-term memory influence online self-appraisal of tasks and the methods that are used. Similarly, new task experiences can update metacognitive knowledge if discrepancies are perceived, leading to adjustments in performance. For example, repeated experiences in getting sidetracked and forgetting important tasks could eventually lead the client in Clinical Example 3.2 to change her behaviors. Although both general and online awareness are inter-related, discrepancies can occur as illustrated with the clinical examples. Impairments in attention, memory, and executive functioning can affect the ability to recognize or recall performance errors within tasks. Therefore, mismatches between pre-injury and current abilities may not be perceived, resulting in a failure to update one's general knowledge. Other factors such as personality, culture, emotions, or context can also contribute to disassociations between general and online awareness.

The disassociation between general awareness and online awareness has been supported by several studies that included people with multiple sclerosis, traumatic brain injury, and stroke (Chen & Toglia, 2018; Goverover et al., 2007; Goverover et al., 2014; O'Keeffe et al., 2007; Robertson & Schmitter-Edgecombe, 2015). There is also evidence that suggests that distinct neuroanatomical systems may underlie these two types of awareness deficits (Hoerold et al., 2012). Online awareness is not typically included within standard assessments, yet in daily life, it may be just as important for successful functioning as the person's cognitive abilities. Therefore, the disassociation has important clinical implications for both assessment and treatment as discussed later in this chapter.

Variations in Awareness across Domains and the Object of Awareness

General and online awareness can both vary across domains (physical, functional, emotional, social, cognitive) as well as within the same domain. Therefore, it is important to clarify and specify the "awareness of what?" or the object of awareness. A person may have awareness of physical and functional difficulties but be unaware of problems in other domains such as social, emotional, or cognitive difficulties (Fleming & Strong, 1999). They might also fail to recognize that the same limitation affects multiple areas. For example, a person might recognize memory difficulties when reading, but may not recognize memory difficulties within social situations. Similarly, within the same domain, a person may have awareness of some abilities but not others. For example, within the functional domain, a person may acknowledge difficulties in dressing or cooking but fail to recognize limitations in financial management (Abreu et al., 2001). Awareness of difficulties that occur in some functional tasks but not others has also been described as task-specific awareness (Goverover et al., 2007). In general, awareness for instrumental activities of daily living (IADL) tasks is more impaired than awareness for basic activities of daily living (ADL) tasks (Rotenberg-Shpigelman et al., 2014). Exhibit 3.1 provides a few examples of different objects of general awareness; however, it is not an inclusive list (e.g., social, interpersonal, emotional).

The majority of literature concentrates on general awareness of impairments and their implications. Awareness of functional abilities across different types of tasks also needs to be considered during an interview (offline) as well as within the context of a task (online). Similarly, the person's perspectives regarding need for support or assistance for functional performance and ability to meet role expectations are important considerations. If the person does not think that they need assistance, they will likely attempt to perform activities without supervision.

Online Awareness of Performance

As mentioned above, online awareness of performance includes metacognitive skills. Exhibit 3.2 outlines subskills within online awareness. It includes anticipatory skills or recognition of the need to plan ahead, knowing when performance is going smoothly versus not smoothly, the effectiveness of the methods used, and the extent that the task outcome meets goals. It also includes understanding the task methods that were most effective in contributing to successful task completion and knowing when to adjust effort, speed, and task strategies or ask for assistance during a task. An understanding of the methods that lead to positive task outcomes appears to be more important in

---

Exhibit 3.1 Different Objects of General Awareness

Awareness of Health Conditions and Impairments or Awareness of

- Illness, diagnosis, disorder, prognosis, or disability
- Strengths and limitations across domains: motor, sensory, cognitive, emotional, social
- Strengths and limitations/symptoms within a specific domain; for example, within a cognitive domain: e.g. concentration, processing speed, ability to keep track of information, control impulses
- Implications or consequences of disorder and/or impairments

Awareness of Function or Awareness of

- Function across domains: e.g., self-care, IADL, leisure, work
- Abilities and limitations within the same functional domain; for example, in IADL: e.g., driving, financial management, cooking
- Need for supports, assistance, or accommodations (in an interview)
- Awareness of functional consequences of limitations (e.g., understands how difficulties in functional tasks such as household/financial management could impact independence)
- Awareness of ability to meet expectations of roles (student, sibling, worker, parent)

> **Exhibit 3.2 Subskills: Online Awareness of Performance**
>
> ### Before Task: Awareness of
>
> - Potential task challenges (parts of the task that will be easy versus hard)
> - Need to use a strategy
>
> ### During Task: Awareness of
>
> - Task difficulty during performance (knows if things are going well or not so well)
> - Need for cues or assistance during a task (knows when help is needed within a task)
> - Challenges during activities
> - Specific errors, incorrect responses, or obstacles
> - Task methods that are effective versus ineffective
> - Task inefficiencies
> - Need to adjust speed, allocation of attention, effort, or methods used within the activity
> - Progress toward goal
>
> ### After Task: Awareness of
>
> - Task challenges (parts of the activity that were easy and parts that were hard)
> - Task methods or strategies that were that are most effective in enhancing performance
> - Task outcome, overall performance, or goal attainment

awareness (Dockree et al., 2015; Goverover et al., 2014; Robertson & Schmitter-Edgecombe, 2015; Villalobos et al., 2019). This highlights the importance of addressing online awareness in both assessment and treatment. Indeed, online awareness is an important target of treatment within the MC approach.

Depth of Awareness

The DCMA also describes how general awareness and online awareness can vary in depth. Figure 3.2 illustrates that level or depth of awareness can vary on a continuum from a pre-conscious or implicit level to full awareness and understanding across tasks and situations.

Knowledge expressed through actions and behaviors during task performance without conscious awareness is described as *implicit or pre-conscious awareness*. For example, a person may deny memory deficits yet at the same time take detailed notes during an activity and re-read instructions or notes excessively. Although the person does not verbally acknowledge memory problems or task challenges, their behaviors indicate that they may still be "aware" of them at some level. *Vague awareness* describes a person who realizes something is wrong but is not sure what is wrong and is unable to provide examples or identify specific errors. They may indicate their thinking is not the same or that they have difficulty concentrating but they cannot explain when or describe how they know this occurs. A vague recognition that something is wrong without understanding why difficulties are occurring or what can be done to improve performance can elevate anxiety, frustration or depression and decrease self-confidence, self-esteem, and self-efficacy.

As previously discussed, awareness can be associated with *specific tasks or situations* but not others. The deepest level of awareness involves recognition of how the same problem manifests *across different situations and activities*. In an interview, someone with good general awareness can identify strengths and limitations, provide specific examples, and describe the conditions that are most likely

promoting functional cognitive performance than general awareness of limitations (Toglia et al., 2010).

There is evidence that suggests that online awareness may be more related to daily functioning than general

Figure 3.2 Different Levels of Self-Awareness

- Self Knowledge and beliefs regarding abilities, limitations and functioning

- Online Awareness and Self-Monitoring

Deeper Levels of Awareness ↓

- Pre-conscious
- Global/Vague
- Specific Tasks
- Across Tasks and Situations

to contribute to performance difficulties. A person with good online awareness anticipates task components that will be challenging, recognizes when performance errors occur, and realistically self-assesses performance within the context of performance.

The key concepts of the DCMA have been reviewed and are summarized in Exhibit 3.3. The next section discusses implications of the DCMA for assessment and treatment. This includes a discussion of denial, clinical manifestations, and the factors that influence impaired awareness and denial.

IMPLICATIONS OF THE DYNAMIC COMPREHENSIVE MODEL OF AWARENESS FOR ASSESSMENT

The DCMA highlights different dimensions of awareness as well as the need to use multiple methods of assessment to examine awareness. The ability to describe one's limitations does not mean that the person can recognize these limitations when they occur. Conversely, the ability to recognize and correct errors within an activity does not guarantee that a person is generally aware of their abilities and limitations. This dissociation between general awareness and online awareness suggests that, regardless of responses within an interview, the person's awareness of their performance should be explored within the context of a wide range of different activities.

Assessing General Awareness

The majority of assessment tools used to investigate self-awareness focus on the use of interview methods outside the context of activity performance and thus assess general awareness. Many use the discrepancy method, by which the person's self-ratings or responses are compared with those of significant others or clinicians, and the difference between them is examined. The greater the discrepancy, the greater the unawareness. Some awareness interviews involve direct clinician ratings of awareness based on client responses (Toglia & Maeir, 2018). For example, the Self-regulation Skills Interview (SRSI) (Ownsworth et al., 2000) is a semi-structured interview that involves investigating the person's perception of difficulties as well as any strategies they have used to help them cope with these difficulties. Client responses are rated based on established criteria. Since the SRSI includes both awareness and strategy use, it is often used in conjunction with the MC approach (see Chapter 12).

It is important to keep in mind that awareness interviews require verbal acknowledgment of problems. Lack of verbal acknowledgment does not always correspond to behavior. Poor awareness during an interview along with excellent use of strategies and self-monitoring behaviors can suggest high levels of implicit awareness. Alternatively, inability to admit to problems can be related to ego, personality variables, mood, or difficulty consciously accepting limitations (see section on Defensive Denial), (Beadle et al., 2018; Ownsworth, 2005; Richardson et al., 2015).

Assessing Online Awareness

The DCMA emphasizes the need to understand awareness within the context of activities, including perceptions before, during, and/or immediately after activity performance. This emphasis is reflected in the metacognitive framework used in the MC approach (Chapter 10). Online monitoring can be assessed by frequency counts of errors and error corrections during an activity, along with nonverbal error detection signs (e.g., verbalizations, gestures, facial grimaces) (Doig, Fleming, and Lin, 2017). In addition, asking a client to anticipate potential task challenges or probing their perceptions of performance immediately after completing an activity can provide important insights into their awareness of performance. These methods are used in the Contextual Memory Test and the Weekly Calendar Planning Activity (Toglia, 2015) described in Chapter 5. Online awareness varies across tasks and therefore should be assessed across different activities.

Prediction and self-estimation of activity performance have also been utilized to examine awareness of performance. Prediction techniques are best used in activities that are familiar so that the person has a benchmark for comparison. It should be kept in mind, however, that prediction or estimation can be affected by one's self-confidence and personality. Some clients may

---

Exhibit 3.3 Key Components of the Dynamic Comprehensive Model of Awareness

- Awareness is multidimensional and nonlinear.
- There can be a disassociation between online awareness within activity performance and general awareness or knowledge of abilities (O'Keeffe et al., 2007).
- Awareness may vary across domains and activities within the same domain depending on task characteristics and other variables.
- Different levels of depth of awareness can be observed in general awareness and online awareness.
- Online awareness of performance is a key target for intervention.

be resistant or hesitant to provide specific task ratings or estimation of accuracy level. Semi-structured interview questions that focus on identifying task challenges and methods used to complete the task or overcome challenges may be perceived as less threatening for some clients. Examples are provided in Chapter 10.

Various assessment methods examine different aspects of awareness. Online awareness has significant consequences for rehabilitation and functional outcome and should be included in assessment. Typically, more than one assessment method is needed to create a comprehensive picture of the client's awareness (Toglia & Maeir, 2018).

IMPLICATIONS OF THE DYNAMIC COMPREHENSIVE MODEL OF AWARENESS FOR TREATMENT

The MC approach intervention process includes helping a person discover and understand their new cognitive strengths and weaknesses. Knowledge about cognitive strengths and weaknesses are accumulated over a lifetime of experiences. Impaired self-awareness as a result of brain injury has been described as a lack of information regarding cognitive strengths and weaknesses or difficulty perceiving impairments (Stuss et al., 2001). Following an acquired brain injury or condition, a person may not recognize the changes that have occurred and continue to approach tasks in the way they did prior to their condition. It takes time to recognize, understand, and adapt to changes in the way the brain processes information. Recovery involves adjusting to and learning about one's cognitive changes and "getting to know oneself" again. This requires a restructuring of one's knowledge and beliefs about one's cognitive abilities and rebuilding a sense of self or self-identity.

Building Self-Efficacy

People with impaired metacognitive skills often overestimate their abilities as discussed earlier. Overestimation creates repeated experiences of unexpected failures that can impact a person's sense of control over performance. The DCMA draws from literature on self-efficacy, such as Bandura's concept of "guided mastery" (Bandura, 1997), which has implications for improving people's awareness and sense of control. The concept of guided mastery suggests that restructuring of knowledge and beliefs is most likely to occur when the individual can recognize or discover errors themselves (Bandura, 1997). Telling someone about problems or pointing out errors for them is often ineffective as it may trigger a defensive response. Instead, treatment should involve structured activity experiences and mediation techniques to help the person discover errors themselves. Self-discovery of errors is most likely to occur when activities are 1) familiar, so that the person has a comparison for evaluating current experiences, and 2) emotionally neutral (Toglia & Kirk, 2000). Familiar activities that are highly valued or associated with one's self-identity may need to be avoided in the early stages of treatment, as they can elicit emotional responses and may be threatening to one's sense of self. Activities also need to be at an optimal level of challenge (not too easy and not too hard). If an activity is beyond the person's processing abilities, the experience is less likely to be assimilated and integrated because cognitive processing resources are fully directed toward trying to understand and execute the task without leaving mental resources for self-monitoring.

As awareness emerges, it is important to foster a sense of perceived control and mastery over performance (Toglia & Kirk, 2000). This includes creating a supportive, non-confrontational atmosphere that empowers and supports the person in recognizing and managing cognitive symptoms so that they can stay a step ahead. The focus is not on awareness of impairments but on online awareness and task methods that promote success. Techniques used to build self-efficacy along with self-awareness represent an important part of the MC approach and are included in Exhibit 3.4.

A Focus on Online Awareness

Different objects or subskills of awareness can be targeted for self-awareness intervention as outlined in Exhibits 3.1 and 3.2. General awareness is typically addressed through psychoeducational techniques such as educational lectures, writing of and reflection on narratives, and individual or group discussion, whereas online awareness, is addressed through error-based learning and metacognitive techniques (see Chapters 9-10) within the context of activities (Toglia & Maeir, 2018). Error-based learning provides the opportunity to learn from one's mistakes and has been associated with greater gains in self-awareness, behavioral competency, and generalization as compared to errorless learning (Ownsworth et al., 2017). Metacognitive strategy techniques and guided questions are used to help the person recognize, monitor, and correct errors themselves. Online awareness of one's performance within an activity is the focus of the MC approach.

The DCMA suggests that changes in aspects of online awareness, such as awareness of difficulties with task components, may be observed first, within specific domains, without any changes in general self-awareness. Repeated experiences with different activities over longer periods of time (to build online awareness) may eventually restructure one's beliefs regarding their strengths and weaknesses and thus enhance general awareness over time.

CHAPTER 3 Self-Awareness, Metacognition, and Self-Efficacy   45

> **Exhibit 3.4 Techniques to Increase Self-Efficacy**
>
> - Build a collaborative, open, non-judgmental, and trusting atmosphere.
> - Use active listening. Validate or summarize the person's statements or restate/rephrase and reframe statements in a constructive and positive manner.
> - Provide opportunities for mastery and success.
> - Focus on "staying a step ahead" and controlling or managing performance errors or cognitive lapses within an activity.
> - Use a warm tone of voice.
> - Provide encouragement and positive feedback on the process (methods or strategies used, perseverance, self-checking, or monitoring attempts) rather than the outcome.
> - Reflect on observation and check client's agreement.
> - Encourage the person to self-discover their errors and generate their own solutions.
> - Avoid cues that "tell what to do."
> - Provide choices of activities whenever possible based on the person's interests.
> - Avoid talking too much, doing too much, or intruding on the process.

This is illustrated in Figure 3.3 and implies that, during treatment, online awareness may initially improve with activity experiences without accompanying changes in general awareness. This is supported by several reports of changes in online awareness within specific tasks without changes in standard awareness interviews (Goverover et al., 2007; O'Keeffe et al., 2007; Ownsworth, Fleming, et al., 2006). For example, Toglia et al. (2010) observed changes in self-monitoring and use of a strategy across different situations without changes in general awareness following an MC intervention. Over time, however, improved online awareness across different tasks has potential to update and restructure general knowledge and beliefs.

The bidirectional arrow between online awareness and general awareness in Figure 3.3 illustrates that for some people, general awareness might also improve from repeated experiences of difficulties in functional tasks. For example, the person might realize that they have difficulty paying bills, but may be unable to use this knowledge to monitor performance or recognize errors during bill-paying activities; however, over time, this knowledge could eventually influence and improve self-monitoring abilities. Changes can occur in both directions.

In general, it may be more important for treatment to focus on recognition of successful and unsuccessful methods employed during performance (e.g., awareness

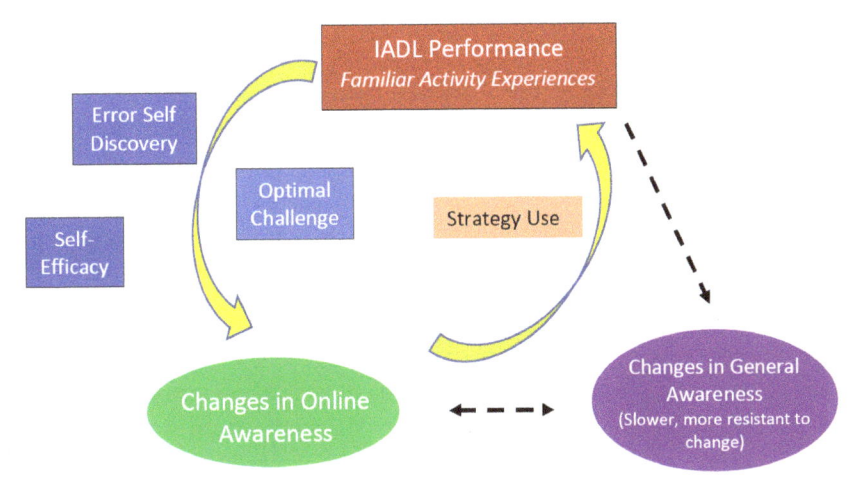

Figure 3.3 Activity Experiences Promote Changes in Self-Awareness

Self-Awareness is a dynamic ability that can be changed

- Error Self Discovery
- Self-Efficacy
- Optimal Challenge
- IADL Performance — *Familiar Activity Experiences*
- Strategy Use
- Changes in Online Awareness
- Changes in General Awareness (Slower, more resistant to change)

of effective strategies) rather than on acknowledgment of limitations. A focus on using efficient task methods rather than on educating or helping the person understand their deficits or problems may be more successful in promoting functional cognitive performance. This premise is supported by studies that have found that metacognitive processes promote strategy use and transfer of skills (Bottiroli et al., 2017; Carrett et al., 2010; Harris & Rempfer, 2020). The DCMA proposes several key guidelines for intervention that are summarized in Exhibit 3.5 and integrated into the metacognitive treatment methods used within the MC approach (Chapters 9-10).

DEFENSIVE DENIAL

In some situations, the person may be aware of their limitations but is unable to accept or acknowledge the changes that have occurred. Individuals with certain premorbid personality traits may minimize problems or reject the notion that there are any performance difficulties, even in the presence of obvious limitations. Defensive denial of disability represents a coping strategy and is more likely to be observed in individuals who have premorbid personality characteristics that include a history of presenting oneself in an overly favorable light, denying inadequacies, resisting help, a need for achievement, and a need to be in control (Ellis & Small, 1993). Denial can be adaptive in the early stages after an injury. It can temporarily protect a person from catastrophic reactions to loss, emotional distress, or overwhelming anxiety, and help to preserve self-image. However, persistent denial can interfere with the adjustment process, result in maladaptive behaviors, and prevent a person from developing realistic goals or plans and moving on with their lives (Ownsworth, 2005). It can also lead to heightened emotional distress and impede participation in rehabilitation (Kortte & Wegener, 2004; Ownsworth, 2005). The difference between defensive denial and impaired self-awareness due to neurological illness or injury is illustrated by Clinical Examples 3.3 and 3.4.

> **Clinical Example 3.3 Aaron**
>
> Aaron is a 43-year-old male who suffered anoxia as a result of a cardiac arrest 5 months ago. He demonstrates significant difficulties in planning, organization, and multitasking. During a computer task that requires following nine steps to obtain information on different websites, Aaron did not anticipate any difficulties but omitted four steps. When he was provided with a self-evaluation checklist, he recognized and acknowledged the omission errors but indicated that he rushed through the task because he was concerned about being late for his next appointment. He indicated that if he had taken his time, he would not have had difficulty. He also stated that the directions were unclear as they did not state that <u>all</u> steps had to be completed. He rated the task as easy.

Exhibit 3.5 Key Guidelines to Promote Self-Awareness

- *Create a close therapeutic alliance* – Create a safe and non-threatening atmosphere that provides support and facilitates the emergence of awareness.
- *Focus on online awareness* (see Exhibit 3.2) – rather than acknowledgment of deficits (general awareness).
- *Optimal level of challenge* – Awareness is most likely to emerge when activities are not too easy and not too hard.
- *Functionally relevant activities* – Awareness is more likely to emerge in activities that are familiar and that are "emotionally neutral."
- *Self-discovery* – Create activity experiences that are structured to allow the client to self-recognize his or her errors.
- Guide self-management of cognitive performance errors and task methods that promote success across different activities.
- Reinforce effective task methods and provide positive comments on the process, parts of the process, or attempts at using strategies (even if inefficient) whenever possible.
- Use metacognitive intervention techniques across activities that help build anticipation, self-generation of strategies, self-monitoring, and self-reflection (see Chapter 10).
- Focus on building self-efficacy and perceived control over functional cognitive performance as awareness emerges. Provide opportunities for "control" and success to minimize anxiety and frustration.

Clinical Example 3.4 Veronica

Veronica had a stroke four weeks ago. She demonstrates difficulties keeping track of information and staying organized within a task. During a computer task involving finding and purchasing items in a simulated online shopping task, she did not anticipate any difficulties and predicted that it would be easy. When she was provided with a self-evaluation, she recognized that she had missed several items and had gone over budget. She was surprised and confused, indicating she did not know what happened as it was a relatively simple task.

Clinical Example 3.3 (Aaron) describes a person with defensive denial. Aaron recognized his performance errors but made excuses for them. Individuals with defensive denial often recognize errors but they reinterpret them in their attempt to cope and may blame external sources such as the task directions, task materials, or other people for performance difficulties. They tend to over-rationalize errors or continually make excuses for performance difficulties. Reactions to feedback or obvious errors are typically met with hostility, anger, and resistance (Kortte & Wegener, 2004; Prigatano & Klonoff, 1998). The person may avoid or refuse to engage in any activity that presents cognitive challenges. In contrast, in Clinical Example 3.4, Veronica demonstrates impaired self-awareness. She was not sure why she had missed items and was both surprised and confused by her performance. Individuals with impaired self-awareness often appear confused, surprised, perplexed, or indifferent when errors are apparent (Prigatano, 2008).

Interaction of Denial Reactions and Impaired Self-Awareness

Denial reactions and impaired self-awareness may interact in the same individual (Kortte & Wegener, 2004; Prigatano & Klonoff, 1998). This is illustrated in Figure 3.4. The same individual can show different responses to varying situations. Multiple factors such as the meaningfulness, value, and context of the task, level of task difficulty, cultural background, interaction with others, and personality can impact the type of response (denial or impaired self-awareness) that is observed (Toglia & Kirk, 2000).

For example, a person may show denial reactions in activities that are highly valued and associated with one's independence such as driving or work, but they may acknowledge performance difficulties with neutral or less important activities. Impaired self-awareness, therefore, can be a combination of partial recognition of limitations and defense coping mechanisms.

Denial and Treatment Implications

Metacognitive strategy interventions may be effective in some individuals with partial denial or implicit awareness. A safe and positive atmosphere that fosters a sense of control can allow awareness to gradually emerge while minimizing defensive reactions. Exhibit 3.6 summarizes strategies for managing clients who have denial responses to activity challenges.

Individuals with high levels of denial and resistance require a focus on gaining acceptance and coping with challenges rather than on increasing awareness. Use of occupation-based activities, motivational interviewing with an emphasis on the person's strengths, and methods

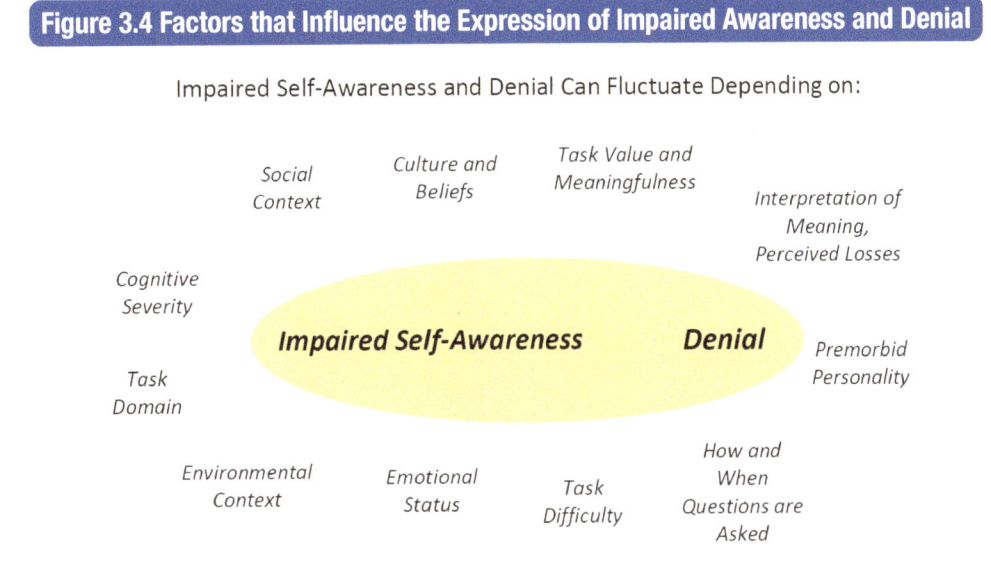

Figure 3.4 Factors that Influence the Expression of Impaired Awareness and Denial

Impaired Self-Awareness and Denial Can Fluctuate Depending on:

- Social Context
- Culture and Beliefs
- Task Value and Meaningfulness
- Interpretation of Meaning, Perceived Losses
- Cognitive Severity
- Task Domain
- **Impaired Self-Awareness / Denial**
- Premorbid Personality
- Environmental Context
- Emotional Status
- Task Difficulty
- How and When Questions are Asked

> **Exhibit 3.6 Strategies for Managing Denial**
>
> - Avoid negative language (problems, difficulties, symptoms, errors).
> - Avoid direct feedback and use of prediction or estimation techniques.
> - Do not argue, confront, or directly point out errors or problems.
> - Be conscious of your tone of voice and nonverbal signals that can convey disagreement.
> - Provide choice and allow control.
> - Observe for implicit awareness.
> - Focus on task methods, increasing task efficiency, and management of task challenges rather than deficits.
> - Use neutral but relevant activities. Recognize that meaningful activities with high value and close ties to one's self-identity may be threatening and elicit more defensive reactions.
> - Develop a close therapeutic alliance first and address other goals (e.g., motor goals) in the initial phase of treatment. Include cognitive tasks within motor activities but place the emphasis on motor goals.
> - Reinforce (e.g., point out and praise) error recognition and self-correction whenever observed.
> - Reinforce any attempts to use strategies, whenever possible.
> - Focus on strengths and successful methods.
> - Listen, understand, and respect the person's perspective, even if it appears contrary to what has been observed.

for successful management of task challenges can be effective for some clients (Medley & Powell, 2010).

A person with strong denial, however, may need to experience repeated failures within the context of their own everyday life before they are ready to accept help or engage in treatment (Toglia & Maeir, 2018). For these individuals, use of structured activities is not advisable, and metacognitive strategy techniques and mediation are typically met with resistance. If attempted, these techniques need to be handled with caution and within the guidelines presented above. The key problem is not self-awareness but acceptance. Other cognitive rehabilitation methods such as errorless learning or task-specific training may be more effective than error-based learning in improving function. Psychological support, a collaborative and consistent multi-disciplinary team approach, and the involvement of significant others are needed to help the person accept their current situation and engage in treatment.

SUMMARY

The concept of self-awareness is complex and multidimensional. Different types of deficits in self-awareness were reviewed in this chapter. Appendix A.7 includes three case scenarios. Review these scenarios and analyze the aspects of self-awareness deficits that are described. Think about treatment implications for each case. An analysis of these cases is presented at the end of Appendix A.

Most of the literature on awareness focuses on general knowledge of one's limitations or cognitive impairments outside the context of an activity (general awareness). Less attention has been paid to online awareness or awareness that is activated within the context of an activity. A person may be able to verbalize strengths and weaknesses yet be unable to use this knowledge to anticipate, monitor, recognize, or correct errors within an activity. The different subskills of online awareness (e.g., anticipation, error recognition, self-correction, need for assistance, awareness of task methods, and task outcome) should be carefully examined. These aspects of awareness appear to be most relevant to everyday functioning and are the focus of intervention within the MC approach.

Limitations in self-awareness are best understood by adopting a holistic perspective and considering the expression of self-awareness limitations within the context of the person's life and their personality. As described by the DCMA, many different factors (e.g., task difficulty or meaningfulness, personality, interaction with others, culture, beliefs) can contribute to a person's responses to feedback or the expression of awareness deficits (see Figure 3.4). Decreased acceptance of one's limitations (i.e., denial) is related to personality characteristics and coping mechanisms and is manifested by denial, resistance, and over-rationalization of errors. Although denial is different than impaired self-awareness, they can co-exist. Those who have a very strong denial reaction may not be responsive to a metacognitive strategy approach because the focus of intervention needs to be on acceptance rather than awareness. Based on the DCMA, awareness intervention requires careful consideration of answers to several key questions:

- How are factors such as personality variables, culture, and values influencing the expression of awareness?
- How are the person's beliefs about capabilities and self-efficacy influencing the expression of self-awareness?
- Are coping skills or difficulty in acceptance influencing the expression of awareness?
- Is depression or anxiety influencing the expression of awareness?
- Does the client's social context hinder or facilitate his or her self-awareness?
- Does the client's living situation hinder or facilitate his or her self-awareness?
- What domains of awareness are areas of strength and/or limitations?
- How do the clients' awareness deficits affect their ability to set realistic goals?
- How do self-awareness deficits affect the ability to self-advocate and ask for help when needed?
- How do self-awareness deficits impact the ability to perform expected activities?
- What is the client's reaction (e.g., surprise, indifference, hostility, anger, or over-rationalization) to errors or feedback?
- Does the client verbally acknowledge cognitive deficits outside the context of an activity (general or vague vs. specific examples)?
- Does the client show implicit behaviors that reflect awareness?
- What is the client's online awareness (before, during, immediately after activities)?
- In which activities does the client show the least versus greatest awareness?
- How does awareness change with activity experiences?

The MC approach involves helping the person recognize cognitive performance changes within the context of functional cognitive activities while simultaneously building awareness of methods that optimize performance.

There is a focus on building self-efficacy in managing cognitive symptoms and challenging tasks. The inter-relationships of self-awareness, metacognition, and self-efficacy are important to understand as a means of helping to promote participation and well-being.

KEY POINTS

- The DCMA integrates and describes the relationship between self-awareness, metacognition, and self-efficacy.
- General awareness is unrelated to specific tasks, is stable, and includes knowledge and beliefs in long-term storage.
- Online awareness is activated within a task, is dynamic, and changes within and across tasks.
- Although online and general awareness are inter-related, discrepancies can be observed.
- Awareness may be specific to a task, task components, strategy, situation/context, or domain.
- Multiple methods are needed to assess awareness.
- Changes in online awareness can occur without changes in general awareness and vice versa.
- Awareness emerges slowly with structured experiences that allow a person to self-discover their own performance errors.
- The focus of the MC approach is on building online awareness and self-efficacy simultaneously.
- The expression of awareness deficits or reactions to errors/feedback varies with the task value, meaningfulness, and difficulty as well as other factors.
- Decreased self-awareness is different from a lack of acceptance or denial reactions.
- Use of occupation-based activities, motivational interviewing, psychological support, and a focus on coping strategies within a non-confrontational team-based approach is recommended for those with strong denial.

Chapter 4

The Dynamic Interactional Model of Cognition: Activity and Environmental Demands

This chapter presents the Dynamic Interactional Model (DIM) of cognition and explains how this conceptualization of cognition and performance is used in clinical assessment and treatment. The Multicontext (MC) approach is based on the DIM. The influence of activity and environmental characteristics on cognition and performance represent one aspect of this model that is the focus of this chapter. Methods for analyzing and adjusting activity and environmental demands to place lesser or greater demands on specific aspects of cognitive performance are described with multiple examples. This provides a foundation for interpreting and analyzing performance during assessment and treatment.

CONTENTS OF CHAPTER 4

Overview of the Dynamic Interactional Model of Cognition
  Conceptualization of Cognition
  Internal and External Factors Influence Cognitive Performance
  Summary of the Dynamic Interactional Model of Cognition
Analyzing and Manipulating Activity and Environment Demands
  The Activity and Cognitive Performance
  • Activity Characteristics that Influence Cognitive Demand
  • Manipulating Activity Characteristics to Influence Cognitive Performance
  • Integrating Cognition into Motor-based Activities
  • Functional Cognitive Activity Sets
  • The Environment and Cognitive Performance
Summary and Key Points

OVERVIEW OF THE DYNAMIC INTERACTIONAL MODEL OF COGNITION

The DIM, influenced by the work of Vygotsky (1978), Feuerstein et al. (2015), and others in Educational Psychology, provides the foundation for performance analysis and the MC approach described in this manual. This section provides a brief overview of the DIM; however, the reader is encouraged to refer to other sources that provide a more comprehensive description to gain a full understanding of the theoretical basis of this model (Toglia, 2011, 2018) and clinical applications (Kaizerman-Dinerman et al., 2018; Zlotnik et al., 2009).

The DIM was developed in 1992 and indicates that cognitive performance is best understood by analyzing the dynamic relationship between the person, activity, and environment. Contemporary descriptions of functional cognition as described in Chapter 1 integrate this foundational concept (Wesson, et al., 2016). A simplified version of the model is illustrated in Figure 4.1. Internal or person factors include: (a) personal context such as life experiences, interests, occupations, general beliefs, values, coping style, personality, emotions, motivation, and self-efficacy; (b) self-awareness and metacognitive skills; (c) cognitive behaviors, process skills, and cognitive strategies (d) processing capacity (Toglia, 1992). External factors include activity and environmental demands or characteristics and will be the focus of this chapter. Activity and environmental demands are often interwoven with each other. Small changes in activity or environmental demands can significantly impact performance. It is important, therefore, to specify activity and environmental features when describing functional cognitive performance.

The DIM indicates that self-awareness and cognitive strategies represent core and malleable aspects of cognitive function that interact dynamically with external factors and other internal factors such as life experiences, beliefs, or values. The strategies that a person uses or the ability to self-monitor performance is not static but instead is influenced by activity demands, environmental features, and other aspects of the person's context (Toglia, 1992; 2018).

The DIM provides a framework for both assessment and treatment. In the area of assessment, the DIM suggests that information should be gathered on personal context, strategy use, and self-awareness, across different activities, environments, or contexts. Functional cognitive performance is not static but is expected to fluctuate with changes in the inter-relationships between the person, activity, and context at any given point in time. Assessment, therefore, needs to capture the range of performance variability and the factors that facilitate or inhibit optimal performance.

For treatment, DIM suggests that functional cognitive performance can be influenced by: (a) facilitating strategy use or metacognitive skills, (b) manipulating activity demands, (c) modifying environmental context, or (d) a combination of these areas. In some situations, functional performance is best facilitated by cues, or task or environmental adaptions by others. In other cases, performance is best facilitated by helping the person modify the task or environment themselves or use strategies across different situations. The DIM presents a broad view of cognition that supports performance analysis, dynamic assessment, and multiple treatment approaches including adaptation, use of technology, task-specific training, and strategy or awareness interventions. Different treatment approaches are not mutually exclusive and can be used simultaneously to support performance across different types of tasks (Toglia, 2018).

The MC approach is rooted within the DIM and its conceptualization of cognition, but it provides a narrower framework with specific guidelines for enhancing self-awareness, metacognition, and cognitive strategy use, while simultaneously analyzing and manipulating external factors so that the activity and environment present the right level of challenge. This chapter will focus on the external factors (activity and environmental demands and characteristics) that influence cognitive performance,

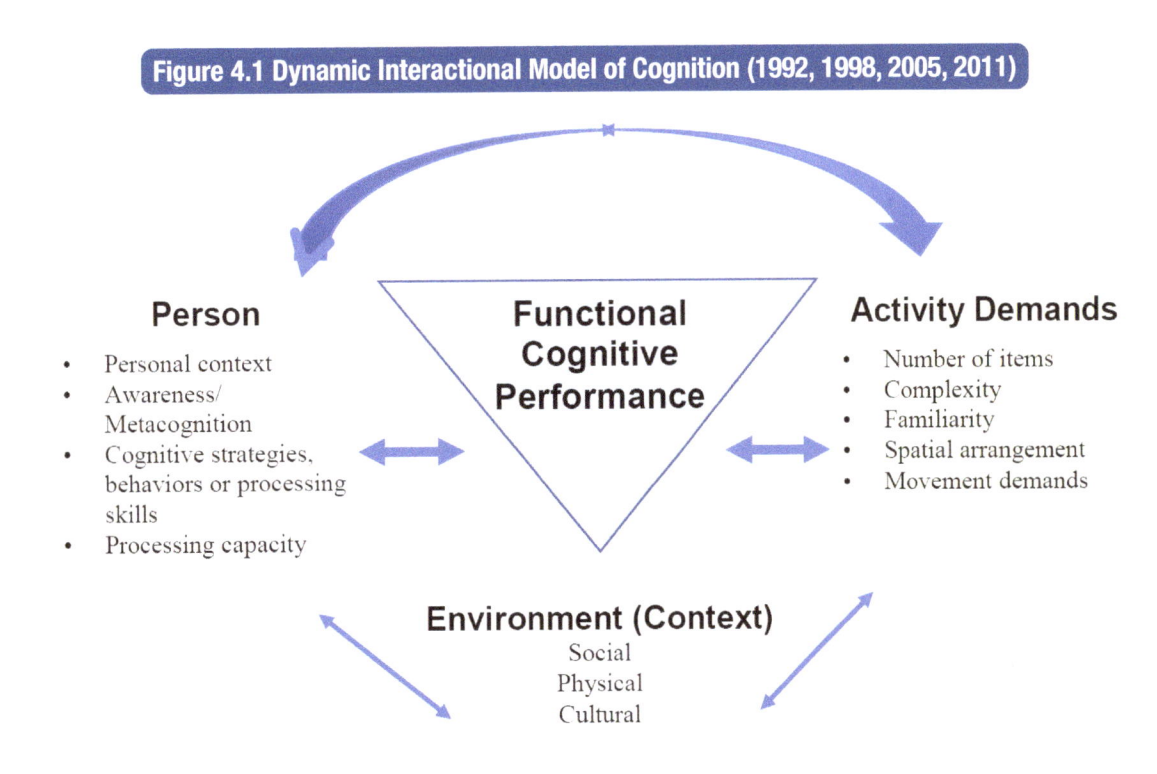

Figure 4.1 Dynamic Interactional Model of Cognition (1992, 1998, 2005, 2011)

Person
- Personal context
- Awareness/Metacognition
- Cognitive strategies, behaviors or processing skills
- Processing capacity

Functional Cognitive Performance

Activity Demands
- Number of items
- Complexity
- Familiarity
- Spatial arrangement
- Movement demands

Environment (Context)
Social
Physical
Cultural

while other chapters focus on strategy use (Chapter 7), self-awareness, and metacognitive skills (Chapters 3,9,10).

Conceptualization of Cognition

The DIM emphasizes the global capacities of cognition. Limits in information processing resources, or their inefficient allocation or use, can underlie many different cognitive performance problems. In the DIM, cognition is defined as a "person's capacity to acquire and use information to adapt to environmental demands" (Toglia, 2018). Cognitive limitations are operationalized as patterns of behaviors or performance errors that negatively affect functional performance across a variety of different activities. For example, a tendency to overfocus on details, omit key information within an activity, or lose track of information represent specific cognitive patterns of behavior that can interfere with functional performance across different situations. Exhibit 4.1 includes common observable behaviors that can also be described as signs of specific cognitive deficits such as deficits in the executive function (EF) components of working memory, initiation, inhibition, and flexibility. However, here the focus of analysis is on specific *observable behaviors* that contribute to performance difficulties, rather than on identification of the type of cognitive deficit.

Typically, a combination of behaviors is observed that contribute to cognitive performance errors. Exhibit 4.2 provides examples of common cognitive performance errors or *task errors* that can be observed during activities. While cognitive behaviors represent discrete or smaller units of observations, task errors can be the result of a combination of behaviors. For example, omissions errors can be related to inability to keep track of what was just done, a tendency to overfocus on parts, and difficulty regulating pace of performance. Performance analysis, therefore, specifies both patterns of observed behaviors and task errors across activities as a foundation for intervention. MC treatment seeks to help a person control or reduce cognitive behaviors and performance errors through use of cognitive strategies.

Internal and External Factors Influence Cognitive Performance

A person who has a specific profile of underlying cognitive deficits often has cognitive performance problems that emerge under certain conditions. As discussed in Chapter 1, internal factors such as anxiety, stress, depression, pain, or fatigue can increase the probability of cognitive performance problems. In addition, external factors can influence the degree of complexity or challenge and, thus, the potential for cognitive performance problems.

Exhibit 4.1 Sample Patterns of Cognitive Behaviors

- Loses track of information, steps, or materials during an activity.
- Gets sidetracked by irrelevant information or stimuli.
- Difficulty persisting to completion.
- Gets stuck on ideas, actions, or task steps and doesn't move on.
- Unable to switch task method, approach, or ideas when expectations are violated, or obstacles are presented.
- Difficulty regulating or pacing timing (too fast/slow).
- Overfocuses on pieces or parts and misses the overall point or picture.
- Does not recognize errors or obstacles.
- Difficulty initiating actions or thoughts or generating ideas.
- Strays away from the activity goal or topic of conversation.
- Haphazard, trial and error, or unsystematic approach.
- Jumps into the activity without pre-planning.
- Difficulty moving from one task component or activity to the next.
- Does not attend to or search the entire activity space or environment.
- Recognizes problems but cannot adjust or modify performance.

Cognitive difficulties are most likely to emerge under external conditions that involve non-routine activities or environments, new or unpredictable situations, multitasking, ambiguity, interruptions, visual and auditory distractions, or a fast rate of presentation because these situations place a high demand on executive control and strategic thinking.

Figure 4.2 illustrates how functional cognitive performance can change depending on a variety of external and internal factors. For example, in a familiar, well-organized kitchen at home, the person may have no difficulty making lunch. However, if the same kitchen is now cluttered from a recent shopping trip, items in cabinets and pantries have been rearranged by a well-meaning relative, the refrigerator shelves are overcrowded, and the telephone or doorbell rings multiple times, the same person may exhibit significant cognitive performance problems. Under these conditions, greater demands are

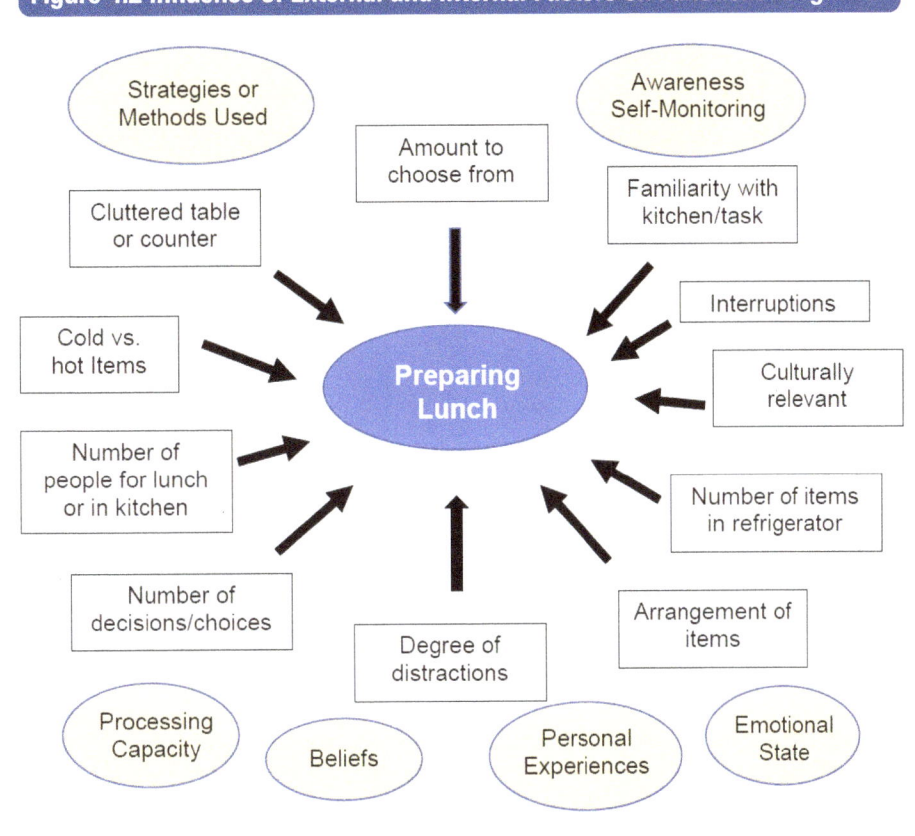

Figure 4.2 Influence of External and Internal Factors on Functional Cognition

Factors influencing **Preparing Lunch**:
- Strategies or Methods Used
- Cluttered table or counter
- Cold vs. hot Items
- Number of people for lunch or in kitchen
- Number of decisions/choices
- Processing Capacity
- Beliefs
- Amount to choose from
- Degree of distractions
- Personal Experiences
- Emotional State
- Arrangement of items
- Number of items in refrigerator
- Culturally relevant
- Interruptions
- Familiarity with kitchen/task
- Awareness Self-Monitoring

Exhibit 4.2 Sample Cognitive Performance Errors

- *Omissions:* misses details, materials, actions, information, or steps
- *Incorrect selection:* chooses or uses wrong items, materials, or information
- *Wrong order:* objects, steps, or actions out of sequence
- *Repetitions:* repeats actions, ideas, steps, or information
- *Inaccuracies:* steps, actions or information do not match directions or goal
- *Incomplete:* steps, actions, or information partial or incomplete
- *Additions:* extra steps, objects, actions, or information added (goal-related)
- *Extraneous actions or information:* irrelevant items, actions, steps, or information included (not goal-related)
- *Misplacements:* items or information in the wrong location

placed on cognitive skills such as the ability to inhibit distractions, visually scan, discriminate, keep track, and organize information. Similarly, a person with impaired balance or weakness may be able to perform a cognitive task such as following a recipe to make a fruit salad in a sitting position without difficulty. The same task, however, may present difficulty if the person performs the task while standing, because movement skills may now require greater attention, which places additional challenges on task performance (Toglia, 2018).

Cognitive performance problems are not always tied to a particular task or context. For some people, they emerge from cumulative effects of multiple activities or particular combinations of activities that place demands on cognitive processing over several hours or a day. A person may have no difficulty during the first 30-60 minutes of an activity but may be unable to process information and may experience mental fatigue or "cognitive overload" after three hours of activities or cognitively demanding tasks (Johansson & Ronnback, 2014). Such fluctuations and variabilities in performance are important to analyze and understand. This indicates that the person's broader daily routines, activity configurations, and lifestyle need to be considered along with the impact of the specific activity and environment characteristics.

Summary of the Dynamic Interactional Model of Cognition

Functional cognitive performance is vulnerable to dynamic fluctuations that result from interactions between personal factors, activity demands, and contexts. For example, cognitive performance with the same task can vary depending on the internal and external conditions. This indicates that descriptions of performance need to specify and describe the conditions under which functional cognition is optimal as well as the conditions under which performance problems are most likely to emerge. This requires observation and analysis of functional performance across a wide range of different situations. The goal is to identify common behaviors and errors that interfere with performance on a number of different tasks and to specify activity and environmental characteristics that increase and decrease cognitive performance problems.

Figure 4.3 summarizes key aspects of the DIM. It illustrates how cognitive performance problems emerge from a combination of cognitive impairments, activity characteristics, environmental demands, and other personal factors (e.g., experience, personality). Strategies can help the person control performance errors or behaviors across different activities. The effectiveness of strategies also depends on the person's abilities and other factors such as task difficulty and the context of the situation (Chapter 7).

ANALYZING AND MANIPULATING ACTIVITY AND ENVIRONMENT DEMANDS

Familiarity with activity and environment characteristics that can increase or decrease demands on specific underlying cognitive processes is important in analyzing and interpreting functional cognitive performance. Analysis of performance requires that the therapist simultaneously consider the activity demands and environment as well as the person's skills. Similarly, the ability to quickly adjust activity features to place either more or less demand on specific cognitive skills

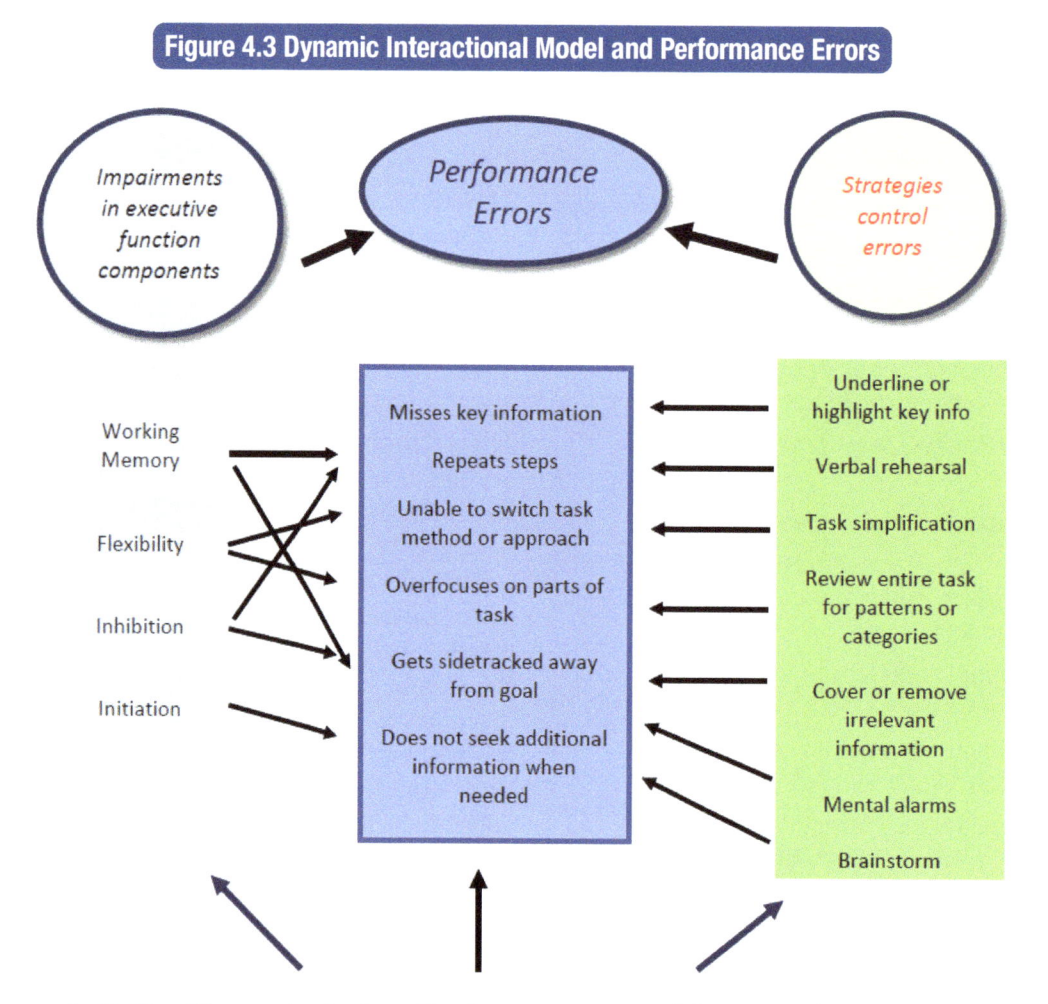

Figure 4.3 Dynamic Interactional Model and Performance Errors

Impairments in executive function components → Performance Errors ← Strategies control errors

Working Memory, Flexibility, Inhibition, Initiation →
- Misses key information
- Repeats steps
- Unable to switch task method or approach
- Overfocuses on parts of task
- Gets sidetracked away from goal
- Does not seek additional information when needed

← Underline or highlight key info
← Verbal rehearsal
← Task simplification
← Review entire task for patterns or categories
← Cover or remove irrelevant information
← Mental alarms
← Brainstorm

Activity Characteristics, Environment, and Personal Context

is important in both assessment and intervention as it can provide insight into the conditions that influence performance.

The Activity and Cognitive Performance

Activity Characteristics that Influence Cognitive Demand

An understanding of functional cognition requires a thorough analysis of cognitive activity demands. This includes understanding how slight variations in directions, materials, number of items or steps, arrangement of materials, or other characteristics of activities can influence functional performance. Cognitive demand can be considered an inherent part of an activity and thus can be used to guide analysis, grading, and manipulation of activities. Below are two lunch preparation activities. Think about how the differences in instructions and materials place different demands on underlying cognitive skills.

Activity Example 1: The person is in an unfamiliar kitchen and is asked, "Make yourself lunch. You can use anything that is in the refrigerator or cabinets."

Activity Example 2: A variety of cold cuts and bread choices are crowded on a table. The person is asked, "Make a ham and cheese sandwich on whole-wheat bread."

Example 1 places high demands on initiation because the person has to generate his or her own ideas for lunch, actively seek information (look for available food options, find utensils, etc.), and decide how they should go about preparing the meal. In contrast, Example 2 places relatively low demands on initiation as it does not require generating ideas, seeking information, or making choices. Instead, it demands inhibition in that the person has to focus on selecting the correct items while ignoring or filtering the irrelevant food items. Appendix A.8 includes a learning activity that requires analyzing how variations in directions place different demands on EF skills.

Figure 4.4 illustrates that the cognitive abilities of a person are separate from the cognitive demands of an activity. A person may have strengths and weaknesses across different cognitive skills. For example, one individual may show stronger working memory or initiation skills than another. At the same time, an activity (separate from the person) can inherently require different types and levels of cognitive skills. A match between the cognitive skills of the person and the cognitive demands of an activity result in successful performance. The importance of creating a fit between the cognitive abilities of the person and the activity demands has also been described by (McCraith & Earhart, 2018).

Table 4.1 summarizes *activity characteristics* that place low or high demands on different components of EF. As an example, activities that are predictable place minimal demands on flexibility, while those that are unpredictable or involve changing rules or circumstances place high demands on flexibility. As performance is analyzed, the activity characteristics that influence specific EF components always needs to be considered and specified.

In addition to Table 4.1, Appendix A.9 demonstrates how task features and complexity level can alter the cognitive components involved in different stages of problem solving. The IDEAL model (Bransford & Stein, 1993) described in Chapter 2 is used to frame the characteristics of simple and complex problem-solving tasks. Appendix A.10 provides examples of different functional cognitive scenarios and asks readers to analyze the differences. Some scenarios are more difficult than others. An analysis is included at the end of Appendix A. These examples illustrate how variations in problems change complexity and cognitive demands.

These examples further illustrate that cognitive components such as working memory, inhibition, flexibility, organization, or problem solving are not all or none but depend on activity demands. Functional cognition requires understanding how activity characteristics impact

Figure 4.4 Executive Function Skills of Person versus Activity or Context Demands

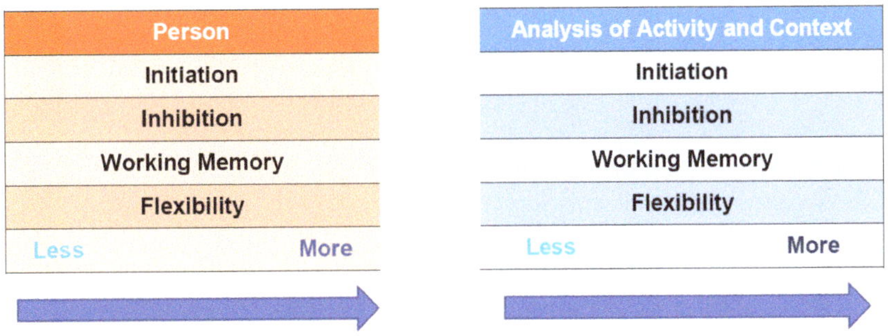

Person	Analysis of Activity and Context
Initiation	Initiation
Inhibition	Inhibition
Working Memory	Working Memory
Flexibility	Flexibility
Less — More	Less — More

Table 4.1 Activity Characteristics: Effect on Executive Function Performance

EF Components	Low Activity Demands / Low EF Requirement	High Activity Demands / High EF Requirements
Initiation — Ability to seek information or materials, ask questions, get started.	• Structured • All needed information, objects, and steps are provided. • Goal is provided.	• Unstructured, ambiguous directions. • The goal may not be clear, or the person may need to identify the goal and steps. • Information seeking is needed.
Inhibition — Ability to ignore irrelevant information or distractions.	• Familiar • No distractions. • Only relevant information is included.	• Extra criteria, rules, salient distractions, visual clutter, extraneous information, interruptions or noise is present.
Working Memory — Ability to keep track of information needed during an activity.	• External or written cues, directions, or lists to reduce memory load.	• Increased number of items or steps to remember during an activity. • Information needs to be compared or constantly updated.
Flexibility — Ability to switch back and forth among stimuli, information, or steps.	• Predictable activity • Minimal alternation • Few steps	• Alternating, switching stimuli. • Changing rules or circumstances are presented. • Unpredictable obstacles
Organization — Organization of materials, time, activity.	• Materials are pre-organized or arranged. • Structured outline, list, sequence, or plan to follow is presented.	• Create an organizational structure. Select and arrange materials, • Decide the order in which the steps should be done. • Determine how much time should be allotted • Maintain organization during an activity. • May need to detect associations or connections to organize materials.

cognitive performance as well as analyzing the fit between the person's abilities and the activity demands (Wesson & Giles, 2019).

Manipulating Activity Characteristics to Influence Cognitive Performance

Knowledge and skill in adjusting activities to vary cognitive demands and thus impact performance provide a foundation for both assessment and intervention. It allows the therapist to identify the types of activities that a person might need supports for, as well as guides the selection, sequence, and grading of treatment activities.

Table 4.2 illustrates how specific functional tasks such as packing a lunch or making coffee can be modified to place different demands on different EF skills by changing key activity characteristics. As in the preparing lunch examples above, the "same" activity can present different cognitive demands and produce different performance problems depending on the directions, set-up, or other activity characteristics.

On the other hand, different activities (e.g., packing a lunch and making coffee or tea) can present similar cognitive demands, thereby resulting in similar cognitive performance errors. For example, in Table 4.2, working memory directions that emphasize "keeping track" are used

Table 4.2 Examples of Functional Tasks: Variations in Activity Demands

EF Components	Activity Characteristics	Packing a Lunch for a Picnic	Making Coffee or Tea
Initiation	Ambiguous directions	Pack a lunch bag for a picnic. *Client has to ask about how many people and their preferences and search for options*	Make coffee and tea for guests. *Client has to ask about how many people and their preferences and search for items.*
Working Memory	Increased number of items and steps	Pack two or three lunch bags. Include beverages, sandwiches, two cookies, bag of potato chips and apple.	Make tea for two or three people, e.g., one herbal tea with two sugars and milk; two plain teas with two tea bags, milk and one sugar.
Inhibition	Rule constraints, cluttered environment with multiple choices, distractions, or interruptions	Identify a drink and a snack for each person. One person has lactose intolerance. One person is on a caffeine-free diet, another has diabetes, and another is vegetarian.	Serve hot drinks to four people. One person prefers either vanilla or hazelnut coffee, one person only likes strong unflavored blends, one person likes herbal decaffeinated teas, while another does not like coffee or tea
Flexibility	Alternating responses, changing rules, or obstacles	Using a list of items for the picnic, check items from the kitchen you are including and circle items on the list that are not included. *Add obstacles:* Run out of foil to wrap sandwiches	Cup and saucer for tea and mugs for coffee located in different cabinets. *Add obstacles:* Not enough mugs.

in two different activities (packing a lunch and making tea). A person that has difficulty keeping track of information will likely show similar errors across both tasks. Therefore, strategies such as using a written list or verbal rehearsal that help a person to keep track would be beneficial for both tasks.

The cognitive skills and type of cognitive strategies required for efficient performance change if the activity or environmental demands change. If the directions are modified so that they are now ambiguous, greater demands are placed on the ability to initiate ideas, ask questions, and seek information (see Table 4.2). With ambiguous directions, the strategy of verbal rehearsal that was effective with more explicit directions that emphasized keeping track is no longer beneficial because strategies that promote generation of ideas or information seeking are now needed.

Table 4.3 demonstrates a detailed analysis of how activity demands can be manipulated to place demands on key aspects of EF using a table setting task. It shows how the activity of setting the table can place more or less demand on the components of EF, depending on how the activity is presented. For example, increasing the number of distractors or interruptions places greater demands on inhibition by increasing competition and disrupting the flow of actions, whereas increasing the number of steps or items needed can place more demands on the ability to keep track of information.

Table 4.3 also illustrates that the same task can result in different types of performance errors, depending on how the task is presented as well as the person's cognitive difficulties. The last row of the table illustrates how the strategies that help a person in an activity may differ depending on the performance error. A blank form for use with other activities is included in Appendix A.13. Analysis of performance errors and strategies are discussed in more depth in Chapters 5 and 7, respectively.

Tables 4.2 and 4.3 illustrate that the same activity can be used in many ways depending on activity characteristics, cognitive difficulties, or performance errors. Blank activity analysis forms are included in Appendix A.12–A.13 and can be used to practice manipulating the cognitive demands of everyday activities.

Table 4.3 Manipulating Task Components to Increase or Decrease Demands on Executive Function

Activity: Setting Table

Scene: Unfamiliar Kitchen

Directions: You have people coming over for tea, coffee, and dessert. Set the table.

	Initiation	Inhibition	Working Memory	Flexibility
Task components that place demands on this skill	Person has to initiate by asking questions (e.g., how many people?), identifying what is needed, and searching for the materials or options.	Choosing relevant items related to goal and ignoring irrelevant materials	Recall items just retrieved	Shifting between items, locations, and place settings
Level of cognitive demand	__None __x Low __ Medium __ High	__None __x Low __ Medium __ High	__ None __x Low __ Medium __ High	__None __x Low __ Medium __ High
Methods to decrease demands (adaptations)	Provide more information in directions Place all needed items on table Set table with fewer number of items (e.g., dessert only) Copy a diagram or template of table setting Familiar kitchen	No distractors Set table with pre-chosen items	Set table using a written checklist Familiar kitchen Set table for 2 people Provide written instructions	Set table with all items on table for 1 person Set table for just dessert or for just tea
Methods to increase demands (*change directions, rules, items, arrangement, distractions etc.*)	Some items not easily found and require questions, seeking, and active searching. Ambiguous directions – "Set the table for people coming over at 3:00" Provide menu and have person decide how to set table.	Increase related number of distractors and interruptions Choose items in crowded, unfamiliar cabinet with salient distractors Add criteria (e.g., only use cups with design)	Provide more complex directions (increase number of items and number of people) Include certain placemat, tablecloth, etc.	2 different place settings: 1 for dinner, 1 for dessert Alternate pattern (e.g., solid then patterned plate or placemat) Obstacles are introduced (cups are in different locations or there are not enough of the same type of cup)
Task errors that might be observed	Does not know where/how to start Stops searching for items prematurely or stops task before it is completed Does not actively search for items or move from step to step	Acts before thinking or hearing all of the directions. Chooses items not needed Gets sidetracked	Forgets what just was just done Loses track of which items were already retrieved or which steps were completed	Repetition of items or steps Becomes stuck if an obstacle is encountered (e.g., not enough cups), does not know what to do
Sample strategy	Alarm signal that prompts self-questions Mental alarm "keep going"	Finger-pointing to control timing	Rehearse keywords List with verbal rehearsal	Talk aloud and self-monitor tendency to repeat

CHAPTER 4 The Dynamic Interactional Model of Cognition

Integrating Cognition into Motor-Based Activities

Often within acute care and inpatient rehabilitation settings, treatment has a focus on physical or motor skills. However, cognitive demands can easily be integrated into traditional physical or motor treatment activities, such as exercises and ambulation, by manipulating influential activity and environmental characteristics. For example, while walking or performing fine motor exercises, the person can be asked to simultaneously perform activities that require the ability to seek or keep track of information, adhere to directions, inhibit distractions, generate alternatives or shift attention. Examples of directions that can increase cognitive demands during ambulation or fine motor exercises are presented in Table 4.4. Also, Table 4.4 includes examples of prospective memory tasks or brief tasks that need to be carried out at specific times or following certain events. Prospective memory tasks can easily be integrated into any task to increase cognitive load or multitasking requirements.

Simultaneous demands on cognitive and motor skills

Table 4.4 Varying Cognitive Demands of Motor Activities by Changing Directions

EF Component	Ambulation	Fine motor (coins) exercises
Initiation	• Find certain locations (seek information) Provide office # or name with no other info • Generate a shopping list to make dinner while walking • Search and locate items from a list, or landmarks, in an unfamiliar environment (can be within a floor of a hospital or room)	*Searching for coins* There are coins in this room in hidden locations. You can ask questions to locate the coins, but I can only answer yes or no.
Working Memory	• Recall office number just passed • Keep track of the number of pictures and/or chairs • Counting change as putting coins in pocket • Read a list/directions and then locate items during a walk • Follow 3-4 step directions to a specific location	Pick up coins and place them in a covered container or piggy bank. Add and keep track of a running total + the number of coins used. You need to pick up coins that add up to 93¢. Keep track of the number of coins you use.
Inhibition	• Deliver mail to only specific locations on a map • Distribute brochures to only certain offices or locations • Find items or locations on a list that meet specific criteria, while following rules	*Coins in rows with written rules* • Only pick up a nickel if it is in between 2 pennies. • Pick up a quarter only if it is before a dime.
Flexibility	• Cross off items on a list that are not located and circle items that are located – then switch rule. • Write down the names of people with even-numbered offices on list 1 and odd-numbered offices on list 2.	*Switching rules* Pick up all of the pennies and add up. Pick up all of the dimes and add up. *Generation of Alternatives* See how many times you can make 93¢ with different numbers of coins (or different combinations of coins). ____
Prospective Memory	• Write the location you are at and the time after 3 minutes, 5 minutes, and 7 minutes (or identify specific times) (time-based). • When you get to the elevator and nursing station, circle the item you are up to on the list (cued). • Drop off this envelope at office #__ at 2:05 p.m. and meet me by the elevator at 2:08. • At 2:11, ask me about your next appointment, and at 2:17, text me to ask me about an important message.	Write down the number of coins that you have after 3 minutes, 5 minutes, and 7 minutes (or identify specific times) (time-based). Once you have picked up 3 quarters in a row or 5 dimes, write down the time. Remember to ask me about your next appointment at 3:02. Send me a text message at 3:10 to remind me to call your physician. *(unrelated to task – more difficult)*

require dual-tasking and simulate the skills needed in many functional activities. A person may not have any difficulty with cognitive tabletop activities or walking down the hall, but as soon as the person is required to move and think simultaneously, performance can quickly deteriorate. This is particularly true if previously automatic motor skills now require extra attention or concentration. Greater attention to balance or motor skills reduces available cognitive resources, and performance can be adversely affected (Cockburn, 1998). Cognitive demands may need to be lessened when motor demands are increased to create the desired level of challenge.

Functional cognitive performance should always be examined under a variety of conditions, including at the person's highest motor level. Of course, the therapist should consider and ensure a person's safety in these dual-tasking situations. Similarly, cognitive demands can be reduced within motor activities to support performance if dual tasking is a problem for the person.

Functional Cognitive Activity Modules

Ready-made functional cognitive activity modules are available that use everyday materials such as menus, schedules, and business name cards in different ways. The sets include lists, cards, and a wide variety of directions that can be used to place demands on different cognitive skills, namely EF components. Exhibit 4.3 illustrates how the same everyday materials (calendars and lists) from the Schedule Module (Toglia, 2017) can be used differently depending on the cognitive focus by changing the directions. The schedules can be placed on a magnetic board and the lists or direction cards can be spread apart or across a room to incorporate motor skills. These activities will be described further in Chapter 8.

The Environment and Cognitive Performance

As with activity characteristics and demands, environment characteristics such as familiarity and predictability, amount, type, and organization of objects, people, or stimuli, level of noise, social expectations, and type of social interactions with others need to be identified and specified when describing functional cognitive performance, as they can all impede or support information processing, learning, and performance. Task complexity, therefore, requires consideration of both the activity demands and the environment (Toglia, 2018). Familiar and routine tasks such as taking a shower, making coffee, or purchasing items in a grocery store may

---

Exhibit 4.3 Schedule Module: Same Activity Places Different Demands on Executive Function by Changing Directions

Classes and Activity Schedule I

	Sunday	Monday	Tuesday	Wednesday	Thursday	Friday	Saturday
9:00–9:30 am	Card Games	Yoga/Pilates Class	Crossword Puzzle Games	IPad Workshop for Beginners	Cardio Tone Exercise	Board Games	Treadmill Exercise
9:30–10:00 am	Scrap Book Class		Stretching Exercises			Nutrition Class	
10:00–10:30 am	Aerobic Exercise	Basic Computer Class	Shuttle to Mall	Arts and Crafts Workshop	Blood Pressure Screening	Chess Club	Aquatic Exercise
10:30–11:00 am	Bread Baking Class			Gardening Club		Golf Outing	
11:00–11:30 am	Bingo Games	Tennis Game	Health and Wellness Class	Cycling Exercise	Income Tax Preparation Class	Ball Room Dance Class	Word Games
11:30–12:00 pm	Digital Camera Workshop	Arthritis Exercises		Shuffleboard Game		Book Club	

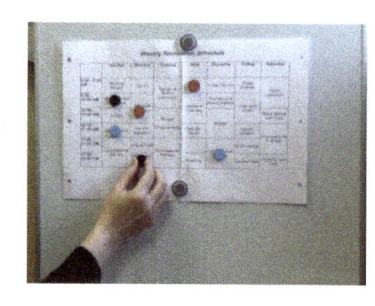

List of Classes and Activities II

Bocce Ball Game
Stairmaster Exercise
Badminton
Garden Club
IPad Workshop for Beginners
Bowling
Cycling Exercise
Arts and Crafts Workshop
Blood Pressure Screening
Horseshoe Tournament
Jewelry Making Class
Music Appreciation Class
Ball Room Dancing
Light Weight Exercises
Jogging
Word Games
Stretching Exercises
Income Tax Preparation Class
Creative Writing Workshop
Choir Practice
Photo Editing Class

Varying Directions (on cards)

1. Find the items on this list that are also on the schedule.
2. Study the list and remember as many items as you can from the list at one time.
3. Underline the Exercise Activities and circle all the Classes.
4. Using a blue marker, put a ✓ on the games; using a green marker, place an ✗ on the Exercise Activities; and using a red marker, circle the Classes.
5. For each Exercise Activity, place an ✗ in the same location on the blank schedule using a red marker.
6. For each Game, place a ✓ in the same location on the blank schedule #2, using a blue marker.

be more cognitively demanding in unfamiliar or new environments.

Similar to activity demands, environmental characteristics can also be manipulated to increase or decrease demand on cognitive skills and, thus, to influence cognitive performance. Table 4.5 includes examples of environmental characteristics that can increase demands on EF skills. These environmental characteristics need to be considered simultaneously with activity characteristics to interpret functional cognitive performance.

If environmental characteristics are influencing cognitive functional performance, adaptations or changes in the environment can be considered to minimize cognitive demands. Care partners can be instructed on ways to change the environment or the therapist can help the client learn how to modify environmental features themselves. Exhibit 4.4 demonstrates ways that the environment can be modified to *reduce* cognitive demands and support cognitive performance.

SUMMARY

The Dynamic Interactional Model of cognition, developed in 1992, describes cognitive performance as an ongoing product of the dynamic interaction among the person, activity, and environment. The term *functional cognition* as described in Chapter 1 integrates this key concept. The Dynamic Interactional Model indicates that observed cognitive errors or behaviors can best be understood by analyzing the interactions between a variety of internal (person) and external (activity and environment) factors. Appendix A.14 provides the reader with the opportunity to practice organization and analysis of clinical case information using the DIM framework. Specific methods for performance analysis using the DIM framework will be described in Chapter 5.

Cognitive deficits are not all or none but represent observable patterns of errors or behaviors that emerge under certain conditions. Functional cognitive performance is vulnerable to dynamic changes in response to various external and internal factors. Descriptions of functional cognition need to specify and analyze the conditions under which performance is optimal as well as the conditions that increase the probability that cognitive errors or symptoms may emerge.

This chapter focused on the external factors of the Dynamic Interactional Model and provided a comprehensive description of the ways that activity and environmental demands can impede or support performance. Assessment and treatment involve analyzing, adjusting, or manipulating activity and environmental characteristics to increase or decrease demands on functional cognition. Examples illustrated how variations

Table 4.5 Physical and Social Environmental Characteristics that Increase Demands on Executive Function Skills.

Contextual Factor	Characteristics that Increase Demand	Link to Executive Functions
Physical Environment	Unfamiliar environment	Novel situations increase demands on EF. Environment is less predictable; contents and location of items in environment are unknown. This places greater demands on initiation, working memory, inhibition, and flexibility.
	Multiple interruptions (e.g., phone calls, important text messages)	Greater demands on flexibility and working memory – requires ability to keep track and switch back and forth.
	High distractions, overstimulating environment (e.g., noise, increased visual stimuli)	Greater demands on inhibition – requires ability to inhibit responding to distractions and remain focused on the task.
	Large environment spread out (e.g., mall, airport)	Greater demands on initiation, information seeking, route finding, using signs or landmarks for navigation.
	Rooms with multiple cabinets, closets, drawers	Greater demands on ability to keep track of where things are that are not within sight.
	Disorganized objects/materials or overcrowded spaces	Greater demands on inhibition – requires ability to filter irrelevant information and attend to what is relevant.
Social Environment	Conversation within a group of people	Less predictability, greater demands on working memory, and flexibility, e.g., ability to keep track of who said what and switch between people and topics.
	Person speaks quickly, uses long sentences	Greater demands on working memory and speed of processing.
	Caregiver is often stressed, frustrated and angry, creating high tension	An environment that creates stress can further inhibit executive functions.

Exhibit 4.4 Environmental Modifications that Facilitate Cognitive Performance

Increasing Saliency

- Increase salient visual cues by using sharp visual contrasts in the environment to attract attention to relevant information, e.g., orange soap and towel in bathroom, red tape on wheelchair brakes; brightly colored key box.
- Create strong context of activity, e.g., run water; put object (washcloth) in person's hand to prompt initiation.
- Place cue signs in visible key locations to remind the individual to perform a task and minimize EF skills, e.g., slow down, read list, take meds, remember keys.

Decreasing Amount of Information Presented Simultaneously

- Limit or reduce clutter, irrelevant information, noise, or salient distractions in the environment. For example, reduce the number of items that are presented within a functional task at any one time (e.g., instead of a crowded food tray, present plate with only one item of food).
- Limit choices (or eliminate if necessary); e.g., clothes pre-chosen, clothes picked out and on the same hanger, closet pre-organized.
- Break up activities into shorter segments (e.g., two 10-minute sessions) or provide
- frequent breaks to reduce demands on sustained attention.
- Pre-organize or pre-select relevant objects needed for task. Pre-gather materials for tasks such as dressing, bathing, items for lunch/dinner, preplanned menu.
- Present tasks or task steps one at a time or present tasks or task steps in order of priority.

Increasing Predictability and Routines

- Decrease the need for planning with predictable, routine tasks.
- Important items in same locations, e.g., key box always by door.
- Establish daily schedule so it becomes easily memorized and automatic.
- Restructure daily or weekly schedule for optimal timing and combination of activities that reduces cognitive demands.

External Cues and Prompts

- Guide care partners on methods of cueing, how to redirect attention, or give instructions, e.g., strategies for cueing memory, such as providing the overall category or theme of a conversation to recall the details, encouraging verbal rehearsal and elaboration.
- Guide care partners on how to prevent disruptive behaviors by symptom monitoring and recognition of warning signs.
- Guide care partners on how to modify instructions, e.g., reduce the length, complexity, and rate of presentations; use short sentences, key words; check for proper understanding by asking the person to repeat instructions.
- Guide care partners on matching cognitive abilities with productive activities.
- Use of technology prompts to support cognition; e.g., use of voice digital assistants to provide daily reminders and messages, preprogrammed automatic text messages or alarm messages (cues client for appointments, to take meds, to do errand, make a phone call, initiate a task, or announce time on an hourly basis).
- Use of picture sequences or video instructions of activities to prompt a specific task sequence.

in specific activity and environmental characteristics place demands on different types of cognitive abilities. Activity analysis forms that can be used to analyze the effect of changes in activity demands on executive function abilities are included in Appendix A.

KEY POINTS

- Cognitive performance is not only a function of a person's cognitive processing skills. Rather, it can vary depending on a combination of internal (e.g., personal context, strategies, self-awareness) and external (activity and environment) factors.
- Cognitive limitations are described as observable patterns of behaviors or performance errors that affect functional performance across a variety of different activities.
- Performance on the same task can vary depending on the conditions. Specification and analysis of both activity and environmental demands are critical for a comprehensive understanding of functional cognitive performance.
- If activity and/or environmental demands change, different levels of cognitive resources, strategies, and self-monitoring skills are required.
- Slight variations in activity characteristics (e.g., directions, materials, number of items or steps, arrangement of materials) or the environment (e.g., familiarity, predictability, people, level of noise, amount of distractions, interruptions, other people, social interactions) can influence the demands placed on cognitive abilities.
- Knowledge of cognitive skills (e.g., EF components) and their interaction with activity and environmental characteristics can be used to manipulate activity and environmental variables so that different demands are placed on functional cognition.
- The same type of activity (e.g., making lunch, scheduling appointments on a calendar) can place different demands on cognitive skills depending on its characteristics and how it is presented (e.g., directions). This suggests the same functional activity can be used in a variety of ways in treatment.
- Knowledge and skill in adjusting activities to vary cognitive demands and thus impact performance provide a foundation for both assessment and intervention.

Chapter 5

Assessing Functional Cognitive Performance

This chapter focuses on how to obtain information on a person's functional cognition from direct observation of performance. Prior to this, therapists should gain an understanding of the client's personal context such as their beliefs, concerns, valued activities, culture, routines, roles, and previous lifestyle as well as the environment and community in which they function. This information can be gathered through questionnaires and interviews of the client, relative, and/or care partner. In addition to a more general occupational history or profile, self and informant report measures can be used to gain an understanding of functional cognition. Questionnaires, formal interviews, and rating scales that can be used to gather this information are described in other sources (Bar-Haim Erez, & Katz, 2018) and Chapter 12. These perspectives of the person's functioning should be combined with information from performance-based assessment of functional cognitive performance, as detailed in this chapter, to provide a comprehensive picture of the person's functional cognition.

CONTENTS OF CHAPTER 5

Methods of Performance-Based Assessment

Performance Analysis Based on the Dynamic Interactional Model of Cognition

   Dynamic Interactional Model Performance Analysis Guide

   General Methods for Observation of Performance and Error Analysis

- Cognitive Performance Observation Tool
- Error Analysis Tools
- Performance-Based Tools for Specific Activities

   Summary of Dynamic Interactional Model-based Performance Analysis

Dynamic Interactional Model and Treatment Planning

Summary and Key Points

METHODS OF PERFORMANCE-BASED ASSESSMENT

Different methods can be used to observe and rate functional cognitive performance. These include (1) breaking a task into discrete steps or components and rating competency in performing each task step or component, (2) rating the level of cues or assistance needed to successfully perform a task or each task step or component, (3) rating underlying cognitive skills or impairments, and (4) analyzing the type of performance errors. These methods can be used alone or in combination. Table 5.1 provides a summary of these methods along with examples of corresponding performance-based instrumental activities of daily living (IADL) measures. Links to standard performance-based functional cognitive tools can be found on the website www.multicontext.net.

The purpose of assessment or the identification of what information is needed determines the rating method to use. For example, to determine the level of assistance someone will need on discharge, performance-based assessment may need to examine the degree of assistance needed to complete an activity and identify adaptations required to support performance. While this provides important information for caregiver training and recommendations for discharge living situations, additional information would be needed to help a person manage their functional cognitive limitations on their own; namely, how or why they are experiencing cognitive performance difficulties. Furthermore, if the person is provided with assistance when they have difficulty, the ability to identify and solve performance problems on one's own is not easily observed.

Observation of performance without cueing provides the opportunity to observe error patterns as well as the person's ability to recognize and cope with obstacles, novelty, or performance challenges. Performance analysis based on the Dynamic Interactional Model of cognition (DIM) involves refraining from providing cues or assistance. Instead, the therapist observes and analyzes cognitive performance errors as well as the process of how a person goes about doing the activity on their own, including their use of strategies and awareness of performance. Awareness of performance is further probed through interview questions before and/or after the activity.

PERFORMANCE ANALYSIS BASED ON THE DYNAMIC INTERACTIONAL MODEL OF COGNITION

Performance analysis based on the DIM focuses on strategy use, self-monitoring abilities, and self-awareness, as well as identification of common behaviors and error patterns that may be contributing to performance difficulties across different functional activities. As discussed in Chapter 4, the activity and environmental conditions that increase or decrease performance difficulties are also described as a part of performance analysis.

This chapter will first describe general, structured methods of observing functional cognitive performance that can be used across any chosen activities. The first method, the DIM Performance Analysis Guide, involves a generic set of questions for the therapist based on the key concepts of the DIM (Toglia, 2018). The next two methods, the Cognitive Performance Observation Tool and Error Analysis Tools, provide general frameworks that can be used to structure performance observation and error analysis. They focus on analysis of cognitive patterns of behavior or performance errors that can be used to guide observations within the performance section of the DIM Performance Analysis Guide. These tools can also be used separately as structured means of recording and identifying error patterns during functional cognitive performance.

These are followed by tools that examine awareness,

Table 5.1 Performance-Based Testing Methods

Performance-Based Assessment Method	IADL Performance-Based Test Example
Competency or accuracy for performing task/task steps are rated (no cues)	• Test of Grocery Shopping Skills (TOGGS) (Brown et al., 2009)
Level of cues/assistance needed to perform task components or task is rated	• Kettle Task (Hartman-Maeir et al., 2009) • Performance Assessment of Self-care Skills (PASS) (Holm & Rogers, 2008) • Executive Function Performance Test (EFPT) (Baum et al., 2008)
Underlying process skills, cognitive abilities, or impairments are rated	• Assessment of Motor and Process Skills (AMPS) (Fisher and Bray Jones, 2012) • EFPT (Baum et al., 2008) • Actual Reality (Goverover et al., 2010; Goverover & DeLuca, 2015)
Types of performance errors are analyzed (no cues)	• Multiple Errands Test (MET) (Knight et al., 2002) • Weekly Calendar Planning Activity (WCPA) (Toglia, 2015)

strategies, and performance within specified activities such as the Weekly Calendar Planning Activity (WCPA), a smartphone task, the Upper Body Dressing Performance Analysis Tool, and the revised Contextual Memory Test (CMT-2). These assessments provide specific information that can be used to supplement information obtained from the general methods.

Dynamic Interactional Model Performance Analysis Guide

A generic set of performance analysis questions for therapists based on the key concepts of the DIM (personal context, activity, and environmental demands, cognitive behaviors and strategies, self-awareness) can be used to structure and record observations of chosen activities and to systematically apply the DIM model to clinical practice (Toglia, 2018). The performance analysis guide is designed to be used with a single activity and includes four sections: (1) Personal context, environment, and activity demands; (2) Performance: Observation of process and outcome; (3) Self-Perceptions and awareness; and (4) Implications for function and treatment. The first step involves choosing a personally relevant activity for performance analysis based on the client's interests, routines, or goals (Toglia, 2018).

The format for the performance analysis guide is provided below (Clinical Example 5.1). The first section of the form begins by briefly summarizing the client's personal context as well as specifying the demands of the chosen activity and environment. This includes the context of the person such as the person's experiences, occupations, familiarity with the selected activity, motivation, and goals, as well as the person's living situation. Next, the activity is described along with the setting or context and the activity/environmental demands as described in Chapter 4.

The "Performance" section includes the performance outcome or results and analysis of performance. The latter requires the therapist to carefully observe and describe the process of how the person went about doing the task. Cognitive behaviors or types of error patterns observed are described (see Chapter 4, Exhibit 4.1, 4.2) along with the task methods or strategies used. The Cognitive Performance Observation Tool or Error Analysis Tools described below can be used to structure observations and provide information for this section.

The "Self-Perceptions and Awareness" section asks the therapist to describe the person's awareness and self-perceptions of task performance. This requires observation of error monitoring behaviors within the activity such as spontaneous error correction or nonverbal signs of error recognition (e.g., shaking head). It may also involve an interview with the client before and/or after the activity to investigate the client's self-perception of task difficulty or performance (see #3). If the activity is less familiar to the client or has elements of novelty, awareness questions before the task can be difficult to interpret and are not used. Similarly, pre-activity awareness questions are avoided if the therapist wants to observe the client's spontaneous performance or self-monitoring skills without questions that might prompt task reflection. An after-task interview asks the client to describe how well they think they did, how they went about doing the activity, the type of challenges they may have encountered, and if they might do anything differently next time. This indicates the person's awareness of performance including the methods used and recognition of performance errors. As discussed in Chapter 3, awareness can vary across tasks. An interview within the context of a specific activity can yield very different results compared to a general awareness interview conducted outside the context of an activity. It is therefore important to investigate the person's self-perception of performance across all activities.

The last part of the performance analysis guide asks the therapist to describe functional and treatment implications. This includes the overall functional impact of limitations as well as identification of the conditions that influence the observed error patterns. The performance analysis guide focuses on describing common behaviors and errors that are not limited to a single task or situation. The same types of errors or behaviors are likely to affect performance across a wide variety of activities.

If the performance analysis guide is used within an initial session or observation, additional functional cognitive observations may be needed. As functional cognitive difficulties are observed, the therapist should always consider additional types of activities and situations in which the same error patterns might also emerge. For example, if the person appears to have difficulties managing three-step directions, a different activity with three-step directions should be observed. Ideally, assessment involves an analysis of performance across a number of different activities and contexts. Implications for treatment depend on the combination of awareness, strategy use, and performance.

The clinical examples in 5.1-5.2 illustrate the use of the DIM Performance Analysis Guide for two clinical cases. Complete assessment results and a treatment plan for Clinical Example 5.1 is also presented in Chapter 15 (Case 1). A blank DIM Performance Analysis Guide is available in Appendix B.3.

General Methods for Observation of Performance and Error Analysis

There are two tools that provide structured methods for observing performance in a selected activity. The first is the Cognitive Performance Observation Tool (Toglia,

Clinical Example 5.1 Analysis of Functional Cognitive Performance Using DIM Performance Analysis Guide (see treatment plan, Chapter 15)

1. Personal Context, Environment, and Activity Demands

Personal context: Fred is 64 years and had a stroke 2 weeks ago. He actively participates in therapy and is motivated to "get better" so he can return to work and living independently in his apartment. He is independent in all self-care activities. Fred describes himself as an organized person that likes to "get things done." Before his stroke, Fred lived alone in an urban setting and worked as an inventory control manager for an electronics company. He reports that he consistently prepared meals and paid his bills without difficulty. Self-identified concerns were only related to physical deficits.

Activity: Paying three bills (simulated bill-paying task)

Environment: Quiet room, tabletop activity, in an inpatient rehabilitation setting. The therapist was the only other person in the room.

Specify activity/environmental demands: Fred was asked to pay three bills. The bills, a checkbook, envelopes, and register were scattered on the table in a quiet room without distractions or interruptions. Fred was able to repeat the activity directions correctly.

2. Performance: Observation of Process and Outcome

a) Performance outcome: Fred only paid two out of three bills. He placed one bill in the wrong envelope and made out a check for the incorrect amount. He also exceeded the amount in his account.

b) What are the cognitive performance error(s) or behaviors? Why do you think the errors occurred?

The error patterns included both omissions and inaccuracies.

Before the therapist had finished her complete instructions, Fred began writing out a check (before he even looked at the bills). With cues, he randomly chose a bill on the table but wrote the check without checking the amount on the bill or his balance. Fred appears to have a tendency to jump into tasks without gathering the needed information (impulsivity). He rushes through tasks without adjusting speed of actions and made several careless mistakes involving omission of information. There is a lack of congruence between the directions or goal and his actions. He appears to act before thinking or before considering all aspects of a situation. At times, performance appeared random and disorganized. He was easily distracted by irrelevant thoughts or by irrelevant stimuli in the environment.

External stimuli may be triggering automatic behaviors (he sees a check and begins writing) in non-routine tasks due to decreased executive or top-down control. Fred's difficulties could also be described as disinhibited or impulsive; however, further specification of behaviors and types of errors are needed for the purposes of intervention.

c) Strategies: What task methods or strategies does the person use during performance?

No strategies were observed. Fred appeared to jump from one part of a task to another as described above.

3. Self-Perceptions and Awareness

What is the client's perspective before and after the task?

Before task: Anticipate possible challenges? Generate strategies?

During task: Recognize challenges? Detect and/or correct performance errors?

After task: Aware of performance, task challenges, task methods that were successful versus unsuccessful? Able to generate alternate strategies?

a) Before task: Did not anticipate the task as difficult and indicated that he pays his bills all the time. He rated the activity as easy and did not identify any challenges.

b) During task: Fred did not notice errors during or immediately after the task. Fred responded to cues to slow down actions but appeared to be unaware that his quick actions were contributing to performance errors.

c) After task: Initially, Fred perceived the task as easy and did not acknowledge performance errors. He rated the activity challenge level as 1 or easy. With a structured self-assessment activity checklist, Fred recognized some of his errors and commented that he should have taken a little more time but was unable to generate specific strategies. He indicated that he always did things quickly.

Clinical Example 5.1 Analysis of Functional Cognitive Performance Using DIM Performance Analysis Guide (see treatment plan, Chapter 15)

4.1 Functional Implications

a) Describe the activity demands and environmental conditions under which the performance error(s) or cognitive behaviors are least likely and most likely to emerge:

Not observed in familiar or routine self-care activities. Appears to be most likely to emerge within new or non-routine activities. Additional observations in new or non-routine activities involving following multiple-step directions of four or more steps are needed to confirm initial observations.

b) Error patterns: If applicable, identify other activities or situations that the same cognitive behaviors or performance errors have been observed:

The physical therapist also reported that Fred tried to get up and start walking before she finished giving him directions on how to use the walker. He attempted to get up by grabbing the middle of the walker in an unsafe manner.

c) How or to what extent do the observed performance error(s) or cognitive behaviors impact overall functional performance?

Directions are not followed accurately. Relevant information to the activity is not attended to, resulting in omissions or errors due to a failure to consider all information. The tendency to act before attending to required task information puts safety at risk and considerably impacts functional performance in all non-routine situations.

4.2. Treatment Implications:

Fred perceived the activity as easy and did not initiate strategy use. Immediately after the activity, he self-identified performance errors with structured methods, indicating that he would be a candidate for a metacognitive strategy approach. In general, Fred tends to jump into tasks quickly without pre-planning. While this may have been part of his pre-morbid style, intervention should be focused on helping him recognize the need to adjust his task methods and style to optimize performance.

Clinical Example 5.2 Analysis of Functional Cognitive Performance Using DIM Performance Analysis Guide

1. Personal Context, Environment, and Activity Demands

Personal context: Marie is 75 years old, 1-month post-stroke. She lives with her husband in a two-bedroom apartment within an independent living center for older adults and is independent in all self-care activities. Before her stroke, Marie was actively involved in attending activities within the center, including movies, lectures, exercise sessions, bingo or card games, and social gatherings, and managed her schedule and medications without difficulty. Although she has a cell phone, she prefers to use a personal planner book to manage her schedule. She uses a computer for e-mail. She describes herself as a "social" person who enjoys being active. Her goal is to return to her apartment and resume her former activities.

Activity: Copying selected activities from the master activity schedule into her planner.

Environment: Clinic, outpatient setting. There were 2 other clients working with therapists in the area.

Specify activity/environmental demands: Marie brought in the activity schedule from her center and her personal planner. The activity schedule was on a crowded monthly schedule. The environment included distractions such as other people talking, walking in and out of the room, and a phone ringing.

2. Performance: Observation of Process and Outcome

a) Performance outcome: Marie completed the schedule incorrectly. 3 appointments were entered more than once, and 2 appointments were missing.

b) What are the Cognitive performance error(s) or behaviors? Why do you think the errors occurred?

Marie wrote some of the same appointments several times without realizing it. On several occasions, she read the name of the appointment correctly and said it aloud but then wrote the name of the previous appointment in the schedule.

Marie is repeating the same actions. She repeats directions correctly out loud but is unable to execute the steps accurately.

> **Clinical Example 5.2 Analysis of Functional Cognitive Performance Using DIM Performance Analysis Guide**
>
> There appears to be a disassociation between saying the right thing and carrying it out. Within the context of an activity, Marie is not able to effectively monitor performance or recognize her repetitive errors, until after it is too late.
>
> *c) Strategies: What task methods or strategies does the person use during performance?*
>
> Marie attempted to go in order sequentially from the beginning of the month to the end of the month and placed a check next to each item she was entering in her planner. On some occasions, she placed a checkmark before she actually entered the appointment, and on other occasions, she placed a checkmark after she entered the activity. She randomly checked some activities twice so that overall, the checkmark system was ineffective in helping her keep track of what she had entered.
>
> ### 3. Self-Perceptions and Awareness
>
> *What is the client's perspective before and after the task?*
>
> *Before task: Anticipate possible challenges? Generate strategies?*
>
> *During task: Recognize challenges? Detect and/or correct performance errors?*
>
> *After task: Aware of performance, task challenges, task methods that were successful versus unsuccessful? Able to generate alternate strategies?*
>
> a) *Before task*: Did not identify any challenges or obstacles; however, she indicated the level of activity challenge as a 3/5.
>
> b) *During task*: Marie did not initially notice errors during the task. Towards the end of the activity, she realized she had placed one activity twice in the same time slot and that she had placed another activity three times in the same week when it was only offered twice. She self-corrected these errors but did not recognize other errors.
>
> c) *After task*: Marie acknowledged some of her errors but was unaware of others. She rated the level of challenge after the activity as a 5, indicating that she was aware the activity was difficult. She indicated that her performance was somewhat changed as compared to before her stroke (3/5). When asked to double-check her work, she detected most of her errors and was surprised and perplexed by them. For example, she made comments such as "I don't know why I wrote that" when she noticed her errors. When asked what she would do differently she indicated that she needed to slow down and pay more attention.
>
> ### 4.1 Functional Implications
>
> *a) Describe the activity demands and environmental conditions under which the performance error(s) or cognitive behaviors are least likely and most likely to emerge:*
>
> Not observed in familiar, routine self-care activities. Appears to be most likely to emerge within new or non-routine activities that involve moving back and forth between stimuli or moving from one step to the next. Has difficulty following two-step directions, copying information from an e-mail, or following a list of 10 items in non-routine tasks.
>
> *b) Error patterns: If applicable, identify other activities or situations where the same cognitive behaviors or performance errors have been observed.*
>
> Similar behaviors were observed in non-distracting environments while copying information into an e-mail, copying an address on an envelope, making coffee, and placing medications into an organizer. In the latter task, she read the directions out loud correctly (take two pills in the morning and one pill in the evening); however, she placed all pills in the same slot. While making coffee, she said out loud that two scoops of coffee were needed but placed four scoops in the container without realizing it.
>
> *c) How or to what extent do the observed performance error(s) or cognitive behaviors or impact overall functional performance?*
>
> Directions are not followed accurately. There is a tendency to get "stuck" in responses and repeat actions without realizing it, resulting in some items being missed or omitted. This could compromise safety (e.g., medication management).
>
> ### 4.2. Treatment Implications:
>
> Marie demonstrates attempts to use strategies and shows awareness that emerges with task experience and guidance. This suggests that she is an excellent candidate for a metacognitive strategy approach.

2017) and the second is the Error Analysis Tools. Either of these tools can be used to complete the Performance section of the DIM Performance Analysis Guide (Section 2, Performance: observation of process and outcome) or to supplement information. Alternatively, either tool can also be used separately to structure observations of performance within any activity.

Cognitive Performance Observation Tool

The Cognitive Performance Observation Tool, included in Appendix B.4 (selected items illustrated in Exhibit 5.1), focuses on analysis of cognitive patterns of behaviors and errors. This tool provides a structured method of documenting observations regarding both negative and positive cognitive patterns of behavior, including performance errors, strategy use, and self-monitoring skills (Toglia, 2017)

Eleven cognitive behaviors are included in the full tool, and there are two blank areas for miscellaneous cognitive areas that can be added (see Appendix B.4). There is space for the therapist to document specific examples of task errors or difficulties within each cognitive behavior on the left side and strengths, strategies, or positive observations within the cognitive area on the right side. This tool highlights the need to focus on a person's cognitive strengths as well as identifying their cognitive weaknesses. This form can also be used to structure observations during treatment.

Depending on the activity, not all behaviors listed will be applicable or observed. Exhibit 5.1 illustrates the partial use of this tool with three cognitive behaviors (out of 11) during a treatment activity (i.e., from a recipe, identify items that are not in the kitchen and create a shopping list).

Error Analysis Tools

The error analysis tools require the therapist to subdivide a selected activity into specific task components or steps and write the steps on the form prior to observation. Any type of functional activity can be chosen. There are 2 different formats available for use: 1) DIM Analysis of Task Errors and 2) DIM Multi-Step Activity Management Error Analysis. Both formats require the therapist to carefully observe performance without interference or cues and record task errors as well as observations regarding error recognition and strategy use. Both formats provide similar information, however, the Multi-Step Management Error Analysis format has slightly less detail. The format used depends on preference and the level of desired analysis. Each format will be described separately.

Dynamic Interactional Model: Analysis of Task Errors

In the DIM Analysis of Task Errors, the steps to a selected task are inserted into the form prior to assessment. As the person performs the activity, accuracy is rated (accurate, inefficient, partially accurate, or inaccurate), and the type

---

Exhibit 5.1 Sample Cognitive Performance Observation Tool *Activity: Gathering items for a new recipe*

Searches or seeks information when needed; Generates alternative ideas	
Specific Observations: Task errors or Difficulties 1. None 2. 3.	*Specific Observations: Strengths/Strategies used* 1. Immediately began the activity after reading instructions without hesitation. 2. Asked therapist questions to clarify directions.
Keeps track of information during an activity	
Specific Observations: Task errors or Difficulties 1. Lost track of items already searched. 2. Missed details on list. 3.	*Specific Observations: Strengths/Strategies used* 1. Verbally rehearsed some item names to self after reading them (but inconsistent). 2. Checked off some items on recipe (but inconsistent).
Stays focused on task/goal – resists distractions or irrelevant info (does not become sidetracked)	
Specific Observations: Task errors or Difficulties 1. Sidetracked by irrelevant information. 2. Began talking about irrelevant topics.	*Specific Observations: Strengths/Strategies used* 1. Eventually re-directed self back to the task after being distracted (without cues).

of task errors observed are documented for each step (Exhibit 5.2). Cues or assistance are not provided. This provides the therapist with the opportunity to fully observe how the person copes with performance challenges. If the individual becomes stuck and cannot complete the activity, the activity is stopped, and the individual's baseline performance or percentage of steps accurately completed is documented.

Error awareness, including error recognition and correction, is carefully observed and documented during activity performance. If a person spontaneously corrects an error, error recognition is assumed. Error recognition, however, can also occur without error correction and may be indicated through gestural signs (shaking head or pointing) or verbal acknowledgment. Errors that are spontaneously self-recognized without obvious problems (e.g. writing an incorrect number when copying an address) are differentiated from those that are recognized after obstacles, visible problems, or feedback from results prompt recognition of errors (e.g. food in oven burns because it was forgotten). The percentage of errors spontaneously recognized (#SR/total errors), recognized with problems (SR-P/total errors), or spontaneously corrected (EC/total errors) can be documented.

The time required for task completion is also noted. After the activity, the type of errors are analyzed and coded using the task error descriptions following the record form (see Appendix B.5, B.6). Therapist hypotheses about why the error may have occurred can also be documented.

This format is illustrated in Exhibit 5.2 with a partial example of a "calling for pizza delivery" task. The directions and recording form for the *pizza phone delivery task* is included in Appendix B.5.

In addition, to the pizza task, a blank form for performance analysis of task errors for a selected task is available in Appendix B.6. The blank form allows the therapist to enter the task steps of an activity that is relevant to the client so that error types, error recognition and correction can be systematically observed and recorded.

Dynamic Interactional Model: Multi-Step Activity Management Error Analysis

This format presented in Exhibit 5.3 also involves analysis of task errors; however, the activity is divided into 3 phases: (1) Task preparation phase; (2) Task implementation phase; and (3) Task completion phase. The same procedure for analysis of task errors (described above) is used, but the format of the form is slightly different and is partially illustrated below using an abbreviated version. The full blank form is included in Appendix B.7.

Prior to the start of the assessment, the therapist lists the task steps of the selected activity within the implementation phase. The therapist highlights or checks off steps that are

Exhibit 5.2 Pizza Phone Delivery Task: Analysis of Task Errors (NO cues or assistance provided)

Activity Steps Calling for pizza delivery	√, I, P X	Task Error or Inefficiency	*Error Awareness	Interpretation Why do you think the error occurred?
1. Initiates searching on phone or electronic device.	I	Initiates searching but gets distracted by weather forecast and looks at other info first. *Irrelevant actions*	NO	Saw weather icon and could not inhibit distraction.
2. Uses appropriate search terms, narrows search appropriately.	P	Initially searches for "pizza" without other qualifying terms (e.g., location). *Inaccurate selection of term*	NO	Found a pizza place without qualifying terms.
3. *Correctly* _X_ Identifies local pizza place _√_ Phone number	P	Pizzeria is more than 30 minutes away. Correctly identifies phone number *Inaccuracies*	SR-P EC	Only recognized error after calling and finding out it was too far for delivery (1 hr. away) and then conducted a new search.
Total Accurate steps completed:		Total # inefficient steps: _____ Total # partial steps: _____	**Time Required for Completion:** _____	

√ = completed accurately, I = accurate but inefficient, P = partially accurate, X = inaccurate;
* SR = Self- Recognition of error, SR-P = Self-recognized error only after obstacle or problem, EC = Error Correction

Exhibit 5.3 Sample of Multi-step Activity Error Analysis

Specify Task: Call for Pizza	Task Errors/Observations	Ineff	Omit	Inacc	Seq	Irrelev Action
1. Task Preparation Phase						
After initial directions, client initiates actions, takes time to review directions and plan ahead, re-clarifies directions or checks understanding if needed, gathers, organizes or re-organizes relevant tools, materials, directions, lists or information	Client does not review directions and jumps into task. No pre-planning or preparation is observed. Client does not ask for pen or pencil.		✓			
2. Task Implementation *Specify Main steps*						
X Searches on phone or electronic device	Initiates searching but gets distracted by weather forecast and looked at other info first.					✓
X Uses appropriate search terms, narrows search appropriately	Initially searches for "pizza" without other qualifying terms (e.g., location). Does not adhere to directions (local area).			✓		
Correctly X Identifies local pizza place √ Phone number	Pizzeria is more than 30 minutes away. Correctly identifies Phone number. Does not adhere to directions (local area).				✓	
3. Task Completion						
Persists until completion, does not stop prematurely or continue aimlessly when finished; self-checks work or compares to initial directions	Does not review directions or self-check that all directions were followed.		✓			

Recall of directions: Adequate, Inadequate **Persistence:** Good, Needs encouragement to persist, Gives up easily
Spontaneous Error Recognition: No error recognition, Slight error recognition, Partial error recognition, Full recognition
Paces Speed: Adequate, Too fast (impulsive), Too slow, Fluctuates – either too fast and too slow

completed accurately. Similar to the analysis of task errors described above, no cues or assistance are provided and task errors for each step are observed, recorded, and then categorized during or immediately after the task.

The most common errors are listed on the form (e.g., inefficiencies, omissions, inaccuracies, sequencing errors or steps performed out of order, and irrelevant actions or actions that are extraneous to the task goal) for ease in identification of general error patterns. Strategy observations are included in the last column (not shown). Observations regarding self-recognition of errors are generally recorded at the bottom of the form based on overall performance, rather than at each task step, along with additional observations on recall of directions, timing, and persistence.

Performance-Based Tools for Specific Activities

Whereas the previous section described methods of performance analysis that could be applied broadly to any chosen activity, this section describes analysis of performance for specified activities or tasks. Consistent with the DIM, the focus across all tasks is on error analysis, task methods or strategy use, and self-perceptions of performance.

Weekly Calendar Planning Activity (WCPA)

The Weekly Calendar Planning Activity (WCPA) (Toglia, 2015) is an example of a standardized performance-based assessment that is derived from the DIM (Toglia & White, 2020). It is used with adolescents and adults, age 12 and above. In addition to accuracy, it focuses on error types, strategies, and awareness. Unlike the performance analysis methods described above, the WCPA involves a pre-selected task involving entering a list of appointments into a weekly schedule while adhering to rules, monitoring time, and managing conflicts. Completion of this task requires the interweaving of executive function (EF) skills.

The WCPA was designed to guide strategy-based treatment such as the MC approach. The WCPA allows for the opportunity to observe and analyze error patterns, task efficiency, adherence to rules, use of strategies, and self-monitoring skills to provide a comprehensive understanding of cognitive performance abilities and deficiencies. A standard after-task interview probes the person's perspective regarding performance, including challenges encountered and task methods or strategies used (Lussier et al., 2019; Toglia, 2018). This type of in-depth analysis of performance provides information that is highly relevant to strategy-based interventions. The WCPA includes normative data so that results can be compared to healthy controls (Toglia, 2015). Additional information and resources including articles and a series of videos on administering and interpreting the WCPA can be found on www.multicontext.net (resources – assessment tools).

A preliminary dynamic test-teach-retest format that provides additional information on learning and carryover of strategies is also described in the WCPA test manual as an option (Toglia, 2015). The test-teach-retest method looks at independent performance before and after a period of mediation or cues (rather than cueing during an activity) to provide an indication of responsiveness to intervention or learning potential. Most clients do better when they are cued within an activity, but it is more important to look at what happens when cues are withdrawn. Consistent with the DIM, the test-teach-retest format provides information on the extent that performance can be changed or modified through mediation by another person or by task modification/adaptation. This information is directly related to treatment and is used when it is unclear if the person would be responsive to a metacognitive strategy approach (Toglia, 2018).

Smart Phone Multiple Tasks

An activity involving a list of tasks that need to be completed with a smartphone is included in Appendix B.8 using a similar format as described in the error analysis tools section. Use of everyday technology is an important part of daily life. This simulated phone task provides information on everyday technology skills as well as the ability to follow a list and keep track of rules. It also shares similarities with both the Multiple Errands Test (MET) (Burgess et al., 2006) and WCPA (Toglia, 2015). This task is presently being piloted with people who have acquired brain injury.

Upper Body Dressing Error Analysis Tool (UBDEA)

Another example of performance analysis of a specific task includes upper body dressing tasks (T-shirt and button-down shirt). Typically, activities of daily living (ADL) are assessed by determining the amount and degree of assistance needed for successful performance. Assistance is automatically provided by the therapist whenever it is needed. In contrast to typical ADL assessments, the UBDEA asks the person to identify when and what type of help they need. Cues are focused on helping the person recognize errors and figure out alternate ways to address any obstacles encountered, rather than telling the person what to do.

The ability to recognize when and what type of help is needed is important in functional tasks. Those who are less aware of when they need assistance are more likely to be at risk for safety problems. If a person does not recognize when they need assistance, they will likely attempt to perform activities on their own even though they may not have the physical or cognitive capacity to do so.

For individuals who struggle with basic ADL, this example illustrates how performance analysis that focuses on error patterns, error recognition, and correction can be used with basic tasks. The person is asked to put on a T-shirt, followed by a button-down shirt. Garments are presented inside out and upside down to observe the way the person goes about recognizing and correcting this. Directions are as follows: "I would like you to put on this shirt by yourself." "If you need any help, please let me know what type of help you need. Try not to ask for help unless there is no other way to put the shirt on." Verbal cues and assistance are not provided unless the person is stuck or cannot progress. Then cues are provided to help the person recognize errors or to help them figure out how to correct errors. This type of cueing is different than direct cues that are focused on task completion. Clinical example 5.3 presents a summary of results and highlights a focus on reasons for difficulty in dressing as well as error recognition and correction.

> **Clinical Example 5.3 Summary of Performance on T-Shirt Task**
>
> Greg was able to complete 4 out of 6 steps independently to put on a T-shirt. He had difficulty orienting and positioning the shirt correctly and placing his affected arm in the sleeve. For both these sub-steps, Greg was aware of difficulties and verbalized what he wanted to do but he was unable to carry it out. He identified errors but could not correct them and did not ask for assistance. Greg was observed to attempt to put the garment on inside out. He recognized this but was unable to figure out how to correct it and position the garment accurately. He repeatedly approached the task the same way, making the same errors (without changing his method), became quickly frustrated, and stopped the task prematurely. Greg was asked if he needed assistance and he agreed that he did. At this point, the therapist guided him in positioning the garment correctly by directing his attention to relevant aspects of the shirt, generating a plan for correction, and helping him recognize that he should place his affected arm in the sleeve first. Once this was done, he was able to carry out the remainder of the steps on his own.

In Clinical Example 5.3, Greg was aware of difficulties but did not initiate asking for assistance because he wanted to complete the task on his own. Instead of jumping in to provide direct assistance or complete task components for Greg, the therapist guided him in figuring out what to do.

Guidelines for cues and directions for completing the forms are presented in more detail in Appendix B.9. Implementation of these guidelines were piloted with video analysis; however, further testing and research is needed. The before- and after-task interview previously described can be used with this task as well.

Revised Contextual Memory Test (CMT-2)

The revised Contextual Memory test (CMT-2) examines immediate and delayed recall of 20 pictures of objects related to a theme (restaurant, morning, or school) for children and adults ages 7 and above (Toglia, 2019). The original CMT included black and white drawings of objects related to the restaurant or morning theme and had norms for adults (Toglia, 1993a). The CMT-2 is web-based and includes colored photos of objects. It also generates an automatic summary of scores and a narrative report organized into the areas of performance, awareness, and strategy use. The original CMT manual describes different result patterns in these areas and treatment implications (Toglia, 1993a). Normative data collection on the revised version is currently in progress across ages 7 to 90.

The use of objects in standard memory tests is typically avoided because such tests were designed to differentiate between verbal and nonverbal memory or to determine brain areas that might be involved in impairment. Everyday memory, however, includes objects and the use of context. The CMT-2 was not designed to be used in isolation or to diagnose memory problems. Consistent with the DIM, the CMT-2 investigates awareness and self-perceptions of memory before and after recall. Strategy use is also probed in a standard after-task interview (Raphael-Greenfield et al., 2020). The CMT-2 is narrower in scope than the performance-based tests described above, but it is similar in that it provides information relevant for treatment.

Summary of Dynamic Interactional Model-based Performance Analysis Tools

The DIM Performance Analysis Guide, as well as the sample performance analysis tools described above, provide structured methods for observation, recording, and analysis of performance that can be used as part of the assessment process. They illustrate how performance analysis can encompass a wide range of activities and levels. All of the examples or sample formats presented place a focus on the process of how someone goes about doing an activity, including the type of performance errors, methods or strategies used, the ability to recognize and correct errors, and the ability to self-assess performance. Questions immediately following activity performance can be used with any of the tools described and provide information on the person's perspective of their performance, including strategies used. Appendix B.10 provides a table that can be used to generally summarize the overall results of assessment including the concerns of the client and others, performance, performance error patterns, activity, and environmental characteristics that influence performance, awareness, and strategy use. Examples of assessment summaries using this table are presented within clinical cases in Chapter 15. As indicated in Chapter 4, individuals with subtle cognitive deficits might not show difficulties in performance within a short (e.g., 1 hour) structured testing environment, but subtle cognitive deficits may emerge after sustained activity participation or as the result of cumulative activities or combinations of activities. In these individuals, participation assessment tools, as well as use of a log that describes the context that cognitive lapses emerge are needed (e.g., when, where, types of activities etc.; see Chapter 14 and Appendix C.19).

DYNAMIC INTERACTION MODEL AND TREATMENT PLANNING

The information derived from performance analysis provides a foundation for using the DIM model for treatment planning and use of the Multicontext (MC) approach. Treatment may involve concurrently adapting activity and environmental demands while promoting awareness and strategy use across activities. For example, some activities may be adapted or modified to ensure safety or enhance function, while strategies and awareness may be promoted in other activities. Activities might also be adapted or modified to ensure that the activity is at the optimal level of challenge for strategy training.

This process is illustrated in the clinical example presented with the DIM treatment planning form in Exhibit 5.4. The DIM treatment planning form is used to help a therapist consider and integrate all aspects of the DIM when planning treatment. The example corresponds to Clinical Example 5.2 that was presented earlier in this chapter. The treatment planning form in Exhibit 5.4 indicates that medication management is an activity that will be adapted by others. The activities of copying information and making coffee include some task or environmental modifications (to make certain that activities are at the optimal level of challenge) but will also be used within a framework of strategy and awareness training (i.e., the

Exhibit 5.4 Sample Dynamic Interactional Model (DIM): Treatment Planning

Person factors: (interests, motivation, experiences, psychosocial, occupations, goals)
See Clinical Example 5.2; manages her medications; uses a cell phone, e-mail, and a personal planner.

Error patterns across tasks: repetition

Awareness: Not aware before or during task. Aware after task with therapist guidance.

Strategy use: Ineffective and inconsistent use observed.

Activity/environment conditions that increase/decrease symptoms: Decrease need to go back and forth between two or more stimuli, decrease number of steps in task to 2-3.

Functional Problem(s)	Specify Activity Demands Identify any Modifications Adaptations Technology	Environment/Context (e.g., environmental cue signs or signals, adaptations, technologies, cues by others)	Person — Strategies Across Situations	Person — Awareness and Self-Monitoring
Medication management	Pillbox is set up by others.	Alarm reminders with voice messages are pre-programmed. Collaboration with significant others on adaptations needed for medication management.	--------	--------
E-mail or copying information	Information to be copied is no longer than 3 or 4 lines (to be an optimal challenge level).	Quiet environment without distractions. Help significant others understand performance errors and collaborate with them on methods of guided questioning to promote performance.	Reads what is written out loud using her finger to point to each word to self-check for "doubles" or repetitions.	Asked to anticipate things she needs to watch out for (e.g., repetitions). Self-checks for repetitions after task.
Making coffee	Uses typical coffee pot with needed items on counter. Only one task at a time.	Kitchen counter uncluttered. Collaborate with significant others as indicated above.	List of written steps. Highlights or checks off list with each scoop and/or step. Talks out loud with each scoop.	Asked to anticipate things she needs to watch out for (e.g., repetitions). Self-checks for repetitions after task.

MC approach, described in Part 2 of this manual). In both of these activities, there is a focus on helping the client monitor her tendency to repeat information. The client is guided in the use of strategies that are applicable across other activities, such as talking out loud or using a list, to control repetition errors. Thus, the example below illustrates how different treatment approaches can be used simultaneously by selecting some tasks that are completely adapted by others and selecting other tasks that involve strategy and awareness training. A blank DIM Treatment planning form is included in Appendix C.1.

SUMMARY

Performance analysis provides information on how a person goes about doing an activity. This requires an understanding of the cognitive demands of the activity as well as the ability to observe and recognize cognitive errors that may be influencing performance. Performance analysis identifies patterns of task errors that impede performance across activities. At the same time, strategy use, self-monitoring skills, and self-awareness of performance are observed, probed, and analyzed. This includes the ability to recognize and detect performance errors, describe task methods used, identify task challenges, and accurately assess performance. Cues are generally avoided during assessment so that the person's ability to cope with cognitive challenges and problem solve can be best observed. If additional information for treatment is needed, a test-teach-retest dynamic assessment format that examines changes in performance after a brief period of mediation, as briefly described within the WCPA, is suggested.

Information on performance errors, self-awareness, and strategy use provides a foundation for treatment planning. Within the Dynamic Interactional Model framework, cognitive performance can be facilitated by changing the task, environment, person's awareness and strategy use, or a combination of approaches. If the person exhibits a total lack of awareness or strategy use during assessment, despite attempts at probing after the task or mediation (test-teach-retest approach), treatment approaches that do not expect change in awareness or learning across different situations may be most appropriate. This includes adaptations by others, care partner collaboration and training, errorless learning, use of the Cognitive Disability Model (McCraith & Earhart, 2018), or the Neurofunctional approach (Giles, 2018).

If the person demonstrates some awareness or strategy use during performance-based assessment, it implies that the person may be a good candidate for strategy-based intervention such as the MC approach, which is described thoroughly in the next section of this manual. The specific information obtained through performance analysis based on the Dynamic Interactional Model provides an important starting point for treatment planning.

KEY POINTS

- Performance-based functional cognitive assessments differ according to methods used and the type of information provided.
- Assessments based on the Dynamic Interactional Model of cognition include analysis of performance errors, awareness, and strategy use. This information is interpreted together to guide treatment.
- Assessments refrain from cues and focus on the process of how a person goes about doing an activity.
- An after-task interview is used to probe the person's perceptions of performance and strategies used across different activities.
- Tools that can support performance analysis based on the Dynamic Interactional Model include:
  - DIM Performance Analysis Guide (broad generic guide for any activity).
  - Cognitive Performance Observation Tool (structures observations for use with any activity).
  - Performance-Based Error Analysis tools (specific analysis of performance errors that can be used with any activity).
  - Specific Performance-Based Assessment Tools (specific activities including the WCPA, Multiple Phone Task, Upper Body Dressing Error Analysis Tool).

PART II

COGNITIVE REHABILITATION INTERVENTION: THE MULTICONTEXT APPROACH

Chapter 6

Introduction to the Multicontext Approach

This chapter introduces the Multicontext (MC) approach to cognitive rehabilitation, including background, theoretical concepts, treatment components, history and evolution, evidence, and criteria for use. Subsequent chapters within this section operationalize the key elements of the MC approach and provide guidelines and resources for clinical practice and research.

CONTENTS OF CHAPTER 6

Overview of the Multicontext Approach
 Characteristics of the Multicontext Approach
 Phases Across the Multicontext Approach
Background of the Multicontext Approach
 History and Evolution of the Multicontext Approach
 A Review of Evidence on the Multicontext Approach
For Whom is the Multicontext Approach Most Appropriate?
Knowledge and Skills Needed to Implement the Multicontext Approach
Summary and Key Points

OVERVIEW OF THE MULTICONTEXT APPROACH

The MC approach was initially developed for adults with acquired brain injury and cognitive limitations who had difficulty learning as well as recognizing and understanding changes that had occurred in their thinking and information processing skills following a traumatic brain injury, stroke or other neurological condition. The treatment principles broadly focus on methods to optimize learning, generalization, and functional outcomes and are therefore applicable across a wide range of conditions.

The MC treatment approach, derived from the Dynamic Interactional Model (DIM) of cognition (Chapter 4) is directed at promoting the person's use of strategies and metacognitive skills so they can control and optimize their cognitive performance across a variety of situations. While the Dynamic Interactional Model presents a broad conceptualization of cognition, the MC approach provides intervention guidelines and methods to help a person learn to recognize, monitor, and manage cognitive symptoms or control error patterns across different activities by using effective strategies. The MC approach emphasizes intervention methods that are directed at the "person" aspect of the Dynamic Interactional Model, while other treatment approaches such as the Cognitive Disability Model (Allen et al., 1992; McCraith & Earhart,

2018) emphasize intervention methods directed at the activity or environmental aspects of the model. Although different aspects of the Dynamic Interactional Model may be emphasized by different treatment approaches, the model suggests that all three components (person, activity, and environment) need to be simultaneously considered in treatment (Toglia, 2018). For example, within the MC approach, activity and environmental demands are consistently analyzed and adapted so that metacognitive strategy intervention methods are used within an optimal level of challenge.

The MC approach provides a broad framework that can be used with different age groups and diagnostic categories to promote strategy use, self-awareness, self-monitoring, self-regulation, and generalization of these skills across everyday activities. Figure 6.1 illustrates how the MC approach simultaneously emphasizes cognitive strategies, self-awareness, and metacognitive skills (e.g., self-monitoring, self-regulation) in an integrated manner across a variety of activities. Four key goals or areas of focus of MC intervention are summarized in Exhibit 6.1.

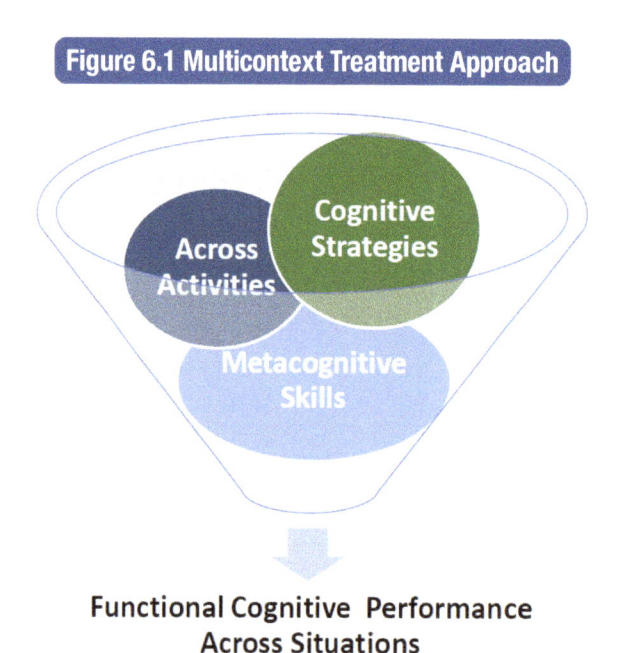

Characteristics of the Multicontext Approach

The MC approach seeks to improve occupational performance by facilitating strategy use, self-monitoring, and self-regulation during functional activities and by explicitly helping clients make connections between activity experiences so they can transfer/generalize strategies. Consistent with the Dynamic Interactional Model, the goal is not to develop cognitive skills or task-specific solutions. Rather, it is to help the person cope with cognitive demands and manage cognitive performance errors by using strategies across situations and within the context of everyday activities. Since an understanding of one's performance strengths and limitations is a key ingredient for effective strategy use, intervention emphasizes self-awareness in the initial treatment stages if needed (Toglia, 2018; Toglia et al., 2020).

The MC approach is a complex and multi-component metacognitive strategy intervention. The focus of therapist-client interaction during the intervention is on the process of how one goes about doing an activity and managing cognitive challenges. Cognitive strategies that are self-generated or selected with therapist mediation and collaboration are used to control cognitive symptoms and performance errors across different activities. The MC approach encompasses a broad range of cognitive strategies depending on the client's abilities, preferences, and pattern of cognitive performance problems (Chapter 7). Strategy intervention is intertwined with metacognition in that each session uses a structured metacognitive framework and guided learning techniques (detailed in Chapter 10) to help a person understand and monitor their performance and generate strategies. There is a focus on building cognitive self-efficacy by helping a person recognize how they can take control of their performance by using strategies (Steinberg and Zlotnik, 2019; Toglia, 2018; Toglia et al., 2020).

Repeated experiences with a variety of activities that present common cognitive challenges provide the client with the opportunity to self-discover patterns of performance errors and practice applying strategies to control performance (Chapter 8). Treatment uses functionally relevant or meaningful activities to motivate

Figure 6.1 Multicontext Treatment Approach

- Across Activities
- Cognitive Strategies
- Metacognitive Skills

↓

Functional Cognitive Performance Across Situations

Exhibit 6.1 Goals of the Multicontext Approach

1. **Optimize strategy use in cognitive functional activities**
   - Ability to generate and select strategies.
   - Initiation, frequency, appropriate timing, and efficiency of strategies in functional cognitive activities.
   - Use of strategies to encode, process, and integrate information needed for learning and successful task completion.
   - Ability to self-manage cognitive lapses or cognitive performance errors.
   - Use of strategies to manage functional cognitive performance challenges.
   - Use of multiple strategies, when needed.

2. **Transfer and generalize cognitive strategies to a variety of situations**
   - Apply strategies to a number of tasks and environments (transfer breadth).
   - Apply strategies to tasks and environments that are very different (physically) than the initial training task (transfer distance).
   - Apply what is learned during treatment sessions to real-life functional cognitive activities and goals.

3. **Increase online self-awareness of performance**
   - Awareness of task or performance challenges.
   - Awareness of strategies or methods that contribute to task success.
   - Ability to self-reflect and self-appraise performance.

4. **Increase self-efficacy or perceived control over cognitive performance**
   - Confidence in the ability to self-manage cognitive performance.
   - Persistence in the face of cognitive challenges,

and engage the client and to facilitate transfer or generalization to real-world performance. Initial phases of treatment focus on self-awareness of cognitive strengths and challenges and self-monitoring of performance. As the person begins to recognize, understand, anticipate, and monitor performance errors, the treatment focus shifts to strategy generation or efficient and effective use of cognitive strategies to regulate performance (Toglia et al., 2010). Throughout this process, the therapist continually analyzes and adjusts activity and environmental features to provide an optimal level of challenge across different situations. Client goals are also continually revisited and adjusted, or new goals emerge as the person gains self-awareness.

Transfer and generalization are promoted by (a) use of functionally relevant activities, (b) multiple contexts for strategy practice, and (c) explicit guidance to help the person make connections across activity experiences and situations. For some clients, particularly those who have difficulty initiating or applying strategies to new activities, treatment activities are structured across a horizontal continuum to make it easier to detect and connect similarities across treatment activities (detailed in Chapter 8) (Toglia, 1991, 2018; Toglia et al., 2010). The key treatment components along with techniques or guidelines for incorporating these components and achieving the goals of the MC approach are listed in Table 6.1.

Phases Across the Multicontext Approach

The MC approach can have different areas of emphasis across a treatment program, depending on the needs of the client. For example, for some clients, the initial phases of MC treatment are focused on helping the person experience and understand their cognitive strengths and weaknesses or identifying performance problems. As awareness emerges or a clearer understanding of the performance problems occurs, treatment places a greater emphasis on generating alternative methods or strategies to cope with task challenges. Strategy use is practiced and

Table 6.1 The Multicontext Approach: Key Treatment Components

Treatment Components	Sample Techniques or Treatment Guidelines
1. Focus on use of cognitive strategies	• Guidance is provided to help the client select, apply, or practice specific cognitive domain strategies and/or non-situational (generic) strategies to manage cognitive performance challenges. • Strategies chosen depend on client needs and preferences.
2. Activities structured to promote transfer and generalization	*Horizontal transfer continuum* - Activities are structured *horizontally* along a transfer continuum from near (similar) to far (dissimilar). • Sideways Learning - Practice and reinforce strategy use across activities at the same level of difficulty before grading complexity. • Structured activities can be used to enhance self-awareness and strategy use in the initial stages of treatment. • A wide variety of activities and contexts are used. • Help the person explicitly recognize connections between activities.
3. Metacognitive framework	*Use of mediated learning techniques and guided questions* • Guided questions and mediated learning techniques are used before, during, and immediately after activities within each session. • "Mediate" and guide rather than "tell" the person what to do. • Periods of "stop and check" or review. • Structured self-assessment techniques that allow self-recognition of errors. (Errors are not pointed out.) • Explicitly help the client make connections between past, present, and future activities through questioning or structured journaling.
Additional Components (not unique)	
4. Therapeutic support focused on enhancing self-efficacy	• Focus on strategies or methods that lead to success and empower the person to understand and manage their cognitive symptoms. • Help a person understand why the strategy works. • Feedback on the process/ strategy use rather than pointing out errors. • Reframe, reflect, build sense of self-competence in managing errors. • Create a collaborative, positive, and supportive atmosphere.
5. Treatment activities are functionally relevant and at an optimal level of challenge	• Consideration of personal context, interests, occupations, lifestyle, and routines. • Treatment includes everyday functional materials or meaningful activities. • Activities are not too easy and not too hard but present a level of challenge that allows for success with strategies or effort.
6. Goal Setting and Revision	• Structured goal setting and goal rating techniques may be used. • Goal revision/adjustment is facilitated as self-awareness emerges.

monitored across activities that have similar demands. The final phases of treatment focus on broad application of strategy use (Toglia et al., 2010). Figure 6.2 illustrates typical phases in treatment; however, these are not fixed treatment stages.

Progression through the phases in Figure 6.2 may vary during treatment. For some individuals, particularly those who have good self-awareness, the treatment program may emphasize strategy generation and effectiveness; while for others, treatment might focus on making connections across experiences. Although the intervention program may spend more or less time on different treatment phases, each session has a consistent "within-session" metacognitive framework (described in Chapter 10).

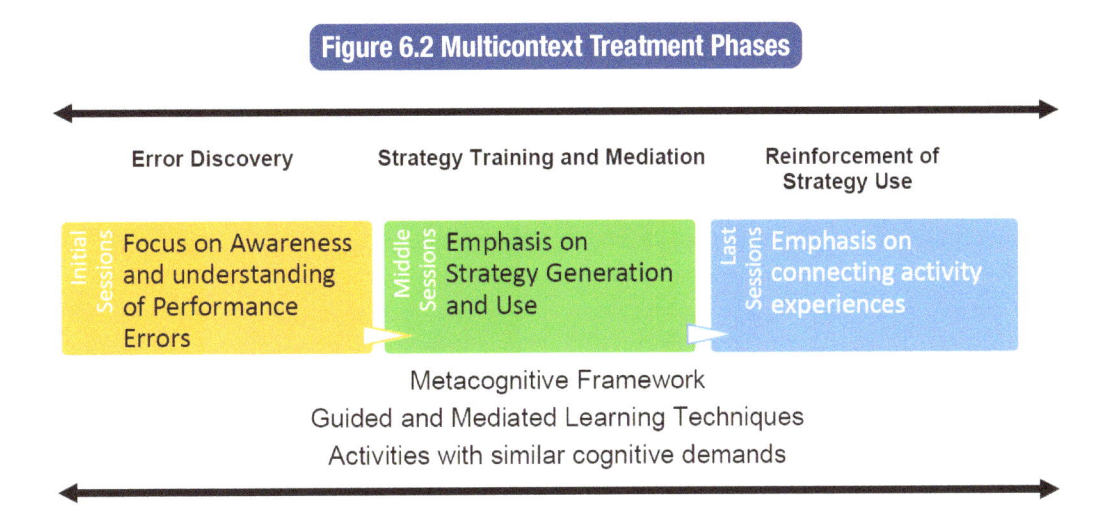

Figure 6.2 Multicontext Treatment Phases

Error Discovery — **Initial Sessions:** Focus on Awareness and understanding of Performance Errors

Strategy Training and Mediation — **Middle Sessions:** Emphasis on Strategy Generation and Use

Reinforcement of Strategy Use — **Last Sessions:** Emphasis on connecting activity experiences

Metacognitive Framework
Guided and Mediated Learning Techniques
Activities with similar cognitive demands

BACKGROUND OF THE MULTICONTEXT APPROACH

History and Evolution of the Multicontext Approach

The MC approach was initially described in 1991 and was heavily influenced by clinical observations of people who had traumatic brain injury. Limitations in self-awareness and a lack of transfer and generalization of skills were identified as barriers to treatment and successful outcomes, however, few or no guidelines addressed these areas in occupational therapy practice or rehabilitation (Toglia, 1991). The MC approach built upon earlier work of Abreu and Toglia (1987) by expanding concepts from educational and cognitive psychology literature on learning and generalization (Feuerstein et al., 2015; Pressley et al., 1990; Salomon & Perkins, 1988; Vygotsky, 1978) and incorporating them into occupational therapy practice and cognitive rehabilitation. Practical guidelines for teaching strategies and transfer of strategic performance were extrapolated from this literature and applied to treatment of people with acquired brain injury as described in this section.

The foundation for the instructional methods used in the MC approach for promoting learning and strategy use were influenced by the seminal work of Michael Pressley and his colleagues on strategy instruction in the special education and educational psychology literature in the 1980s and 1990s (Harris et al., 2008; Pressley et al., 1987; Pressley et al., 1990). Pressley conceived of effective strategy use as good information processing and described several characteristics of good strategy instruction. For example, Pressley described good strategy instruction as providing experiences that help students construct and personalize the strategies they use. This involves collaborating with and empowering students to use procedures that help them accomplish tasks (Harris & Pressley, 1991). The focus is not to develop task-specific strategies but to help the student apply strategies across situations. Pressley highlighted the importance of a focus on metacognitive processes including evaluating strategy effectiveness and helping to increase awareness of when, how, and where strategies should be used. He also emphasized that maintenance and transfer of strategic performance should be planned for and supported rather than assumed to occur (Harris et al., 2008; Pressley & Harris, 2009). Pressley argued that strategy instruction that was metacognitively rich was needed to obtain durability and generalization of strategies. All of these principles were later integrated into several evidence-based educational programs as well as into the MC approach.

The MC approach combined foundational literature on strategy instruction with the work of Vygotsky (1978) (zone of proximal development) and Feuerstein et al. (2015) in mediated learning experiences to provide guidelines on how to interact, cue, and use questioning to facilitate performance. Vygotsky described the zone of proximal development (ZPD) as the area between what a learner can do independently (mastery) and what can be accomplished with the assistance of a competent other person. The ZPD represents skills that are just beneath the surface or that have the potential for change. Intervention is best when it takes place within the ZPD. Scaffolding techniques derived from Vygotsky are instructional methods for promoting learning within the ZPD. Learning is scaffolded by structuring the task, jointly participating in problem-solving, or focusing the person's attention when needed. Scaffolding involves the gradual release of responsibility to the learner (Frey & Fisher, 2010). Similarly, Feuerstein, et al.'s (2015) mediated learning experience (MLE) is a structured and interactional approach to learning in which another person or mediating agent interposes themselves between stimuli and the learner to assist the learner in processing and integrating information. The literature on scaffolding techniques and Feuerstein's MLE was assimilated into guided learning techniques used in the MC approach and described in Chapter 10.

Literature on teaching for transfer (McKeough et al., 2013; Salomon & Perkins, 1988) and evidence on the conditions that are most likely to increase the probability of strategic transfer also influenced the development of the MC approach. Some people (e.g., individuals with brain injury) may need more help in transferring the effects of learning than others. The MC approach views transfer on a continuum (from near transfer to very far transfer) and suggests that treatment can be designed in a manner that increases the likelihood, durability, and breadth of strategic transfer (Toglia, 1991, 2018). This is described in Chapter 8.

At the time that the MC approach was introduced in the early 1990s, the focus of cognitive rehabilitation was on remedial or deficit-specific approaches. Treatment targeted separate cognitive impairments using tabletop cognitive activities, worksheets, or computerized exercises, graded from simple to complex. The success of this type of treatment, which focused on improving cognitive skills, was measured by standardized cognitive tests. In contrast, the MC approach was a complex, multi-component intervention that targeted changes in self-awareness, strategy use, and function (Toglia, 2018). This represented a paradigm shift, as the focus on metacognition and strategy use was not well accepted or integrated into clinical practice at the time. As such, empirical investigation of the MC approach presented challenges and obstacles given the available (or lack of available) assessment tools at the time. It has not been until the last decade that the use of metacognitive strategy approaches has received greater acceptance and popularity in occupational therapy and rehabilitation (Cicerone et al., 2019).

Similar to this manual, the initial manuscript on the MC approach (1991) discussed the need to integrate metacognitive and strategy training together to promote generalization and transfer. It urged therapists to focus on the *process* of how a person goes about doing a task rather than the results, outcomes, or errors: "Feedback that provides information about results may be ineffective in improving performance unless the patient understands why the error occurred" (p. 510). It also focused on self-monitoring and self-awareness and described several different metacognitive training techniques to promote awareness, as exemplified by the statement, "The patient must learn how to monitor and evaluate his or her own performance" (p. 510). Modification of a person's perception concerning his or her own performance was described as a key component that affects the subsequent course of treatment and outcomes. The concepts of self-awareness and cognitive strategies were further defined, clarified, and expanded in subsequent publications (Toglia & Kirk, 2000; Toglia et al., 2012).

The core concepts of the MC approach today are the same as they were in 1991. The MC treatment components described in 1991 included a focus on metacognition and processing strategies, use of multiple activities and environments, structuring treatment along a transfer continuum or establishing criteria for transfer, and using methods to connect new information to previous knowledge or experiences. Although these concepts remain the same, current descriptions of the MC approach have reframed and condensed them into the three main components identified in Table 6.1 (previous table). Table 6.2 summarizes the core treatment components and key statements from the initial publications on the MC approach in 1991 and 1992 and compares them to current MC practices and guidelines to illustrate the evolution as well as the consistency of the approach over the years.

A Review of Evidence on the Multicontext Approach

A number of studies strongly support the core components of the MC approach, such as strategy training (Haskins et al., 2012; Cicerone et al., 2019), awareness training (Engel et al., 2017; Goverover et al., 2007), and practice in different contexts (Waldum et al., 2016). For example, a systematic review provides preliminary evidence that the use of interventions directed at increasing awareness improves everyday performance and enhances functional outcomes at both an activity and participation level. Specifically, they found support for metacognitive strategy intervention and guided discussion within the context of experiential participation and functional tasks (Engel et al., 2017).

Umanath et al. (2016) describe a pilot study demonstrating the superiority of the use of a metacognitive framework over explicit strategy instruction in older adults. Similarly, Bottiroli et al. (2017) found that a self-guided strategy adaptation approach that used questioning to encourage older adults to analyze tasks and self-generate strategies resulted in wider transfer effects than those typically observed in cognitive training studies. These studies support the essential ingredients of the MC approach.

The MC approach specifically has been described for clients with posterior cortical atrophy, object recognition difficulties or Balint syndrome (Perez et al., 1996; Toglia, 1989), spatial neglect (Chen & Toglia, 2019; Golisz, 1998; Toglia & Chen, 2020), people with acquired brain injury and executive dysfunction (Landa-Gonzalez, 2001; Toglia et al., 2011; Jaywant et al., 2020), women with lupus (Harrison et al., 2005), children with learning difficulties or attention deficit hyperactivity disorder (Cermak, 2018; Waldman-Levi & Steinmann Obermeyer, 2018), and people with schizophrenia (Josman & Regev, 2018;

Table 6.2 Comparison of Core Multicontext Treatment Components Over Time

Treatment Components	Then . . . (1991–1998)	. . . and NOW
Use of multiple environments	Transfer of information is facilitated when the person is required to apply the newly learned skill or strategy to multiple contexts or environments. The terms "context" and "environment" were used interchangeably. "Transfer is part of learning and should be required during treatment rather than at the end of treatment" (Toglia, 1991, p. 507).	The focus on variability and application of a strategy across multiple contexts, environments, or activities during treatment remains the same. However, this component is included within the concept of the *horizontal transfer continuum*.
Establishment of criteria for transfer (near, intermediate, far, very far)	"Transfer of learning is not an all-or-none phenomenon. It occurs in different degrees along a continuum. Establishment of criteria is appropriate for the determination of when and to what extent transfer of learning has taken place" (Toglia, 1991, p. 507). Transfer criteria are established by identifying a graded series of tasks that display decreasing degrees of physical similarity (surface characteristics) to the original learning situation (Toglia, 1991).	The principle of a horizontal transfer continuum and the need to identify activities that represent different degrees of transfer distance remains the same. Current publications describe the transfer continuum as a general guide for activity progression, rather than representing distinct categories of transfer. The degree of physical similarity is emphasized rather than transfer categories (near, intermediate, etc.).
Metacognitive training	Treatment techniques that aim to help the person detect errors, predict outcomes, estimate task difficulty, and evaluate performance outcome were suggested to increase self-monitoring skills and self-awareness. Self-estimation, role reversal, self-questioning, self-evaluation were all described (Toglia, 1991, p. 510). "Simultaneously, metacognitive training techniques that emphasize the ability to anticipate and detect errors are employed to assist the patient in developing the self-monitoring skills necessary to move from a cued to an uncued condition" (Toglia, 1991, p. 514). There was a focus on providing cues from general to specific and on helping to identify ways cueing could be transferred from the therapist to the client. Examples of guided questions focused on the process were included in case descriptions in, (e.g., Explain how the cards go together or how did you try to remember?) (Toglia, 1992). In 1998, the use of strategy investigation questions that helped clients reflect on how they went about doing an activity was described (Toglia 1998). At this time, the focus of anticipation changed from predicting errors or outcome to anticipating potential obstacles or whether a strategy might be needed (Toglia, 1998).	Metacognition and self-awareness remain a major area of emphasis; however, the conceptualization of self-awareness has been further expanded and described, and the distinction between awareness outside and within the context of an activity has been highlighted (Toglia & Kirk, 2000). Metacognitive training techniques have been further specified, clarified and organized into a framework, while the focus on self-prediction and estimation of task performance has decreased (Toglia, 2018). Direct cues are avoided. Guided questioning techniques and guidelines have been expanded and specified. Questioning is faded as the client learns to anticipate, self-generate strategies, and self-evaluate performance themselves. Questions to build anticipation and strategy generation prior to task performance have been further specified and included within the metacognitive framework.

Treatment Components	Then... (1991-1998)	...and NOW
Processing strategies, continued	Processing strategies are organized approaches, tactics, or rules that operate either unconsciously or consciously. Situational strategies (e.g., rehearsal, imagery, association) operate in certain tasks and environments, whereas non-situational strategies (e.g., planning ahead, removing distractions or irrelevant material) are effective in a wide range of tasks and environments (Toglia, 1991, pp. 510-511). Strategies help the individual select relevant information from the environment and guide the organization of incoming material for information processing (Toglia, 1991). Initially, the therapist selected and taught strategies to the client. The same strategy was practiced with a variety of carefully selected tasks, movement patterns, and environments. The surface similarities of treatment tasks were gradually changed, whereas the underlying skills and strategies required for performance of the task remained consistent across varied conditions (Toglia, 1991).	Strategies continue to be described by their range of application (generic vs. more specific to a domain, task or situation), however, the conceptualization of strategies has been further expanded and defined (Toglia et al., 2012). The role of strategies in supporting and enhancing performance is more clearly described. Current practice involves helping clients self-generate strategies, when feasible, rather than providing them for the client.
Connecting new information to previously learned knowledge or skills	"Information is better learned and better retained when the person can relate new information to previously learned skills or knowledge. Information that cannot be connected to experience is devoid of meaning. A few words or questions that show how the new materials relate to previous experiences or knowledge can substantially increase learning and recall" (Toglia, 1991, p. 511). "Both novel and familiar activities should be used in treatment, but the patient needs to understand the relevance of the activity and be able to connect it to other experiences" (Toglia, 1991, pp. 511-512). Activities are therapist chosen and depend on the client interests and experiences (Toglia 1992, 1998). If the person does not understand the relevance of an activity, it should be discarded.	These concepts remain the same, but techniques and methods for helping a person make connections between activities have been further described and operationalized and included within the metacognitive framework. This remains the same except that although initial cognitive treatment activities may be therapist chosen (with consideration of the client's personal context or physical and functional goals), the client is encouraged to identify or choose treatment activities and goals as awareness emerges and treatment progresses.
Additional Components		
Self-efficacy	The importance of self-efficacy was acknowledged: "The more an individual believes her or she has control over a situation, the better he or she will perform" (Toglia, 1992, p. 111).	The importance of self-efficacy has expanded and techniques or methods to build and foster self-efficacy are described.
Goals	Goals were therapist driven. Concrete feedback on strategy use or self-monitoring behaviors (e.g. spontaneous self-checking or initiating use of a strategy) through frequency counts, points, or graphs was described (Toglia, 1992, 1998).	Client-centeredness of goals and goal setting is viewed on a continuum. Goals are discussed collaboratively, but specific techniques to structure the goal-setting process are often needed (Chapter 12). Goal adjustment and revision across treatment may be an indicator of increased awareness.

Kaizerman-Dinerman et al., 2018). It has also served as a foundation for development of the Cog-Fun approach (Maeir et al., 2018).

The metacognitive framework used in the MC approach was initially examined in a randomized controlled trial to enhance self-awareness among people with acquired brain injury (Goverover et al., 2007). Twenty participants with acquired brain injury were randomly assigned to either the control or intervention group. Both groups participated in six treatment sessions with the same instrumental activities of daily living (IADL) activities. The intervention group also included metacognitive strategy questions before and after activities. For example, participants in the treatment group were asked to predict task performance, anticipate and preplan for any type of error or obstacle expected during task performance, choose a strategy to circumvent difficulties, and self-assess performance using structured self-evaluation methods immediately after the task. After the discussion, participants were asked to write in a journal about their experience performing the task (Goverover et al., 2007). Compared to the control group, the intervention group significantly improved IADL performance and self-regulation.

Subsequently, this metacognitive framework was modified to place less of an emphasis on self-ratings and prediction of accuracy and a greater focus on analysis and identification of task challenges and self-generation of strategies. Toglia et al. (2010) identified and defined specific key components of the metacognitive framework used within each session, including guided anticipation of challenges, guided strategy generation, mediation during the activity to guide error discovery, session self-evaluation, and structured journaling. These components were examined in a pilot study of the MC approach with single cases of participants who had chronic traumatic brain injury (TBI). The implementation of the MC approach included eight individual sessions; the first four sessions included the same pre-chosen functional cognitive activities for all four clients and the last four sessions consisted of different activities that were self-selected and tailored to participant's needs and preferences. Descriptive analysis of proximal and distal measures of awareness and executive functioning revealed changes in specific awareness and transfer of strategy across similar tasks and to everyday life (Toglia et al., 2010).

Foster et al. (2017) tested the feasibility of MC components, including the metacognitive framework, in seven people with Parkinson's disease. Results supported the feasibility and potential efficacy of the intervention for individuals with Parkinson's disease. Currently, a pilot randomized controlled trial assessing the effectiveness of the MC approach is being conducted for people who have mild to moderate Parkinson's disease and self-identified cognitive deficits.

Recently, the preliminary efficacy of the MC approach was tested in an inpatient rehabilitation setting with people with acquired brain injury. Results indicated that MC intervention was associated with significant improvements in awareness, strategy use, and executive functioning. Participants with acquired brain injury found the treatment to be satisfying and engaging, and they perceived subjective improvement in their ability to use cognitive strategies to facilitate performance in everyday activities (Jaywant et al., 2020). This project is also in the process of being expanded to a pilot randomized controlled trial.

FOR WHOM IS THE MULTICONTEXT APPROACH MOST APPROPRIATE?

As can be seen from the above literature, the MC approach provides broad treatment guidelines that can be used across ages and diagnostic categories for persons who have difficulty learning or successfully performing functional cognitive activities. In general, the MC approach is most appropriate for those who show at least minimal awareness of difficulties or who have potential for increased awareness. It is not appropriate for individuals with global cognitive deficits, severe memory deficits, significant aphasia or language comprehension deficits, or high levels of defensive denial (Steinberg & Zlotnik, 2019). Exhibit 6.2 presents some characteristics that may render a person a good candidate for the MC approach:

Exhibit 6.2 Who is Best Suited for the Multicontext Approach?

- At least minimal self-awareness of cognitive performance difficulties OR potential for increased awareness with activity experiences.
- Demonstrates some responsiveness or openness to mediation or guided questions.
- Recalls previous experiences (with prompts or memory supports if needed).
- Good language comprehension
- Mild-moderate cognitive deficits
- Severe deficits in circumscribed areas

Note: Poor awareness in an interview does not preclude use of the MC approach as the focus is on online awareness of performance.

KNOWLEDGE AND SKILLS NEEDED TO IMPLEMENT THE MULTICONTEXT APPROACH

Implementation of the MC approach requires the ability to analyze performance, including patterns of cognitive performance errors as well as task methods or strategies used; select, structure, and sequence cognitive functional activities along a horizontal transfer continuum; and use mediation to facilitate self-awareness, monitoring, strategy generation, and use, and performance (Steinberg & Zlotnik, 2019). To do this, the therapist needs to have knowledge and understanding of the below areas:

1. Typical cognitive symptoms, performance errors, and activity and environmental characteristics that influence cognitive performance (Chapters 1-2,4)
2. Self-awareness, metacognitive skills, and self-efficacy (Chapter 3)
3. Performance analysis (Chapter 5)
4. Cognitive strategies (Chapter 7)
5. Transfer and generalization principles (Chapter 8)
6. Mediated learning and guided questioning techniques (Chapters 9-10)

situations or resist the tendency to become sidetracked across activities. The reader is referred to other sources for an overview of different treatment approaches used in cognitive rehabilitation (Goverover, 2018; Toglia et al., 2018).

This book provides in-depth information on the MC approach treatment components and how to apply these methods in practice; however, it is not all-inclusive. Treatment of cognitive impairments requires a holistic overall program that addresses psychosocial skills, social participation, interpersonal skills, engagement in meaningful activities, and subjective well-being or quality of life. The MC approach can be applied broadly, but it is viewed as one aspect of a comprehensive treatment program that aims to help a person achieve optimal functional outcomes.

The next several chapters (7-10) build on the information presented in this chapter and the first section of this book and explain how to help a person recognize and manage cognitive performance errors by using strategies, manipulating activity and environment demands, and mediating performance with guided learning methods. Optional goal-setting methods are presented in Chapter 12. Although these key components of the MC approach are presented in separate chapters, they are integrated together during treatment as discussed in Chapters 11 and 13.

SUMMARY

This chapter provided a broad description of the MC approach, including intervention focus, key characteristics, background and evolution, and a review of studies applying the MC approach in clinical practice. The MC approach is a complex multi-component metacognitive strategy intervention based on the Dynamic Interactional Model of cognition. It has a focus on simultaneously building self-awareness, strategy use, and self-efficacy while structuring treatment activities to facilitate transfer and generalization across situations. The MC approach is not mutually exclusive, and it is not appropriate for all clients. For example, the MC approach would not be beneficial for those with significant denial, severe global cognitive impairments, or aphasia. Additionally, within the same client, there may be some areas of function where the MC approach is useful and other areas of function where other treatment approaches or task-specific functional training would be more beneficial. For example, task-specific training or adaptations might be appropriate to help a person learn the procedure for setting an alarm on their smartphone. At the same time, the same person may require strategies to effectively follow a list across

KEY POINTS

- The MC approach is based on the Dynamic Interactional Model of cognition (described in Chapter 4). It focuses on optimizing the *person's* self-awareness, self-monitoring skills, and strategy use while simultaneously adapting *activity and environmental demands* so that activities are at an optimal level of difficulty.

- The MC approach was initially described in 1991 and was based on literature from cognitive and educational psychology, neuropsychology, and occupational therapy.

- The core components and goals of the MC approach have not changed since 1991, however, the principles have been further clarified, operationalized, and refined and in some instances expanded over time.

- The goals of the MC approach include enhanced self-awareness and self-monitoring of cognitive performance, strategy use across cognitive functional activities, transfer and generalization of cognitive strategies to a variety of situations,

- and increased self-efficacy or perceived control over cognitive performance.
- Three key MC approach treatment components include: (1) focus on cognitive strategies; (2) structuring treatment activities horizontally to promote transfer and generalization; and (3) metacognitive framework and guided learning methods. Additional treatment components include therapeutic support focused on enhancing self-efficacy, the use of functionally relevant treatment activities that are at an optimal level of challenge, and goal setting and revision.
- Treatment with the MC approach can have different areas of emphasis depending on the client.
- The MC approach has broad clinical applications. It has been applied across a wide variety of clinical problems including spatial neglect, visual object recognition disorders, and executive dysfunction as well as diagnoses (e.g., Parkinson's disease, stroke, traumatic brain injury, learning disability, schizophrenia).

Chapter 7

Cognitive Strategies

The Multicontext (MC) approach utilizes a broad range of cognitive strategies within the context of a structured metacognitive framework. This chapter defines and describes general characteristics of strategies including important things to think about when using strategies in intervention. Examples of strategies for various cognitive performance problems and domains are provided. The latter part of this chapter discusses how strategies are used specifically in the MC approach.

CONTENTS OF CHAPTER 7
What are Strategies?
- Classifying Strategies
- Multiple Uses of Domain-Specific Cognitive Strategies
- General Cognitive Strategies
- Summary of Strategies and Their Use

Strategy Use in the Multicontext Approach
- Distinguishing the Multicontext Approach from Other Strategy-based Intervention Approaches
- Strategy Selection
- Observation of Strategy Use
- Insights from Strategy Development
- Implications for Intervention: Clinical Examples

Summary and Key Points

WHAT ARE STRATEGIES?

Strategies are often described as compensatory or as serving the purpose of circumventing cognitive limitations (Ihle et al., 2018). In the MC approach, cognitive strategies are not just compensatory. Rather, they are considered to be an inherent part of normal cognition, learning, and performance. They include task methods, tactics, or mental tools that people use to help manage cognitive resources, enhance information processing, and cope effectively with performance challenges (Toglia et al., 2012). Strategies can be described as mental routines, mind tools, or mind habits that can be used before, during, or immediately after a task to enhance learning or performance. Figure 7.1 demonstrates this conceptualization of strategies.

Healthy people have a wide repertoire of strategies that can be combined, adjusted, or modified to help them cope with cognitive challenges, prevent or manage cognitive lapses, and support functioning. Cognitive strategies, therefore, are an inherent part of healthy functioning and performance. In challenging activities, people typically use multiple strategies to enhance cognitive performance (Toglia et al., 2012).

Lower or inefficient strategy use compared to healthy controls has been linked to poorer performance across a wide variety of ages and populations that experience cognitive difficulties including people with mild traumatic

Figure 7.1 Conceptualizing and Defining Strategies

- Inherent part of skill acquisition and learning
- Mind habits or mental routines "mind tools"
- Part of normal cognition
- Cope with cognitively challenging activities
- Enhance depth of information processing
- Inherent part of occupational performance
- Monitor and control cognitive lapses

brain injury (TBI) (Geary et al., 2011), schizophrenia (Kaizerman-Dinerman et al., 2019), Parkinson's disease (Johnson et al., 2005) mild cognitive impairment (Brum et al., 2013), at-risk youth (Toglia & Berg, 2013) and children with learning disabilities (Swanson et al., 2015). For example, Bottari et al. (2014) found that the element that distinguished the highest functioning participant with TBI from others while performing a real-world shopping task was the effective use of multiple self-generated internal and external strategies. Also, changes in the effective use of strategies after strategy training has been linked to changes in neural activation in the brain (Han et al., 2017; Lepping et al., 2015). This literature highlights the importance of using methods to promote effective strategy use as a means of optimizing cognitive functional performance.

Classifying Strategies

Strategy-based interventions require analyzing and specifying how a strategy is being used. There are many ways that strategies can be grouped or described. For example, strategies are often labeled as external or internal. They are also commonly classified according to their domain. Both of these common methods of characterizing strategies have limitations that are described below.

Commonly used Dichotomies for Strategy Classification
External versus Internal Strategies

External strategies are those that are apparent to another person such as making notes or lists, finger-pointing, or physically covering or removing information. Internal strategies are those that are not apparent to others such as mentally repeating things to oneself or mentally visualizing information. People use a combination of internal and external strategies in everyday life. External strategies can be gradually internalized. For example, talking out loud can be internalized into mental self-talk. The distinction between external and internal strategies is not always clear and represents an over-simplification. For example, a person may look for external cues to trigger mental ideas, create a checklist of things they need to do or seek information by asking others. While these strategies can be observed, they have been initiated internally by the person. Due to this overlap, the common distinction between internal and external strategies is not completely adequate.

Task- or Domain-specific versus General or Non-situational Strategies

Strategies can be linked to specific situations, contexts, tasks, or domains or they can be non-situational or generic. For example, a checklist of the steps to set an alarm for a person's watch is a task-specific strategy. Reading or listening strategies represent strategies that are useful in specific domains of function. Similarly, strategies that are associated with cognitive domains (e.g., memory, problem-solving, or organization) are helpful when used within tasks that place demands on the respective cognitive domain. In contrast, nonspecific or non-situational strategies can be used across a wide range of tasks or situations. For example, self-regulation or self-monitoring strategies such as self-checking are useful across many different types of tasks and domains. Once again, however, these differences are not sharply defined. For some people, a generic strategy such as self-checking can be tied to a specific task or domain. Similarly, a memory strategy such as verbal rehearsal can also enhance performance in other domains or across a wide range of tasks or situations that require memory.

A Strategy Framework: Defining Multiple Attributes

Given the difficulty in clearly grouping strategies into mutually exclusive subtypes, Toglia, Rodger and Polatajko (2012) suggest that strategies should be described and analyzed according to multiple attributes. They proposed a framework with seven strategy *attributes* (strategy outcome, strategy purpose, range of application, visibility, permanence, performance phase, strategy target) that can be used to more precisely define strategies. See Table 7.1.

This framework can be used in strategy interventions such as the MC approach to help therapists analyze and select strategies that match the person's performance problem, abilities, and goal. It may be helpful for the therapist to use a worksheet to clearly describe and define the targeted strategy and how it is being used in treatment. An example of a blank worksheet based on Table 7.1 and Table 7.2 can be found in Appendix B.11.

Table 7.2 uses the framework proposed by Toglia et al. (2012) to illustrate how the performance problem, outcome, and strategy (e.g., using a list) can be similar across each example, yet the same strategy can differ across other multiple attributes (strategy purpose, range, visibility, and permanence).

Multiple Uses of Domain-Specific Cognitive Strategies

Before we provide specific strategies, it is important to think more generally about how strategies can be used.

The Same Strategy: Variations in Purpose and Cognitive Skills Required

Table 7.2 illustrates how a simple everyday tool such as a list can vary widely in type and purpose. Closer analysis indicates that these different uses also require different cognitive abilities. Precise definition and analysis of strategies and their cognitive requirements can thus help explain discrepancies in strategy use and effectiveness. For example, a person may be able to use a list to find items in the kitchen but be unable to follow a list of steps because the cognitive skills required for these two lists differ. Therefore, strategies need to be carefully analyzed and matched with the person's cognitive abilities. This is further explained in the section below.

Table 7.1 Strategy Attributes

Strategy Attributes	Description
Strategy outcome	Desired outcome can include the acquisition or re-acquisition of task skills.
Strategy purpose	The purpose of strategies can be broadly grouped into those that are directed towards (1) improving efficiency, quality or accuracy of performance; (2) optimize learning or information processing; or (3) self-regulation/self-monitoring.
Range of application	Extent that strategies are applicable across different activities or contexts. Strategies can generally be (1) task-specific and trained only within a specific task or context; (2) situational or used in certain situations and contexts; or (3) used across a variety of different tasks and situations.
Timing of use (performance phase)	Strategies can be used immediately before activity performance (preparation phase), during performance, after activity completion (self-evaluate), or a combination of all three.
Visibility	Strategies may be overt or readily observable and visible or they may be internalized, covert, or hidden.
Permanence	Strategies can be temporary or used to facilitate the acquisition of skills or routines and then faded, or they can be used permanently to support performance. They can also be activated as needed.
Strategy target	Strategies can be directed at changing the task or environment (modifying or adjusting task/environment features or demands) or they can be directed toward changing the person's behavior, ability to process information, monitor, or regulate performance.

Toglia, J., Rodger, S. A., and Polatajko, H. J. (2012).

Table 7.2 Strategy Attribute Worksheet Example

Performance problem	Desired Outcome	Strategy and Example	Strategy Purpose	Range	Timing of Use	Visibility	Permanence
Often misses steps, leaves out key ingredients	Independence in cooking tasks	**List: Self-checking** Client uses a list to double-check that all steps were completed.	Cope with challenge	Across all cooking tasks	After task	Overt then covert	Temporary or Permanent
Often misses steps, leaves out key items	Independence in preparing coffee, toast, and cereal	**List: How-to** List of items and steps needed to make a specific type of breakfast is provided.	Re-Learning	Specific	During	Overt	Temporary Will be faded
Often misses steps, leaves out key items	Independence in multi-step tasks	**List: Planning** Client creates a written list of steps before multistep activities such as cooking to pre-plan needed items, steps, and time.	Optimize Performance	General Across all multi-step tasks	Before and during	Overt	Temporary or permanent
Often misses steps, leaves out key items	Independence in multi-step tasks	**List: Mental Planning** Client visualizes himself performing activity and goes through mental checklist of items needed before starting.	Optimize Performance	General Across all multi-step tasks	Before	Covert	Permanent

Toglia, J., Rodger, S. A., and Polatajko, H. J. (2012).

In addition to lists, other strategies such as verbal mediation or mental imagery are also often erroneously described as single strategies. However, similar to the list example, closer inspection reveals differences in cognitive skills required and multiple uses. For example, strategies can be tied to a specific task or situation or they can be used as a general strategy across situations. Differences in cognitive requirements and ways that the same strategy can be used are further illustrated in this section continuing with the example of a list and also with verbal mediation and mental imagery.

Lists

A list is a common tool that is embedded in everyday routines and activities; however, as previously described, a list is not a single strategy. In addition to variations in the strategy attributes described in Table 7.2, lists can also vary in the cognitive skills required for their use, and in the methods needed for effective use. Although a list is often described as a compensatory strategy, closer analysis indicates that a list is not always compensatory. For example, sometimes a list is not used as a strategy but is an inherent part of an activity that requires cognitive skills to use (e.g., taking inventory, using an address list). Different types of lists require different cognitive skills. Lists can be cognitively challenging to use, and in some situations, multiple strategies are required to use a list effectively. Exhibit 7.1 provides examples of different types of lists and shows how lists are used in a variety of ways to accomplish different goals in everyday life. The wide range of ways that a list is used, as well as the cognitive abilities required to use a list, are described below and need to be kept in mind when planning or describing treatment.

Lists for checking and verification require gathering items or comparison of a list against items in a kitchen or closet. This involves searching and locating items while keeping in mind the items that are being searched. As one looks away from the list to gather items or check for items in a closet, they need to mentally keep track of what they were looking for and which item or step they were at. Additional strategies such as repeating keywords to oneself after looking away from the list or crossing or checking off items after they have been completed may be needed. Rearrangement or re-organization of the list may be needed to gather items efficiently. Problems can occur if the person checks the item off the list before the item is located or forgets to check off an item that has been completed.

Lists for copying information such as addresses, or phone numbers require greater attention to detail. In this type of list, the items are similar (all phone numbers or all addresses). A strategy such as finger-pointing or highlighting details to focus visual attention may be helpful. Those who are prone to repetition of stimuli or perseveration may also show more difficulties with less difference between stimuli.

"To-do" lists are commonly used to keep track of things that need to be done including errands, assignments, purchases, appointments, or phone calls. Although written or digital lists may be used, mental checklists of things that need to be done are also frequently used. To-do lists help people carry out intentions and require planning, prioritization, organization, frequent review, and prospective memory. Effective to-do lists are organized by clustering associated tasks together by type of task, importance, proximity or location, and estimating or assigning times for task completion. Simple to-do lists can involve daily errands and fixed items or those that need to be carried out at a specific time. Complex to-do lists include a wide range of items that can be carried out anytime within the next few weeks or months. The latter requires greater prioritization, initiation, organization, and prospective memory.

Following a list of steps to a task requires completing steps in a fixed order and translating written instructions into action. The person needs to understand how each step is connected to the others and the larger goal. This requires shifting from one substep to the next, keeping track of what step was just done and what needs to be done next, and adhering to the overall goal.

Creating task lists requires the ability to initiate and

Exhibit 7.1 Examples of Types of Lists

- Gather, locate items: e.g., shopping list, travel/packing list
- Checking, verification, or comparison of task components against a list: e.g., compare inventory list of office or cleaning supplies against actual items
- Copy information from list: e.g., address cards, send invitations, or make phone calls
- List of information for reference: e.g., playlist of songs, names in a directory, upcoming events, list of apps, list of accomplishments, list of goals
- To-do lists: e.g., errands, list of work tasks to be done
- Follow a list of steps/directions to complete a task: e.g., list of directions for arts and craft project
- Break down complex activities or directions into a list (task simplification)
- Create a list of steps to follow in a multi-step task project
- Create a list of things that one does not want to forget (may be a mental list of items)
- Brainstorm ideas: e.g., list of meals to make for dinner, list of possible places to take a visitor, list of ideas for a web page
- Agenda: e.g., list of topics to discuss, list of questions

generate ideas. Task guidance checklists that involve general steps to an activity can be created broadly so that they can be used in different situations. For example, generic lists that involve packing for a trip, travel planning, holiday dinner planning or party planning can be used anytime the situation arises. Lists can also be specific to a certain task or situation, such as the steps to make a particular recipe or to find a specific file on your computer. Creating broad or specific task checklists involves internally generating a list of steps to a task or situation based on prior experiences. Mental practice or imagining oneself performing each step of the activity can help create checklists that can be used to guide task performance. If the person has difficulty creating a list, visual supports such as observing a video or another person performing the activity may be needed. This reduces demands on initiating or generating ideas. The person either writes down the steps as they perform the activity themselves or as they watch another person performing the activity.

Brainstorming lists can be used to generate ideas for activities, projects, or events as well as to aid planning or problem solving. Brainstorming lists require initiation, flexibility of thinking, and abstraction or thinking beyond the "here and now." For example, in planning a website or a brochure, one may initially brainstorm all the ideas that come to mind. Generating broad categories before specific details is most effective. As the written list of ideas is reviewed, redundant items can be eliminated and items that are associated can be categorized, grouped, re-organized or re-ordered. Grouping items helps to reduce and simplify information. Planning and problem solving often proceeds from brainstorming lists to categorizing or grouping items on the list to ordering or examining relationships between items. Lists, therefore, can be a tool for solving problems and can help in identifying relationships and solutions.

Lists to simplify directions can be used to break down complex instructions for multiple-step activities. This can also be described as task simplification. It requires the ability to identify key information and divide large chunks of information into smaller sub-steps while keeping the overall goal of the activity in mind. Strategies such as previewing the directions and highlighting the most relevant information as a first step may be useful.

Self-Verbalization Strategies

Self-verbalization strategies can involve talking aloud or it can include inner self-talk for many different purposes (Toglia et al., 2012). For example, verbal rehearsal of key words, steps or procedures helps one focus attention, keep track, or retain information. Self-talk or repetition of key phrases can help a person cue themselves during a task (e.g. go slowly) or self-monitor behavior. Self-verbalization can also be used to connect information to previous knowledge or to help manage and solve problems. Vygotsky (1962) described inner speech as the primary vehicle for thought and self-direction. Methods of self-instruction, verbal self-guidance, and self-talk have been described that help people systematically talk themselves through ways to overcome obstacles or effectively solve problems during activities (Meichenbaum, 1975, 1977; Meichenbaum & Goodman, 1971). Examples of different ways that self-verbalization strategies can be used are listed in Exhibit 7.2.

Exhibit 7.2 Self-Verbalization or Self-Talk Strategies

- Mental alarm – Instruct self to "Stop and Review" at periodic times
- Repetition – Repeat keywords or directions several times, silently or out loud before or during task execution
- Rehearse a script or a phrase – "Lock brakes before I stand"
- Rehearse task goals
- Verbal self-guidance or self-instruction – Self-talk through a task or problem, verbalize thought processes as a problem is considered, plan or state each task step before or as performing it
- Self-cues – Remember to slow down, focus
- Self-questions – Monitoring. Self-questions, e.g. Am I double-checking?
- Verbally identify key features to pay careful attention to during performance
- Knowledge – Verbally identify what one knows before beginning
- Anticipate – Verbally identify potential obstacles or challenges
- Plan – Make a verbal or written plan
- Elaborate or associate information for retention

Mental Imagery

Mental imagery involves mental representations of images, scenes, or sensory information without a direct external stimulus. It includes visualization, mental practice, reconstruction of previous events, imagination of future events, mental association, or manipulation of information in one's mind (Pearson et al., 2015). Mental imagery of future or past situations is created from stored representations in memory and goes beyond the visual representation of images. Images can involve other modalities such as imagining sounds, smells, or emotions in the context or environment where the situation or activity occurs/occurred (Pearson et al., 2013).

The use of visual imagery for mental practice or rehearsing an activity mentally as if it were actually being performed before an activity has been demonstrated to enhance task performance (Liu et al., 2004; Liu et al., 2009). Mental imagery strategies can be supported by external aids, pictures, or video clips. For example, in the initial stages of mental practice, the person can be shown a video clip of a task prior to imagining it or they can be shown pictures of the first and last steps of a task and asked to mentally imagine the rest. The person can also be asked to visualize obstacles or challenges they might encounter in each step of an activity or situation and imagine how they might manage challenges successfully (Liu et al., 2004; Liu et al., 2009). In a randomized controlled trial, Liu and colleagues demonstrated that mental practice with people who had a stroke enhanced relearning of daily activities on both trained and untrained functional tasks (Liu et al., 2009). They observed that the mental imagery strategy enhanced planning skills and generalized to other daily tasks.

Visual imagery strategies have also been found to enhance prospective memory in people with acquired brain injury. Training involves asking the person to imagine themselves completing a future activity at the correct time or in response to the correct cue. The person is asked to imagine where they will be at a certain time and to vividly picture the context and the cues in the environment that will serve as a trigger to carry out the intended actions or activity (Raskin et al., 2019).

Mental imagery strategies have been used for a wide range of purposes across different ages and populations including those with stroke, traumatic brain injury, multiple sclerosis, Parkinson's disease, and learning disabilities. For example, visual imagery strategies have been reported to be effective in increasing reading comprehension and literacy in both adults (Hock & Mellard, 2005) and children (Harris & Pressley, 1991). Other uses of mental imagery strategies including alleviating anxiety by rehearsing a situation beforehand, facilitating learning of a skill through mental practice, increasing awareness of intentions to be performed, and enhancing problem solving, visual working memory, self-regulation, or memory of past and future events (Ernst et al., 2015; Haskins et al., 2012; Pearson et al., 2015; Raskin et al., 2019; Tamir et al., 2007). Considerable evidence exists that mental practice assists learning in a broad range of motor, perceptuo-motor, cognitive and functional skills (Ginns, 2005). Exhibit 7.3 provides examples of the different ways that mental imagery can be used to enhance thinking and performance.

Exhibit 7.3 Mental Imagery or Mental Practice Strategies

- Mental practice – Mentally imagine or rehearse performing an activity before doing the activity; visualize incorrect versus correct performance.
- Mental problem solving – Visualize obstacles or problems that could be encountered during task performance and mentally practice alternative ways of solving problems or coping with obstacles.
- Mental visual associations or mnemonic techniques – Creating images and associations; e.g., remembering the name Angela Price by imagining an angel embedding with a $ sign.
- Mental anticipation – Visualize (mentally rehearse) how, where, and when the desired activity will be completed in the future (Raskin et al., 2019).
- Mental reconstruction – Visualize past experience; e.g., before performing an activity, mentally visualize a specific time and place where you performed the same or similar activity (Hewitt et al., 2006).
- Mental translation (words into pictures) – When reading directions such as "Place 2 eggs in a bowl," translate this to a picture in your mind of two eggs in a bowl.
- Create a strong mental representation of the goal or "problem space" or create a mental picture of the task outcome. Draw a picture of the goal, i.e., What will it look like if I successfully complete the activity or accomplish my goal?
- Snapshot technique or movie technique – Take a mental picture or snapshot of information one is trying to learn or play a movie of the information in one's mind for retention (Green, 2012)

Combining Strategies

Multiple strategies are typically used in combination with each other. For example, repeating information, visualizing it, and writing it down may all be used to help remember information. Acronyms can be used to help a person use a combination of different strategies simultaneously. Although creating an acronym for information to be recalled is a common mnemonic strategy in and of itself, acronyms can also be used to group different strategies together. Exhibit 7.4 illustrates common acronyms for strategy use in memory, reading, or listening. Some common acronyms for remembering people's names are listed in Appendix D.1. Acronyms associated with an image or picture may be easier to recall for some people.

General Cognitive Strategies

There are many strategies that can be used alone or in combination with each other to address certain cognitive domains or to control certain types of cognitive symptoms and performance errors. Examples of strategies organized by cognitive domains are listed in Appendix D.1. The below section describes more general strategies for managing complex activities. These examples illustrate the wide variety and range of strategies or "mind tools" that people use every day when faced with cognitive challenges. Since, as discussed above, the same strategy can be used for a variety of purposes, can require different cognitive skills, and can be used in combination with other strategies, these features should be specified using the strategy attribute framework for a particular client to ensure appropriate selection and application.

Global Activity Management Strategies

Several strategies provide structured frameworks to help a person manage multi-step activities and cope with obstacles or problems. These strategies are similar because they provide a structured system for approaching multi-step activities or problems and thereby replace the impulsive, disorganized, and unsystematic approach that many people with executive function impairments use. We use the term *activity management strategies* as a way of grouping these strategies together because they all provide a general structure that helps a person plan, problem solve, or manage multi-step and complex activities. Exhibit 7.5 provides examples of these strategies.

A wide number of activity management strategies have been identified that use easy to remember acronyms such as STAR, STOP, or IDEA. Some of these strategies place an emphasis on deeply encoding the goal prior to the activity. Goals provide direction, organization, and structure for actions. In people with executive dysfunction, the goal can often fade away as the person becomes involved in "doing" an activity (termed goal neglect) (Krasny-Pacini et al., 2014). If the goal is not maintained in mind, actions lack purpose, and performance disintegrates. Strategies that involve rehearsing or visualizing task goals or end products can be effective in organizing and driving task performance. Other strategies provide a systematic method for coping with obstacles or problems that may occur within an activity, while others focus on managing or simplifying a complex activity.

Several of these strategies have been used and are beginning to amass evidence for their use in cognitive rehabilitation or occupational therapy practice. For example, Ylvisaker et al. (1998) described the Goal, Plan, Do, Review (GPDR) global strategy and developed worksheets to structure and reflect on performance within a task. A GPDR app and worksheets are readily available (see Resource section). The Cognitive Orientation to Daily Occupational Performance (CO-OP) approach uses a similar Goal-Plan-Do-Check strategy that also

Exhibit 7.4 Examples of Strategies with Acronyms			
Reading or listening	***Memory**	**Reading** (Wilson, 2009)	***Memory**
S = Summarize I = Identify main points N = Never mind the details G = Get the gist	T = Translate into your own words R = Repeat it to yourself 5 times A = Associate it with something familiar or ask yourself what the main idea is P = Picture it S = **S**elf-Test	P = Preview material Q = Question self R = Review S = Summarize T = Test self	R = Repeat I = Imagine P = Put it together

*http://www.ldonline.org/article/5602,

emphasizes verbal self-instruction. Although the global strategy is nearly identical, a key difference is that the CO-OP approach embeds this same strategy within a client-centered framework (Dawson et al., 2009; Polatajko & Mandich, 2004). Goal management training (GMT) uses multiple strategies that include cessation of ongoing activity "STOP," breaking down goals into manageable sub-steps and self-checking strategies (Levine et al., 2000).

All of the activity management strategies in Exhibit 7.5 focus on self-monitoring, self-checking, or metacognitive skills. These frameworks can be developed into worksheets to help structure thinking and performance. Visual cues or icons can be placed in prominent locations and used to help the person initiate or adopt use of the activity management strategy as a mental habit. By using content-free cues or acronyms such as IDEA or STOP, automatic text message reminders can be set (if needed) to be sent periodically throughout a day to facilitate strategy use to help the person to stop and self-monitor actions (Fish et al., 2007; Hart, Vaccaro, et al., 2019).

Implementation Intentions and Action Plans

Similar to activity management strategies, implementation intentions and action plans also represent generic strategies that can be applied to a wide range of problems, situations, or activities. Both strategies are designed to help people who have difficulty carrying out intentions or goals due to poor planning. They have a strong emphasis on deep encoding of the goal through methods such as elaboration, specification, rehearsal, and visualization.

Implementation Intentions

This strategy involves creating an explicit link between a specific cue, situation or context, and an intended behavior or action (Brom & Kliegel, 2014; Gollwitzer, 1999; Radomski et al., 2018). The person specifies when, where, and how to act in a given situation and then creates an if-then statement. For example, "If I encounter situation X, then I will initiate action Y." The statement can then be repeated (aloud or internally) and the entire situation (i.e., encountering the cue or context and executing the action) can be visualized. Implementation intentions can serve a variety of purposes. They can serve as a cue for specific actions or use of learned strategies (e.g., before I go out the door, I need to check the list on the refrigerator) or they can help one cope with problems or obstacles (e.g., if it is raining, I will take the bus). Implementation intention phrases are rehearsed and practiced so that they become a habit of mind. Automatic daily text messages have been used to remind or cue people with acquired brain injury to use targeted implementation intentions (Hart & Vaccaro, 2017).

It is hypothesized that the creation of a strong link between an environmental cue or mental representation of a situation and the desired action prompts automatic recall of the action when the cue or situation occurs, thereby decreasing cognitive resources or executive control required to initiate the action at the appropriate moment (Wieber et al., 2015). Although implementation intentions can be task or context-specific, they can also be used to cue strategies using strategy-specific or

---

Exhibit 7.5 Activity Management Strategies

- PAC – Prepare/Plan, Act, and Check
- FAR – Focus and plan, Act, and Reflect (Kable et al., 2016)
- GPDR – Goal, Plan, Do, Review (Ylvisaker et al., 1998)
- GOPDR – Goal, (obstacle) Plan, Predict, Do, and Review
- GPDC – Goal, Plan, Do, Check (Polatajko & Mandich, 2004)
- STOP – Stop, Think, Organize, Plan (Fish et al., 2007)
- STAR – Stop, Think, Act, and Review
- S and S – Stop and Split
- Stop, Plan, Review
- Stop, Define, List, Learn, Monitor (Do it, Check) (GMT)
- SWAPS – 1. Stop! Is there a problem? 2. What is the problem? 3. Alternatives and options to solve the problem 4. Pick and plan the chosen option 5. Satisfied with the outcome of the plan? (Cantor et al., 2014)
- KISS-R – Keep it simple, split and remove
- IDEA – **I**dentify challenges, **D**escribe method/strategy, **E**xecute, **A**ssess results, methods and challenges
- IDEAL – **I**dentify problem, **D**efine problem, **E**xplore possible strategies, **A**ct and carry out plan, **L**ook at effects or self-evaluate (Bransford et al., 1987; Bransford & Stein, 1993)

situational-specific strategy training as described later in this chapter.

Action Plans

Action plans share common elements with implementation intentions and are often used interchangeably, but they can also involve more detailed, deliberate, and conscious planning that may include multiple cues, complex plans, or responses (Hagger & Luszczynska, 2014). For example: *To help me keep track of information during a conversation with others or when I am reading new information, I will repeat keywords to myself and summarize what I have just heard or read in my own words. If it is a noisy or distracting environment, I will ask for a quieter location.* Action plans include cues to action ("when," "where"), similar to implementation intentions, but also steps to action ("how") and plans for coping with potential challenges or obstacles. They are more complex and require more conscious control and effort to create and use than implementation intentions. Sample blank action plan forms are included in Appendix C.16-17.

Emotional Self-Regulation Strategies

Emotional self-regulation is the ability to monitor, adjust, and manage one's feelings or emotions such as anger, distress, frustration, anxiety, sadness, or feelings of being overwhelmed. People with acquired brain injury who are aware that they are having difficulty in daily tasks that were once very easy may have negative emotional reactions that can impede processing and further contribute to task difficulties. Emotional overreactions tend to overwhelm cognitive processes and lead to inaction (Rath et al., 2003). The person may feel as if their brain is "flooded" or "overloaded" and that they cannot think. Alternatively, emotional reactions can lead to impulsive actions or decisions, self-defeating dialogue, and "thinking traps," or appraising a situation as worse than it really is (Champion, 2006). Exhibit 7.6 provides examples of thinking traps or negative thinking.

> **Exhibit 7.6 Examples of Negative Beliefs and Thinking**
>
> - I will never get this.
> - I don't know what I am doing. I can't do this. It's too hard.
> - My brain is messed up.
> - I am a complete failure. I'm useless.
> - Everyone will think I'm stupid.
> - I should be able to do this easily. I can't cope.

Such "thinking traps" can lead to low mood or diminished self-efficacy and negatively affect performance. As a result, the person may begin to withdraw from or avoid activities in which they previously engaged.

Emotional self-regulation strategies help a person recognize warning signs or triggers for negative emotional reactions, reframe negative thoughts with positive internal statements, or manage emotions in a manner that is consistent with one's goals. The first step is to help a person monitor their feelings and emotions and recognize triggers or precursors to a loss of emotional control (Cantor et al., 2014). The person can be asked to identify their mood or self-rate their emotions (e.g., level of frustration or anxiety on a scale of 1 to 10) before, during, and after an activity. If the person easily experiences information overload, they can be asked to rate their level of "overload" during a task. This can help the person become more aware of their mood or feelings and how they affect performance. In addition, the therapist can guide the person in developing an action plan to help a person learn to identify and monitor the warning signs and cue the person to use methods that help them manage emotions. Exhibit 7.7 provides a sample of an action plan to help a person cope with frustration and anger during a task. A blank action plan for emotional regulation is also included in Appendix C.18.

Several of the strategies described previously can be used to manage emotions. For example, strategies that help a person break down a task into more manageable components (activity management strategies) can decrease anxiety and help increase comfort in approaching challenging tasks or problems. Exhibit 7.8 lists additional examples of strategies aimed at regulating emotions. Emotional regulation strategies may need to be addressed before or concurrently with strategies focused on managing cognitive performance errors.

Summary of Strategies and Their Use

We have reviewed general concepts related to strategies and their use. We have also provided examples of strategies that serve domain- or problem-specific purposes and others designed to support functional performance more generally through activity management, planning, and emotional or self-regulation. The therapist should be familiar with the range of strategies that people might use.

It is important to remember that the same strategy can be used for different purposes and, depending on how it's used or its attributes, can require different cognitive skills. This implies that although two interventions might indicate use of the same strategy, the treatments could look significantly different. Thus, therapists should be able to provide a precise and thorough description of a strategy's purpose, attributes, and use for a client. A worksheet for

Exhibit 7.7 Action Plan to Manage Frustration and Anger	
Identifying Triggers: What are the warning signs?	What is my plan to stay in control? *If others notice...what can they do to help?*
• Voice gets louder • Can't focus • Can't sit still • Feel like throwing something	• Think of "lowering the temperature" • Take 3 deep breaths • Ask to take a break • Use my relaxation app • Imagine petting my dog • Listen to my favorite song • *Others can say "Time to lower the temperature"*

analysis of strategy attributes is available in Appendix B.11 for therapists to use in planning, selecting, and specifying how a strategy is used in treatment.

In addition, the therapist should carefully observe the *type* of strategies used during treatment. A sample therapist worksheet that includes a list of commonly used strategies is included in Appendix B.12 to help structure and document observations regarding the *type* of spontaneous strategies observed during activities. The next section describes how the MC approach teaches strategies.

STRATEGY USE IN THE MULTICONTEXT APPROACH

There are many ways to go about promoting strategy use, and strategy-based interventions can differ considerably. In this section, we describe some key features of the way strategies are trained, analyzed, and used in the MC approach.

Distinguishing the Multicontext Approach from Other Strategy-based Intervention Approaches

We provide an overview of some of the distinguishing characteristics of the MC approach here. These are described in further detail throughout the manual.

What Strategies are Taught

Many strategy interventions use *task-specific* strategy training, which involves systematic and repetitive practice of the same task and strategy in the same context with gradually fading cues or supports. A strategy is used, but the focus is on improving performance of a specific task, rather than on learning and using a strategy that can

Exhibit 7.8 Emotional Regulation Strategies
• S.T.A.R. – Smile, Take a deep breath, And Relax
• SRR = Stop—Relax—Refocus (Loya et al., 2017)
• Use or create a personal mental image or use a picture/icon for self-regulation (e.g., stop sign, calm ocean)
• Positive self-coaching – Using positive thinking or statements, e.g., "I am capable of doing this; I did it before and succeeded."
• Watch out for "thinking traps."
• Re-frame the problem – Instead of saying "This is difficult," say "This is a challenge. I know I can do this if I take my time, simplify the directions, and break up the task into steps" (Champion, 2006)
• Mental Rehearsal – Imagining oneself performing a task before actually performing it can decrease anxiety and increase self-confidence
• Implementation Intentions: When I feel ___, I will do ___ ; e.g., "When I feel anxious, I will use my deep breathing techniques and think of a calm ocean."

be applied to different situations. As task performance improves with practice, strategy use may be faded. Task-specific strategies can be practiced until they become habitual or "proceduralized."

An example includes learning to operate a microwave oven. The person may be encouraged to refer to a list and/or repeat the steps out loud during task performance. Awareness or the ability to recognize task challenges is not required because the activity itself can cue automatic use of the strategy. As the task becomes easier with practice, strategies are gradually faded. Task-specific strategy training can be used with errorless learning or spaced retrieval methods for individuals who have difficulty learning or retaining information. It is appropriate for individuals with moderate-to-severe cognitive deficits as well as for higher-level individuals who have identified a specific task that is important for everyday function (Toglia & Golisz, 2018).

In contrast, the MC approach aims to promote strategy use beyond a single task or context and does not advocate use of one type of strategy. Any of the strategies or different types of strategies described above can be used during treatment. Single strategies or combinations of strategies are incorporated into MC treatment through skilled guidance and facilitation of strategy use described in Chapter 10. The type and number of strategies used in treatment depend on the type of performance errors or difficulties the person is experiencing, their metacognitive skills, and their choice, preferences, and abilities. The goal in the MC approach is to increase function across multiple tasks or situations. In the MC approach, a person learns to anticipate, generate, and use the same strategy across a variety of activities. Intervention can be *strategy specific* or *situational specific* or it can aim to promote strategy use across a variety of situations (*flexible*), depending on the abilities of the client.

Strategy-specific intervention is most appropriate for lower-functioning clients and involves practice of the same strategy across different situations. The person learns to anticipate, generate, execute, and self-monitor use of a single strategy that broadly enhances performance. Repetition and practice of the same strategy across situations increase accessibility and initiation of the strategy so that it requires less conscious control and effort. Toglia, et al. (2011) describes an adult female with chronic traumatic brain injury who learned to initiate and effectively use lists to gather needed items and follow steps across a variety of activities. Although the person did not acknowledge cognitive deficits in an interview, she learned to anticipate difficulties in using lists (e.g., skipping over an item or forgetting to check off an item) and carefully self-monitor her performance. The awareness that emerged was specific to the use of a list, but it was effective in optimizing use of a list across situations. Although single strategy intervention can increase functional performance, it can be limiting because a single strategy is not effective for every situation.

Situational-specific strategy intervention involves helping a person learn to anticipate and use a strategy under certain situations. This is exemplified in the use of the implementation intentions to prompt strategy use. For example, "If there is an activity with a lot of directions, I will ask for a list." Activities with a lot of directions represent the general situation under which the person will use a specific strategy (a list). In this way, situational-specific intervention results in more refined strategy use than strategy-specific intervention because the person has an understanding of the specific circumstances under which a particular strategy is appropriate, rather than just applying the strategy to all tasks.

Independent function, however, requires a wide repertoire of strategies and the ability to recognize when different strategies are most and least effective. The highest level of intervention aims for the *flexible* use of combinations of multiple strategies in challenging everyday situations to optimize performance (Toglia et al., 2012). Strategies are adjusted when needed, and different strategies are used at different times during the task or as task demands change. Table 7.3 compares the different types of strategy-based interventions.

How Strategies Are Taught

In addition to the differing content of strategy interventions as described above, there are other variations in strategy interventions; namely, in the teaching and learning methods used to promote strategy use. For example, whereas many interventions use a more explicit or directed mode of strategy instruction (i.e., the therapist tells the client which strategy or strategies to use under which circumstances), the MC approach uses guided or mediated learning (described in Chapters 9,10). In addition, the type and variety of treatment activities as well as how those activities are sequenced and presented, vary across interventions. The MC approach uses a horizontal or sideways approach to learning to facilitate practice, transfer and generalization of strategy use. This is in contrast to typical rehabilitation approaches that gradually increase difficulty of activities or grade vertically.

Strategy training involves changing the method of how someone goes about doing a task. This can involve adjusting or creating new mental habits. Treatment, therefore, needs to be structured to provide ample opportunity to use and practice the same strategies within activities. Although strategies can include a deliberate or conscious aspect, they also involve a procedural component for execution. Frequent strategy practice is

Table 7.3 Types of Strategy-Based Intervention

	Task/Context Specific	Strategy Specific*	Situational *	Flexible Strategy Use*
Number of strategies	Single	Single	Single or few	Multiple
Awareness required	No Awareness	Awareness is tied to strategy	Awareness of errors under certain conditions	Awareness across task contexts
Strategy Transfer	No Transfer	Application of same strategy across tasks	Use of strategy applied under certain situations	Anticipates or recognizes when difficulty is encountered
Intervention context and domain for practice	Single task domain and context Rote Practice	Practice of same strategy across tasks – may need faded signals	Practice recognizing conditions	Practice anticipation and error detection
Examples	Client follows a list to operate a microwave oven	Client uses a list across tasks, whenever possible	Client uses a list in household tasks with more than 4 steps. Use of a list may be combined with verbal rehearsal, underlining key words etc.	Client determines when a list or other strategy is needed
Examples	Client verbally rehearses the steps to make coffee	Client uses verbal rehearsal across tasks whenever possible.	Client verbally rehearses keywords when directions of two or more steps are presented. Other strategies may also be used.	Client determines when a verbal rehearsal or other strategies are needed

* Types of strategies used in the MC approach

needed to reduce cognitive load and increase efficiency and effectiveness of implementing strategies (similar to habit training). A horizontal approach, detailed in Chapter 8, provides a person with repeated opportunities to practice the same strategy (or strategies) at the same difficulty level across situations.

Finally, the extent to which metacognition is emphasized within strategy interventions also varies widely. Metacognition is a core focus of the MC approach and is embedded within methods to promote strategy use (Chapters 9-10). All these aspects are incorporated into the MC approach to promote the most independent, flexible, and generalizable strategy use possible.

Strategy Selection

This section highlights some key points to consider at the outset of intervention to support the identification or selection of strategies for a particular client and task.

Pre-requisites for Independent Strategy Use

Strategies are easily observed if a client is cued to use them. A challenge in treatment is to help clients spontaneously initiate strategy use. Strategy training requires at least a vague awareness of performance difficulties, knowledge of strategies, and an understanding of how they can help performance. Motivation for change and responsiveness to therapist mediation are also required for strategy training. Strategies can increase cognitive load, particularly if the task is difficult for the client as discussed below. Therefore, client ability needs to be considered along with task difficulty and client goals.

The individual's perception of task difficulty in relation to their abilities as well as beliefs about strategies influence strategy use. If a person incorrectly assesses a task as "easy" and fails to anticipate challenges or recognize errors, strategies may not be initiated or used because the person does not perceive the need to do so. The ability to anticipate and recognize performance challenges is an important prerequisite to independent and flexible strategy use (Toglia, 2018).

On the other hand, if an activity is perceived as too difficult or overwhelming, the person may also fail to initiate strategies because they believe that strategies will not help. Negative statements such as "I'll never be able to do this; this is too hard for me; my brain doesn't work right; I can't do this" will inhibit use of strategies. Similarly, emotional reactions such as anxiety or feeling overwhelmed can negatively impact information processing and the selection of strategies (Rath et al., 2011). Table 7.4 presents a list of some common obstacles to strategy use and suggestions for addressing them.

Self-Generated Strategies

There is substantial evidence that self-generated information, is better learned or remembered than that which is provided (Goverover et al., 2017; O'Brien et al., 2007). This implies that in the context of strategy interventions, clients will be more ready and able to initiate, use, and remember strategies that they have come up with on their own compared to strategies provided to them by the therapist. Although it may be easier for the therapist to tell a person what strategy they should use and instruct them on how to use it, the MC approach capitalizes on the "generation effect" to optimize learning and application of strategies. The process of guiding and facilitating strategy selection and generation requires therapist skill and practice and is described in Chapter 10.

Strategy Use and Task Difficulty (Bray et al., 1999).

Strategies are most effective when activities are at an optimal level of challenge or within an ability range that is not too easy and not too hard. If an activity is too easy, strategies are typically not needed because the task can be performed relatively automatically. The need for strategies increases with task difficulty, but if an activity is beyond the person's abilities, strategies are typically ineffective. This is because strategy use requires cognitive resources that can compete with the cognitive resources required to complete the task itself. If a task is too difficult, all available cognitive resources may be used to understand and complete the activity, and there may not be enough resources available for executing and monitoring strategies. Strategies that are too effortful often hinder performance (Waters & Kunnmann, 2010).

The number of strategies used also varies with the degree of task challenge. Typically, people use multiple strategies to cope with a challenging activity. For example, in the Weekly Calendar Planning Activity (WCPA) (Toglia, 2015), people used an average of 4-5 strategies to complete the activity. A paucity of strategies as well as excessive use of strategies both negatively impacted performance. Excessive use of strategies (9-10) requires increased effort

Table 7.4 Obstacles to Strategy Use

Obstacle	Recommendations
General lack of initiation	Cues in environment, alarms reminders, automatic text message reminders, implementation intentions (if-then).
Poor memory for strategies	Cues in environment, consider errorless learning for strategy-specific training or strategy practice and repetition to proceduralize strategy learning.
Activity beyond person's optimal level of challenge	Adjust level of activity.
The person does not anticipate or recognize task challenges or performance errors	Focus on enhancing self-awareness of performance prior to strategy generation or use.
Beliefs that strategies will not help (negative self-statements, low self-efficacy)	Use a supportive and positive approach with a focus on increasing perceived sense of control or self-efficacy; compare performance with and without strategies to show effectiveness; provide positive reinforcement for strategies or task methods that promote success.
The person acknowledges challenges but is resistant to changing ineffective task methods	Let the person experience activities themselves, using their own methods. Gradually guide them in modifying or refining existing methods rather than suggest new methods. Encourage the person to always have a "plan A" and a "plan B". Use role reversal or ask the client to critique methods used by another person performing the same activities to encourage alternate strategies. If the person is resistant to mediation, a different approach may be needed.
Person is overwhelmed and does not know how or where to begin.	The person can be encouraged or empowered to think about what they can do to simplify the activity or make it less overwhelming. Alternatively, the activity demands can be decreased if necessary.

and resources and is inefficient, while too few strategies place greater demands on the ability to keep track of information.

The relationship between strategy use and task difficulty needs to be considered during assessment and intervention. Strategy use varies with the level of task challenge for that particular person. The number and type of strategies used as well as the degree of effort required to use the strategies should be carefully observed across the course of an activity (Toglia et al., 2012). Intervention is most effective when the person can experience success with strategy use. This requires choosing activities and strategies that are balanced to create an optimal challenge point. Exhibit 7.9 summarizes key points to keep in mind about strategies.

> **Exhibit 7.9 Strategies and Difficulty Level**
>
> - Strategy use depends on task difficulty
> - Too easy – No strategies used
> - Too hard – Strategies can become too resource-demanding (ineffective)
> - Strategy training – needs to be at an optimal level of challenge

Observation of Strategy Use

Observing strategies involves analyzing how a person goes about doing an activity. For example, where does the person begin, how do they proceed, and how do they cope with task challenges? Observation of strategy use involves examining both the number, type, and degree of effort of strategies as described earlier, as well as when and how often strategies are used. In some situations, strategies may be used before the activity (e.g., creating a list of steps), rather than during the activity. The type or need for strategies may change during the activity. For example, the person may not need to use strategies within the initial phase of the activity or the first 5 to 10 minutes. During the middle or end of the activity, challenges may increase, and strategies may be required. In other situations, strategies are needed after the activity is completed to self-check work. Finally, the ability to use strategies flexibly and adjust them as needed is also an important aspect of strategy use (Toglia et al., 2012). A person may jump into an activity without a plan, thinking it will be easy. As they encounter difficulties, they may realize that a different approach is needed. This requires the ability to change task methods and approach the task differently. Optimally, it is best to observe and analyze methods used by several healthy people to complete a task before observing a person with cognitive limitations to understand what represents typical/normal patterns of strategy use versus not.

A person's strategy use also needs to be analyzed across different activities. Since strategy use varies with task difficulty, strategy use is best observed when an activity is at an optimal level of challenge. Although careful observation of performance can provide insights into the person's strategy use, an after-task interview should be used to confirm observations and to probe for strategies that cannot be easily observed. For example, the Weekly Calendar Planning Activity (WCPA) uses an after-task interview that includes questions such as "Tell me how you went about doing this activity? What methods did you use? How did you begin?" to probe for strategy use. These questions provide rich insight into performance and supplement direct observations. The metacognitive framework (Chapter 10) provides other examples of techniques for probing and guiding strategy use.

Characteristics that affect the quality of strategy use and should be considered or observed during performance are summarized in Table 7.5. A brief therapist checklist for observation and analysis of strategy use is included in Appendix B.13. Also, Toglia et al. (2012) provides a more in-depth clinical reasoning tool for observing and analyzing strategy use.

Insights from Strategy Development

The developmental process of strategies provides useful insights that might partially explain the process of relearning or learning new strategies for adults and may help guide intervention. For example, the development of strategies generally follows the below sequence (Flavell et al., 2002):

- Strategy not available due to either a lack of knowledge or lack of capacity to use it.
- Strategy used only when cued (production deficiency).
- Inability to carry out strategy efficiently or skillfully (production inefficiency).
- Strategy used but not always beneficial (utilization deficiency).
- Efficient strategy use.

Many of these same phases are often observed in adults, although they might not always follow the same sequence. During strategy training, adults often fail to use a strategy unless cued. Once the strategy is used, it is not always used efficiently or effectively. Learning to use a new strategy or relearning to use strategies is not as simple as showing or telling a person the strategy and expecting

Table 7.5 Characteristics that Affect the Quality of Strategy Use

Characteristic	Observations	Analysis
Type of strategy used	Is the type of strategy selected appropriate to the performance problem?	Strategies may be used but may be ineffective because the strategy selected does not match the performance problem.
Number of strategies used simultaneously	How many different strategies are used?	An optimal number of strategies should be used. Too many strategies or too few strategies can influence performance.
Frequency	How often the strategy is used? Does the frequency match the performance need?	Overuse of a strategy can be resource or energy-consuming. Under-use of a strategy can also hinder performance. If a task is easy, strategies may not be needed.
Timing	When are strategies used? (Before, during, or after? If during an activity, is it initial, mid, or late stage of activity?)	Strategies used too late or too early can affect strategy effectiveness.
Degree of effort required to use strategy	The degree of extra effort and concentration needed to use a strategy is important to consider.	If strategies are too effortful or resources too demanding to use, they can be ineffective.
Adjustment of strategies	Is the person able to adjust or switch to a different strategy when needed?	Persistent use of the same strategy when it is not working often creates frustration and anxiety.

that they will use it. Rather, it takes time and practice. Once a strategy is learned and used, it still might not be beneficial. This has been described as a strategy utilization deficiency (UD) (Miller, 1990). A person can produce an appropriate strategy but cannot yet benefit from the strategy during performance. UDs are thought to be more common when a strategy is first acquired and diminishes as the strategy is practiced and becomes less resource-demanding. UD also appears during strategy transfer (Clerc et al., 2014).

During strategy development, it has been suggested that strategy training begins at a level that is well within the child's ability so that enough cognitive resources are available for strategies to be learned and used before application to more challenging activities (Waters & Schneider, 2010). This might be also true of adults who are relearning or learning strategies. If a strategy appears to be too effortful, the activity may need to be simplified so that the strategy can be used with less effort. Reducing strategy effort may also require increasing practice opportunities or intensity.

Implications for Intervention: Clinical Examples

Strategy intervention involves consideration of the prerequisites required for strategy use, analysis of strategy execution, and specification of purpose and range of strategy use (Toglia et al., 2012). Clinical example 7.1 illustrates how this information can guide intervention. It summarizes two clients who both have trouble completing multiple-step activities (e.g., cooking, bill paying, making phone calls, managing medications) due to the inability to keep track of steps that have been completed. Using a list is the strategy selected for both clients, but it involves a different process and outcomes for each client.

In Clinical Example 7.1, Antonio (Client 1) uses a list when cued but he does not self-generate strategies and does not initiate using the list on his own. This may be related to an inability to perceive the need for a strategy, as he does not anticipate task challenges and perceives the task as easy. As a first step, treatment needs to help Antonio recognize and anticipate task challenges. If this is not feasible, an alternative is to use a task-specific or strategy-specific approach. For example, Antonio can be taught to use the same strategy (list) across all multiple-step activities. In contrast to Antonio, Ben (Client 2) does initiate using a list, but the quality of strategy use is poor. It may be that the activity is above the optimal challenge level and needs to be graded down until smooth execution of the strategy is observed. Alternatively, treatment can focus on improving the effectiveness and efficiency of strategy use or helping Ben self-generate and use alternate strategies to enhance performance.

Clinical Example 7.1 Comparison of Two Clients and Differences in Strategy Use

Client	Prerequisites	Execution	Treatment Implications
Client 1 Antonio	Overestimates performance before activities. Does not anticipate any challenges or difficulties. Perceives tasks as easy. No self-generation of strategies but agrees to use a list.	No spontaneous initiation of use of the list. Able to use strategies effectively (e.g., list) when cued.	Focus intervention on recognizing and anticipating the need to use a strategy across situations. OR Practice using the same strategy repeatedly within a single task (task-specific) or across tasks (strategy specific) so that it is initiated automatically or habitually.
Client 2 Ben	Anticipates difficulties in keeping track of information. Initiates strategies (e.g., using a list).	Often misses key details on lists and checks off steps before they are completed.	Decrease task demands (e.g., fewer steps) to enhance the effectiveness of strategy execution. OR Help client discover and use additional strategies to enhance attention to details. OR Practice/work on using the list more effectively.

SUMMARY

Strategy-based intervention is not as simple as showing or telling a person a strategy and expecting them to automatically use it. The time, effort, support, and practice needed for someone, particularly someone with cognitive dysfunction, to effectively use strategies are often underestimated in clinical practice. Strategy intervention requires understanding the client's specific performance problems, characteristics of strategies, different strategy intervention approaches, and the ability to analyze strategy use. Different types and combinations of strategies will be appropriate for different clients, even if they appear to demonstrate the same cognitive performance errors.

Strategy intervention can be tied to specific activities or contexts. Task-specific methods such as *practice with fading cues* or *errorless learning* can increase automaticity of strategy use within a particular task. In contrast, the MC approach focuses on practicing either single or multiple strategies across a variety of activities or situations.

Obstacles to strategy use may first need to be identified and addressed before expecting a person to implement a learned strategy. In addition, a person may be more likely to implement strategies they have generated on their own, than those provided to them by a therapist. The appropriateness of strategies and quality of strategy use needs to be carefully observed during the performance of a variety of activities. The relationship between task challenge and strategy use is particularly important in interpreting and analyzing performance. It may be that a person can learn to use strategies within activities that are at a certain cognitive level, but beyond that level, strategies become ineffective. The MC approach uses specific teaching and learning methods such as guided or mediated learning (Chapter 9), practice across horizontally structured treatment activities (Chapter 8), and a metacognitive framework (Chapter 10) to facilitate strategy self-generation, anticipation, and application.

KEY POINTS

- Cognitive strategies are conceptualized as an inherent part of healthy cognitive functioning and performance. They are used to help us manage or cope with challenges and prevent cognitive lapses.

- The same strategy (e.g., lists or mental imagery) can have different attributes, be used for different purposes, and can require different cognitive skills. Methods for more precisely defining, analyzing, and classifying strategies were described.

- Strategies need to be considered within the context of task difficulty level. Strategies are not needed when tasks are easy and are ineffective if the task is too difficult. Effective strategy use requires an optimal level of challenge.

- Strategies such as lists, self-verbalization, mental imagery, global activity management, implementation intentions, and action plans were reviewed in this chapter. Emotional regulation strategies were also discussed. Additional strategies are listed in Appendix D.1.

- There are four different types of strategy training (1) task-specific, (2) strategy specific, (3) situational specific, (3) flexible strategy use. The MC approach focuses on promoting strategy use across situations (#2-4).

- Obstacles to strategy use include decreased initiation, poor recall for strategies, decreased anticipation or recognition of performance challenges, and low self-efficacy.

- Quality of strategy use needs to be carefully observed including the type of strategy, number, frequency, timing, degree of effort, and ability to adjust strategies when needed.

- Strategy use may break down for several different reasons. Careful observation and analysis that includes consideration of task difficulty level, prerequisite skills as well as analysis of quality of strategy execution are needed.

Chapter 8

Structuring Treatment Activities to Promote Awareness and Strategy Transfer

Generalization, or the ability to apply what has been learned to a variety of situations and environments, including everyday life situations, is a major challenge in treatment for people with acquired brain injury. Strategy *transfer,* or carryover of strategy use from one activity or context to another, is often used interchangeably with generalization; however, it is narrower in scope and can be directly observed within or across intervention sessions. This chapter provides an overview of the principles of generalization and transfer including methods and treatment ingredients that facilitate positive transfer. A horizontal continuum of treatment activities that represent gradual increases in transfer distance is described as a way of promoting transfer for those who have difficulty recognizing connections between activity experiences. Generalization and transfer, therefore, can be facilitated through techniques utilized by the therapist, as well as by structuring the progression of treatment activities in a sideways manner.

Sideways Learning: The Horizontal Activity Transfer Continuum
  Structuring Treatment Across Activity Themes
  - Activities with Consistent Cognitive Demands
  - Treatment Activities and Materials
  - Multicontext Activity Modules

  The Horizontal Activity Transfer Continuum: Considerations
  - The Activity Transfer Continuum Does Not Represent a Fixed Progression
  - Treatment Using the Activity Transfer Continuum Can Also Progress "Vertically"
  - The Activity Transfer Continuum is Not Necessary for All Clients
  - Client-Centered Practice and Structured Activities

Summary and Key Points

CONTENTS OF CHAPTER 8

Overview of Generalization and Transfer
Promoting Generalization and Transfer
  Treatment Techniques to Promote Transfer

OVERVIEW OF GENERALIZATION AND TRANSFER

The occurrence of generalization and transfer of learned strategies is critical because strategies acquired in treatment activities are useless unless they are applied to everyday activities (Toglia, 2018). Transfer involves identifying *what* is being transferred, *how* it is transferred, and the *distance and breadth* of transfer. In the Multicontext (MC) approach, the content of transfer (what) involves self-monitoring, metacognitive skills, and strategies. Mechanisms of transfer are discussed below, whereas the distance and breadth of transfer are discussed in the section on sideways learning.

Generalization and transfer of learning involve the ability to detect similarities or abstract key attributes from situations and recognize that a previously learned or used strategy applies to a new activity or situation. Recognition of similarities between situations can occur at an automatic level (low road transfer) or a conscious level (high road transfer), depending on what is being transferred, the complexity of the task, and the context or physical similarities to the original learning situation. Low road transfer is automatic and involves well-practiced routines that are triggered effortlessly by conditions similar to the learning context. It is most commonly observed in near transfer tasks or tasks that look alike. High road transfer is conscious, effortful, and involves abstracting the critical attributes of a situation. It depends on metacognitive skills and involves the application and deliberate search for connections between previous or novel situations. Transfer typically involves a combination of both mechanisms, although some situations primarily involve low road transfer mechanisms, whereas others require high road transfer mechanisms (Salomon & Perkins, 1988; Perkins & Salomon, 1992, 2012). Regardless of the transfer mechanisms involved, failure to identify relevant cues in a new setting that would trigger use of a previously learned strategy results in a failure to initiate strategy use, so strategies that the person knows remain inactivated or inaccessible.

Generalization and transfer involve the ability to differentiate the strategy from the activity or environment in which it was learned. Difficulty in transfer occurs when information is tightly associated with the specific task or context in which it was learned (Bjork & Richardson-Klavehn, 1989; Haskell, 2001; Perkins & Salomon, 1992, 2012). For example, if a therapist encourages a person to stop and review a list of steps before transferring from a wheelchair to a chair, the person may learn to use that method with that particular therapist in the clinic environment. Performance and methods used may not carry over to a different therapist or environment. Similarly, if a person learns to use a verbal rehearsal strategy to keep track of where they are in a computerized working memory game, they may get better at the working memory game but continue to have difficulty in other tasks such as online shopping or cooking that require keeping track of what was just done. Therefore, strategy transfer is especially difficult if a person is taught a strategy in a single context because the strategy may only be activated in that context (Bjork & Richardson-Klavehn, 1989). The person is unable to recognize cues, attributes, or similarities that would trigger application of the strategy.

Treatment programs typically assume that transfer and generalization occur automatically. In other words, that people will spontaneously or independently apply strategies or information learned during treatment to their real-world everyday activities. However, evidence from experimental and clinical studies indicates that this is not the case (Bottiroli et al., 2017; Gick & Holyoak, 1987; Sala et al., 2019). Rather, generalization and transfer must be planned for in advance, explicitly addressed, and continually probed and tested throughout treatment if it is to be expected to occur.

PROMOTING GENERALIZATION AND TRANSFER

The MC approach has long emphasized the need to integrate principles of transfer within treatment rather than "hoping and praying it will occur" (Toglia, 1991). Treatment can facilitate improved transfer by designing and structuring activity experiences in a way that supports the process of transfer (Perkins & Salomon, 1992). The therapist needs to think about what strategy is being targeted for transfer, the extent of transfer expected (distance and breadth), what should trigger strategy use across situations, how to set up treatment activities and use guided questions to promote transfer, and how they will know when strategy transfer has occurred. Exhibit 8.1 provides guidelines for what therapists should consider when planning, implementing and monitoring treatment to ensure they are explicitly addressing transfer.

Treatment Techniques to Promote Transfer

The literature has identified several treatment techniques that are effective in facilitating transfer. These are listed in Exhibit 8.2 and are incorporated into the MC approach.

Variability in practice activities and an emphasis on *metacognitive skills* have been most consistently cited as key ingredients for learning and transfer (Bailey et al., 2010; Bransford et al., 2000; Mestre, 2002; Perkins & Salomon, 1992). As mentioned above, skills can become tied to the context in which they were learned, which can interfere with generalization or transfer across situations. Variability in learning contexts and tasks reduces this hyper-specificity of learning, especially when introduced during the earlier stages of learning (Goode et al., 2008; Stokes et al., 2008; Vakil & Heled, 2016). Variability can help the person differentiate critical elements across situations. As the activity and context continually change,

> **Exhibit 8.1 Explicitly Addressing Transfer during Treatment: Guidelines for Therapists**
>
> - How will you know that or when transfer has occurred? What will you observe?
> - Specify the tasks among which transfer will be expected to occur. For example, will transfer tasks be variations of the same task (e.g., making a sandwich) or within a task category (e.g., meal preparation) within similar or different environments? Or will transfer be expected to occur across very different tasks within similar or different environments?
> - What will be the indicators of transfer? Specify the behaviors indicative of transfer such as changes in strategy initiation, generation, quality, or in error recognition and self-monitoring skills that would be observed.
> - What type of strategy is being targeted for transfer (e.g., specific or general, self-generated or provided, single or multiple strategies)?
> - Think about what should trigger the connection:
> - Is the strategy always used regardless of task or situation or is it used under certain conditions?
> - How will a person know to use the strategy? What supports might be needed within the task or environment to help the person "detect" and "connect" (Perkins & Salomon, 2012)?
> - Think about transfer distance (near, intermediate, far) and how treatment activities can be structured to facilitate recognition of similarities (set up activities so transfer can be immediately tested).

the elements that are important and remain consistent are accentuated and reinforced. Multiple contexts and examples that require wide application of a strategy promote flexible learning (Bransford et al., 2000; Butler et al., 2017; Gick & Holyoak, 1983) and sensitize people to common, general or overarching conditions under which a strategy is applicable. This promotes strategy activation across situations (Stokes et al., 2008). This technique is a key component of the MC approach (it's in the name!) and is operationalized in the structuring of treatment activities across a horizontal continuum (described below).

The use of a *metacognitive framework* is also a key component of the MC approach and is discussed in depth in Chapter 10. Briefly, this framework includes prompts or questions before, during, and after a task to help a person anticipate, monitor, evaluate, and reflect upon their cognitive performance. A focus on generating one's own strategies, task methods or solutions is embedded within this framework. Guided questions that facilitate this strategic thinking are used consistently across treatment (Toglia, 2018). This is in line with Bransford's view of transfer as a dynamic process that requires a

> **Exhibit 8.2 Treatment Methods to Promote Positive Transfer**
>
> - ** Variability in application and practice of the same strategies to a wide array of activities and contexts.
> - ** Metacognition: Self-regulation, self-monitoring (including self-testing), and self-reflection.
> - Self-generation of strategies.
> - Guided mediation to facilitate metacognition and self-generation.
> - ** Explicitly help people abstract key patterns or similarities, see connections (detect similarities), and recognize differences among situations.
> - Use elements of actual, real-world, everyday situations that are meaningful to the person within the learning environment.
> - Focus on building self-efficacy: Treatment activities that are within an "optimal challenge level" or at a desirable level of difficulty and allow successful strategy application to promote self-efficacy.
> - Convey the meaning and value of what is being learned to promote the client's active engagement/motivation.
>
> ** *most consistently identified in the literature*

person to be actively involved in choosing and evaluating strategies (Bransford et al., 2000). It is also supported by evidence that has shown that metacognitive approaches to instruction and rehabilitation increase the degree to which people transfer learning to new situations without the need for explicit prompting (Bottiroli et al., 2017; Cella et al., 2015; Zepeda et al., 2015).

The MC approach further addresses transfer and generalization by explicitly helping people see *connections between activity experiences* and/or new and prior experiences (seeing the "old" in the "new"). This has been described as *bridging* by Perkins and Salomon (1992) and involves high road transfer mechanisms. Connections are facilitated through prompts, guided questions, expansive framing of contexts (Engle et al., 2012), and by structuring activities along a horizontal activity continuum (described below) so that similarities between them are easier to notice. Throughout treatment, the person is encouraged to identify commonalities and patterns as well as differences among activities and experiences (Perkins & Salomon, 2012). This includes practice in determining the application of a strategy as well as identifying activities or conditions to which a strategy does and does not apply.

In addition, the use of *functionally relevant materials and activities* that share similarities with everyday situations in which strategies are expected to be used increases the likelihood of strategy transfer to real-world functioning. The use of everyday materials and activities also enhances engagement and motivation in treatment because the person sees the meaning, value, and relationship to their real-world function (Toglia et al., 2010). Perkins and Salomon (1992) describe this as *hugging* or approximating learning situations to those where the desired performance will be used. Situations that share obvious similarities are thought to capitalize on automatic or low road transfer mechanisms. The combination of both methods together (hugging and bridging) has been postulated by Perkins and Salomon (1992) to promote rich transfer.

Finally, activities that are within an *optimal level of challenge* (not too easy and not too difficult) are important for promoting effective strategy use, motivation, and self-efficacy. The optimal level of challenge has also been framed as the desirable level of difficulty (Maddox & Balota, 2015) and is similar to Vygotsky's concept of the zone of proximal development (Vygotsky, 1978) discussed in Chapter 6. The optimal level of challenge is relative to the ability of the client and varies with task characteristics. Tasks that are too easy are boring while those that are too difficult cause frustration. Tasks at the optimal or desirable level of difficulty provide positive experiences in using strategies effectively to successfully meet task challenges (discussed further in Chapter 7). This helps to build a sense of mastery over performance and self-efficacy. As discussed in Chapter 1, self-efficacy is positively related to learning and strategy use (Aurah, 2013) as well as to transfer and generalization (Bandura, 1982; Burke and Hutchins, 2007; Issurin, 2013). If a person believes that they can use a particular cognitive strategy to help their performance, they are more likely to use that strategy across different situations.

SIDEWAYS LEARNING: THE HORIZONTAL ACTIVITY TRANSFER CONTINUUM

In the MC approach, treatment activities and programs can be structured in a way that capitalizes on the principles of variability and facilitates the ability to make connections between activity experiences to facilitate strategy transfer. Many individuals with cognitive limitations have difficulty detecting and connecting similarities in activity experiences, including failing to recognize that similar errors or cognitive behaviors are hindering performance across situations. In these cases, it can be helpful to structure treatment activities in a "horizontal" manner. This involves setting up a series of activities that are at the same level of cognitive difficulty but that gradually differ in surface features or physical characteristics. This provides the client with the opportunity to experience, identify, and manage similar cognitive challenges across different situations (Steinberg & Zlotnik, 2019; Toglia, 1991, 2018).

Activities along the horizontal continuum represent *transfer distance*. Distance of cognitive transfer can be defined as the degree of physical difference between the tasks or contexts. The more physically similar the tasks (e.g., two almost identical or alternate activities), the nearer the transfer; the more different the tasks (e.g., using a schedule and then a menu), the farther the transfer (Toglia et al., 2010). The extent of transfer can also be described in terms of the generality or *breadth of transfer*, that is, the number and type of different tasks, domains, and contexts to which original learning is successfully applied (McKeough et al., 2013). Transfer, therefore, includes both transfer distance and breadth. Figure 8.1 illustrates the use of a sideways learning approach to treatment as a way to facilitate strategy transfer across activities, both in distance and breadth.

A horizontal approach to structuring treatment programs may require a shift in thinking for many therapists. Typically, activities in rehabilitation are structured "vertically" in the process of grading. If the individual can successfully complete an activity, activities are increased in difficulty. The result is that the individual often gets better at the activities that are practiced, but there is limited transfer and generalization of learning. The use of a horizontal structure of treatment activities in the MC approach facilitates the ability to make connections and apply strategies across activities. It also provides continual opportunity to observe and probe for carryover of learning

Figure 8.1 Increasing Transfer Distance: The Appearance of Activities is Gradually Changed

Very Similar ⇄ Somewhat Similar ⇄ Different ⇄ Completely Different

A Horizontal and Reversible Continuum

⟷

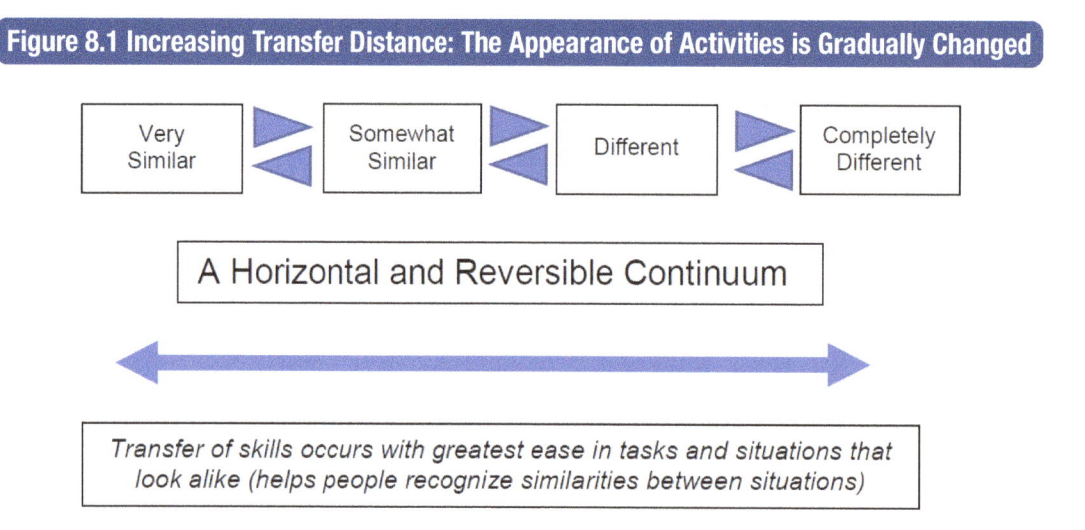

Transfer of skills occurs with greatest ease in tasks and situations that look alike (helps people recognize similarities between situations)

and transfer within and across treatment sessions, before difficulty level is increased (Toglia, 2017, 2018).

Structuring Treatment Across Activity Themes

Activities with Consistent Cognitive Demands

Transfer of learning between tasks is related to the degree to which they share common elements, however, the common elements need to be detected or abstracted (Bransford et al., 2000, p.78). Transfer requires recognizing underlying similarities in cognitive demands of tasks and contexts that are physically different (Lobato et al., 2012). Recognition of similarities across tasks or situations activates the consistent application of strategies that are effective in managing similar cognitive demands. For example, recognizing that two tasks both require keeping track of information, even though one task involves searching for and keeping track of items on a calendar while the other involves locating and keeping track of items in an online store, could prompt initiation of the same "checking off" strategy to facilitate keeping track in both tasks.

In the MC approach, a series of activities that have common activity characteristics and underlying cognitive demands are grouped in *activity themes*. Activities within activity themes are at the same level of cognitive difficulty and are presented along a horizontal continuum (i.e., gradually vary in surface features). Performance within the activity themes provides the person with repeated opportunity to discover that the same difficulties are interfering with performance across situations. Similarly, it also allows for practice in using the same strategies across activities. This helps the person gain awareness of and anticipate activity characteristics that may pose performance challenges. It also helps the person understand that the same strategy can be effective in managing performance challenges across different tasks (Toglia, 2017).

The first step in using the horizontal activity transfer continuum is to identify activity themes or key activity characteristics that remain constant and that also keep relevant cognitive demands consistent across activities. Exhibit 8.3 illustrates an activity theme that involves use of a list to search and locate ten items using a variety of materials such as schedules, menus, catalogs, closets, or materials on the computer, etc. The number of items on the list and the directions remains the same, while the materials change. Activities at the beginning of the continuum represent near transfer tasks. They have similar physical features and represent alternate versions of the same task. Strategy transfer under near transfer conditions tends to be fast and automatic in healthy adults (low road transfer). People with moderate or severe acquired brain injury, however, may require greater practice to achieve near transfer (Ownsworth et al. 2017).

The activities in Exhibit 8.3 gradually differ in physical characteristics and context along the continuum so that those at the end of the continuum represent far transfer from the initial learning context (Toglia, 1991). The first two activities include using a 10-item list to find food items. The activities in the middle of the continuum involve using a 10-item list in contexts such as a schedule or menu, while the last activity involves using a 10-item list to find items in a bathroom to pack a toiletry bag. The underlying cognitive demands remain generally constant across the continuum (Toglia, 2017). Therefore, application of the same strategy facilitates functional cognitive performance across the continuum.

The use of varying materials at the same level of complexity helps the person differentiate strategies from the specific task and context in which it was learned.

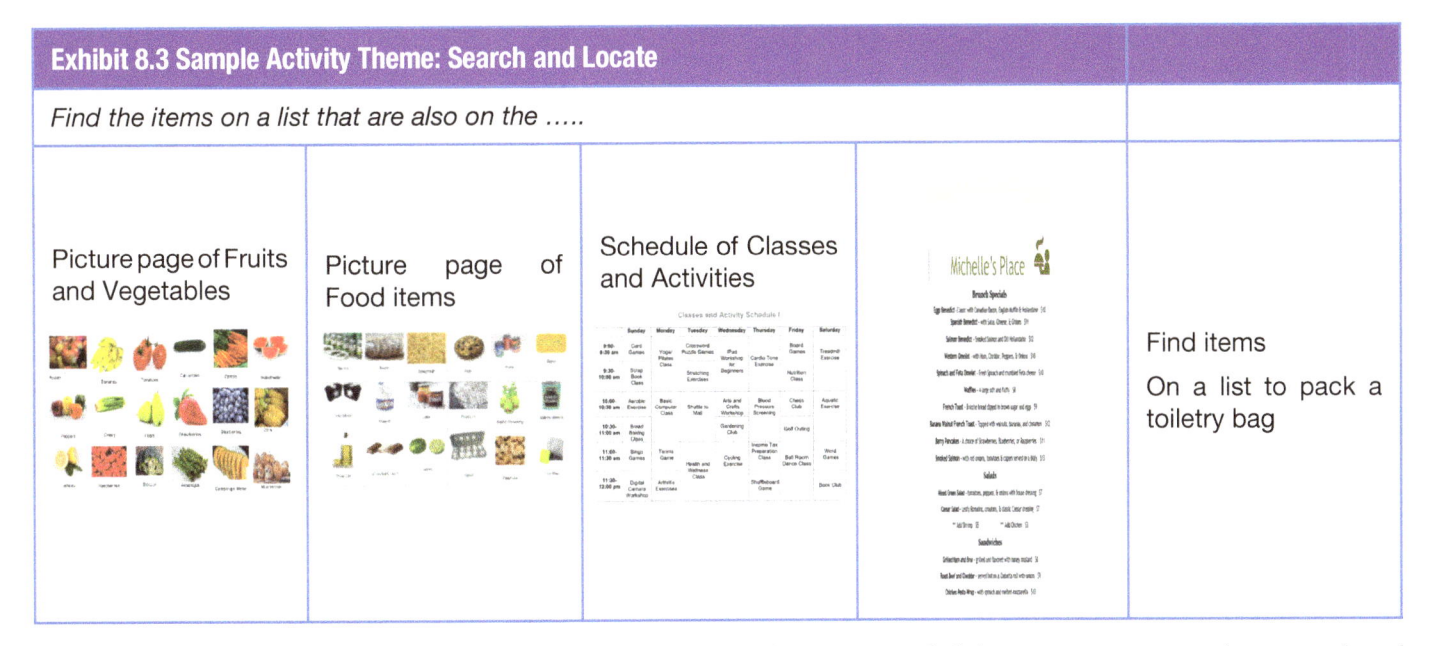

Exhibit 8.3 Sample Activity Theme: Search and Locate

Find the items on a list that are also on the .....

Picture page of Fruits and Vegetables	Picture page of Food items	Schedule of Classes and Activities	Michelle's Place (menu)	Find items On a list to pack a toiletry bag

From Toglia, J. (2017). *Schedule activity module: Functional cognitive rehabilitation activities and strategy-based intervention.* NY: MC CogRehab Resources, LLC.

This treatment structure is designed to promote flexible application and strategy transfer by helping the person recognize and understand the essential attribute (Toglia et al., 2010). The person learns that the strategy is not only applicable to one task but is helpful across many tasks. It should be noted that single strategy training such as practice using a list across a variety of multi-step activities has greater dependence on low road automatic transfer mechanisms whereas multiple strategy use or cognitively complex activities rely more on high road transfer mechanisms that require metacognitive skills.

Different performance errors can be observed during the activities above, depending on the client and their cognitive abilities. For example, the person may lose track of what they were looking for as soon as they look away from the list. They may start in the middle of the list and proceed in a haphazard or disorganized manner, or they might become sidetracked by irrelevant information that triggers ideas or past experiences. The same activities, therefore, can be used with different clients to elicit distinct patterns of cognitive performance errors and to provide the context for the generation and use of varying strategies. This is because the appropriate strategy will depend on the type of cognitive performance error. It is not the activities themselves but the ability to effectively manage the same performance error across situations that is the target of treatment (Toglia, 2017).

Examples of activity themes are presented in Appendix D.2. As described earlier, activity themes describe general cognitive characteristics or requirements that remain consistent across a sequence of activities as the physical appearance, materials, or contexts are gradually varied. For example, an activity theme may be a series of activities that involve comparing or contrasting information, searching for items that meet multiple criteria, or identifying the most relevant information. Activities within these themes are selected so that they have the same level of difficulty and require common cognitive skills, although they might be physically different. Since the activities contain common cognitive demands, the same strategies are effective across tasks. Activity themes are chosen based on analysis of the client's cognitive error patterns that are observed across different activities as well as consideration of their interests and experiences.

Treatment Activities and Materials

Once an appropriate activity theme is identified for a client, the second step is to generate a list of activities that use everyday materials related to the theme. The person's lifestyle, interests, and experiences need to be considered when brainstorming and selecting activities to promote motivation, engagement, and relevance to their everyday life. A wide variety of everyday materials and activities can be used during intervention. When using the MC approach, it is important to ensure that treatment materials are well organized so that relevant everyday activities can present cognitive challenges for different levels of ability and that materials for different interests are readily available. Appendix D.3 presents a list of everyday materials that might be helpful to have available in a clinic to use in treatment activities; however, the materials that are assembled will vary depending on the general interests, occupations, culture, and/or location of the population served. Alternatively, as described in the next section, pre-made structured MC activity modules are also available.

The complexity or number of items, degree of distractions, arrangement of items as well as other activity characteristics need to be further specified by the therapist to provide the optimal level of cognitive challenge and to ensure they remain constant across the continuum (or can be graded up if appropriate). At the same time, the task context, type of stimuli, movement requirements, and environment can vary. An activity worksheet for increasing transfer distance of activities along the horizontal continuum is included in Appendix C.4 and a sample is illustrated in Exhibit 8.4.

In general, it is suggested that two activities be used within one treatment session when feasible to allow for the opportunity to observe carryover and transfer from one activity to the next within a treatment session. Typically, a minimum of 6 to 8 structured activities are used across 3 to 5 treatment sessions; however, more or fewer structured activities may be needed depending on the client.

Multicontext Activity Modules

A series of MC Activity modules that use functionally relevant materials and are designed to be tailored to different levels of ability and patterns of cognitive performance errors are available for purchase separately (www.multicontext.net). They were developed using the principles described in Chapter 4. In addition, Appendix D.4 includes brief descriptions of each module. The MC Activity modules include similar activity themes and directions, but they use different functional contexts.

Exhibit 8.4 Multicontext Treatment Activity Planning Worksheet: Increasing Transfer Distance

Activity Theme (characteristics that stay constant): All activities require adhering to 3-4 criteria while completing or assembling 6-8 photos or pieces of information or searching and locating 6–8 pieces of information

Error Patterns: Jumps into tasks without preplanning, gets sidetracked, loses track.

Processing Strategy/Behavior to control errors: 1) "stop and plan" 2) visualize the end goal/outcome before beginning

	Initial Activity	Very Similar	Somewhat Similar	Different
	Make a photo collage of 8 pictures on the computer following 3-4 rules/criteria.	Make an invitation or sign on the computer following 3-4 rules (involves importing pictures). Create a greeting card with photo on the computer following 3-4 rules.	Follow 3-4 rules to make a brief PowerPoint presentation with 8 pictures. Catalog shopping: Find 8 items within a certain price range following 3-4 criteria.	Gift Shop: Find 6 items that meet 3 criteria. Café: Identify 2-3 meals that meet three different criteria. *Note: each meal should contain a beverage, main dish, and dessert.*

Characteristics that may vary across activities:

Task context	Computer *Leisure*	Computer *IADL/Leisure*	Computer *Work and IADL*	*IADL*
Type of Stimuli	Photos	Digital cards photo	PowerPoint Catalogs	Items on crowded shelves or menus
Directions or rules	Follow 3-4 steps and criteria	Follow 3-4 steps and criteria	Follow steps and 3-4 criteria	Search and locate Follow 3-4 criteria
Movement Requirements	Fine motor	Fine motor	Fine motor	Walking
Environment	Clinic quiet room	Clinic quiet room	Clinic – open area	Real-world environments
Other				

Treatment along a horizontal continuum: At the same level of difficulty, gradually change.

Presently, there are three different MC Activity modules: 1) schedule module, 2) menu module and 3) business activity module. Each module includes a wide variety of activities, materials, or directions that vary in complexity (detail, number of items, distractors) and cognitive demands; however, as can be seen from their names, all of the activities within a single module use the same functional context (e.g., schedules). Activities *across* the different modules have parallel features (e.g., activity themes), so they can be combined and arranged across the activity transfer continuum. The features of an individual module will be described first, followed by ways that modules can be combined.

Single Multicontext Activity Module

Each module includes directions and materials that are carefully manipulated to place different demands on cognitive abilities such as keeping track of information while searching, selecting relevant information while ignoring distractions, shifting between rules or task components, organizing information, and multitasking. For example, the menu module includes a variety of menus (picture and written) and lists of food items that differ in detail and number of items. In addition to differences in complexity of materials, the directions and questions that accompany the materials also vary in level of structure, length, and cognitive demands. The menu activities can be increased in difficulty by using more detailed materials (e.g., menus) or by using the same materials and changing the directions. For example, two different directions that can be used with the same materials – a list and a menu – are as follows:

1. *Remember 3 food items on the list and then find the items on the menu.*
2. *Circle all of the items on the list that are below $8.00 on the menu and check off items that are above $12.00.*

Direction #1 requires basic immediate recall of information while #2 requires the ability to keep track of two different rules, shift back and forth between materials, and respond differently based on criteria. In this example, both activities use the same materials, but the different directions alter their cognitive demands as discussed in Chapter 4. Alternatively, the same directions can be used with more detailed menus and longer lists.

Each MC activity module also includes different types of activities that reflect a wide range of ability levels and cognitive skills within the same functional context. Single modules contain activities grouped within three levels of difficulty that differ in quantity and level of detail so that they can be tailored to the client's ability level. Level 1 activities are brief (10 minutes) and can be used in an inpatient setting or with people who have moderate-to-severe cognitive deficits. For example, within the menu module, there are basic activities that involve matching pictures of individual food items to items on a written or picture menu or searching for and locating specific items on a simplified picture menu. Level 2 activities include about twice as much information as Level 1 activities, but the questions are similar. They can be used with higher-level inpatients or in outpatient settings. Level 3 activities are detailed or complex and include the integration of executive function (EF) skills including planning, multitasking, shifting between different sources of information, and organization. They are most appropriate for those with subtle cognitive difficulties that are typically seen in an outpatient or community setting. For example, Level 3 activities in the menu module involve choosing restaurants based on multiple criteria or selecting, planning, and organizing meals using a combination of different menus.

Activities at all levels include the same materials (schedules or menus etc.); however, the activity features are manipulated to place more or less demand on different cognitive functional skills. This allows the therapist to choose the activity characteristics and difficulty level that are best suited for the client's ability and performance problems. The modules also provide alternate versions of the same activity, which allows the therapist to examine carryover of strategies to similar activities (i.e., transfer).

Combining Multicontext Activity Modules

Each MC activity module includes parallel themes, directions, and difficulty levels, despite differences in materials or functional context. Activities from different modules with similar directions (activity theme) and difficulty level are designed so they can be combined and arranged across a horizontal continuum to promote awareness and strategy transfer.

Exhibits 8.5. and 8.6. illustrate how similar activities from each of the three activity modules can be combined to create horizontal transfer continuums of treatment activities. The first example involves basic cognitive skills and can be used within an inpatient setting, while the second example involves higher-level activities for people with subtle cognitive difficulties. These two examples are each further specified in Appendices D.5 and D.6, showing a sample sequence of eight treatment sessions.

In Exhibit 8.5, all activities involve searching for and locating information from a 10-item list (activity theme). Since the person tends to lose track of information, the directions and activities are chosen to place demands on the ability to hold and keep track of information while searching. The activity is at an optimal level of challenge

Exhibit 8.5 Sample Multicontext Horizontal Activity Structure Across Treatment Sessions: Basic (search and locate)

Similar activity theme across activities: Finding and locating information from a 10-item list.

Performance error: Loses track of information on the list (e.g., forgets items being searched; loses place).

Sample strategy to control performance error across all activities: Verbal rehearsal of keywords during searching (can progress from talking aloud, to whispering, to talking to self).

Sample directions across activities: *Remember the first 3 items from the list and see if they are in or on the….*

Schedule Module	Schedule Module	Menu Module	Business Module	Schedule Module
Class and activity weekly schedule	TV program schedule	Picture Menu	Business Name Cards Or on both lists	*Supplementary Activities*
Sightseeing activities and events schedule	Things to do schedule or calendar	Written Menu		Kitchen cabinets
				Bathroom
				Office supply closet

Initial Task ←————————→ *Similar* ←————————→ *Different*

From Toglia, J. (2019). *Business Card Activity Module: The Multicontext Approach.* NY: MC CogRehab Resources, LLC.

Exhibit 8.6 Sample Multicontext Horizontal Activity Structure Across Treatment Sessions: Complex Activity

Similar activity theme across activities: All activities involve using and synthesizing information from two different sources, selecting relevant information, and identifying options based on multiple criteria.

Typical performance error: Jumps into higher-level activities without fully attending to all directions or pre-planning.

Sample strategy to control performance error across all activities: Planning ahead or breaking down information and creating a list of key information.

Similar directions across activities: *Identify a list of possible options based on criteria (days, times, preferences, location, price, etc).*

Schedule Module- Complex Questions	Schedule Module- Complex Questions	Menu Module	Business Module	Supplementary Module Activities
Based on criteria, identify a list of…	Based on criteria, identify a list of…	Based on criteria, identify a list of…	Use business name cards and registration lists to identify and sort attendees to a conference based on criteria.	*Online Shopping*
• "Class and Activity" options from schedule and information sheet.	• TV viewing options from schedule and information sheet.	• Restaurant options from cards and information sheet.		Select products based on criteria and compare prices across websites.
• "Sightseeing and Event" options from schedule and information sheet.	• "Things to Do" options from schedule and information sheet.	• Meal options from multiple menus.		*Planning a Trip*
				Based on criteria, identify a list of options for airline flights.

Initial Task ←————————→ *Similar* ←————————→ *Different*

Adapted from Toglia, J. (2019). *Business Card Activity Module: The Multicontext Approach.* NY: MC CogRehab Resources, LLC (not too easy and not too hard) and allows for success with effective strategies. The initial activities are very similar and represent alternate forms of the same activity, making it easier to detect and connect activity experiences. The activities gradually become physically more dissimilar, but the cognitive demands remain the same in that the activities repeatedly require the person to keep track of and find three items from a 10-item list. These consistent cognitive demands across activities help the person recognize and practice managing the same error (losing track) across situations. Once the person can successfully use strategies to effectively keep track of three items, the complexity or difficulty (e.g., number of items or degree of detail) can be increased and strategies may be expanded or adjusted.

Each activity set also includes higher-level activities, as in Exhibit 8.6. This example illustrates how the same materials described above (schedules, menus, business cards) can be used to place higher cognitive demands on the ability to adhere to rules or criteria, inhibit distractions, and keep track of information by altering directions and increasing the number of items and detail presented simultaneously. In this example, all activities involve selecting relevant information and identifying possible options using two different sources of information and multiple criteria (activity theme). Similar to Exhibit 8.5, the directions and cognitive demands are consistent while the physical similarity of activities gradually decreases across the continuum. The person is provided with repeated opportunity to restrain impulsive tendencies, plan ahead and simplify or break down the activity.

To summarize, the MC Activity modules provide parallel structured activities within different functional contexts. Each module includes different activities within the same functional context that range in difficulty level and cognitive demands. The combination of activities *across* the modules or functional contexts provides the opportunity to structure treatment activities horizontally. This can facilitate connections between activity experiences and contribute to promoting strategy transfer.

The Horizontal Activity Transfer Continuum: Considerations

The Activity Transfer Continuum Does Not Represent a Fixed Progression

The progression of treatment activities depends on the client's ability to transfer strategy use and perceive connections between activities. In some situations, activities can jump from similar to different (near to far transfer) within the same treatment session, whereas in other situations, treatment activities may need to progress slowly in terms of transfer distance. The common cognitive demands of activities across the horizontal continuum provide the opportunity to analyze, observe, and probe carryover and transfer of awareness and strategies across activities. If carryover of strategies is not observed, the transfer continuum progresses more slowly, and a greater number of alternate activities (physically similar) are used. On the other hand, if the person readily perceives connections between activities and recognizes the application of strategies, treatment jumps to a variety of intermediate or far transfer activities (physically dissimilar).

Treatment Using the Activity Transfer Continuum Can Also Progress "Vertically"

As mentioned above, once strategy use is observed across a variety of activities, activity demands can be added or changed to increase difficulty level. In this way, treatment progresses in both a sideways or horizontal manner as well as in a vertical or graded manner, like a staircase, as illustrated in Figure 8.2. As with progressing across the horizontal continuum, the amount of time spent at the same level of difficulty varies depending on the client's ability to apply strategies across tasks. Figure 8.2 shows that for some clients, activities can be graded up or changed quickly while others require a slower progression.

As difficulty level or activity complexity increases, the same strategies that were previously successful may become ineffective. New strategies may be needed, or previous strategies may need to be revised, adjusted, or expanded. In some situations, strategy use may only be effective at a certain level of task difficulty or within certain activity characteristics. If activity type is changed or complexity is increased, strategy use can fall apart. The therapist needs to recognize this and specify the situations under which certain strategies are most and least effective.

The Activity Transfer Continuum is Not Necessary for All Clients

The horizontal activity transfer continuum provides therapists with a guide for sequencing and structuring activities across a treatment program when an individual has limited awareness or difficulties detecting and connecting similarities between activity experiences. It is particularly helpful in facilitating awareness of performance errors because it provides the person with repeated experience in encountering similar performance challenges. Performance is embedded within a metacognitive framework that involves repeated practice in identifying task challenges, generating solutions, monitoring, and self-assessing performance (see Chapter 10). These techniques are used within activities that, while different in surface features, present consistent cognitive challenges. As the ability to recognize and monitor errors emerges, strategy use and

Figure 8.2 Sideways Learning

Short Horizontal Continuum
2 activities at same level

Long Horizontal Continuum
8 activities at same level

Increased difficulty - Horizontal Continuum is Repeated at higher difficulty level

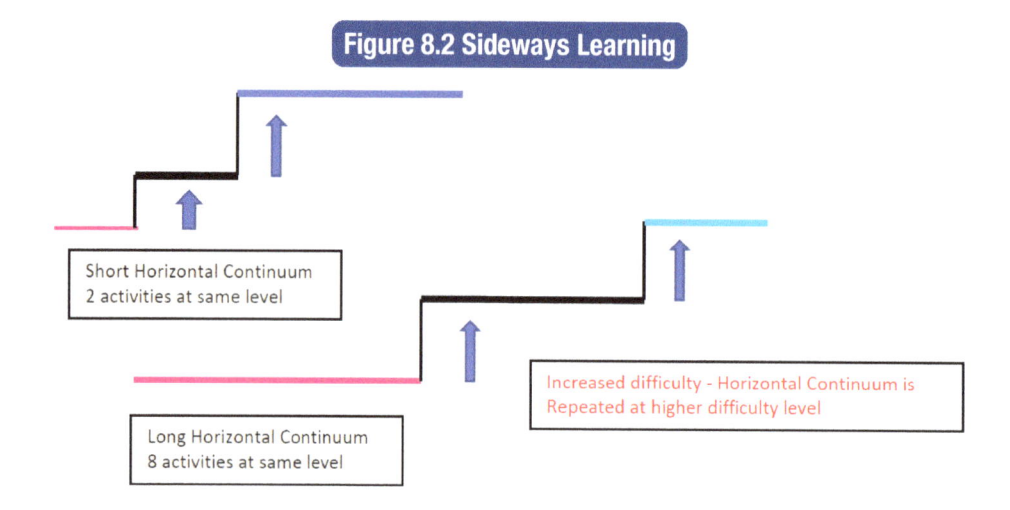

Activities are not graded up (vertically) in difficulty until evidence of horizontal transfer (application of the strategy across situations at the same level of difficulty) is observed.

performance are enhanced. This increases engagement in treatment and fosters the ability to identify more specific and realistic goals. Treatment gradually moves away from structured activities and toward client-directed activities as self-awareness and cognitive goals emerge.

The horizontal activity transfer continuum is not necessary in all cases. Some individuals have good awareness and understanding of their performance and can immediately recognize connections between activities and apply learning to varied situations. For these individuals, self-chosen activities that vary widely or require distant transfer from each other can be used. In these cases, the focus may be on increasing the breadth of transfer rather than increasing transfer distance. Regardless of whether the activity transfer continuum is used, the focus is always on helping a person generate effective strategies to control performance errors across activities.

Client-Centered Practice and Structured Activities

Client-centered practice is viewed on a continuum within the MC approach. If awareness is limited, incomplete, or at a superficial level, the therapist may take a greater role in choosing and structuring functional cognitive treatment activities and goals in the initial stages of treatment. This is particularly true if the person is in an inpatient setting and has not had the opportunity to experience functional cognitive activities. If the client only identifies physical goals, functional cognitive activities are used to address these goals within the context of motor activities. This occurs by manipulating placement of materials to reinforce motor skills such as reaching, fine motor coordination, standing balance, or ambulation (see Chapter 4). For example, a list might be on a table while a menu with prices is placed on a bulletin board on the other side of the room. The person may be asked to recall the prices of items on the menu (on the bulletin board) while they walk back to the table and write the prices next to the items on the list. This addresses the client's physical goals while at the same time increasing awareness of functional cognitive limitations (Jaywant et. al, 2020).

There are a wide variety of activities that can be used to address cognitive limitations, so it is important to use activities that fit the person's interests, lifestyle, and physical goals. If the person does not perceive the relevance of an activity, it should not be used. The emergence of self-awareness and strategy use requires active participation and engagement within treatment activities.

As self-awareness emerges, the person may begin to identify goals related to cognition. Goal adjustment can be one indicator of increased self-awareness as described in Chapter 12. Functional cognitive activities progress from those that are therapist directed or pre-chosen within the context of the person's physical goals, to client self-chosen, functional cognitive activities and goals. This is summarized in Figure 8.3. Typically, structured activities are recommended for the first 3 to 5 sessions or for a minimum of 6 to 8 activities. The client is then encouraged to choose their own activities that would provide similar levels of cognitive challenge.

If clients have difficulty identifying or generating activities for treatment sessions on their own, they can be asked to choose activities from a pre-established activity list. The list should be based on knowledge of the person's interests, experiences, and goals. A structured list can also stimulate ideas and help a client generate other activities

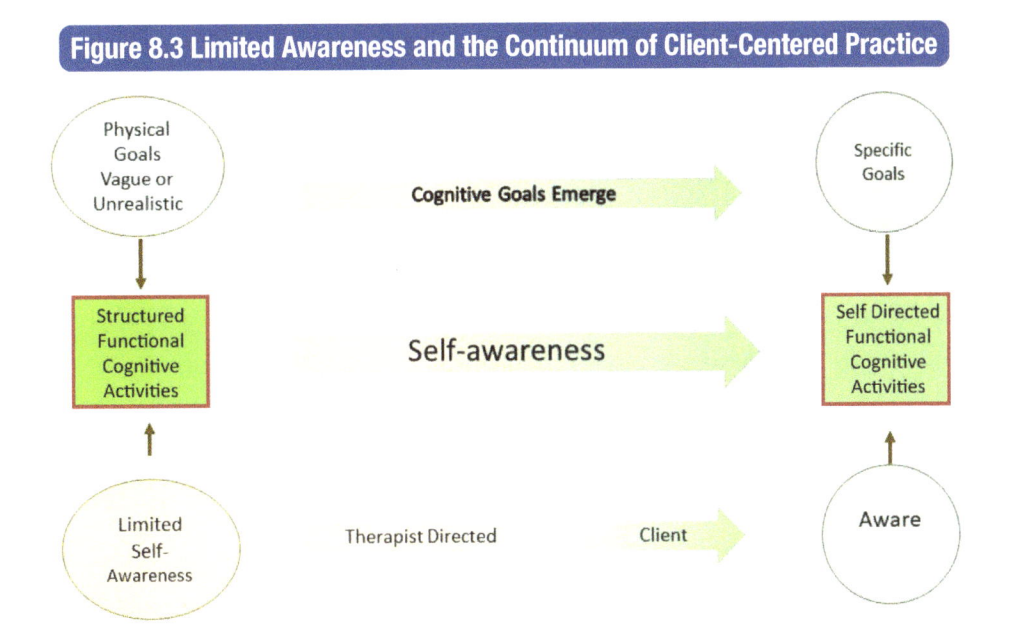

Figure 8.3 Limited Awareness and the Continuum of Client-Centered Practice

and goals themselves. Appendix C.5 includes sample lists of activities that could be presented to a client to help them choose or select relevant activities and goals.

It should be emphasized that if the person is fully aware of their cognitive performance difficulties or identifies specific goals from the start of treatment, then intervention begins with client self-selected goals. Activities and structured activities arranged along a horizontal continuum as described earlier are often not needed in higher-level clients that show a full understanding of their cognitive abilities and areas of weakness and can anticipate or recognize the need to use strategies across situations. In these situations, treatment goals and activities are client-directed from the beginning of treatment. Intervention focuses more on strategy generation, execution, and effectiveness across a wide variety of activities.

SUMMARY

The MC approach emphasizes the need to integrate and structure treatment to promote transfer and generalization. Principles of transfer described in the literature have been incorporated into MC treatment and include the following key features: (1) variability in practice activities and contexts, (2) a focus on metacognitive skills, (3) use of functionally relevant materials that share similarities to situations in which strategies are expected to be used, and (4) explicitly helping people see connections between current activity experiences and future or prior activities (see Exhibit 8.2).

A horizontal structure of treatment activities is used in the MC approach to facilitate the ability to detect connections between activities. Activities with common cognitive requirements are arranged along a continuum from those that are physically very similar (near transfer) to those that are physically dissimilar (far transfer). This provides the opportunity for the person to repeatedly apply the same strategy across activities that represent different levels of transfer distance. Sideways learning is promoted by requiring strategy application across a variety of different activities while keeping cognitive complexity constant. Activities are not graded in difficulty until evidence of strategy transfer has been observed across situations.

Pre-made MC activity modules that are organized into activity themes provide the opportunity to target different error patterns across activities. These activities were briefly described in this chapter and are available separately (www.multicontext.net).

The horizontal activity transfer continuum provides therapists with a guide for the sequence, structure, and progression of activities across a treatment program, however, it is not fixed. It is most applicable when an individual has difficulties detecting and connecting similarities between activity experiences; however, the extent that it is used depends on the person's awareness and ability to carry over learning.

Structured cognitive functional activities are typically chosen by the therapist if the person has limited awareness. Initially, activities might focus on the client's motor goals, while simultaneously incorporating structured cognitive functional activities to build self-awareness. As self-awareness emerges, the client takes greater responsibility for choosing cognitive functional activities.

KEY POINTS

- Structure treatment activities in a sideways manner along the horizontal transfer continuum to facilitate the ability to perceive connections between activity experiences or situations, thus promoting transfer of strategy use.
- Activities along the horizontal continuum represent increasing levels of transfer distance. Underlying cognitive demands remain consistent while physical appearance, materials, or context gradually change.
- Structuring activities across the transfer continuum increases the likelihood that the same error pattern will emerge. This provides the opportunity to (1) build awareness, (2) practice the same strategy so that it becomes more habitual, and (3) help people make connections between activity experiences.
- Explicit repeated practice across a variety of situations is required so that less effort is needed to activate and execute the strategy. This supports strategy transfer.
- Once spontaneous strategy use is observed across activities, activity demands can be increased (i.e., graded vertically).
- If the client demonstrates awareness, initiation of strategies, and/or readily perceives similarities between activities, the horizontal activity transfer continuum may not be needed.
- The MC activity modules provide pre-made parallel structured activities that can be combined to create horizontal activity transfer continuums for a variety of clients.
- Some specific guidelines for using structured activities:
  - Use within a Metacognitive Framework (see Chapter 10).
  - Try to use two activities within one treatment session to allow for the opportunity to observe carryover of metacognitive skills and strategies.
  - Use a minimum of 6-8 structured activities from across the continuum over 3-5 treatment sessions.
  - Arrange activity materials to address physical goals when appropriate.
  - As awareness emerges, transition to client-chosen and real-life activities and contexts.

Chapter 9

Introduction to Metacognitive Strategy Interventions and Guided Learning

This chapter introduces and explains differences between metacognitive strategy interventions with a focus on the distinction between direct strategy methods and guided learning methods. The way that the Multicontext (MC) approach uses guided or mediated learning techniques is explained and general mediation guidelines are presented. Type and content of guided questions used within the MC treatment are distinguished from those that have a task-specific focus. The use of mediated learning methods to promote self-awareness and self-efficacy for management of cognitive performance errors is discussed. Chapters 10 and 11 further expand upon the concepts and information presented in this chapter and operationalize the procedures for using and assessing metacognitive methods.

CONTENTS OF CHAPTER 9

Metacognitive Strategy Intervention
Instructional Approaches in Metacognitive Strategy Interventions
    Therapist-Directed
    Guided Learning
- *Application of Guided Learning: Mediation Methods in the Multicontext Approach*
- *General Therapeutic Techniques*

Summary and Key Points

METACOGNITIVE STRATEGY INTERVENTION

Metacognitive strategy intervention is a broad term to describe interventions that focus on helping a person think about their own thinking. Several different studies, as outlined in Exhibit 9.1, support the effectiveness of metacognitive strategy-based approaches within the context of functional activities to optimize executive functions (EF) and self-awareness (Cicerone et al., 2019, Haskins et al., 2012; Radomski et al., 2016). Metacognitive strategy interventions have been identified as evidenced-based and recommended for treatment of mild-moderate deficits in EF after traumatic brain injury (practice standard) and stroke (practice guideline) (Cicerone et al., 2019).

Although all metacognitive strategy interventions share a focus on structured methods for managing multiple-step activities and using strategies, there can be key differences in skills emphasized, degree of client centeredness, and teaching and learning methods used. For example, some metacognitive strategy interventions such as the MC approach emphasize online self-awareness of performance (Goverover et al., 2007; Toglia, 2018); others emphasize goal management and problem-solving strategies, (Dawson, Binns, et al., 2013; Stamenova & Levine, 2019), and others include a focus on emotional regulation (Cicerone et al., 2008; Tornas et al., 2016).

121

Exhibit 9.1 Evidence for Metacognitive Strategy Intervention

- Short-Term Executive Plus (STEP) (Cantor et al., 2014)
- Goal Management Training (Stamenova & Levine, 2019)
- CO-OP Approach (Dawson et al., 2009; Dawson, Richardson, et al., 2013; McEwen et al., 2018)
- CogSMART (Caplan et al., 2015; Kannan et al., 2017)
- Time Pressure Management (Winkens et al., 2009)
- Multicontext Approach (Toglia et al., 2010; Toglia et al., 2011; Toglia, 2018; Jaywant et al., 2020; Toglia et al., 2020)

Similarly, some metacognitive strategy interventions provide direct instruction on strategy use (Kennedy & Coelho, 2005; Sohlberg & Turkstra, 2011) while others use guided learning to facilitate strategy generation and problem-solving (Skidmore et al., 2015; Toglia et al., 2010), described in more detail below. In addition, strategies can be directed toward methods for specific tasks or toward general strategies for detecting and managing cognitive performance errors that are applicable across tasks (discussed in Chapter 7). The variability and ambiguity in what constitutes metacognitive strategy intervention can make it difficult for practitioners to implement such an approach in clinical practice.

INSTRUCTIONAL APPROACHES IN METACOGNITIVE STRATEGY INTERVENTIONS

There are two general approaches to strategy instruction: therapist-directed and guided or mediated learning. These approaches are summarized in Figure 9.1. The blue shaded boxes on the left side of Figure 9.1 represent therapist-directed instruction and use of direct cueing methods, whereas the yellow shaded boxes on the right side represent a guided or mediated learning approach. These approaches will be introduced in this section, and then the guided or mediated learning method, which is used in the MC approach, is further explained below and in Chapter 10.

Therapist-Directed

Therapist-directed methods focus on educating or instructing the person on particular methods to perform a task. The therapist uses their expertise to identify barriers hindering performance and provides strategies or solutions for the client to overcome these barriers. Strategies or methods to enhance functional performance are taught to the client and practiced (Skidmore et al., 2017). This is typical in rehabilitation, where teaching person-specific skills such as how to use equipment, perform a transfer, or use one-handed techniques is commonplace. If the person has difficulty, cues that provide hints, feedback, or corrective action or instruct the person on what to do are used to facilitate performance. Cues may be auditory, verbal, visual, gestural, tactile, or a combination.

A graded sequence of cues may be used within therapist-directed methods. Table 9.1 presents one example of a cue sequence that is arranged from general to specific and progresses from least to most assistance. This method is

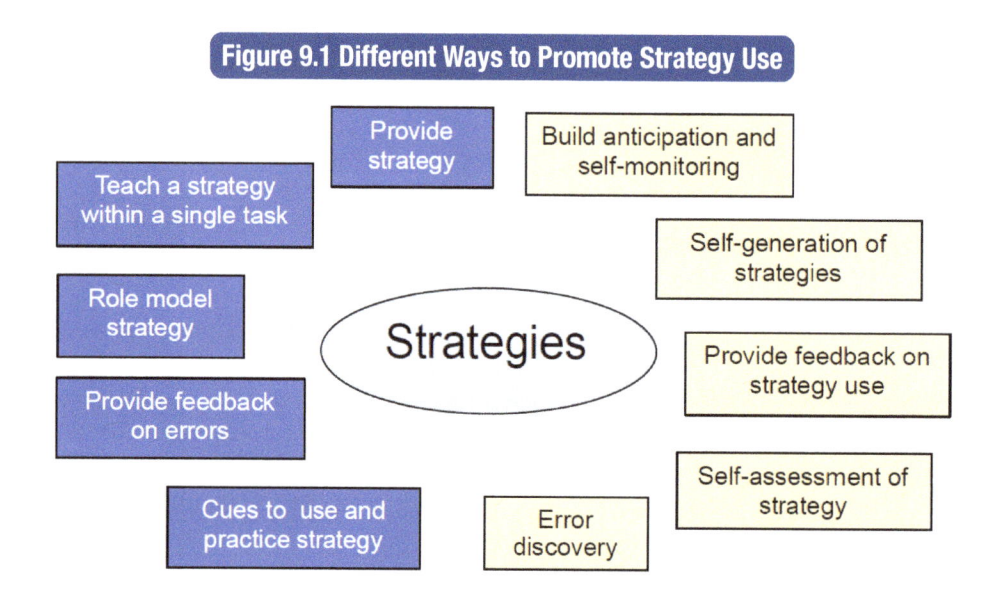

Figure 9.1 Different Ways to Promote Strategy Use

Therapist-directed (blue):
- Teach a strategy within a single task
- Provide strategy
- Role model strategy
- Provide feedback on errors
- Cues to use and practice strategy

Guided/mediated (yellow):
- Build anticipation and self-monitoring
- Self-generation of strategies
- Provide feedback on strategy use
- Self-assessment of strategy
- Error discovery

Table 9.1 Hierarchical Cues From Least to Most Assistance

Types of Cues	Example of Cues
General Feedback	"You are not quite finished. Look again; double-check yourself"
Specific Feedback	"Look here; the appointment is in the wrong location." "You are getting distracted; look here and try to stay focused on this task."
Provide Strategy	"Try making a list before you begin." "Try crossing off each item on the list once you do it." "Try underlining or circling keywords." "Try repeating the directions to yourself."
Direct Cues or Instruction	*Verbal:* "Put the appointment here," "Push your arm through the sleeve," or "Get the milk from the refrigerator." *Visual:* Therapist points to brakes as a cue to lock brakes. *Auditory:* Therapist taps to draw attention to a particular area.
Demonstrate	Therapist demonstrates or shows client next step or demonstrates task methods.
Task Adaptations or Physical Assist	Task is adapted or simplified (e.g., Directions shortened, items re-arranged, amount of information or number of items is reduced), or physical assist is provided to complete a task step or component.

often used within the context of assessment to provide information on the amount of assistance needed to successfully complete a task (Toglia, 2018). It is also used in rehabilitation interventions to provide encouragement and gradual assistance for task performance as it is needed. This method (least to most) can avoid over cueing or the provision of too much assistance too quickly.

In addition to systematic or graded cue sequences, direct cues and feedback are perhaps most commonly used in everyday clinical practice to teach the person a functional skill or task. Direct cues or feedback can produce fast results and quickly improve performance. This provides an advantage when there are time constraints. However, the limitations of direct cues need to be kept in mind. Driven by a desire to help others, health professionals tend to "over cue" or provide more cues than the client needs. In addition, while the majority of individuals with cognitive impairments show improved performance when direct cues are provided by others (Harrison et al., 2019), maintenance of performance when cues are withdrawn is often non-existent, short-lived, or tied to the specific task and context of training. It is important to recognize that therapist-directed cues are passive. The therapist is the one providing the cues, pointing out the errors, or telling the person what to do and therefore has all of the control (Harris & Pressley, 1991). People with brain injury can easily become "cue dependent" and continually look to others for the next cue rather than trying to figure out what to do on their own (Toglia et al., 2011). Direct cues can therefore create a sense of "learned helplessness." The client stops trying to think or figure out things on their own and waits until they are directed by others. Therefore, it is not enough to know that a person can follow a cue or carry out a strategy that is provided by someone else.

Direct corrective feedback has been commonly used to increase self-awareness in clinical practice and has been recommended as a practice guideline in individuals with TBI (Tate et al., 2014). Evidence on the effectiveness and efficacy of direct verbal feedback, however, is limited. Clinical experience has found that direct feedback or making a person aware of an error is often ineffective in changing awareness of performance and may elicit a denial response. This is supported by the findings of Richardson et al. (2015) who reported that although 60% of individuals with TBI were able to recognize errors once they were brought to their attention, they showed low levels of acceptance or acknowledgment in response to direct feedback. Similarly, Fleming and colleagues (2019) found no effects of direct verbal feedback in improving self-awareness over and above the benefits of experiential feedback.

Many individuals can recognize errors when they are pointed out or execute a strategy when told to do so but are unable to self-monitor performance or spontaneously initiate and apply cued strategies in everyday life. Optimizing performance involves helping the person understand why the error occurred as well as to select, try, and evaluate strategies rather than telling the person the strategies that they should use.

Guided Learning

An alternative to therapist-directed instruction is the use of guided learning. *Guided learning* is a broad approach that is described as a collaborative, interactive, or give-and-take exchange process between a learner and facilitator. It provides an opportunity for the person to take an active role in monitoring and managing their cognitive symptoms. The facilitator provides structure, gradual prompts, scaffolds, mediation, or Socratic questions to support and guide the person's quality of thinking, learning, and performance (Campione and Brown, 1990; Frey and Fisher, 2010). The focus is on the *process* of how someone goes about doing the task rather than on the *outcome*. A key feature is that guidance is individualized and gradually diminishes as competence increases. Table 9.2 provides a summary and comparison of therapist-directed instruction and guided learning methods (Harris & Pressley, 1991; Swanson & Sachse-Lee, 2000).

Although there is limited information on the effectiveness of different types of cues for persons with cognitive impairments, available evidence suggests that guided learning methods lead to positive rehabilitation outcomes in those with stroke and may be more beneficial than therapist-directed instruction for those who have potential for learning (Skidmore et al., 2017).

Application of Guided Learning: Mediation Methods in the Multicontext Approach

Guided learning is a broad term that encompasses a variety of different methods, while mediated learning methods represent a specific application of guided learning concepts. The guided and mediated learning methods used within the MC approach and detailed in Chapter 10 are adapted from the work of Vygotsky (1978), Feuerstein et al. (2015), and Harris and Pressley (1991). Mediated learning is described as a special way of interacting that affects the person's learning and processing of information. It refers to the quality of interaction between the learner (e.g., client) and mediator (e.g., therapist). There is an intention on the part of the

Table 9.2 Comparison of Therapist-Directed versus Guided Learning Methods

Therapist-Directed Instruction	Guided Learning Methods
Provide direct commands or step-by-step directions that instruct the person on what to do.	Back and forth interactive discussion.
Focus on task subskills and the task outcome. Discrete task subskills are taught in sequence. Discussion of the task processes is minimal.	Focus on the task process rather than the outcome or results.
Provide direct cues, verbal hints or prompts as needed, whenever a person has trouble.	The person is encouraged to stop and review performance. Questions are asked that encourage the person to monitor and reflect on the methods that they are using.
Provide direct or immediate corrective feedback on errors.	The person is encouraged to self-assess performance. Structured methods of self-evaluation may be used. Observations on the process are shared and re-interpreted rather than focusing on the outcome.
Provide strategy or method (e.g., try making a list). If needed, the therapist models or demonstrates the strategy or method first.	The person is encouraged to think of their own strategies. If needed, the therapist provides choices and models a strategy; however, the person is encouraged to personalize the strategy.
Encouragement and positive reinforcement for accurate actions or responses.	Encouragement and positive reinforcement for task methods such as self-checking behaviors or strategy use.
Learner is a passive participant. Therapist is the manager and possesses expertise or knowledge.	Learner is actively involved in treatment. Control of performance is in the hands of the learner.

mediator to help the person reach a different level of understanding beyond what the person could achieve by performing or practicing the task alone (Feuerstein et al., 2015).

Mediated interactions include summarizing, questioning, probing, clarifying, rephrasing, reframing, or re-interpreting observations rather than transmitting information through conventional instruction. The mediator provides experiences and questions that help the person construct and personalize strategies, self-evaluate performance, and make connections beyond the immediate experience to facilitate learning and transfer. This has also been termed "transcendence" by Feuerstein et al. (2015). Mediated learning aims to change or modify a person's approach to tasks or situations by encouraging strategic thinking and self-monitoring.

Mediated learning techniques such as open-ended statements, reflection of observations, and guided questions help the person focus attention on key information, notice similarities and differences, interpret information, adjust strategies, recognize connections or associations, plan ahead, and make comparisons. The mediator helps a person figure out methods that they can use to solve problems or manage challenges and optimize their performance. Guided questions ask "how," "what," or "why" to facilitate thinking. Questions that can be answered by "yes" or "no" are typically avoided. General guidelines for mediation that are used consistently throughout MC treatment are outlined in Table 9.3.

It is important to recognize that the content of guided questions can have different areas of focus. Guided questions can be broad and directed toward helping a person evaluate or self-reflect on performance. They can also be directed toward helping a person self-monitor and manage cognitive performance errors or symptoms. These types of questions apply to a wide range of tasks or situations and are therefore generalizable. In contrast,

Table 9.3 General Mediation Guidelines

AVOID	Instead, DO	IF…
Jumping right into activities without discussion. (Unless the person is fully aware and able to independently generate strategies)	Encourage the person to think about how the activity is similar to previous activity experiences. Encourage the person to "size up the activity" and identify potential challenges. Encourage the person to think about methods (strategies) that will enhance activity success (see sample questions).	If no connections are identified, provide clues. E.g., "What about the ___ activity. Do you see any similarities?" If no challenges are identified, gently bring attention to task components that could be challenging.
Using negative words: Problem, difficulty	Use neutral words that focus on activity performance: Challenge, obstacles, things you might need to watch out for, aspects of the task that might be tricky.	If person perceives task as easy, proceed with the activity experience and mediate during the activity if needed.
Focusing on the person's problems.	Focus on task components or aspects of the task that might be easy versus challenging.	If person perceives task as easy, draw attention to task components that could be challenging and guide analysis of activity demands.
Questions that can be answered by yes/no.	Use how, why, describe, tell me, what can you do to__? How can you be sure that __? E.g., "Tell me how you are going about this" "Why do you think that happened?" "Can you think of a way to help___?"	If answers are vague, prompt with more structured questions.
Telling the person what to do.	Help the person figure out what to do. Guide the person in self-generating their own strategies and solutions. Focus on strategies or methods to increase activity efficiency, time, smooth activity performance, or methods to keep track of activity components.	If the person cannot self-generate strategies, focus on increasing awareness and understanding of performance errors. OR Provide choices of strategies.

Table 9.3 General Mediation Guidelines *(continued)*

AVOID	Instead, DO	IF…
Over-focusing on accuracy, task completion, or the task product.	Focus on how the person goes about the activity. Use questions aimed at methods or the process used, rather than on accuracy (right vs. wrong). Provide positive reinforcement for efficient task methods.	If the person inaccurately completes a task or recalls information that is inaccurate, ask them how they could be sure. Focus on methods for self-checking, monitoring, or preventing errors.
Hierarchical cues that proceed from general to specific levels of assistance.	Use questions that empower the person to generate their own solutions.	If the person is unable to generate solutions, focus on helping the person understand why performance errors occur and/or provide strategy choices.
Jumping in too quickly. **Cueing or mediation as soon as a problem occurs.**	Wait at least 25-30 seconds before providing a mediation question. In some situations, it is better to wait for 60 seconds.	In early stages of intervention, it may be best to let the person experience the activity themselves without mediation and self-evaluate/reflect on the activity experience at the end of the activity.
Adapting the task or providing cues as soon as the person has difficulty or is overwhelmed.	Investigate the person's perceptions of task performance if needed. Guide the person in figuring out how to adapt or simplify the activity themselves (or make it less overwhelming).	If the person is unaware of difficulties and does not understand the concept of the activity or the directions, the activity may need to be adapted. If the person is overwhelmed or showing signs of frustration and cannot think of ways to simplify the activity, provide choices or suggestions.
Over-cueing or talking too much.	Activities need to be at the "optimal level of challenge" to promote strategy use. Cues or mediation should not be provided for more than 25–30% of the activity.	If the activity is too difficult and the person cannot simplify it themselves, the activity level needs to be adjusted.
Pointing out errors or telling/showing the person what is wrong.	Structure activity experiences and questions to help the person self-discover errors themselves. Use questions that facilitate self-checking, self-monitoring or awareness of performance errors.	If the person is unaware of errors during an activity, use "stop and check" questions. If there is vague recognition that something is not quite right, share your observations and/or interpretations. E.g., "Seems like you are stuck. Let's try to figure this out."
Guiding awareness of errors without strategy mediation.	As soon as some recognition of performance error emerges, guide strategy generation. E.g., "Let's think about ways to make it easier to keep track of everything."	If the person is aware of errors but unable to generate strategies, provide strategy suggestions.
Asking the person "How did you do?" or "How did it go?"	Break down the process of self-assessment or provide structured methods for self-evaluation.	
Ending the session without reflection on the activity experience.	Ask questions that encourage self-evaluation of performance, self-generation of alternate strategies, or what they would do differently.	If time is limited, have the person complete a self-reflection questionnaire or journal reflecting on the activity experience, if they are able.

AVOID	Instead, DO	IF…
Assuming that transfer and generalization will occur.	Guide the person in the process of detecting and connecting activity experiences. Encourage the person to think of how the target activity relates to other activity experiences in their everyday life.	If the person is not able to detect or see connections individually, consider structuring treatment activities to facilitate the connection (see transfer guidelines).
Trying to educate the person on "impairments or deficits."	Focus on awareness of activity performance and the methods that facilitate success or are inefficient.	If the person does not acknowledge difficulties, do not push for "awareness" by telling or pointing out errors. Awareness emerges slowly through structured activity experiences.
Taking too much control. Disagreements.	Maintain a supportive, non-threatening atmosphere. • Focus on methods for "efficient or smooth" activity performance and not on deficits or "problems." • Provide activity choices.	If the person does not acknowledge difficulties, over-rationalizes errors, or only identifies physical goals, it is best to focus on their physical goals and work at their highest physical level. Cognitive demands can be integrated into physical activities. As a safe and therapeutic relationship is formed, the person may be more willing to explore or engage in cognitively challenging activities with time.

guided questions can also be narrowly focused on specific tasks or task components. Task-oriented questions facilitate performance in a particular task, but they are likely ineffective in promoting metacognitive skills across tasks.

In the MC approach, mediation techniques, including guided questions, avoid a task-specific focus whenever possible. The emphasis is on helping the person self-monitor and evaluate performance while learning to effectively manage cognitive performance errors. Questions are initially general but can be followed up with questions that are more specific when needed. Task-specific questions are only used if more general or performance-focused questions are ineffective in facilitating awareness or strategy generation. If task-specific questions are used, the goal is to progress to broader questions as soon as it is appropriate. Individuals with greater deficits in self-awareness may require task-focused questions in the initial stages of treatment. Gradually the content of questions moves from task components to cognitive errors or symptoms to more general questions.

Table 9.4 outlines differences in the type and content of guided questions. The reader is encouraged to carefully examine the type of questions (yes/no is avoided) and the distinction between task-specific questions (last column) and other questions within the table.

General Therapeutic Techniques

A critical component of treatment and effective mediation involves creating a non-threatening, safe, and supportive atmosphere so that a person can experience and recognize errors themselves and at the same time gain self-confidence and a sense of control over performance (Toglia & Kirk, 2000). This involves use of an even, calm, and encouraging tone that avoids negative language (e.g., problem, error, difficulties) and focuses on what the person can do. The message conveyed during mediated learning needs to be positive, with an emphasis on "staying a step ahead" by using strategies. Treatment involves encouraging the person to believe that they can be successful with the right strategies or task methods and helping them recognize that managing cognitive errors is within their control. Use of mediation to optimize use of strategies and increase self-management of activity demands has been described as one of the most direct means of changing self-efficacy beliefs and subsequent performance (Cicerone, Azulay. 2007). Therefore, it is more important to focus on recognition and understanding of successful methods employed during performance (e.g., awareness of effective strategies) rather than on acknowledgment of limitations or deficits. Interventions that allow the person to experience success and mastery can have a powerful influence on building self-efficacy, particularly when there is a trusting relationship between the client and therapist

Table 9.4 Differences in Type and Content of Guided Questions

Content of Guided Questions	General	Performance or Symptom-specific	Task-Specific
Directed at error awareness/self-monitoring or self-evaluation	Let's take a look at this. How can you be sure that everything is completed?	How can you be sure that all steps have been completed in the right order? How will you know if everything is in the right order?	How many bills need to be paid? How many checks do you have?
Encourage solutions/ strategy generation	What are some special methods, tricks, or strategies that might help?	Let's think of a way to help you keep track of things. What could you do to help keep track of everything you need to? What can you do to remind you of which step is next?	What could you do to help you remember which bill is next?
Encourage planning	Tell me how you are going about this? Tell me how you plan to do this. How will you know if the (strategy) is working?	Let's think of a plan to help you keep track of all the information as you do this task.	What could you do to keep track of each bill that you have paid?
Encourage connections, missing links	How do these relate to each other?	Let's take a look at this and see if there is any information that can be grouped together to help make things more manageable.	Which bills have similar due dates?
Facilitating problem solving	Tell me what is happening.	Seems like you have hit an obstacle (roadblock). Let's try to figure this out. What other ways can you go about this?	If you only have $200.00 left, which bills can you pay?
Breaking apart the task, identifying the steps, or stimuli reduction	What can be done to make it less confusing?	How can we simplify things? What could be removed or covered to make it easier to focus? Why/how does that help?	Let's look at how we can break down the steps (or make a list). What are the first 2-3 things you need to do before you pay the first bill?
Attention to key information **Focusing on parts versus whole**	How can you be sure that all the key information has been included? What can you do to be sure…?	How can you make sure that all parts (pieces of information) have been considered? How can you make sure that you attended to all of the right details?	How can you be sure that the check was made out correctly?
Sequence	How can you be sure that everything is in the right order?	What can you do to help keep track of what step you have just completed?	Let's think about what you need to do to pay this bill and write down the steps in order.

Exhibit 9.2 General Therapeutic Methods

- *Positive, Supportive Atmosphere:* Create a collaborative, supportive, open, non-judgmental, and trusting atmosphere, where it is OK to make mistakes.
- *Provide positive feedback or reinforcement* on the process, methods, or strategies used, including self-checking or monitoring attempts.
- *Supportive Tone:* Use a neutral, warm, and supportive tone of voice. Avoid negative language (problems, errors, difficulties, "you didn't").
- *Use positive comments* encouraging patience, perseverance, acknowledging efforts, and positive attributes.
- *Focus on successful activity experiences:* The process of learning and coping with challenges is more important than accuracy. De-emphasize accurate task completion. If the person learned about themselves and the strategies they used within the activity, it is framed as a successful experience with positive feedback as per above.
- *Focus on Methods to Enhance Success:* Empower the person to control their own cognitive performance errors. For example, use the term "*Staying a step ahead*" to help the person prevent performance errors.
- *Focus of Helping the Person Figure Out Problems:* Convey confidence in the client's ability to achieve successful performance.
- *Reflection and Reframing of Observations*: Reframe or interpret client statements or reflect on observations and check client agreement. Use the client's own words whenever possible in reflecting back.
- *Uses active listening*. Validate or summarize the person's statements or restate, rephrase, statements in a constructive and positive manner.
- If client blames the task or therapist directions (denial), do not disagree (see Chapter 3).

(Cicerone & Azulay, 2007). Exhibit 9.2 summarizes general therapeutic methods that are emphasized in the MC approach. Some of these methods were previously discussed in Chapter 3 (Exhibit 3.4).

SUMMARY

This chapter highlights the broad nature of metacognitive strategy interventions and describes dimensions along which they can differ. Therapist-directed instructional methods that involve corrective feedback and direct cues are contrasted with guided learning methods that are consistent with the MC approach (Table 9.2). Within guided learning, differences in the type and content of questions used to prompt performance were summarized in Table 9.4, and general guidelines for mediated learning techniques are presented in Table 9.3. The metacognitive framework used in the MC approach uses mediated learning techniques (guided questions, reflection of observations, re-stating, reframing, rephrasing or interpretation of client statements) before, during, and/or after treatment activities. The next chapter (10) provides specific examples and guidelines for implementation of the MC metacognitive framework.

KEY POINTS

- All metacognitive strategy interventions used in cognitive rehabilitation use error-based learning (learning from one's mistakes) and strategies. However, the treatment focus, types of activities, and instructional methods used differ across approaches.
- Directed instruction or graduated cues are commonly used in clinical practice to enhance functional cognitive performance.
- In contrast to direct instruction, guided learning is a broad approach that is described as a collaborative, interactive, or give-and-take exchange process between a learner and facilitator.
- Multicontext treatment sessions use mediated learning techniques (a specific application of guided learning concepts).
- Task-specific guided questions are differentiated from those that focus on error patterns, symptoms, or general investigative questions. The MC approach avoids a task-specific focus, when feasible because it aims to promote transfer and generalization.

- Specific mediation guidelines include avoiding questions that can be answered by yes or no, negative language, a focus on deficits, or task outcome (rather than the process of how a task is performed), and adaptation of the task as soon as difficulty is experienced (Table 9.3). Instead, there is a focus on empowering the person to recognize and work through challenges as well as emphasizing the methods that contribute to successful performance.
- A critical component of effective mediation involves creating a non-threatening, safe, and supportive atmosphere so that a person can experience and recognize errors themselves and at the same time gain self-confidence and perceived control over performance.

Chapter 10

The Metacognitive Framework: Guidelines for Mediated Learning within Multicontext Treatment Sessions

This chapter builds on the general guidelines for mediated learning described in Chapter 9 and provides specific examples and methods for implementing mediated learning techniques within the structured metacognitive framework used in the Multicontext (MC) approach. This framework focuses on identifying aspects of activities that are challenging and generating methods to stay a step ahead. It involves questions that encourage the person to self-generate strategies and anticipate, monitor and evaluate performance.

CONTENTS OF CHAPTER 10

Pre-Activity Discussion
    Pre-Activity Discussion: When is it Used?
    Guidelines for the Pre-Activity Discussion
    Summary of Pre-Activity Discussion
During-Activity Mediation
    Mediation Relies on Observation of Performance
    The Art of Mediation
    Guidelines for Mediation in the Multicontext Approach
    Summary of Mediation During Activity Performance
    Alternatives to Mediation
Post-Activity Discussion
    Structured Self-Evaluation Methods
    Guidelines for the Post-Activity Guided Questions
    Summary of Post-Activity Discussion
End of Session: Methods to Enhance Connections to Everyday Life
    Guided Questions for Strategy Bridging
    Journaling or Structured Logs
    Cognitive Strategy Action Plans and Strategy Worksheets
Summary and Key Points

The metacognitive framework and mediation techniques are designed to help a person reflect on their performance, control cognitive symptoms during functional activities, and promote autonomy. A focus is placed on online awareness of performance (see Chapter 3) and methods used to obtain a successful outcome rather than on cognitive deficits. Helping a person learn to anticipate, monitor, regulate, and manage challenges themselves builds self-efficacy and promotes effective performance as described in Chapter 9 (Mentis et al., 2008).

MC treatment sessions involve four phases of mediated learning that occur within the context of functional cognitive activities. These include (1) Pre-activity questions, (2) During-activity mediation, (3) Post-activity self-assessment and questions, (4) End of session strategy bridging methods (Toglia et al., 2010; Toglia, 2018). These phases are summarized in Figure 10.1.

The first three phases of guided mediation (before, during, and immediately after activities) can be repeated for each activity within a treatment session whereas strategy bridging methods that help a person make connections between treatment activities and everyday life are used at the end of a session. The extent that the first three phases of mediation are utilized can vary within a treatment session or across a treatment program (beginning, middle, or end of treatment), and depend on the client's cognitive abilities and level of awareness. In general, the post-activity discussion is used most consistently within and across treatment. The pre-activity discussion is skipped in the first activity and may be minimal across the first several sessions. The pre-activity discussion often increases toward the middle of treatment and may be faded by the end of the treatment program. Mediation during the task may or may not be used, especially during the initial treatment sessions when the person needs to experience cognitive activities and self-assess their performance. At the same time, if the person does not accurately self-assess performance after the task and/or is struggling during a task, mediation during the task might offer the best opportunity to help them figure out what is wrong and generate their own solutions on the spot.

Throughout treatment, there is a consistent focus on building anticipation, strategy generation, self-monitoring, and self-assessment across a variety of functional cognitive activities. Detailed mediation guidelines for each of the phases (pre-activity, during, post-activity, end of session) within the metacognitive framework are presented below. The extent of questioning and prompts depends on client responses.

I. PRE-ACTIVITY DISCUSSION

The pre-activity discussion uses guided questions to help the person (1) recognize the connection between the current activity and past activity experiences, (2) identify activity challenges, and (3) self-generate strategies. These three components are summarized in Exhibit 10.1

> **Exhibit 10.1 Components of the Pre-Activity Discussion**
>
> 1. Connection to previous activity experiences (optional);
> 2. Anticipation and identification of activity challenges;
> 3. Self-generation of strategies, task methods, or an activity plan to optimize performance.

Prior to the discussion, the person is presented with the activity and its instructions. As an option, the therapist can ask the person to identify similarities between the current activity and activities completed in previous sessions. This is followed by pre-activity *anticipation* questions. These questions are designed to help the person stop and think about the activity and analyze the activity characteristics and demands before jumping into the task. Next, *strategy generation* questions are used to empower clients to generate their own solutions. Initially, client responses to the pre-activity questions are often non-existent or vague. Repeated experience with the same questions across different activities promotes online awareness of performance and provides a structure for approaching activities (Toglia, 2018). Exhibit 10.2 presents a summary of pre-activity questions that reflect the three main components described above. These questions are followed up with more structured questions if needed, as detailed in the guidelines presented in the following sections.

Figure 10.1 Metacognitive Framework

Before Task
- Appraise task and connect with previous tasks
- Anticipate potential challenges
- Self-generate strategies

During Task
- Recognize and manage errors
- Evaluate and adjust strategies

After Task
- Self-evaluate performance
- Reflect on strategies used and challenges encountered
- Self-generate alternative strategies

End of Session
- Strategy Bridging
- Conect to past and/or future activities

> **Exhibit 10.2 Pre-Activity Discussion: Examples of General Questions**
>
> 1. How is this activity similar to the other activities we have done together? (optional)
> 2. What types of challenges could you encounter as you do this activity?
> 3. What are some special methods or strategies you could use to help you complete everything you need to do?

Pre-Activity Discussion: When is it Used?

Typically, the pre-activity questions are not used in the first or second treatment sessions (only post-questions are used). This provides an opportunity for the therapist to observe the client's ability to spontaneously recognize challenges and initiate strategies. The person may need to first experience different activities, self-assess performance errors, and learn about their new strengths and limitations before building anticipation and strategy generation skills. Therefore, during the early phase of treatment, there may be a greater focus on guided questions after the task. As treatment progresses, the use of the pre-activity questions can be increased and then gradually faded or reduced to a self-selected cue or phrase such as "Prepare and plan" or "Size it up" or "Anticipate." Alternatively, a client-selected mental or physical image such as a picture of railroad tracks to signify "stay on track" or a stop sign to signify, "stop, think, organize and plan" can be used to prompt anticipation and strategy generation (without questions).

Pre-activity discussion questions can also be reduced or eliminated if the person (a) shows good self-awareness, (b) can immediately identify potential task challenges, or (c) spontaneously verbalizes strategies themselves. In these situations, the focus of treatment may be on other areas such as monitoring or assessing the quality and effectiveness of strategy execution during activities. Guidelines and examples of each of the three components of the pre-activity discussion are provided in the following sections, but the extent to which the pre-activity questions are used and the type of questions used depends on the client and their response. Exhibit 10.3 summarizes indications for use of the pre-activity discussion.

Guidelines for the Pre-Activity Discussion

The pre-activity guided questions presented in this section are arranged in order from those that are general or require greater initiation of ideas from the client to those that provide more structure and cues for responses. Several examples of questions are redundant to illustrate different ways in which the pre-activity questions can be worded. As discussed above, questions should provide the least amount of structure needed. If the client has difficulty responding to general questions, more structure is gradually provided.

In general, individuals with significant limitations in self-awareness may show greater levels of awareness for questions directed at task-specific components compared to general questions or questions related to cognitive symptoms. Although specific questions or mediation techniques may be initially used to facilitate identification of challenges or strategy generation, the aim is to progress to broader questions that help the person understand how the same performance problem interferes with different activities. As this goal is achieved and the client can fully respond to general questions, the pre-activity questions can be faded. Appendix C.7 provides a sample form that can be used during treatment sessions to guide and record responses to pre-activity questions. Each of the three pre-activity discussion components is discussed below.

1. Connecting to Previous Activity Experiences

The pre-activity discussion includes helping the person detect similarities between the current activity and previous activities or sessions (these questions are skipped if it is the first session). Recognition of similarities between activities and situations activates previous knowledge or learning experiences and is the key to strategy transfer. If the person understands how the present activity is similar to previous activity experiences, it is more likely that they will apply the skills learned from prior experiences to the current, new situation (Toglia, 2018).

Typically, the therapist waits and observes to see if the client recognizes similarities between the current activity and previous activities. Answers to questions related to identification of challenges or strategy generation indicate the person's ability to connect and draw upon previous activities or treatment sessions. If the person has difficulty, prompts can be used to help the person make connections. These prompts are discussed under questions 2 (challenge identification) and 3 (strategy generation).

There are some situations, however, where the therapist chooses to start with questions that prompt connections to previous activities. Exhibit 10.4 includes examples of questions that can be used. These questions are particularly useful if it is unclear whether the person recalls the previous session or if the person has demonstrated repeated difficulty spontaneously recognizing similarities between activities. If needed, previous activities can be shown to the client to prompt recall or comparisons.

2. Identification of Challenges

The ability to recognize potential task challenges requires analysis of task demands and an understanding of one's

Exhibit 10.3 Pre-Activity Discussion: Indications for Use

When is Pre-Activity Discussion Not Used?

- *First or second treatment session:* Person needs to experience activity challenges.
- *Poor awareness:* Person does not perceive any problems or need to use strategies, so the focus of treatment is on helping person recognize performance errors *during* or immediately *after* activities as an initial phase in treatment.

Person appears defensive or resistant to questioning.

- *Good strategy generation*: Person generates good strategies prior to the task (implies awareness of challenges).
- *Second activity within the same treatment session:* If the therapist wants to observe spontaneous carryover of strategy use.
- *Late phase of treatment:* Toward the end of intervention, pre-activity questions may be faded as the person learns to identify challenges and generate strategies on their own.

When is the Pre-Activity Discussion Typically Used?

- *After session 1 or 2:* Typically, the pre-activity discussion questions are used most often after initial sessions through the mid-phase of treatment.
- If the person generally recognizes challenges, difficulties, or the need to use alternate strategies immediately *after* activity experiences (but not before).
- Treatment focus is on building anticipation, estimating activity challenge level, and initiating effective strategies.

When are Only Parts of the Pre-Activity Discussion Used?

- *Spontaneous transfer or generalization:* The initial question about connection of the current activity to previous activities is eliminated if the person is showing spontaneous carryover of strategy use or if the therapist wants to assess if the person can spontaneously carryover learning and make connections between activities themselves (typically the second activity within a single session or during mid-late phases of treatment).
- *Good awareness:* Identification of challenge questions are eliminated if the person recognizes challenges or appears defensive to questions, or if the therapist wants to assess if the person spontaneously recognizes the need for strategies.
- *No challenge identification:* Strategy generation questions may be eliminated if the person does not identify any challenges and does not perceive the need to use strategies or appears resistant to strategy questions.

Exhibit 10.4 Pre-Activity Questions to Prompt Connections to Previous Activities (Optional)

- How is this activity similar to the other activities we have done together? What did we learn from those activities?" or "What methods helped you as you did that activity?
- Summarize or tell me about the last activity we did together? How is this activity similar? What worked well with the last activity? What challenges did you encounter with the last activity? What things do you want to keep in mind as you do this activity?
- How is this activity similar to an activity you have recently done?" (Show activity if needed). "What do they both have in common? What methods worked well that might be applicable here?
- This (previous) activity had a lot of criteria to keep track of while shopping online." (Show activity.) How does that compare with this (current) activity?

abilities and limitations. If a task is perceived as easy, there is no need to use special methods or strategies. The ability to "size up" an activity and recognize task challenges is an important prerequisite for spontaneous, flexible, and independent strategy use (Toglia, 2018).

If the person is very aware of their cognitive difficulties and consistently anticipates challenges or if it is the mid-phase/end of treatment, the therapist may want to proceed directly to strategy generation questions (3) or the activity itself to observe whether the person spontaneously uses strategies without prompts or questions. If a lack of initiation of strategies has been observed, pre-activity questions that help the person recognize task challenges can create a context and motivation for strategy use.

The initial *identification of task challenge* questions are general. Examples of questions that can be used are presented in Exhibit 10.5. General probes such as "Tell me more about that" or "Give me an example" or "Tell me why that would be challenging" may be used to encourage the person to expand upon responses.

> **Exhibit 10.5 Pre-Activity General Questions for Identification of Challenges**
>
> "Before we begin, let's think about this activity" or "Let's look over this activity carefully and analyze it" or "Let's look at what is required."
>
> - "What types of challenges (or obstacles) do you think you could run into as you do this activity?"
> - "What parts of the task might be easy? What parts might be tricky/hard?"
> - "What are some of the things you might need to watch out for as you do this activity?"
> - "What areas should (might) you pay special attention to as you do this activity?"

Mediation of Identification of Challenges

Follow-up questions or therapist actions depend on the client's initial response to general questions (Exhibit 10.5). Guidelines for handling different types of client responses to the initial general questions are outlined below.

2a. Client-Identified Challenges

If the person recognizes specific challenges, the challenge areas identified can be used within the strategy generation questions as described below (3a). The discussion should move ahead to helping the person generate strategies or methods for managing the identified challenges.

2b. Vague or Incomplete Challenges Identified

In some cases, the client might identify vague, incomplete, or partial task challenges. For example, the client might state that "sorting" or "getting the instructions right" will be challenging. Probing questions that ask the client to explain why these task attributes will be challenging should be asked. For example, "Tell me why it might be challenging to get all of the instructions right?" Also, the therapist can ask the client about other task features. For example, "In addition to 'sorting' what other aspects of the task might be challenging?" If necessary, the therapist can suggest additional task challenges as described below (2d).

Similarly, if the client mentions vague cognitive challenges (e.g., paying attention, concentrating, my mind is not working right), the therapist should probe for specifics, like "Tell me more about that" or "How would you know if your concentration is slipping?" For example, if the client says they have to watch out for things getting "jumbled up," the therapist can ask them to explain what "jumbled up" means or to provide an example. If the client is unable to explain or provide examples, the therapist can try to re-interpret what the client might be trying to articulate based on observations of performance to see if the client agrees. For example, "It sounds like you are saying that some of the information might get confusing or overwhelming; does that sound right?"

The therapist can also use one of the methods described below (2d) or choose to proceed to strategy generation questions (3).

2c. Task-Specific Responses

Clients often identify challenges that are specific to the task or simply restate the task directions. For example, in an online shopping activity, the person might say, "I need to remember to choose a blue men's shirt in a size large and keep track of my $75.00 budget." In this situation, the therapist can re-state, interpret, or reframe what the person is describing in broader terms before proceeding to strategy generation questions. For example, the therapist might say, "So it seems like there are a lot of details to keep track of" or "It sounds like what you are saying is that noticing or keeping track of all the details might be challenging." This can be immediately followed by a strategy generation question related to the specified task challenge as described below (3).

2d. Appropriate Challenges are Not Identified

It is common for clients to have difficulty anticipating task challenges at the start of treatment, particularly if they are in an inpatient setting and have had limited experiences with activities since the injury or illness. If the task is perceived as very easy or it is the first or second session, it is best to let the person experience the activity without further questions so that the client can discover activity challenges themselves. Intervention may need to focus on increasing recognition of performance errors during or after they occur, before trying to build up anticipation before the activity.

Some clients may identify challenges that are irrelevant or focused on physical challenges. For example, the client may state that "the scissors may be hard to cut with" or "the cookie dough will be sticky." The therapist can ask, "In addition to the physical challenges you mentioned, what else might be challenging?"

Strategy generation will likely be limited if the person does not perceive relevant challenges. The therapist can provide support in identifying challenges by *prompting connections to previous activity experiences*. For example, "Let's think about the last time you did an activity similar to this (e.g., when there was also a lot of information, there were a lot of details). What was challenging about it? What did you need to pay special attention to?" or "What parts were most challenging?" The therapist can also *suggest or draw attention to challenging aspects of the activity*. For example, "There seems to be a lot of information in front of you (can point)," or "There is a lot to keep track of. What do you think about that?" or "How could all of this information make things challenging?" Identification of task challenges by the therapist provides a context for facilitating strategy generation. This is elaborated further below (3a, 3c).

Lack of verbal acknowledgment of challenges, however, does not necessarily reflect unawareness of challenges. As discussed in Chapter 3, personality variables and lack of acceptance may contribute to decreased ability to admit to potential problems, particularly if the person perceives the activity as one that he or she should not have any difficulty with.

If the person is unable to identify challenges but generates effective strategies, it suggests that the person may have difficulty acknowledging or accepting limitations and is more prone to denial responses. Treatment that focuses on awareness of methods that promote efficient performance or success and avoids discussion of problems, difficulties, or challenges might be effective in changing performance without changes in verbal acknowledgment of challenges. With this type of client, questions that involve discussion of task challenges may need to be eliminated, and it is appropriate to proceed to strategy generation questions even though the person does not verbally identify task challenges.

3. *Strategy Generation*

Questions that encourage the person to think of task methods that will help them be most successful and prevent performance errors are used to guide strategy generation (Toglia, 2018). In some situations, the person is aware of challenges but cannot generate strategies, even with guided questions. If the person is unable to identify a strategy and it is the early phase of treatment, it is important to let the person experience the activity without further questioning, as strategies often emerge from the activity experience.

As with the initial identification of challenge questions, strategy generation questions typically begin with general questions that are presented in Exhibit 10.6. Different words can be used as a substitute for the word "strategy." For example, some people relate better to words such as "trick," "tip," "tool," "plan of attack," or "method." The ability to identify effective strategies with general questions suggests that the person recognizes task challenges (even if they were unable to verbalize them).

Strategies generated that are vague, ambiguous, or overly general should be probed further as they may lack the specificity needed to effectively carry out the strategy. For example, if the person states that they will use an "organized approach," probing for more specifics is recommended. For example, "Tell me more about that" or "Give me an example" or "Tell me how you will use an organized approach – what will you do first, second, etc.?"

Exhibit 10.6 Pre-Activity General Questions for Strategy Generation

- "Before we start, let's think of the best way to go about doing this. Can you think of some strategies (tricks, methods, special approaches) that you could use to help you complete everything you need to do (or successfully complete everything)?"

- "What are some methods (strategies) that you can use to help complete this activity efficiently (effectively or successfully)?"

General Probe:

- "Tell me about your plan – where will you start and how do you plan to go about this activity?"

Mediation of Strategy Generation

If the person is unable to think of strategies with general questions and probes and it is after the first or second treatment session, strategy generation can be facilitated by asking more structured questions that, (3a) use the client's identified task challenges, (3b) facilitate connections to previous activities, (3c) target observed cognitive symptoms or behaviors, (3d) target task steps or components, or if necessary, (3e) provide strategy choices or suggestions. Questions progress from those that are less structured and require more initiation of strategies from the client to those that are more structured and provide greater cues or hints for strategy generation. These strategy generation mediation techniques are outlined below and are presented in order from less to more structured. It is important to note that they are not mutually exclusive and one or more of these techniques may be combined or used.

3a. Use Challenge Identified by Client

If the person has identified appropriate cognitive challenges in the previous question (even if re-framing by the therapist was used), these challenges can be used as the context for facilitating strategy generation. The following are three examples:

Example 1: If the client indicates that they need to watch out for the tendency to "go too fast"

- *Less structured*: "What could help remind you to keep a slow and steady pace or control that tendency to go too fast?"
- *More structured*: "What *mental picture* (words, saying) could help remind you to keep a 'just right' pace?"

Example 2: If the client indicates that a challenge will be to "pay attention to the key details"

- *Less structured*: "What can you do to help make it easier to attend to the key details?"
- *More structured*: "What can you do to make it easier to *notice* the key details (help the details to stand out)?" or "How can you be sure that you have noticed all of the key details?" or "What could you do to double-check yourself?"

Example 3: If the client says that a challenge may be "feeling overwhelmed"

- *Less structured*: "What can you do if that overwhelming feeling is starting to build up? What are the warning signs? What can you do to help make the task less confusing or overwhelming?"
- *More structured*: "What are some ways you can *simplify the task* to make it less overwhelming? How can you break up the task into substeps?"

In all of the examples above, the person accurately anticipated relevant challenges, and guided questions were used to help them generate methods for managing those challenges. More commonly, however, the person is unable to anticipate relevant or appropriate task challenges. In these cases, other mediation techniques are used as described below.

3b. Prompt Strategy Connections to Previous Activities

Strategy generation can be facilitated by helping the person recognize similarities with previous activities. This can be combined with other questions or used individually. For example:

- "Think about other activities we have done and the methods or strategies that were helpful. What might be applicable here? What methods have you used previously that could help here as well?"
- "Let's think about some of the special methods that have been useful in other activities. How could some of those methods be helpful in this activity?"
- "Think about other activities that we have done together (e.g., where there was a lot of information or details to keep track of, there were a lot of parts to organize). What methods did you use (or what methods/strategies seemed to help)? How could those same methods apply here?"

3c. Use Observed Performance or Symptoms

Strategy generation can be facilitated by using guided questions that focus on cognitive performance errors, symptoms, or behaviors observed by the therapist. If the client was previously unable to identify task challenges (question 2), the therapist may need to provide greater support by suggesting, drawing attention to, or directly identifying potential task challenges that relate to observed symptoms. This is illustrated below. The therapist should *proceed directly to the activity* if the client does not agree with task challenges identified by the therapist or continues to perceive the activity as very easy.

Less-Structured Examples:

- "What methods can you use/do to (insert main symptoms; e.g., remind you of which step is next? locate everything? keep track of everything you need to do?) as you do this task?"
- "Let's think of special things that can you do to help you (go slower, be more careful, pay attention to all of the details, stay focused, remember what you need to do)."
- "What can you do to help *keep track* of everything that needs to be done?"

- "What can you do to help you *remember*?"
- "What can you do to help *stay focused (or organized)* as you do this activity?"
- "What can you do to resist the tendency to get distracted and sidetracked by other things as you do this activity?"
- "What are some special methods or strategies that might help you keep your materials organized as you do this activity so that it is easier to find what you need?"

More-Structured Examples (providing task challenges):

- "Let's look closely at the materials and everything that needs to get done. There is a lot of information in these directions. It might be tricky to keep track of it all. Can you think of a method that will help you keep track of all of these steps?"
- "There are a lot of directions and task steps all jumbled together. What could you do to make sure each step is followed? What could you do to break down the activity directions?"
- "This activity is complicated. It has a lot of steps and involves doing a lot of different things. What could you do to simplify the activity?"
- "There is a lot of information on one page. It looks like it could get confusing. What could you do to make it less confusing?"
- "There is a lot of information to keep track of during this activity. What could you do to help you remember everything?"
- "There are a lot of details to watch out for. What could you do to make sure that you pay attention to all of the details?"

3d. Use Task-Specific Mediation

Task-specific mediation questions focus on methods to manage steps or components of a particular task.

Less-Structured Examples:

- "What can you do can do to help (insert task component; e.g., remember which items on the list you have already completed)?"
- "How can you make sure that you remember to get the cookies out of the oven at the right time?"
- "What methods can you use to make sure the right pill is put in the correct slot?"
- "What could you do to make it easier to find the items on this shopping list before you go to the store?"
- "What can you do to make sure that you do not go above $75.00 as you do this shopping task?"

More-Structured Examples (specifically define task features):

- "There are ten different appointments on this list. What strategies can you use to keep track of which appointments have already been entered? What methods can you use to make sure that the right appointment is placed on the right day and time slot?"
- "This activity involves paying three bills. There are a lot of details to pay attention to and a lot of steps to keep track of."
  - "What can you do to organize the checks, bills, and envelopes before you begin?"
  - "What can you do to be sure you have written out all three checks for the correct amount?"
  - "What can you do to be sure that the right bill is in the right envelope?"

3e. Provide Strategy Suggestion or Choice

If the person is unable to generate strategies after questions or prompts, it is best to move forward with the activity as it is easier to generate strategies during or immediately after activity experiences. On occasion, there are some situations where strategy suggestions or choices might be offered before the task. For example, if the person can generate strategies during or after activities but has difficulty with strategy generation before activities. In these cases, the therapist should try to guide the person toward strategies that are effective for the performance errors that the person is exhibiting. If needed, the therapist can model or demonstrate different strategies and encourage the person to choose the method that they think would be most useful. This should be used as a last resort.

- "What do you think about repeating it to yourself or writing it down?"
- "There may be some methods that can help. Do you think it would be better to 1) rehearse or repeat the steps in your mind; 2) make a list or write the steps down; or 3) just commit them to memory, without doing anything special?"

Strategy Generation versus Strategy Use

It is important to note that verbalization of a strategy before an activity does not necessarily mean that an individual will initiate or use strategies effectively during an activity. During treatment, it has been observed that individuals are often able to verbalize strategies before they can effectively use them. Strategy execution requires a different set of skills (see Chapter 7). If strategy generation is good but strategy execution is limited or of poor quality, the pre-activity discussion may be minimized or eliminated, and mediation during or after the activity is emphasized. Intervention then focuses on how the individual initiates, uses and adjusts strategies within the context of an activity. Mediation questions can be directed towards enhancing execution, quality, and effectiveness of strategy use during or immediately after activity performance as described in the below sections.

Summary of Pre-Activity Discussion

The extent to which the pre-activity questions are used will depend on (a) if it is the first few sessions (pre-activity discussion questions may be skipped in the first couple of sessions), as well as (b) the client's level of awareness. Questions that prompt the person to identify connections between the current activity and previous activity experiences are optional and can be used to begin the pre-activity discussion. Alternatively, the therapist can delay or skip this question (i.e., connections with previous activity) and ask it later in the discussion if the person has difficulty identifying challenges or strategies. Identification of challenge questions encourage the person to "size up" or analyze the activity and anticipate potential areas that might be most challenging. Figure 10.2 summarizes different responses to the identification of challenges question and demonstrates how these responses can influence follow up strategy generation questions. If the person is unable to generate strategies, it is best to move to the activity because strategies can be generated from activity experiences as discussed in subsequent sections.

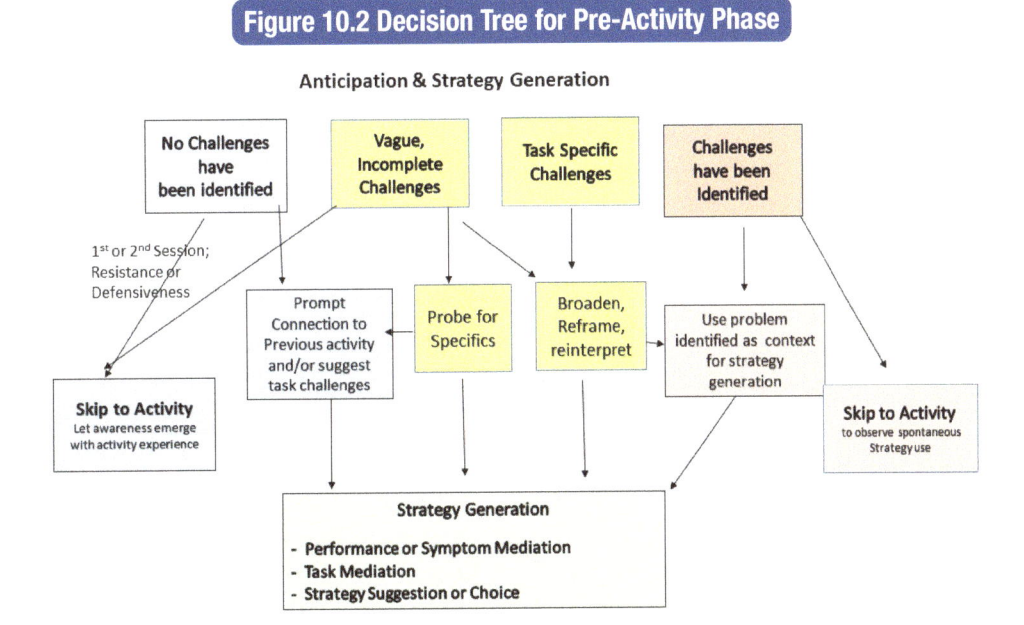

II. DURING-ACTIVITY MEDIATION

Mediation Relies on Observation of Performance

During the activity, the therapist observes how the person is going about doing the activity. The focus is not on the task *product* but on the task *process*. Task strategies and self-monitoring skills should be observed within the context of an activity (Toglia, 2018). For example, notice whether the client uses strategies to help keep track of information, recognizes errors or obstacles, or shows nonverbal signs of error recognition such as shaking their head or putting their hand on their forehead. Also, observe whether the client uses self-checking strategies such as crossing off items completed, double-checking, or reviewing work. Appendix C.10 includes a checklist that can be used to structure therapist observations of activity performance within treatment and quickly record the types of strategies and performance errors that may be observed. Chapter 5 also has additional tools to support performance observation. A series of questions that therapists can ask themselves as they observe the process of performance is presented in Exhibit 10.7.

Figure 10.2 Decision Tree for Pre-Activity Phase

Anticipation & Strategy Generation

- No Challenges have been identified
  - 1st or 2nd Session; Resistance or Defensiveness → Skip to Activity (Let awareness emerge with activity experience)
  - → Prompt Connection to Previous activity and/or suggest task challenges
- Vague, Incomplete Challenges → Probe for Specifics
- Task Specific Challenges → Broaden, Reframe, reinterpret
- Challenges have been Identified
  - → Use problem identified as context for strategy generation
  - → Skip to Activity (to observe spontaneous Strategy use)

Strategy Generation
- Performance or Symptom Mediation
- Task Mediation
- Strategy Suggestion or Choice

> **Exhibit 10.7 During Activity Mediation: Observe the Process of Activity Performance**
> - How is the person going about the activity?
> - What are the task methods? How does the person begin? How do they proceed?
> - What are the task errors and why might they be occurring?
> - Is the person monitoring performance? Do they recognize performance errors?
> - Is performance efficient? Are there extra steps, poor timing, redundancy, or extra efforts?
> - Is there anything the person could do differently to help control the errors or improve performance?

The Art of Mediation

Mediation during activity performance serves as a means to an end. Interactions are mediational when they promote learning and executive functioning skills and aim to help the person learn to manage performance challenges themselves (Feuerstein et al., 2015; Lidz, 2002). When another person successfully mediates or structures incoming information, the person may begin to internalize this external structuring and adopt regulatory activities on his or her own (Brown & Ferrara, 1985).

General mediation guidelines are summarized in Chapter 9, Table 9.3; however, mediation is an art and goes beyond following guidelines. Mediation takes practice on the part of the therapist. The therapist has to recognize when to sit back and let the person struggle with problems that may arise during an activity and when to step in to guide performance, based on the client's response, personality, and any emotional factors. It is important for the therapist to resist the urge to jump in and help as soon as difficulties are observed. Adequate time needs to be provided to observe how the person manages errors and solves problems that are encountered unless negative emotions such as frustration are rising. In this latter situation, the therapist should quickly intervene to prevent negative emotions from increasing and inhibiting performance. The therapist has to be mindful of their tone of voice and their nonverbal reactions as they observe errors. In addition to reflecting on how a question is asked, the therapist needs to pay attention to the content and purpose of the questions (elaborated below in the Guidelines for Mediation in the MC Approach).

During-Activity Mediation: When is it Used?

Mediation is not always needed or used during an activity. In the MC approach, it is typically not used in the initial 1-3 treatment sessions to allow the person to experience activity challenges and discover performance errors themselves. It tends to be used the most in the middle phases of a treatment program and then is gradually faded because the goal is for the person to internalize the questions and self-monitor or self-regulate performance. General indications or situations for when mediation should and should not be used during performance are described in the following paragraphs and summarized in Exhibit 10.8.

There are many situations in which the therapist may decide *not* to mediate or intervene during an activity. For example, individuals who are in the early stages of treatment, have experienced a recent neurological injury or illness, and/or who have very poor self-awareness may need to experience activities themselves. Awareness emerges slowly with repeated experiences within the context of activity performance. Therefore, the therapist may choose to remain silent, especially during the first several sessions, and allow errors to occur without mediation or interruption. For example, if the person is cooking brownies and omits ingredients or forgets to put the timer on, the therapist may not intervene (unless safety is of concern). Then at the end of the activity, the therapist can have the person assess task outcome using a structured means of self-evaluation to help them discover performance errors themselves. This can be paired with a supportive discussion on error prevention methods and strategies to enhance success (see Post-Activity Discussion).

Higher-level clients that can recognize performance errors may also benefit from experiencing an activity themselves and self-assessing their experience once the activity is completed. Therefore, in many cases mediation during activities is not used at all within the MC approach because the pre- and post-activity discussions are adequate in building awareness and effective strategy use. Additionally, some clients may be resistant to mediation due to personality factors. Clients who may not respond well to mediation are those that are less flexible, resistant to change, like to do things their way or are closed-minded. In addition, some activities may not lend themselves to mediation. Mediation should also not be used if it interrupts the flow of the activity or is otherwise disruptive.

Mediation offers the opportunity to help a person figure out what is wrong in the moment and generate their own solutions for successful task completion. It can be used to promote error recognition *within* an activity for people

> **Exhibit 10.8 During Activity Mediation: When is it Used?**
>
> **When is Mediation Not used?**
> - Typically not in the first and last few sessions (unless one of the conditions below is met).
> - When it disrupts the activity.
>
> When the person…
> - Makes some errors (may omit steps) but is progressing in the activity.
> - Is resistant.
> - Can reflect on performance and recognize errors after the activity with self-assessment.
> - Generates alternate methods or shows learning from activity experiences.
>
> **When is Mediation used?**
>
> When the person…
> - Is not progressing in an activity, spending a long time but "getting nowhere," or "spinning their wheels."
> - Is stuck or over-fixates on parts.
> - Is sidetracked or exhibiting goal neglect.
> - Appears to have completely misunderstood the directions.
> - Shows nonverbal or verbal signs of being overwhelmed, anxious, or frustrated.
> - Makes negative self-statements (e.g., I can't get this).
> - Does not recognize errors when they occur.
> - Does not accurately identify challenges after the activity.
> - Is aware of difficulties but persists with the same inefficient or ineffective methods.
> - Is unable to reflect back or accurately assess performance after the task.
> - Uses inefficient methods that are taking excessive time.

who do not recognize errors *during* performance. The person may be able to recognize errors afterward, but they are unaware of errors at the time that they occur. Mediation can also be used to build self-monitoring habits to avoid errors, such as stopping and self-checking or pacing speed within activities.

Mediation may be necessary if a person is unable to progress in an activity or to help a person get back on track. For example, someone who cannot figure out how to start or proceed, gets sidetracked, spends extra time attending to extraneous or irrelevant information, or shows goal neglect that persists for more than 1-2 minutes may benefit from mediation. In addition, mediation during an activity is useful to promote adjustment of strategy use; for example, if the person recognizes that something is wrong but persists with the same methods or uses inefficient methods that are taking excessive time. Mediation should also be used if the person is exhibiting negative emotional reactions during task performance.

Guidelines for Mediation in the Multicontext Approach

As with the pre-activity questions, during-activity mediation questions can be general and applicable to many different situations or they can be narrower in scope and focused on cognitive performance challenges (e.g., keeping track of information, following steps in order, or organizing information) or task components. In addition to varying questions in terms of specificity, the content of questions can vary depending on the goal. In the MC approach, mediation during an activity involves two major areas of focus: (1) enhancing *error recognition*, or (2) assisting the person in *strategy execution and effectiveness*. Exhibit 10.9 presents examples of general questions that reflect these different areas of focus. Mediation can be used during an activity at set intervals or as necessary to help a person self-recognize errors or assess the effectiveness of strategy use. As awareness of performance and error recognition emerges, mediation gradually becomes directed more toward strategy use and effectiveness. If the person already demonstrates good awareness of performance at the start of intervention, mediation focuses exclusively on strategy

> **Exhibit 10.9 During Activity: Examples of General Mediation Questions**
>
> - "Let's stop. How can you go about double-checking everything?"
> - "Tell me how you are going about this activity. What methods you are using?"
> - "How well is your plan (strategies or methods) working?"

generation, execution, and effectiveness. The next section further elaborates on types of mediation within an activity based on these two areas of focus.

1. Focus on Error Recognition

If awareness is limited, mediation can focus on recognition of performance errors through "stop and check" or "stop and review" periods and questions that prompt reflection or review of performance. The activity is interrupted at periodic intervals using methods to help the person pause and examine their performance. Questions gently cue the person to check their work to promote self-recognition of errors. The type of mediation questions asked depend on the level of awareness of the client and the type of performance errors observed, as described below. Mediation is faded as the person's self-monitoring skills increase or as they learn to use more efficient strategies and their performance improves.

1a. Mediation for Poor Awareness

If the person shows limited awareness of performance errors during an activity, questions should promote general self-checking or self-monitoring. ("Let's stop and check.") For example, asking the person to stop and describe how they are going about the activity prompts the person to pause and re-examine their work. Examples of general questions to promote error recognition are presented in Exhibit 10.10. If the person is unable to recognize errors using general "stop and review" periods, the therapist can provide further structure and suggestions by using questions that are specific to the person's cognitive performance errors or the task as listed below.

Performance or Symptom Mediation:

- "How can you be sure that all the directions are followed?"
- "How can you be sure that all the key information has been included?"
- "How can you check to make sure you have included all the details?"
- "How can you be sure that you have all the items that you need?"
- "Let's stop and check. What can you do to be sure that you have completed each step in the right order?"

Task-Specific Mediation:

- "Let's think of a way to make sure that all the ingredients on the list have been gathered. Can you think of a fool-proof method so that when you look at the list you will know which items you have already found? What do you think about circling each item on the list that you have located, or can you think of a different method?"
- "Let's take a look at the number of bills that need to be paid. And let's check it against the number of checks that you wrote. Why do you think that you missed one bill? What could you do differently next time?"
- "Let's take a look at the recipe. There are five ingredients. How many ingredients do you have? Let's check. How can you be sure that they match? It is not easy to keep track of everything. What can you do to make sure that you have gathered all the materials that are needed, before starting an activity?"

1b. Mediation for Vague or General Awareness

Partial awareness occurs if the person recognizes some errors but not others, or if the person is vaguely aware of difficulties but is unable to recognize errors or the source of difficulties. If the person generally recognizes that something is wrong (e.g., attempts to self-correct, uses trial and error, nonverbal signs such as shaking head, negative comments), the therapist should use guiding questions

> **Exhibit 10.10 During Activity: General Mediation Questions for Error Recognition (poor awareness)**
>
> - "Let's stop and review. What methods could you use to make sure everything is on track?"
> - "Before you move on, how could you check that everything is done the way it is supposed to be?"
> - "Let's stop and review. Tell me how you are going about this."

to help the person understand the problem and figure out solutions. Error recognition without knowledge of why the error occurred or without being able to correct performance can lead to anxiety and frustration. These emotional responses can present additional obstacles to problem-solving. Exhibit 10.11 includes general questions that can be used during an activity to help a person identify the reasons for difficulties.

> **Exhibit 10.11 During Activity: General Mediation Questions for Error Recognition (Partial Awareness)**
>
> - "Let's stop and review. Tell me how things are going. What is happening?"
> - "Let's try to figure out what is happening. What things are going well and what things are going not so well (or what things are confusing)?"
> - "Seems like you've hit an obstacle (or roadblock). Let's try to figure this out (or figure out why this is happening)."

The use of reflection and gentle interpretation of observations can help validate or describe what the client is experiencing and stimulate further discussion. Exhibit 10.12 provides examples of general observations shared by the therapist that can help the person recognize factors that might be influencing performance. Once problems are identified and understood, immediate guidance in generating solutions or strategies to address those problems should be provided.

> **Exhibit 10.12 During Activity: General Reflection on Performance Observations**
>
> "It seems like ...
> - "Things are getting a bit confusing (mixed up)."
> - "You might be 'stuck.' I see that you are trying the same method but it doesn't seem to be getting you anywhere."
> - "You are struggling to keep your attention strong and steady."
> - "It is getting challenging to keep track of all the information as you are doing this."
> - "Some of the details (or information) are getting lost."
>
> "Let's try to figure this out."

Reflection on Cognitive Performance Observations with Performance or Symptom Mediation:

- "It seems that you are getting 'stuck.' Let's go through the steps and figure out what has gone wrong" or "Let's go through the steps to figure out what you do next." Or "What could help you know what to do?" (If needed, the therapist can repeat what the client just said or did.)
- "I can see some frustration. Let's stop and check each item at a time." If errors are detected, ask "Why do you think that may have happened? If you did this activity again, what could you do to prevent that from happening?"
- "It seems as though this is getting overwhelming (confusing). Let's try to figure out what is making it feel overwhelming." Other possible remarks: "Let's think of what we can do to make it less overwhelming or confusing" or "What can we do to simplify this activity? Let's take a look at this and see if some of the information or materials can be removed to make it less confusing."
- "It seems like it is tough to keep focused. Let's try to think of some things that you can do to help stay focused."
- "It seems like you are having a hard time keeping track of all the information, details, or steps. What can you do to make it easier to keep track of everything?"
- "It seems like as you became involved in the activity, other things started to pull you away and you got sidetracked a bit. What can you do to try to stay focused and resist that tendency to wander away from the task?"
- "Seems like it is tough for you to get started. Would you agree? Let's try to think about things that might help to get you started more easily."

Task-Specific Mediation:

- "The amount is not adding up. What could we do to figure out what is wrong?"
- "The alarm did not go off. Let's figure out why the alarm didn't go off."
- "There are six bills to pay. How can you make sure all the bills have been paid?"

2. Focus on Strategy Execution and Effectiveness: Managing Performance Errors

A person may be well aware of performance errors but be unable to use strategies effectively. Excessive use of strategies or underutilization of strategies can contribute to performance difficulties. Similarly, the quality of strategies can be poor. For example, the strategies used may require extra steps or too much effort or time. Strategy execution can be incomplete, restricted, or overly rigid so that the person is unable to adjust methods when faced with an obstacle. The timing of strategies used may be inconsistent, too late, or the strategy might be abandoned halfway through the task.

In these situations, mediation is directed at helping a person assess how well a strategy is working, adjust strategies to optimize their effectiveness, and generate new or alternative strategies. If general questions (Exhibit 10.13) do not facilitate performance, more structured questions (performance or symptom mediation) can focus on strategy initiation, optimizing strategy use, or as a last resort, task-specific mediation.

The therapist can share their observations on strategy use for verification and determine if the client agrees. These reflections can help the client become more aware of the strategies or methods that he or she is using. The aim is for the person to learn about the task methods or strategies that are contributing to success versus those that are ineffective.

Exhibit 10.13 During Activity: General Mediation Questions that Focus on Strategy Execution and Effectiveness

- "Tell me what methods you are using? How are the methods working?"
- "How well is your plan is working? What parts are working and what parts are not working?"
- "Tell me how you are going about doing this."
- "Let's try to think about other ways that you can go about doing this activity. What could you do to help make things go faster (more smoothly)?"
- "Let's try to think of methods that might be more efficient or take up less time."

Performance or Symptom Mediation: Initiating a Strategy:

- "Let's take a look at this and see if there is any information that can be grouped together to help make things more manageable."
- "Let's take a look at this and try to figure out a way to simplify things. What could you do to make this more manageable?"
- "How could the activity be organized differently? What could you do to help keep track of everything you need to?"
- "What could be removed or covered to make it easier to focus?"
- "Tell me how you are keeping track of what step you are up to. Can you think of a plan to help make it easier to keep track?"

Performance or Symptom Mediation: Optimizing Strategy Use:

- "I see that some of the items are crossed off the list, but some are not. Tell me more about that? Why did you decide to cross some of the items off the list? How could crossing items off make it easier to keep track? Why do you think you stopped crossing off the items?"
- "Tell me what you were doing to try to remember everything. I noticed that sometimes you were repeating the items to be remembered. How did that help?"
- "I noticed that sometimes you circled or underlined these words in the directions. Tell me more about that. How did that help?"
- "I noticed that you were talking out loud during the beginning of the activity but then you stopped. How did the talking out loud help?"
- "Let's take a look at how you are using the list. How is the list helping you? What could you do differently? What can we do to make it more helpful?"
- "How well is the "talking aloud" (repeating the items, etc.) method working?"
- "Let's review how well the (strategy; e.g., list) is working."

Task-Specific Mediation:

- "Can you think of a way to help you remember which bill is next?"
- "Can you think of a way to help you pay attention to the exact amounts on the recipe?"
- "Can you think of something that will help remind you that the brownies are in the oven?"
- "I see that you circled the balance on the bill. Let's take a look at that more closely. Is there

another amount that you might want to circle (amount due) instead of the entire balance?"

- "I see that you re-wrote the entire list of appointments according to the day of the week before putting them in the calendar. Can you think of another way to organize the appointments on the list without re-writing the list?"

Positive Reinforcement of Strategy Use

Effective strategy use should be positively reinforced when it is observed. Positive comments and feedback for spontaneous initiation of strategies heightens awareness of task methods and helps the person recognize how the methods might be contributing to successful performance. For example, "It is great that you decided to make a list before beginning. How is that helping?" or "It is great that you decided to underline the keywords in the directions. Why did you decide to do that?" These comments can emphasize positive, desired, or expected behaviors and promote a sense of competence.

Summary of Mediation During Activity Performance

Mediation is directed at helping the person (1) discover performance errors and (2) initiate, evaluate, and adjust strategies to manage performance errors. Guidelines about when mediation is most appropriate to use during an activity are summarized in Figure 10.3.

Mediation helps the person stop and review their task progress as well as reflect how they are going about the activity. During-activity mediation is not easy because it is done "on the spot" depending on the client's performance errors and responses. The therapist must observe performance, generate hypotheses about what might be interfering, determine if and when they should jump in, and figure out what to say simultaneously. This requires practice such as role-playing with others and/or recording and reviewing of treatment videos.

Alternatives to Mediation

Alternatives to verbal mediation include the use of everyday technology apps that allow for multiple pre-programmed reminders or automatic text messages to provide personalized cues for strategy use and self-monitoring or "stop and review" during activities. Similarly, a set of self-questions or prompts can be pre-programmed at specified time intervals within an activity. The therapist observes the type of questions or prompts that facilitate performance and then uses technology such as pre-programmed talking reminders, photo reminders, or text messages to replace verbal questions or

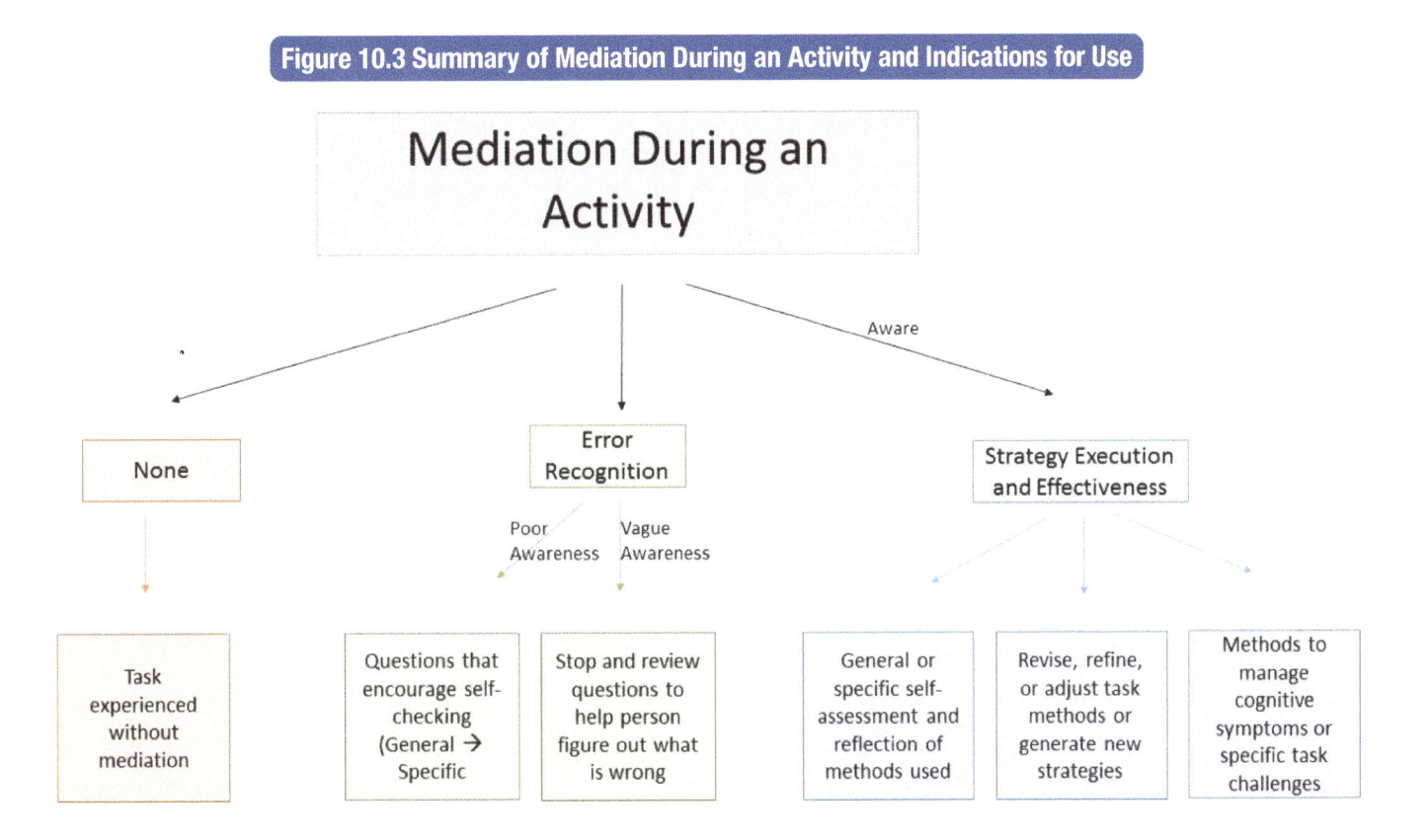

Figure 10.3 Summary of Mediation During an Activity and Indications for Use

Mediation During an Activity

- **None** → Task experienced without mediation
- **Error Recognition**
  - Poor Awareness → Questions that encourage self-checking (General → Specific)
  - Vague Awareness → Stop and review questions to help person figure out what is wrong
- **Aware: Strategy Execution and Effectiveness**
  - General or specific self-assessment and reflection of methods used
  - Revise, refine, or adjust task methods or generate new strategies
  - Methods to manage cognitive symptoms or specific task challenges

mediation from the therapist if needed. This is discussed further in Chapter 14. In addition, apps are emerging, such as swapmymood that guides the user through the steps in problem solving or regulating emotions (www.livewellrerc.org/swapmymood).

III. POST-ACTIVITY DISCUSSION

The post-activity phase involves helping the person reflect on activity experiences through self-evaluation and discussion of strategies or methods used, challenges encountered, and alternate strategies. Structured self-evaluation methods help the person detect their performance errors, while self-ratings, guided questions, and the sharing of observations help the person evaluate their performance, reflect on the effectiveness of strategies that were used, and investigate their perceptions of the task experience. The post-activity discussion needs to go beyond identifying the strategies used to help the person understand why or how a strategy may have helped or hindered performance.

These methods are typically used immediately after each activity within a treatment session and are summarized in Exhibit 10.14. Structured self-evaluation methods are used when the focus of treatment is on promoting self-awareness or recognition of errors. Post-activity guided questions are consistently used; however, the type of questions used can depend on the treatment focus. The following section describes these methods in further detail.

Exhibit 10.14 Components of the Post-Activity Phase

1. Structured self-evaluation methods and optional self-ratings
2. Post-activity guided questions for awareness and strategy generation
   - Awareness of strategy use or task methods
   - Identification of activity challenges
   - Self-generation of alternate strategies or task methods

It should be noted that some clients may have difficulty with the retrospective recall or analysis of performance that is required in the post-activity discussion. In these situations, mediation *within* the activity may be emphasized to a greater extent than the post-activity discussion. Gradually, mediation within the task can be decreased, while the post-activity discussion can be increased and then faded as treatment progresses.

Structured Self-Evaluation Methods

Structured methods of self-evaluation involve breaking down an activity into component parts or providing the person with tools that can be used to self-evaluate their work so that they can detect performance errors themselves or identify areas that could be improved. These methods are not used if the person is already aware of their performance errors. General questions such as "How did you do?" are often met with responses such as "good" and should be avoided because they do not facilitate the process of self-evaluation. The self-assessment process can be structured by using any of the below methods:

- A generic checklist or list of questions that the person can use after a variety of different activities (e.g., Did I review the directions carefully? Did I take enough time to make a plan before beginning? Did I double-check my work?). See Appendix C.20 for an example.

- Use of a correctly completed task, worksheet, or model so that the person can compare their completed activity to that of the model or answer sheet.

- A task-specific structured checklist may be helpful for those with low awareness. The person can review and self-assess each task step or component. Completion of task steps is more concrete and readily apparent. A partial example of a task-specific checklist for making cookies is presented in Table 10.1. This checklist can be further adapted by presenting only one step at a time to focus attention on each task component.

- *Video Review*. Verbal discussion after an activity may be ineffective for some clients because they have difficulty recalling or reflecting back on how they performed the activity. In these situations, video review of activity performance may be beneficial. Video review can help the person retrospectively identify and assess performance errors and/or generate alternate task strategies. The combination of structured self-observation through video and guided questioning can help some clients gain a better understanding of their strengths and weaknesses compared to verbal discussion alone (Schmidt, et al., 2013). See Chapter 14 (treatment considerations) for additional explanation.

Self-Ratings (Optional)

The client can also be asked to self-rate different aspects of performance either as a substitute for the above self-

Table 10.1 Task-Specific Assessment for Making Cookies

How did I do on…?	Needs Improvement	Adequate
• Gathering the correct ingredients		
• Using and measuring the correct amounts		
• Looking at the list		
• Following the list		
• Setting a timer to help keep track of the cookies in the oven		

evaluation methods or in addition to one of the above methods. This can include rating satisfaction with the activity, level of performance, targeted cognitive behaviors, or ability to manage cognitive or activity challenges. Unlike the self-evaluations described above, self-ratings require the person to choose a definitive numerical judgment on a scale from low to high. A disadvantage of self-ratings is that they can be perceived as threatening to some individuals. If the client resists self-ratings or does not appear to be taking them seriously, self-ratings should be avoided.

Self-ratings can be particularly helpful for increasing online monitoring of targeted cognitive behavior or symptoms. For example, the person can be asked to rate their timing or pacing (too slow, just right, too fast), level of mental energy, anxiety or mood (low, medium, high), before, during, or immediately after an activity (see examples in Appendices C.21-C.22). The extent that the person uses strategies to manage cognitive symptoms can also be rated (Appendix C.23). This can further reinforce the focus of treatment on the strategies or methods used.

When using self-ratings, it is important to consider that some people with moderate cognitive impairment may have difficulties making decisions or may feel overwhelmed with a large number of choices. In these situations, the rating scale should be simplified. For example, a vertical rating scale (from low to high) is a more concrete representation of the numerical scale and simplifies ratings. In addition, the person can be asked to respond to questions that only involve two choices, rather than the typical scales of 1 to 4 or 1 to 10. The type of self-rating scale should be tailored to the cognitive abilities of the client. A scale of 1 to 10 should generally be avoided in those with moderate cognitive difficulties. The number of questions presented simultaneously should also be considered. A piece of paper can be used to expose only one question at a time on a page if needed. The use of card sort activities where each item is presented one at a time on a card and the person is asked to sort the cards into two or three piles (yes, no, maybe) is also an alternate format that may be better suited for those with moderate cognitive limitations. Appendix C.20- C.23 includes samples of self-rating scales that can be used within treatment.

While self-ratings can be a tool to increase monitoring of targeted symptoms, the post-activity guided questions described below provide more comprehensive information about the person's perspectives and self-awareness.

Guidelines for the Post-Activity Guided Questions

The therapist can use guided questions to review how the person went about the activity and what was learned from the activity experience. As with the pre-activity questions and during-activity mediation, the focus is on the *process* rather than on the end product or task outcome. Questions proceed from general to specific as described within the previous sections. The questions have three areas of focus: (1) awareness of strategy use, (2) identification of activity challenges, and (3) generation of alternative strategies or methods. Exhibit 10.15 provides examples of general post-activity questions that correspond to these three components, whereas the section below further describes each area of focus and provides examples of structured questions. Appendix C.8 provides a sample form that can be used during treatment to guide and record responses to the post-activity questions.

Exhibit 10.15 Post-Activity Questions: Examples of General Questions

- "Tell me how you went about doing this activity. What was your method?"
- "What types of challenges (roadblocks) did you experience as you did this activity?"
- "What could you do differently next time?"

1. Awareness of Strategy Use

The client is asked questions that require reflection about the activity process and task methods used. Awareness of the effectiveness of task methods, including identification of methods that contributed to successful performance as well as those that were ineffective, is critical for learning and for recognizing how performance might be improved. It is not enough to recognize that the task outcome was successful or unsuccessful. The person needs to recognize when, why, and how success or failure is related to the methods or strategies used.

The client may believe that improved or successful performance was due to luck, an easier task, or just general effort. Similarly, they may believe that task failure was related to faulty directions, bad luck, or other attributes that are out of their control. The therapist needs to help heighten the client's awareness of the methods or strategies that they used as well as how these methods influenced task outcome.

Those who recognize and believe that strategies help performance will be more motivated and likely to use strategies. Questions should therefore help the person identify the strategies used as well as understand the reasons why the strategies may have helped. Helping a person to discover why their strategic solution was successful has been hypothesized to enhance transfer of learning (Barnett & Ceci, 2002). Exhibit 10.16 includes examples of general questions that can help the person reflect upon the methods and process used to complete the task. If needed, this is followed by more structured questions and/or strategy reflections as listed below, consistent with the sequence of guided questioning described throughout this chapter.

> **Exhibit 10.16 Post-Activity Questions: General Questions for Awareness of Strategy Use**
>
> - "Let's review the activity. Tell me what you did and how you went about it."
> - "Tell me how you went about doing this activity. What was your method (plan, strategy, approach)? Where did you begin and how did you proceed?"
> - "What did you do that helped things go so smoothly this time (as compared to last session)? How was your method of going about this task different than the last time? (Why do you think it was better?)"

Mediation of Awareness of Strategy Use

1a. Performance or Symptom-Specific Strategy Use Questions

- "How did you manage to (insert cognitive symptoms, e.g., organize everything, locate or find everything, stay focused, keep track of everything you needed to do, remember all of the steps)?"

1b. Task-Specific Strategy Use Questions

- "Tell me how you managed to (insert task component; e.g., keep track of which bill was already paid, remember to take the cookies out of the oven)?"

1c. Reflecting on and Interpreting Strategy Observations to Promote Strategy Awareness

The therapist should provide encouragement and positive feedback if effective or efficient strategy use is observed or described. If the person has difficulty identifying strategies used or does not mention all of the strategies that were observed, the therapist should share his or her strategy observations. Comments that reflect on strategy observations raise awareness of the task methods used. Once the person is aware of the strategies or methods used, it is important to help the person recognize how the task methods contributed to or inhibited successful performance as described above.

If the client is not able to identify why a particular strategy was effective (or ineffective) with questioning, the therapist can offer an explanation or interpretation on why and how the strategy contributed to task outcome, to see if the person agrees. Some examples are provided below.

- "I noticed when you used the list and crossed off each step, it made things easier. Why do you think that helped?"
  - *If explanation is needed:* "It seemed to help you keep better track of the step that you were up to. That was an excellent idea."
- One thing I saw you doing was talking out loud. How (Why) do you think that helped?
  - *If explanation is needed:* It seemed that talking out loud helped you stay focused on the goal" or "I noticed that when you repeated things out loud, it seemed to help you keep track of information."
- "I noticed that in this activity, you used your finger as you were reading. Why do you think that helped?"
  - *If explanation is needed:* "It seems that using your finger helped you to slow down (pace your timing). You took more time to review the directions and did not miss any of the details."
- "Why do you think mentally rehearsing the steps first made it easier to perform the task?"

- "You did a great job of remembering to check off the list. It seemed to really help. Why do you think things went more smoothly this time?"
- "I noticed that whenever you remembered to go back to the list, it seemed to help. Why?"
- "I noticed that you went in order and grouped the items that were similar together. That was a great idea. Tell me more about that."
- "I noticed when you used the bill-paying checklist, it really seemed to help."
- "I notice you work best (things seem easier) when you take a rest break."

2. Identification of Activity Challenges

It is important to investigate the person's perceptions of task challenges. For example, can the person identify some task components that may have been more challenging than other parts of the task? If the person is unable to recognize task challenges, it will be difficult for them to generate alternative methods or strategies. Exhibit 10.17 presents examples of general questions that can be used to investigate perceived task challenges. This is followed by additional mediation questions and methods to reframe or re-interpret responses.

> **Exhibit 10.17 Post-Activity Questions: General Questions for Identification of Challenges**
>
> - "What types of challenges (obstacles, roadblocks, or difficulties) did you experience as you did this activity?"
> - "What parts were easy and what parts were a little trickier (difficult, challenging, unexpected)?"
> - "What parts did you need to pay special attention to or which parts required extra concentration and thinking?"

Mediation of Identification of Challenges

2a. Performance or Symptom Mediation

- "There were a lot of details. How did this present challenges?"
- "There was a lot of information to keep organized. How did this present challenges?"

2b. Task-Specific Mediation: Therapist Identifies Specific Task Challenges

- "There were four different menus and a list of different food items. How did this present challenges?"
- "Some days and times of events conflicted with others. How did this present challenges?"

2c. Reframing Responses and Observations

If the person identifies challenges that are overly specific to the task, the therapist should re-frame or re-interpret the challenge at a broader level. For example, if the client states that they missed the size or price of a bottle of shampoo during an online shopping activity, the therapist might re-interpret or re-phrase this as, "It sounds like attending to all the details can be challenging." Consistent reframing of task-specific errors into a more generalizable error pattern helps the person begin to see connections between activity experiences. If the person does not perceive any task challenges, the therapist can gently suggest challenges that were observed to probe for awareness. (e.g., "It seems like the amount of information was a bit overwhelming. It was a lot to keep track of.")

3. Strategy Generation

Similar to the pre-activity discussion, the identification of task challenges should lead to a discussion about how to manage or cope with challenges in future tasks. This may involve adjusting, adapting, or modifying the current strategy to match task demands or generating alternative task methods. As the person experiences successes and recognizes that effective strategies are contributing to positive outcomes, the person will be more motivated to generate future strategy plans on their own. Exhibit 10.18 includes general strategy generation questions followed by

> **Exhibit 10.18 Post-Activity: General Questions for Strategy Generation**
>
> - "What would you do differently next time? Would you change the way you went about the task in any way? What other strategies or methods could you use?"
> - "Let's think of a plan to help this type of activity go more smoothly next time."
> - "Let's identify some things (strategies, methods) that might help make it easier next time."
> - "What special methods or strategies could you use the next time you do this activity?"

mediation questions and examples of methods to reframe responses.

Mediation of Strategy Generation

3a. Performance or Symptom Mediation

- "What do you think you could do to help control (manage) (insert symptom; e.g., that tendency to get sidetracked)?"
- "What could you do to prevent (insert symptom; e.g., getting stuck) from happening again?"
- "What do you think you could say to yourself to help remember to slow down?"

3b. Task-Specific Mediation

- "What do you think you need to do to help (insert task component; e.g., remember how many eggs you added; ignore the names on the list that you don't need)?"

3c. Reframing Responses

If the person only identifies a task-specific strategy, the therapist should re-frame or re-interpret the strategy more generally as discussed previously (under task challenges). For example, if the client states that they need to underline the days that events need to occur before putting them into a calendar, the therapist might reframe this more broadly as "Planning ahead and identifying the key details first is a great idea."

3d. Provide Strategy Suggestion or Choice

As a last resort, strategy suggestions or choices can be offered, particularly if this is not the first or second treatment session. For example, "There may be some other methods that can help. What are your thoughts about rehearsing or repeating the steps in your mind or writing a list of keywords before you start?"

Summary of Post-Activity Discussion

The post-activity discussion is used consistently across treatment; however, in some clients, the discussion is minimized, and a greater emphasis is placed on mediation *within* the activity. The focus of the post-activity discussion is on helping the person self-evaluate and reflect upon performance as well as generate alternate strategies that can be used in future activities. In some situations, such as with poor recall or awareness of performance, this process may be more effective when used in conjunction with video review (see Chapter 14).

IV. END OF SESSION: METHODS TO ENHANCE CONNECTIONS TO EVERYDAY LIFE

At the end of the treatment session, the therapist can use several different techniques including guided questions, journaling, structured logs, or use of a strategy action plan to help the person identify how the activity experience or strategies from the treatment session can be used to promote success in everyday life or future activities and to make connections between past, current and future activity experiences. This is termed "bridging," and it fosters transfer of learning because it helps the person make connections between the strategy and everyday life situations that the strategy can be used with (Perkins & Salomon, 1988). Exhibit 10.19 summarizes strategy bridging methods that can be used at the end of a treatment session. Guided questions may be used alone as an extension of the post-activity discussion or in combination with journaling or strategy worksheets. At least one of the below methods should be used. If the focus of treatment is on building awareness, guided questions on strategy bridging can be too premature. In these situations, a simplified structured journal is the best option as it involves recording the activity or what was learned and can help the person recognize error patterns across activities. As treatment progresses and the person begins to use strategies, strategy bridging methods can be introduced. Each method of strategy bridging is summarized in Exhibit 10.19 and described below.

> **Exhibit 10.19 End of Session: Strategy Bridging Methods**
>
> - Guided Questions for Strategy Bridging
> - *Example:* "Tell me how the methods or strategies you used today might be helpful in other everyday activities that you do."
> - Journaling, Structured Logs
> - Cognitive Strategy Action Plans, Strategy Worksheet

Guided Questions for Strategy Bridging

Guided questions ask the person to relate the treatment session activities and strategies used to past activity experiences or future situations to promote generalization. These questions can be combined with journaling or use of the cognitive strategy action plan (described below) as they may prompt thoughts and discussion during these activities. Examples of general guided strategy bridging questions are listed in Exhibit 10.20 followed by mediation questions.

> **Exhibit 10.20 End of Session: General Strategy Bridging Questions**
>
> - "How were today's activities similar to other activities you have done in the past?"
> - "How did the methods or strategies you used today compare to what you have done in other activities (sessions)?"
> - "Tell me how the methods or strategies you used today might be helpful in other everyday activities that you do."
> - "Let's think about other activities that you can use these same strategies (or task methods)."

Mediation of Strategy Bridging

Performance or Symptom-Specific Mediation

- "Let's think about other activities that involve following a list."
- "Let's think of other activities that require keeping track of a lot of information or organization of materials? How can the same methods used in this activity apply?"

Task-Specific Mediation

- "What do you think about (suggest activity; e.g., meal planning)? How would the same methods or strategies apply?"

Journaling or Structured Logs

The post-activity discussion can conclude by asking the person to write about their activity experience in a journal (i.e., obstacles encountered, methods they used to ensure task completion, and their strengths and weaknesses). The journal can be structured with pre-set questions, or it can be left unstructured for higher-level clients. In the former situation, the journal questions can be used as the guided discussion and responses recorded by the client or therapist (for lower-level clients).

A journal may be used to record activities that were completed during treatment (writing a letter, planning a meal, following a new recipe), summarize what was learned from the experience and/or what might be done differently next time, identify other situations in which the strategies used during treatment might be helpful, and identify thoughts, emotions or feelings during the activities. Journaling can include asking the client to rate the effectiveness of strategies used within a session and comparison of performance with previous sessions. A journal can also be used to establish goals for the next session, and to help the person make connections or bridges to previous and future activity experiences (Toglia et al., 2010). See examples of a structured journal page that can be used with a client in Appendix C.9 and simplified journal formats in Appendix C.14.

Structured logs can also be used by higher-level clients or care partners to record functional cognitive challenges or cognitive lapses that occur in everyday life. This is described further in Chapter 14.

Cognitive Strategy Action Plans and Strategy Worksheets

A cognitive strategy action plan can be developed at the end of the treatment session to more explicitly facilitate strategy application to everyday life. A simplified strategy action plan involves using strategy cards or worksheets to record the strategy (or strategies) that the person identified or used within the treatment session. The person is then asked to list other everyday activities or situations in which the strategy can be used or practiced. For homework, the person is asked to try the strategies within the context of real-life activities and record how well the strategies worked. An example of a strategy worksheet that can be used with clients is included in Appendix C.15.

A more detailed cognitive strategy action plan can ask the person to identify a performance problem as well as tasks or situations where the problem might arise. The person then identifies strategies that can be used to manage the performance problem. Similar to the above, the person is asked to carry out the cognitive strategy plan in between treatment sessions and evaluate the effectiveness of the strategies. Blank cognitive strategy action plan forms are included in Appendices C.16 – C.18.

Summary of End of Session Methods

At the end of the session, the therapist uses methods that are designed to help the person make connections between treatment activities and everyday life activities. This can include guided questions focused on strategy bridging, structured journals or logs, strategy worksheets, or cognitive action plans. In the early phase of treatment, guided strategy bridging questions or journaling is used most frequently. As treatment progresses and the person begins to use strategies more consistently, the methods used at the end of the session are expanded and emphasized to promote generalization to everyday life.

Exhibit 10.21 Clinician Guide: Multicontext Metacognitive Framework Summary

PHASES	CLINICIAN
Pre-Activity Questions *Anticipation*	Let's take a look at this activity. What types of challenges (obstacles or difficulties) do you think you might run into as you do this activity? **Optional Probes:** What do you think you might want to watch out for (or pay special attention to), as you do this activity? Can you give me some examples? What parts (of this activity) could be (most) challenging and what parts will be easy?
Strategy Generation	Before we start, let's think of the best way to go about doing this. Can you think of some special methods (plan or strategies) that you could use to help you complete everything you need to do?
Mediation During Activity	Let's stop for a moment. Tell me how you are going about this. *Mediate as appropriate using guided questioning.*
Post-Activity *Self-Evaluation*	Guide self-checking if necessary to structure the self-assessment process.
Guided Questions for Strategy Awareness and Perception of Challenge	Tell me how you went about doing this activity. What was your method (plan, strategy)? What types of challenges (obstacles or difficulties) did you experience as you did this activity? OR What parts were most challenging (unexpected, difficult)? What parts were easy and what parts were a little trickier (difficulty, challenging)? **Symptom Specific:** Tell me how you managed (insert main symptom or challenge). **Task-Specific:** Tell me how you managed to (insert task component).
Guided Questions for Strategy Generation	What special methods or strategies could you use the next time if you did this activity again? OR What would you do differently next time? **Symptom Specific:** What do you think you could do to help (control, manage) (insert symptom)? **Task-Specific:** What do you think you need to do to help (or manage) (insert task component)?
End of Session *Strategy Bridging*	**Mediation Questions** e.g., What other activities (or situations) could that strategy be helpful in? Journaling of activity experience, cognitive strategy action plan, strategy worksheet

SUMMARY

The MC metacognitive framework is designed to help a person (1) analyze tasks demands or identify task conditions that present cognitive challenges, (2) generate task methods or strategies to control cognitive symptoms or prevent performance errors, (3) self-reflect and assess the effectiveness and efficiency of methods used, and (4) make connections between activity experiences. Exhibit 10.21 provides a quick summary of the metacognitive framework components and samples of key guided questions.

The person is actively engaged in the generation, modification, evaluation, and construction of personalized strategies across treatment sessions. Initiation of strategy use or self-checking behaviors are consistently encouraged and positively reinforced. The goal is not to use strategies when told to do so but to learn when and where to use them, and how and why they work. Strategy training and metacognitive questions are integrated with a focus on increasing perceived competence and control over functional cognitive performance.

The treatment atmosphere needs to be one where it is okay to make errors or mistakes. During mediation, the emphasis is not on task accuracy but on recognizing or knowing when things are not going well and empowering the person to figure out performance problems and generate alternate solutions themselves. This is essential in building cognitive self-efficacy and always needs to be kept in mind during mediation

Specific examples of guided questions and mediated learning methods that could be used to promote awareness of performance and strategy use were provided in this chapter, and Appendix C includes multiple worksheets and forms that can be used within treatment. However, mediated learning methods must be responsive and adapted to the needs of the person. Although the metacognitive framework includes a before-, during- and after-task discussion, the use of these phases is not fixed but represents a guide to be used as needed. It may vary across a treatment program or clients, depending on needs. Appendix D.7 provides a summary for the therapist that includes problems that can be encountered during use of the metacognitive framework and methods for managing them. Additionally, Appendix D.8 provides a "cheat sheet" or things to remember and a summary of common phrases used during mediated learning that may be helpful for the therapist.

During treatment, guided questions are faded as the person begins to utilize more efficient mental habits. For example, as the person begins to plan ahead and size up a task before beginning, pre-task questions may be skipped. Similarly, as the person automatically self-checks work, structured self-assessment can be faded, and a greater focus may be placed on strategy action plans or journaling to facilitate generalization to everyday activities.

The metacognitive framework can be applied broadly across varied levels of functioning, treatment contexts, and different types of cognitive performance problems or activities as described in Chapter 14. Methods for measuring and documenting changes in treatment targets and functional goals within and across treatment sessions are described in Chapters 11 and 12.

KEY POINTS

- The MC approach uses a metacognitive framework that provides guidelines for questions and mediated learning techniques that can be used before, during, and after treatment activities.

- The extent that metacognitive questions or discussion phases (pre, during, post) are used varies across the treatment program and needs of the client. For example, only the post-discussion is typically used in the first or second treatment sessions.

- If answers are vague during questioning, ask for further elaboration or examples (e.g., tell me more about that).

- The pre-activity discussion focuses on helping the person (1) recognize the connection between the current activity and past activity experiences (optional), (2) identify activity challenges, and (3) self-generate strategies.

- Mediation during the activity is directed at helping the person (1) discover performance errors and (2) initiate, evaluate, and adjust strategies to manage performance errors.

- The post-activity discussion guides the person in self-assessment of methods used, challenges encountered, and generation of alternate strategies.

- Guided questions and methods such as journaling, strategy worksheets, structured logs, or cognitive strategy action plans are used at the end of every treatment session to help the client make connections between treatment activities and everyday life.

- Review Appendix C. Appendix C includes a variety of treatment forms to help therapists implement this approach, including a sample treatment activity with pre and post discussion questions (Appendix C.6), pre and post-activity question forms (Appendix C.7-C.8), as well as client strategy worksheets, action plans, and sample self-ratings.

- Tables 9.3 and 9.4 (Chapter 9) and Appendices D.7 and D.8 provide additional mediation guidelines.

Chapter 11

The Multicontext Approach: Assessing Treatment Delivery and Client Response

This chapter begins by summarizing the key features of the Multicontext (MC) approach that have been reviewed in Chapters 6-10 and compares these features to those of conventional practice. The key ingredients of the MC approach are described within the framework of the Rehabilitation Treatment Specification System (RTSS). A treatment fidelity tool that is based on this framework and that can be used as a tool for research and clinical practice to monitor therapist adherence and quality of MC treatment delivery is described and included in Appendix C.13 (Toglia et al., 2020). Methods of monitoring, analyzing and documenting client awareness, strategy use, and generalization within and across individual MC treatment sessions will be presented. This includes structured methods for describing and rating client responses to metacognitive questions. A variety of worksheets and rating scales for assessing and summarizing responses to individual treatment sessions are included in Appendix B and C.

CONTENTS OF CHAPTER 11

The Multicontext Approach and Treatment Fidelity
   Multicontext Treatment Specification
   Multicontext Treatment Delivery: The Multicontext Treatment
      Fidelity Tool

Client Response to Treatment Sessions: Observing, Tracking, and Documenting Progress
   Selecting Treatment Targets
   Observing and Tracking Progress Within and Across
      Treatment Sessions
- *Level of Task Challenge*
- *Strategy Use*
- *Awareness of Challenges, Awareness of Strategy Use, and Strategy Generation*
- *Tracking Progress across Treatment Activities*
- *Other Indicators of Progress*

   Using the Metacognitive Framework to Write Progress Notes

Summary and Key Points

THE MULTICONTEXT APPROACH AND TREATMENT FIDELITY

The MC approach is a complex multicomponent intervention that differs from conventional cognitive rehabilitation practices in several ways. For example, rather than improving specific cognitive skills or providing strategies for improving performance on specific activities, the MC approach aims to help a person use cognitive strategies across activities to manage performance errors. This requires shifting from a focus on task outcome or accuracy to a focus on the task process. It also requires changing how treatment activities progress. In the MC approach, treatment activities are structured horizontally with explicit techniques to expand strategy transfer across activities before increasing difficulty. This differs from usual practice, which typically involves increasing difficulty level (vertically) as soon as performance improves. The MC approach also asks therapists to move away from traditional direct instruction methods and toward guided learning methods. This requires changes in the way therapists cue and interact with clients. Table 11.1 summarizes the areas that require practice shifts from conventional practices to the MC approach.

Multicontext Treatment Specification

The core treatment elements of the MC approach have been summarized and specified within the Rehabilitation Treatment Specification System (RTSS) framework (Hart et al., 2019; Van Stan et al., 2019) (Appendix D.10). The RTSS was designed to provide a standardized way to clearly describe, specify, and classify rehabilitation interventions across disciplines. Fasoli et al. (2019) urged occupational therapy (OT) practitioners to consider using the RTSS to more carefully describe the content and process of OT interventions so that they can be more clearly distinguished. Use of a comprehensive framework that specifies treatment elements and intended targets is necessary for examining how active treatment ingredients bring about therapeutic change and affect the target of treatment. This is essential for designing, replicating, communicating, and comparing treatment approaches and outcomes (Fasoli et al., 2019).

Table 11.1 Side-by-Side Comparison of Routine and Multicontext Treatment

Treatment Guideline	Typical Treatment	Multicontext Treatment
Focus of treatment	Focus is on improving performance of targeted tasks. Strategies are practiced within a specific task.	Focus is on monitoring and managing performance errors or using similar strategies effectively across a variety of different tasks.
Self-awareness	Focus is on educating the person about their cognitive deficits and providing feedback on errors or task results.	Focus is on "awareness of performance" or the task methods or strategies that produce success.
Grading or progression of activities	Functional activities are graded in difficulty once the person achieves success.	Functional activities are not graded in difficulty until transfer of strategies across activities at similar level of complexity is observed.
Within session framework	No particular sequence or structure to sessions.	Structured session framework as detailed in Chapter 10.
Strategy instruction methods	Strategies are directly instructed or provided by the therapist.	Emphasis is on helping a person recognize the need for strategies and self-generate strategies.
Questioning	Questions regarding awareness and strategies are asked informally and inconsistently throughout treatment, depending on the therapist.	The same pre- and post-activity questions are asked consistently across treatment sessions and responses are recorded.
Use of cues and prompts	Cues provided are typically direct and tell the person what to do or how to do it. The cues are focused on the task. The person is readily assisted, or the task is adapted for the person if they have difficulty.	Mediated learning and guided questions are provided that support the person in figuring out problems and solutions. Prompts or questions are focused on error recognition and strategy use rather on the task itself. If the person has difficulty, they are encouraged to figure out how to simplify or adapt the task themselves (before the therapist does it for them).

The RTSS framework is a systematic approach based on treatment theory. It includes three connected elements that together define a treatment component. The three elements include: (1) the active treatment ingredients or what the therapist does to bring about change, (2) the mechanism of action that explains the process by which the ingredients influence change, and (3) the target or measurable treatment outcomes that result from the active treatment ingredients or therapist actions. Within the RTSS framework, the MC approach is classified as "volitional" because it requires participant engagement and effort for positive outcomes (Whyte et al., 2018; Whyte et al., 2019). Additionally, within the RTSS framework, the mechanisms of action of the MC approach can be described as training *skills and habits* through practice and doing as well as changing *internal representations* such as attitudes, beliefs, self-perceptions or knowledge through cognitive/affective information processing (Hart, Djikers, et al., 2019).

Information on the key MC treatment ingredients (metacognitive framework, focus on strategy use, horizontal structure of activities, therapeutic support, functionally relevant activities, optimal level of challenge), are presented in the RTSS table along with the hypothesized mechanisms of action and treatment targets. The MC approach metacognitive framework is subdivided into six components within the RTSS table (Appendix D.10) so that treatment targets for each component can be clearly differentiated. Additional information is presented that briefly summarizes the underlying rationale and provides examples of treatment procedures that would *not* align with the MC approach. This table further elaborates on the information presented in Chapter 6 and provides a more detailed understanding of active ingredients of treatment and the intended treatment targets. Because it specifies and operationalizes the intervention elements and hypothesized active ingredients that affect outcome, the MC RTSS table provides a foundation for use of the MC approach in practice, education, and research.

The treatment guidelines in this manual reflect the MC RTSS framework. The RTSS framework dissects MC treatment elements and provides a theory-driven approach to examining therapeutic change. Assessment of client progress and outcomes as well as the quality of therapist treatment delivery are based on the MC RTSS framework. For example, the MC treatment fidelity tool (described below) was based on the framework and designed to measure the extent that the MC approach is carried out as intended by therapists.

Multicontext Treatment Delivery: The Multicontext Treatment Fidelity Tool

The success of the MC approach is dependent on the quality of therapist-client interactions. The guided learning methods outlined in Chapters 9 and 10 depend on client responses and needs. The therapist observes and analyzes the process of performance, makes hypotheses about difficulties and error patterns, and at the same time is required to make on-the-spot decisions about how to best guide performance. Client responses can be unpredictable and at times surprising. The therapist may need to make adjustments at the moment to the activity, guided learning methods, or therapeutic support. This requires skill and training on the part of the therapist (Toglia et al., 2020).

In our experience, implementation of the metacognitive framework and guided learning techniques within the MC approach is the most challenging treatment component, particularly for therapists who have conventionally used a direct instruction approach. If the therapist has typically used direct cues within clinical practice, it takes time to change habits and integrate a different style of cueing into practice. It can be difficult to resist the tendency to jump in and help when problems arise, as it is often easier and faster to tell a person what to do and how to do it than to sit back and let a person try to figure it out on their own (Toglia et al., 2020). However, it is hypothesized that the effects of direct instruction are short-lived and that a person is more likely to use strategies when they have thought of those strategies themselves.

As discussed above, the use of the MC approach requires shifts in practice methods, habits, and clinical reasoning. Experience has shown us that a therapist's knowledge of mediation guidelines is not enough to be able to easily implement mediation effectively. Therapists who have used the MC approach have indicated that it is one thing to know and understand the metacognitive framework and mediation guidelines and another thing to use them on the spot during treatment. Exhibit 11.1 has a list of common errors that have been observed in clinical practice by therapists who are inexperienced in using the MC approach.

Guided learning techniques require therapist practice and self-reflection. Metacognitive questions and prompts need to become automatic so that the words flow smoothly. Guided questions should be part of a discussion, rather than perceived as an interview. Therefore, it is suggested that therapist's practice, record themselves, and critique their own mediation methods multiple times to become proficient. Appendix A.15 includes a learning activity for therapists involving brief scenarios that involve thinking about what you would say or do in a challenging guided learning situation. Role plays with colleagues who act out typical cognitive performance errors can provide additional

CHAPTER 11 The Multicontext Approach: Assessing Treatment Delivery and Client Response

Exhibit 11.1 Common Therapist Errors in Implementing Multicontext Treatment Treatment approach

- Automatically adapts tasks when client has difficulty.
- Grades tasks in difficulty too quickly (before observing strategy transfer)
- Directions/activities are too structured.
- Lack of explicit connections between activities and sessions.
- Emphasis on task results or accuracy rather than the task methods or process.
- Awareness is not adequately addressed.
- Strategies are immediately provided without providing an opportunity for the individual to generate strategies.
- *Question or cue frequency*: Tendency to jump in and help or cue too quickly/frequently when a person experiences errors or difficulties.
- *Question content:* Cues or guided questions are over-focused on the task.
- *Question type:* Asks yes/no questions rather than what, how, or why questions
- Feedback is too direct.
- Talks too much.
- Falls into instruction mode, rather than helping to facilitate thinking and reflection.
- Does not re-frame, re-interpret statements, or reflect on observations.
- Uses negative language without realizing it (difficulties, problems, symptoms, errors).

opportunities to practice mediation (see Appendix A.16). Therapists are encouraged to video or audiotape treatment sessions for review, analysis, and self-reflection. Appendix C.12 includes a therapist self-reflection form that can be used for self-analysis of mediated learning methods that were used during a treatment session. In addition, supervision or mentoring from a knowledgeable or more experienced therapist can facilitate professional growth and proficiency by provoking reflection and insight and helping the therapist expand their repertoire of prompts, questions, or therapeutic techniques.

To assist in knowledge translation to practice, an MC treatment fidelity tool has been developed and is included in Appendix C.13. This tool is based on the core components of the MC approach and can be used for therapist supervision and training or for therapist self-assessment in carrying out the MC approach. It focuses on implementation of the metacognitive framework and guided learning methods described in Chapter 10 and further operationalizes the actions of the therapist within treatment. Criteria for competency in the use of guided learning methods are specified so that adherence to guidelines and quality of therapist-client interactions during MC treatment can be evaluated. A sample script of mediated learning along with analysis and ratings using the treatment fidelity guidelines is included in Appendix D.9. The development of this tool and its inter-rater reliability are described elsewhere (Toglia et al., 2020). In addition to serving as a guide to clinical practice, this tool can be used in research to assess the extent to which the MC approach is delivered as intended.

CLIENT RESPONSE TO TREATMENT SESSIONS: OBSERVING, TRACKING, AND DOCUMENTING PROGRESS

Selecting Treatment Targets

The treatment process within the RTSS approach begins by identifying targets for intervention and selecting treatment ingredients to bring about the change. Within the MC approach, specific client behaviors and skills that are targeted for change within individual treatment sessions are summarized in Exhibit 11.2 and reflect the MC RTSS framework in Appendix D.10. As previously described, MC treatment sessions can focus on one or any combination of the key treatment elements (awareness of performance, strategy use, or transfer and generalization) as a means of enhancing functional cognition.

The therapist should choose the areas and specific behaviors from Exhibit 11.2 that are the targets of change for a client within a treatment session, based on assessment (Chapter 5). The target for change is the measurable change that is intended to be brought about by treatment. Once the target(s) of change are identified, treatment ingredients or actions, activities, and techniques that will bring about the change are selected, based on hypothesized

> **Exhibit 11.2 Key Multicontext Treatment Session Targets**
>
> *Awareness of Performance Challenges and Strategies*
> - Accurately appraises task demands prior to an activity.
> - Anticipation: Identifies task or performance challenges.
> - Awareness of the need to use a strategy (before, during, or after tasks).
> - Recognition of performance errors (error detection) or inefficient methods.
> - Spontaneously self-corrects errors or adjusts methods as needed.
> - Spontaneous self-checking or self-assessment across tasks.
> - Accurate self-assessment or recognition of challenges after the task.
> - Accurate self-appraisal of performance after the task.
> - Aware of task methods used.
> - Identifies methods or factors that helped or hindered performance.
>
> *Effective Strategy Use*
> - Identifies or generates effective strategies prior to task.
> - Spontaneously initiates strategy use when needed.
> - Selects an appropriate strategy or combination of strategies for the task.
> - Frequency, timing, and execution of strategies are appropriate.
> - Strategy use is efficient and effective in reducing performance errors or managing cognitive symptoms.
> - Explains methods/strategies used (after tasks) and how or why they helped.
> - Identifies or generates alternate strategies after the task.
>
> *Transfer and Generalization*
> - Recognizes that the same error patterns have occurred in previous tasks.
> - Recognizes similarities between activity and previous activities before or after the task.
> - Recognizes application of the strategy to previous or future daily life activities.
> - Spontaneously initiates strategy use in a similar activity (near transfer).
> - Spontaneously applies strategies to intermediate/far transfer tasks.
> - Spontaneously uses strategies in everyday life (generalization).
> - Increases in the number of activities to which strategies are applied.
> - Increases in the breadth (type/contexts) of activities to which strategies are applied.
>
> *Self-Efficacy*
> - Expresses positive attitude or commitment to self-manage cognitive challenges.
> - Increased effort and engagement in treatment
> - Increased persistence in the face of cognitive challenges.

mechanisms of action and theoretical concepts of the MC approach. Multiple targets and treatment ingredients are typically selected at once. These target behaviors guide observations within sessions and should be reflected within communication and documentation of progress.

It is important to note that the RTSS distinguishes between *treatment theory*, which explains changes in targets of treatment as in Exhibit 11.2, and *enablement theory*, which explains distal goals that address activity limitation and participation outcomes or aims (see Chapter 12). In addition to and consistent with the treatment session targets, goals within the MC approach can incorporate awareness and strategy use into more distal functional cognitive goals identified by the client or significant others as prerequisites for independence in functional activities. The principles of the MC approach can be incorporated into standard rehabilitation and OT methods of goal setting and planning as described in Chapter 12. Modifications and adjustments to the goal-setting process based on the person's cognitive limitations and awareness level are also described in Chapter 12.

Observing and Tracking Progress Within and Across Treatment Sessions

The MC metacognitive framework involves semi-structured questions asked before, during, and after performance as detailed in Chapter 10. Responses to these questions can be monitored, analyzed, and summarized within each treatment activity or treatment session and compared over time across treatment sessions. Worksheets that document client responses in the areas of anticipation, error recognition and correction, strategy generation and use, self-assessment, and ability to make connections to other situations can be used to assess progress. This provides the opportunity to observe patterns and small changes within and across treatment sessions that might not always be obvious. For example, Table 11.2 illustrates client responses to guided questions for two treatment activities.

Level of Task Challenge

The first step in analyzing client awareness and strategy use within a session is to consider task difficulty or level of challenge of the task in relation to the person's ability. As discussed previously, strategies are not needed when a task is easy and are ineffective when a task is too difficult (Chapters 7-8). The therapist needs to ensure that any inconsistencies in strategy use or awareness across treatment activities are not related to the complexity of the treatment task. In the MC approach, task complexity should be at an optimal level of challenge and remain consistent across activities. However, it is not always easy to present treatment activities within an *optimal* challenge level, especially because client performance and abilities can fluctuate with fatigue, emotional status, and other factors (Chapter 1). Therefore, immediately following a treatment session, the therapist is encouraged to determine if the level of task challenge was optimal. Task challenge is specified and classified by using the *treatment activity level of challenge scale* that is included at the end of the therapist fidelity tool rating criteria (Appendix C.13).

Strategy Use

Within treatment, the quality of strategies used *during* performance can be monitored, analyzed, and documented by describing the type, frequency, efficiency, and effectiveness of strategies across different treatment activities and sessions as discussed and summarized in Chapter 7 (Table 7.5). A checklist for observation and analysis of strategy use is included in Appendix B.13 for use by the therapist during or immediately after treatment activities. This worksheet is particularly helpful if the focus of intervention is on improving the efficiency and effectiveness of strategy use.

Awareness of Challenges, Awareness of Strategy Use, and Strategy Generation

Responses to selected guided questions asked immediately before and after a treatment activity can be rated and compared across activities and sessions using rating scales in Appendix (B.14-B.16). The *Identification of Challenges* scale rates client responses to the pre- and post-activity questions that ask about challenges anticipated or encountered. The second scale rates client responses to *Strategy Generation* questions (before and after activities), and the third scale examines *Strategy Awareness* after the task. Anticipatory awareness can be described and characterized by completing the identification of challenges and strategy generation scales based on responses before the activity. Emergent awareness of performance can be described and characterized by rating questions after the task involving identification of challenges, strategy awareness, and strategy generation.

The scales include descriptions and criteria for numerical ratings of responses for awareness and strategy questions that may help monitor progress across treatment sessions. They can also be useful in structuring observations as well as writing and documenting progress in an objective and standardized manner. For example, responses to the Identification of Challenges scale are categorized into levels ranging from 1 to 9 (1 = cognitive challenges anticipated with explanation provided, 9 = unable to identify challenges) or that can be condensed into four broad categories (good, partial, limited, or unable to identify challenges). The rating scales are based on independent responses, but if mediation is used to obtain responses, the scales can also be coded so that responses with and without mediation can be compared.

Tracking Progress across Treatment Activities

In addition to rating responses to questions for each treatment activity, a client's awareness, strategy use, strategy generation, and ability to generalize to other situations can be recorded across different treatment activities, as presented in Table 11.2. Using this worksheet, the client's actual responses to metacognitive questions can be documented with or without the numerical ratings from the scales described above. The first two blue-shaded columns represent the pre-activity discussion responses; the next two columns indicate self-monitoring *during* the activity; and the last three columns, shaded in gray, represent the post-activity discussion responses. In the presented example, the numerical ratings for awareness and strategy generation are included (in parentheses) to facilitate comparison. In the first session, the client's awareness and strategy generation improved from pre to post activity. The second activity was done in the second session, and the table shows carryover from the first session in both awareness and strategy generation, as well as improved recognition of the connection between activities and strategies. An alternative form or worksheet for summarizing treatment activities within each session is presented in Appendix C.11. This worksheet is more comprehensive than Table 11.2 and can be completed after each treatment session. It is useful in monitoring, analyzing, and summarizing progress in the key target areas (awareness, strategy use, and generalization) across different activities and sessions.

Other Indicators of Progress

Changes in the areas of awareness are also are reflected in greater consistency between the client's assessment of performance or task outcome and that of the therapist or others, greater engagement in goal setting, and adjustment of goals (see Chapter 12). Application of strategies across a wider range of activities, situations, or contexts can be documented by identifying the number of different activities to which a strategy is applied as well as decreased assistance or increased time and efficiency in performing untrained functional tasks. Changes in self-efficacy across treatment sessions can be evidenced by a decrease in negative self-statements (e.g., this is too hard, my brain is messed up). Qualitative analysis of client journal entries, strategy worksheets (e.g., Chapter 10), or cognitive logs (Chapter 14) can also provide evidence of changes in awareness, strategy generation, and self-efficacy. Clinically we have observed that clients' journals, logs, or action plans are initially overly general and ambiguous. Over the course of treatment, greater specificity of challenges encountered, plans, and strategies can be observed. In addition, entries can reflect changes in beliefs about strategies and the ability to successfully manage cognitive symptoms within activities.

Using the Metacognitive Framework to Write Progress Notes

The MC metacognitive framework and tracking worksheets can be used to structure documentation of treatment sessions and progress notes. For example, progress notes can have subheadings such as "Prior to Task," "During Task," and "After Task." Additional subheadings such as "Observed carryover" or "Connection to other activities" can also be included. A sample progress note using this format is illustrated in Clinical Example 11.1.

Table 11.2 Tracking Progress Across Treatment Activities

Activity	Pre-Activity Discussion		During Activity Monitoring		Post-Activity Discussion		
	Identification of Challenges	Strategy Generation	Error Recognition During Performance	Mediation Provided	Identification of Challenges	Strategy generation	Connection to other activities
1. TV calendar Level 1	None (9)	Pay attention (4)	None	None	I missed some (3)	Mark them off the list (2)	Not sure
2. Classes Calendar	The calendar looks different than mine (6)	Mark them off the list (3)	None	None	Sometimes I forgot to mark the list (2)	Remember to double-check myself (2)	When I am using a shopping list

> **Clinical Example 11.1: Sample Progress Note 1 (Full case presented in Chapter 15)**
>
> *Activity:* Use of a ten-item list to retrieve items from the kitchen as a prerequisite to meal preparation and other everyday activities such as following a recipe, ordering a list of items online, managing appointments, and medications.
>
> *Prior to Task:* Client did not anticipate any difficulties or need to use a strategy and quickly jumped into the activity.
>
> *During the task*: Client did not initiate any strategies such as marking items off the list and took items out of the closet quickly without checking the list. He became distracted by relevant items and took out several items that were not on the list while omitting others.
>
> *Task outcome*: Client omitted three items and retrieved three additional, irrelevant items
>
> *After the task:* Client self-recognized difficulties with structured guidance from the therapist to self-check his work and stated that the next time he would change his task methods, use a more systematic approach, check off each item after it was retrieved, and go more slowly.
>
> *Observed carryover:* With a similar activity in the same session (using a different ten-item list involving kitchen supplies), client spontaneously used the strategies identified above 50% of the time, and performance improved. Only 1/10 items were omitted, and only one extra item was retrieved.
>
> *Summary:* Client self-recognized errors with guidance, generated alternate strategies, and partially applied the strategies to a similar functional task. This represents a significant change from the previous session when the client remained unaware of performance errors and failed to generate or apply alternate strategies with therapist guidance. It also signifies increased self-awareness of performance, which is linked to improved functional outcomes (Villalobos et al., 2019).
>
> *Plan:* Continue use of metacognitive strategy methods within functionally relevant activities to enhance awareness of performance, manage impulsivity, and optimize the ability to successfully manage a ten-item list across two different IADL activities and contexts (ordering a list of grocery items online and gathering needed items to pack an overnight bag).

Alternatively, the traditional SOAP (subjective, objective, assessment, and plan) note format can be used to document MC treatment progress as presented in Clinical Example 11.2. Progress notes should explicitly compare the present level of function to the baseline level or the previous progress note to demonstrate areas of progress or change. The comparison between functional cognitive performance observed during a treatment session (current status), and baseline function is particularly important for reimbursement.

> **Clinical Example 11.2: Progress Note 2: SOAP Note Format**
>
> *Activity:* Make coffee and toast.
>
> *Subjective:* Client did not anticipate any challenges or difficulties before the activity and did not identify the need to use strategies. After the activity, client recognized performance errors and indicated "I need to pay attention more." Client was engaged in the activity and appeared to be surprised by his errors.
>
> *Objective:* Client required mediation and guidance to self-recognize performance errors within the activity (put water in coffee pot and turned on machine without the coffee, placed bread in toaster without recognizing the plug was not on and then completely forgot about the toast).
>
> *Assessment:* Ability to recognize performance errors within an activity is critical for safety and independent functional performance. Client demonstrated changes in the ability to identify performance errors during the treatment session as noted by changes in rating of awareness before (9) and after a functional task (6). This demonstrates improvement from the previous session where awareness of performance errors was not observed with cues.
>
> *Plan:* Continue use of metacognitive strategy methods within functional activities to enhance awareness of performance, and initiate use of strategies to manage the ability to keep track of information for independence in routine five-step IADL activities such as making coffee and toast.

The two progress notes in Clinical Examples 11.1 and 11.2 each use different formats; however, both use the MC approach metacognitive framework as a guide to documenting functional cognitive performance within treatment sessions. The first note describes awareness of performance, strategy use, and application of strategies to a similar (near transfer) activity, while the second note focuses entirely on self-recognition of performance errors within an activity. Both notes reflect and communicate the key MC treatment targets as outlined in Exhibit 11.2.

SUMMARY

This chapter further operationalizes the MC approach by specifying essential MC treatment ingredients within the Rehabilitation Treatment Specification System (RTSS) (See Appendix D.10). The MC components were deconstructed so that its treatment targets were clearly described and linked with treatment techniques and hypothesized mechanisms of action. The RTSS framework provides guidance for assessing therapist adherence and quality of treatment delivery as well as measuring client progress (Hart et al., 2019). A treatment fidelity tool consistent with the MC RTSS framework was introduced as a way of guiding accurate and consistent use of the MC approach in clinical practice and research (see Appendix C.13). This tool can be used in training and supervision and to assess and monitor the quality of implementation of MC treatment procedures (Toglia et al., 2020). Methods for observing, analyzing, and documenting client response to treatment and changes in treatment targets were also described. Examples of worksheets for summarizing client awareness, strategy use, and generalization skills within and across treatment sessions are provided in Appendix C.

KEY POINTS

- The MC approach is a complex multicomponent metacognitive strategy intervention that differs from conventional cognitive rehabilitation in several ways: (1) use of cognitive strategies across situations, (2) focus on the process rather than the outcome, (3) treatment is structured horizontally with explicit techniques to expand strategy transfer across activities before increasing difficulty, and (4) use of guided learning methods.

- Success of the MC approach depends on quality delivery, which may require a shift in practice methods and takes practice and self-reflection on the part of the therapist.

- Clear specification of MC treatment components promotes quality treatment delivery, the ability to track client change, and assists in consistent communication of treatment content, process, and progress.

- Key MC treatment targets are related to awareness of performance challenges or limitations, strategy awareness, strategy use, and transfer or generalization.

- Progress in relation to treatment targets can be tracked within and across treatment sessions, and MC treatment documentation can fit within traditional rehabilitation and OT goals setting and documentation practices.

- Treatment targets that are directly influenced by MC intervention components contribute to achieving larger, functional goals (see Chapter 12).

Chapter 12

Goal Setting and Measuring Functional Outcomes

Collaborative client-centered goal setting, goal adjustment, careful monitoring, and documentation of progress toward functional goals are foundational practices in occupational therapy (OT) and cognitive rehabilitation. This chapter discusses special considerations and techniques to optimize these practices within the MC approach. It discusses the impact of cognition and self-awareness on the goal-setting process and provides suggestions for maximizing client engagement in goal setting and adjustment during treatment. In the MC approach, treatment fosters the process of goal setting and goal adjustment by increasing self-awareness. Thus, engagement in goal setting and identification of realistic and attainable goals are viewed as positive outcomes of treatment. This chapter then discusses monitoring and documentation of functional goals for the MC approach. The use of goal rating, goal attainment scaling, and standardized outcome measures to track progress and measure functional outcomes of MC intervention is reviewed.

CONTENTS OF CHAPTER 12

Goal Setting and Adjustment for People with Cognitive Impairment
- Cognitive Impairment and Considerations in Goal Setting
  - *Breaking Down Goals: Sub-goaling*
- Reduced Self-Awareness and Considerations in Goal Setting
  - *Partial or Vague Awareness*
- The Process of Goal Adjustment

Documenting Functional Goals and Progress
- Goal Rating and Monitoring
  - *Goal Attainment Scaling*
  - *Bangor Goal Setting Interview*
  - *Informal Goal Rating Within the Multicontext Approach*

Assessing Outcomes
- Proximal Outcome Measures
  - *Awareness*
  - *Strategy Use*
  - *Cognition*
  - *Cognitive Self-Efficacy*
- Distal Outcome Measures

Summary and Key Points

GOAL SETTING AND ADJUSTMENT FOR PEOPLE WITH COGNITIVE IMPAIRMENT

Cognitive impairments and decreased awareness can compromise the ability to participate in goal setting and planning. Every effort should be made to engage the client and/or significant others in setting goals for treatment as well as monitoring and adjusting them across treatment (Turner-Stokes et al., 2015). To develop client-centered goals, the therapist must take time to understand a person's life history, experiences, personality, and interests. The process of goal setting needs to be tailored to an individual's needs and preferences, cognitive abilities, and levels of awareness, which can change over time or across treatment (Plant et al., 2016). In this way, goal setting is conceptualized as a dynamic process. Goals are continuously revised during recovery or the course of treatment with changes in cognition and/or self-awareness.

Close collaborations with families or significant others in goal setting and monitoring is particularly important in optimizing outcomes. This includes helping significant others recognize and understand cognitive performance errors and behaviors as well as methods to manage them. Turner-Stokes et al. (2015) developed a scale for rating the level of both client and family engagement in goal setting that is freely available for use (see resource section). Since engagement in goal setting can emerge and change during the course of treatment, this scale may be useful in measuring progress.

Cognitive Impairment and Considerations in Goal Setting

The ability to respond to open-ended questions, set priorities, estimate time frames, understand cause and effect, look beyond the here and now, or comprehend how small goals are connected to larger goals and to each other, can all be limited by cognitive impairments. Thus, therapists may need to use a range of strategies to facilitate engagement in goal setting with their clients with cognitive impairment (Plant et al., 2016).

Open-ended questions that ask a person to identify concerns may be particularly difficult for individuals with cognitive impairments because they require the person to initiate ideas and organize or structure thoughts. When asked open-ended questions, it may seem as though the person completely lacks awareness; however, when questions are structured or focused on specific task components, more informative responses may be elicited (Sherer et al., 1998). Clinical example 12.1 illustrates how differences in reported function can be observed in a person with cognitive limitations (Craig) with different forms of questioning.

Clinical Example 12.1: General and Specific Interview Questions

Therapist:	Tell me about some of the difficulties you are experiencing?
Craig:	Walking.
Therapist:	As you think about your daily life, what activities do you presently need assistance with?
Craig:	Just walking.
Therapist:	What about getting ready in the morning?
Craig:	No difficulties.
Therapist:	What about getting dressed?
Craig:	No difficulties.
Therapist:	What about buttoning your shirt?
Craig:	Someone else buttons it for me.

In Clinical Example 12.1, Craig denied difficulties in dressing or getting ready in the morning but acknowledged assistance needed for buttoning. Structured questions break down larger areas of function into task substeps and focus the person's attention on each step. These questions can elicit more informative responses as compared to open-ended questions in people with cognitive impairment. To simultaneously develop goals and gain an understanding of the client's level of awareness, the therapist should vary the types of questions asked and pay special attention to the responses elicited by different wording and specificity of questions. Vague or one-word responses to questions can indicate that the question may need to be reworded, rephrased, or narrowed. In addition, responses to questions may need to be repeated, summarized, and probed for expansion or clarification.

The Bangor Goal-Setting Interview version 2 (BGSI-2) (Clare et al., 2016) and the Canadian Occupational Performance Measure (COPM) (Law et al., 2014) both offer a flexible and semi-structured interview format for eliciting individual goals (see resource section). Questions to elicit goals typically begin with broad questions regarding difficulties with everyday activities; however, questions can be further structured or focused on specific areas, as suggested above, for clients with cognitive difficulties. Both the COPM and the BGSI-2 break down questions into categories such as self-care, household, leisure, or social activities. Questions within these areas can also be further narrowed to addressing tasks and task components. This may take increased time but should be considered part of intervention. Both the COPM and BGSI-2 ask the client to self-rate abilities and importance of identified goals, but difficulty making decisions and dealing with the abstract nature of such rating scales can present challenges for people with cognitive impairments. Scale options, therefore, may need to be adapted (e.g., shortened or with visual cues or explicit/descriptive anchors at each response option).

If the person has difficulty initiating or generating goals, it can be helpful to encourage them to make a list of their interests or the things they like to do as well as the daily activities they need to do. If needed, structure for this brainstorming can be provided by giving the person a worksheet with categories such as "things I like to do with my friends," "things that I do on my own," "sports," "tasks I need to do at work," etc. The use of categories can help a person with initiation difficulties generate ideas. Once interests are identified, it may be easier for the person to self-identify goals. Alternatively, the person can be provided with examples of goals (Plant et al., 2016). Reviewing a list of pre-made goals can help the person initiate ideas of their own or help them identify areas that they had not thought of. See sample pre-made list of goals in Appendix C.24.

Clients with moderate to severe cognitive limitations can have trouble choosing priorities and making decisions about which goals to pursue, particularly when presented with a lot of information at once. They might have difficulty paying attention, holding more than two or three ideas in their minds at once, keeping track of options, processing all parts of a question, or remembering information presented to them. Over-attention to some information can result in missing other important aspects of instructions or situations. In these cases, the process of choosing goals needs to be simplified. It may be best to ask significant others to narrow down priorities and then ask the person to choose between two key goals presented at one time. Presentation of information should be both visual (e.g., pictures) and auditory and confined to short sentences or keywords in an environment that is free from distraction.

An alternative to verbal goal discussions or interviews is the use of card sort methods that involve identifying or sorting pictures of activities into groups based on current and desired or preferred level of engagement. This method has important advantages for those with moderate cognitive impairments or communication difficulties. For example, the *Life Interests and Values Cards* (LiV) asks clients to look at cards depicting activities, one at a time, and identify those activities that they would like to do more. The presentation of one picture card at a time focuses attention, provides visual prompts of activities, stimulates recollection of experiences, and decreases demands on initiation, attention, memory, and language (Haley et al., 2013). Similarly, the Activity Card Sort (ACS) (Baum & Edwards, 2008) involves sorting colored photographs of activities into groups such as those that the person is currently doing, has given up, does less, or has not previously done. The use of pictures or visual cues by the LiV or ACS supports cognitive skills and facilitates active involvement in identifying desired activities (see resource section).

Memory impairment can cause the person to forget goals that were discussed or identified in previous evaluation or treatment sessions (Evans, 2012). In this situation, the use of a goal book that includes the person's interests and strengths, areas targeted for improvement, and goals can be created and placed prominently in a person's room for frequent review. This also allows for reinforcement and comments by relatives, friends, and other team members. A goal book is also helpful for those without memory impairments because it helps to structure and focus the goal-setting process and provides an explicit roadmap for treatment. See sample page from a goal book in Appendix C.25.

Alternatively, everyday technology using a smartphone or virtual assistant can be used to remind a person of their key goals with daily pre-programmed voice or text messages, or alarms with visual cues or pictures. Daily goal reminders support recollection or learning of goals and have been found to enhance goal focus and motivation in both inpatient and outpatient settings (Culley & Evans, 2010; Evans, 2012).

Breaking Down Goals: Sub-goaling

Cognitive limitations can make it hard for a person to understand how activities and goals within treatment relate to their broader personal goals such as returning to work. Concrete thinking results in difficulty thinking beyond the here and now and simultaneously considering all aspects of a situation. The person may recognize memory problems but be unable to see the connection between memory difficulties and return to work or independent living. Although they can identify goals (e.g., return to work, driving), the person may be unable to break down a large or long-term goal into smaller attainable shorter-term goals or substeps (Prescott et al., 2018). In this situation, sub-goaling techniques can be used to help the person break down larger goals into subcomponents. Sub-goaling methods can use a table, a ladder diagram, a goal map, or other visual representations to facilitate understanding of the connections between smaller and larger goals or the links between impairments (e.g., memory limitations) and functional activities (Toglia & Golisz, 2012).

As an example of a sub-goaling method, the staircase in Figure 12.1 provides a concrete illustration and representation of the skills needed for independent living. In this example, the goal is broad, and the staircase does not represent a fixed sequence but rather shows the

Figure 12.1 Sub-goal Ladder

Living independently requires….

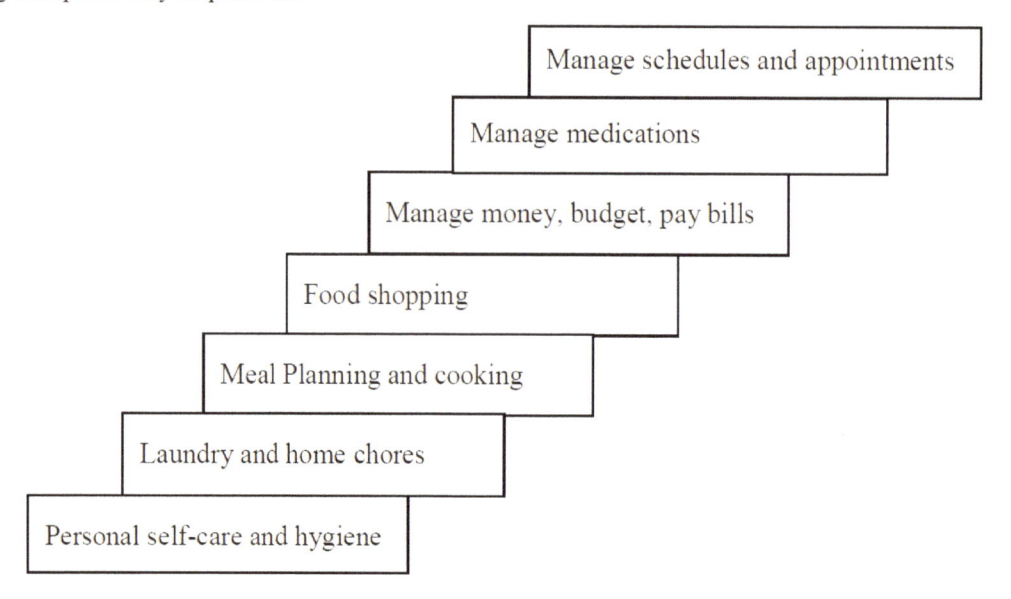

- Manage schedules and appointments
- Manage medications
- Manage money, budget, pay bills
- Food shopping
- Meal Planning and cooking
- Laundry and home chores
- Personal self-care and hygiene

activities required for independent living using the analogy of climbing a staircase.

The sub-goal ladder provides a concrete representation of the premise that steps are required before getting to the top and attaining the goal of living independently. Each area on the staircase such as laundry, meal planning, or food shopping could be further broken down into smaller steps and can represent its own staircase. A goal map can also be used as illustrated in Figure 12.2; however, a goal map is more abstract and can be visually confusing for some clients. Both methods can assist the person in understanding connections between smaller, immediate tasks and a broad functional goal.

Sub-goaling methods can be combined with goal

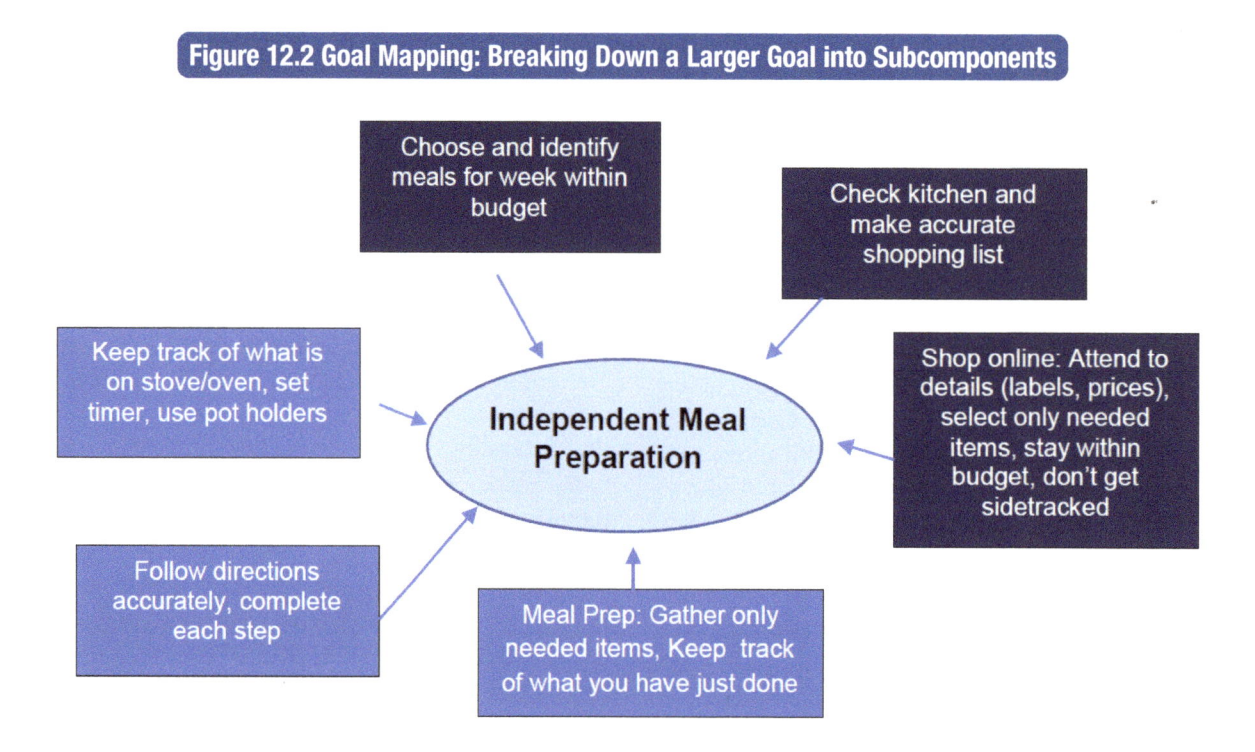

Figure 12.2 Goal Mapping: Breaking Down a Larger Goal into Subcomponents

Independent Meal Preparation
- Choose and identify meals for week within budget
- Check kitchen and make accurate shopping list
- Shop online: Attend to details (labels, prices), select only needed items, stay within budget, don't get sidetracked
- Meal Prep: Gather only needed items, Keep track of what you have just done
- Follow directions accurately, complete each step
- Keep track of what is on stove/oven, set timer, use pot holders

planning. Once a subgoal is identified (e.g., food shopping), a goal plan can be created that identifies the action steps toward achieving that goal, including strategies, methods, and/or activities that can help the person reach their goal. The format of sub-goaling and/or goal plans should be commensurate with the client's abilities. Regardless of the format, the client and significant others should be involved whenever feasible in generating sub-goals and goal plans. This process can take extra time and often requires guided questions and facilitation by the therapist. If the therapist generates task substeps as a starting point, they should be reviewed with the client and agreement should be reached. Additional examples of sub-goaling and goal planning are presented in Appendices D.13-D.15, and blank forms for use within treatment are in Appendices C.26-C.27.

In summary, promoting engagement in goal setting for persons with cognitive impairment often requires structuring the goal-setting process to support difficulties in initiation, memory, attention, and executive function (EF). This may require altering and varying the wording of questions, using pre-made goal lists, pictures, a goal book, goal reminders, sub-goaling, and goal planning methods (Plant et al., 2016). If self-awareness is limited, use of these goal-setting techniques may require additional time, multiple sessions, and extensive guidance from the therapist. If this is the case, techniques such as sub-goaling may be more effective when used therapeutically during treatment as awareness emerges rather than at the start of treatment.

The MC approach views engagement in goal setting on a continuum. As treatment progresses, indicators of increased awareness and acceptance include greater engagement by the client in the goal-setting process. This is further described in the sections below.

Reduced Self-Awareness and Considerations in Goal Setting

In addition to cognitive impairments, impaired self-awareness presents a significant obstacle to realistic goal setting and treatment planning. Sub-goaling techniques may be ineffective or overly time-consuming in individuals with poor self-awareness. In the initial phases of treatment, the person may not recognize or accept changes that have occurred in thinking skills. If a person does not recognize cognitive functional difficulties, it can be difficult to engage them in treatment. Clinical Example 12.2 illustrates the challenges in goal setting with a person that lacks self-awareness.

> **Clinical Example 12.2 Poor Self-Awareness**
>
> Maria is five years post-traumatic brain injury (TBI) and ambulates independently with a cane. She has significant EF and memory deficits and lives with a 24-hour aide in the community. When asked about her goals, Maria stated she wanted to live independently. At the same time, when specific questions were asked, Maria's goals did not include cooking skills, laundry, or paying bills, even though her aide completed these activities for her. Instead, when given a choice about activities in treatment, she chose computer games. She spent most of her days playing computer games. When asked what she thought she needed to do to be able to live independently, she indicated she needed to have better balance so that she could ambulate without a cane. She denied any difficulties in thinking or memory.

In Clinical Example 12.2, the combination of Maria's cognitive limitations and her decreased awareness made it difficult for her to engage in setting realistic goals and identifying appropriate treatment activities. Sub-goaling techniques were ineffective at the start of treatment because Maria did not recognize her difficulties. In this case, enhancing self-awareness through structured activity experiences was the initial focus of treatment (see Chapters 3 and 10). Throughout treatment, Maria continued to deny difficulties in thinking or memory; however, her ability to recognize and monitor performance errors (online awareness) increased. For example, with repeated experiences, she recognized the tendency to miss details and get sidetracked across different activities. As online awareness increased, sub-goaling was re-introduced using the staircase in Figure 12.1. The concrete visual representation was placed in her daily planner and was effective in helping Maria choose realistic treatment activities and goals. As awareness emerged, she gradually began to express goals related to meal preparation and laundry, rather than computer games.

In some cases, a client's self-identified goals may be limited to motor or physical skills and unconnected to observed functional cognitive problems. In these situations, treatment activities should focus on the client's motor goals while at the same time incorporating cognitive skills by manipulating directions (Chapter 4) and using the metacognitive framework and guided learning methods described in Chapters 9 and 10. As the person is working on motor goals within the context of physical activities that also place demands on cognitive skills, awareness of cognitive lapses (e.g., losing track of information or difficulty concentrating) may gradually emerge. This is an indirect way of addressing cognitive abilities and allows time to build a therapeutic alliance necessary to facilitate self-awareness.

Partial or Vague Awareness

In some situations, the person identifies changes in thinking, but awareness is still limited. The person may generally recognize that their mind is not as sharp as it was before or that they have difficulty concentrating or remembering, but they may not fully understand the changes that have occurred. Similarly, a person may be able to provide examples of functional cognitive difficulties but be unaware of performance errors within the context of activities (i.e., awareness of performance). As described in Chapter 3, acknowledgment of cognitive difficulties in an interview does not necessarily mean that the person can recognize performance errors when they occur or explain how they impact performance. As a result, the person's goals may be vague, overly general (e.g., get better, improve my memory, return to work), or unconnected to observed performance. This is illustrated in Clinical Example 12.3.

> **Clinical Example 12.3 Discrepancy between General and Online Awareness**
>
> Laura stated her goal was to improve her attention. She explained that she has difficulty concentrating. She gave examples of performance errors in everyday life such as omitting an ingredient when following a recipe and misreading an appointment time on her calendar. During a complex activity involving making a schedule of possible events for a visitor from out of town according to certain days, times, and costs within a budget, Laura found events on the correct days and times but did not pay attention to the cost. She did not refer back to the written directions and did not double-check her work. She stated the activity was easy. When she was provided with an answer sheet to check her work, she was surprised at the errors that were made and stated, "I can't understand why that happened, I need to improve my attention."

In Clinical Example 12.3, Laura acknowledged general problems in attention during an interview. Although she was aware of functional cognitive performance errors, she did not have a complete understanding of why errors may have occurred. Within the context of an activity, she was unable to use her general knowledge of difficulties to anticipate, monitor, and self-recognize performance errors (poor online awareness of performance). As a result, her goal was overly broad and vague. Although Laura appears to have good awareness of her deficits, she is a good candidate for use of the MC metacognitive framework because her awareness was incomplete. MC intervention can help a person gain a deeper understanding of their cognitive strengths and weaknesses within the context of performance so that more specific goals can emerge.

People who are generally aware of cognitive concerns may also exhibit poor self-efficacy that further compounds difficulties. For example, a person may indicate that they are having difficulties keeping track of information or organizing information, but they believe that these symptoms "just happen unpredictably" and that there is nothing that they can do.

MC intervention can help a person identify the conditions that are most likely to impact cognitive symptoms and performance. A full understanding of why and when cognitive lapses are likely to occur promotes effective strategy use, self-management of cognitive symptoms, and builds self-efficacy. Increased self-efficacy has been linked with increased motivation to work toward goals (Cizman Staba et al., 2020). As self-efficacy and understanding of cognitive limitations and abilities increase, more specific goals emerge. Previous goals and priorities may be revised or changed entirely as treatment progresses. This is further discussed in the next section.

The Process of Goal Adjustment

As discussed above, goal setting, cognitive function, and self-awareness are intertwined. At the start of treatment, people with impaired self-awareness typically identify unrealistic goals. There is a large discrepancy between the person's performance capabilities and the identified goals. The person's goals and priorities should be validated and acknowledged, even if the therapist and others believe that the goals are unattainable. Attempts to dissuade a person from pursuing an identified goal (because it is unrealistic) should be avoided because it will only create tension that negatively impacts the therapeutic relationship. Rather, the therapist should recognize that the person's perception of their situation may be different from reality because they have not fully processed or recognized the performance changes that have occurred.

An aim of treatment, then, would be to narrow the discrepancy between the person's perceptions of their performance and that observed by others. Key aspects of MC intervention involve structuring activity experiences and providing the person with opportunities so that they can self-discover their own performance problems (Toglia & Kirk, 2000). As the person begins to recognize and understand cognitive performance challenges and errors, more specific goals and realistic plans will emerge. Increases in self-awareness naturally result in modifications, revisions, or refinements to initial goals or the choosing of completely new goals. This is illustrated in Clinical Example 12.4.

> **Clinical Example 12.4 Goal Adjustment**
>
> James had a goal of returning to work four weeks after his bicycle accident. As the fourth week was approaching, James realized that he was having difficulty staying focused on tasks within a treatment session. He recognized that he was not yet ready to return to work. At this point, with guidance from his therapist, he revised his goals so that they were smaller, more specific, and attainable. He changed the timeframe of returning to work to four months. His therapist thought that this timeframe was still unrealistic but did not say this to him. The therapist knew that her role was to help James understand his new strengths and weaknesses and not to make decisions for him. As his awareness and acceptance continue to emerge, his goals will likely be adjusted.

Fostering goal adjustment is an inherent part of awareness interventions like the MC approach. In the MC approach, goal setting is a dynamic process that occurs continuously across treatment. Goal adjustment often signifies that the person recognizes the discrepancy between their performance and goals or realizes that goals are unattainable within the time frame they had expected (Brands et al., 2015). New goals emerge or previous goals are modified so that they are more realistic or specific as self-awareness improves. In this way, goal adjustment can be considered an indicator of improved awareness in response to MC treatment and, therefore, is an important and positive outcome of treatment. Appendix C.28 includes a worksheet that can be used to track goal adjustments during treatment. It is important to note that goal adjustments may also occur for reasons that are unrelated to awareness as described below.

The MC approach to goal setting contrasts with conventional goal setting, where goals identified by the client at the start of treatment are used to measure treatment progress and outcome throughout. This approach can be problematic because unrealistic goals result in goal failures or unsuccessful goal attainment. In Clinical Example 12.4, if James' awareness had remained poor at four weeks, there would have been adverse consequences, as premature return to work without recognition of limitations would have resulted in his inability to meet work responsibilities. Goal failures lower self-efficacy and negatively impact emotional well-being (Brands et al., 2015). If a person continuously holds on to goals that are out of reach or cannot be successfully attained, frustration, depression, or decreased motivation can occur. Pursuit of unrealistic goals prevents the person from adapting to their situation and moving on with their life. In contrast, success in pursuing attainable goals increases well-being and positively influences recovery (Brands et al., 2015; Van Bost et al., 2019).

Admittedly, the process of goal adjustment during intervention needs further attention in the literature and investigation. Although increases in the ability to identify realistic goals have been observed as a result of intervention, studies have not adequately documented and examined how goals are adjusted during treatment with changes in awareness.

Finally, while we have focused on the role of cognition and self-awareness, it should be kept in mind that psychosocial issues, personality, and contextual factors can also influence the setting and pursuit of realistic goals (Turner et al., 2008). Abandonment or constant revision of goals can reflect lack of self-confidence, fear of failure, or depression as well as changes in personal needs or circumstances. Also, lack of acceptance of the reality of one's situation and poor coping skills can contribute to unrealistic goal setting in a person who is aware of their limitations (Van Bost et al., 2019). In these situations, treatment focuses on building acceptance, self-efficacy, and the ability to cope with cognitive challenges. Goal adjustments or the identification of new goals can therefore also signify flexible or adaptive coping skills and represent increased acceptance of one's limitations in people who are already aware of their limitations. The reasons for goal adjustment need to be considered and fully explored by the clinician.

DOCUMENTING FUNCTIONAL GOALS AND PROGRESS

The American Occupational Therapy Association documentation guidelines require that goals be measurable, meaningful and directly related to a client's ability and need to engage in desired occupations (American Occupational Therapy Association, 2018). In general, for services to be reimbursed, goals should be related to functional activities, safety, and return to prior level of function. Goals should conform to the SMART principles. This means that they should be **S**pecific, **M**easurable, **A**ttainable, **R**elevant/**R**easonable, and **T**ime-bound. Documentation should also reflect the need for skilled care. Documentation of progress should demonstrate a connection between how occupational therapy (OT) interventions have led to progress in meeting the client's functional goals.

Some specific examples of short-term goals in line with the MC approach are in Exhibit 12.1 below; additional examples are listed in Appendix D.16. While inclusion of strategy use or awareness is not required for documentation of functional goals, doing so may help to demonstrate the need for skilled service or the complexity and clinical reasoning involved in providing services to a person

> **Exhibit 12.1 Sample Short-term Goals Consistent with the Multicontext Approach**
>
> Within 1 week…
>
> 1. Client will consistently prepare a cold lunch independently without verbal cues by using a verbal rehearsal strategy to optimize ability to keep track of steps.
> 2. Client will accurately place one online order for a meal delivery service without verbal cues by following a four-step written list to optimize ability to keep track of steps.
> 3. As a prerequisite to independence with medication management, client will be able to spontaneously recognize errors in placement of pills within a medication organizer 90% of the time.
> 4. Client will make coffee and toast without verbal cues by self-generating one strategy prior to the task to self-manage impulsivity.
> 5. Verbal cues will be decreased from moderate to minimum across two different, five-step IADL activities (making a sandwich, entering an appointment into a calendar), through use of a list strategy.
> 6. Client will accurately use a ten-item list to gather kitchen items, as a prerequisite to meal preparation, by self-generating a strategy to manage distractibility.
> 7. Client will pay one bill accurately with minimum verbal cues to self-recognize and correct performance errors.

with cognitive limitations. It also conveys how cognitive limitations may be contributing to difficulties in functional performance.

Goal Rating and Monitoring

Goal rating is one way to track and report progress toward functional goals across treatment. It can also provide a person-centered outcome measure and be used to enhance or monitor the client's awareness. Goal rating includes scoring the extent to which a client's individual goals are achieved. It involves operationalizing personal goals and establishing criteria for different levels of attainment. Goals need to be transformed into observable, objective levels of attainment so that the extent to which the goal is met can be rated or scored during treatment. This allows for systematic examination of progress (Turner-Stokes, 2009).

The therapist can define the levels of goal attainment and present them to the client and/or family for refinement and agreement. Alternatively, the client or family can be involved in establishing individualized goal attainment criteria. As discussed earlier in this chapter, engagement in goal setting, rating, and adjustment can vary across treatment or with the person's level of awareness and cognitive abilities. Improved engagement in goal ratings may emerge as a result of intervention and can occur towards the middle or end of treatment for some clients.

Goal ratings can be used with both clients and informants. Large discrepancies between ratings of the client and others can create tensions in relationships and may be related to difficulties in coping with deficits or represent limitations in awareness as previously described. Discrepancies between ratings of the client and that of others can be reviewed and discussed to narrow or eliminate the gap between the client's perceptions of performance and that of others; in other words, enhancing the client's awareness.

Several different methods can be used to rate goals. These include goal attainment scaling (GAS), the Bangor Goal Setting Interview version 2 (BGSI-2), or informally rating and tracking goal attainment based on the extent to which a goal is met in terms that are most appropriate for the client's level of understanding.

Goal Attainment Scaling

Goal attainment scaling (GAS) provides a method for using goal attainment scores as an outcome measure that allows determination of a client's goal attainment as well as comparison of goal attainment across clients with different goals. Each goal scale should represent a single dimension of change (Krasny-Pacini et al., 2016; Turner-Stokes, 2009). An example of the GAS numerical scale is included in Table 12.1 (third column), where the baseline level of performance is typically represented by a score of -1. If the client or family is involved in goal rating, it is advisable to convert the goal rating score into a Likert scale of 1 to 5 (last column) for easier interpretation on their part. The ratings can then be converted into the conventional GAS numerical scale for statistical comparison. Ratings are scored in a standardized manner and converted to T scores to allow for statistical analysis and comparison between clients (Turner-Stokes, 2009). Typically, three to five goals are rated, weighted according to importance

Table 12.1 Conventional 5-point Goal Attainment Scale (Turner-Stokes, 2009)

Goal Met	Criteria	GAS Rating Scale	Client/Informant Rating Scale
Goal Achieved	A lot more than expected	+2	5
Goal Achieved	A little more than expected	+1	4
Goal Achieved	As expected	0	3
Goal Not Met	Same as baseline	-1	2
Goal Not Met	Got worse	-2	1

and difficulty, and combined into a goal attainment composite standardized score using a formula identified by Kiresuk and Sherman (1968). Further information on GAS including how to calculate a goal attainment score is included in the resource section.

Alternatively, a simplified 3-point goal rating scale can be used (Table 12.2). This latter scale is easier for people with cognitive difficulties, but it cannot be used with Kirusek and Sherman's (1968) formula.

Bangor Goal Setting Interview (BGSI-2) (Clare et al., 2016)

The conventional GAS 5-point scale may be difficult for individuals with cognitive difficulties to understand and rate. The BGSI-2 (Clare et al., 2016), introduced earlier in the chapter, uses a structured process that involves collaboration with clients to identify levels of goal attainment on a 5-point scale (0%, 25%, 50%, 75%, or 100%) and create an action plan for goal attainment. Although an advantage of GAS is the use of standardized scores, the BGSI-2 method may be easier to implement. In the BGSI-2, clients are asked to rate their current ability to perform the activity (attainment score), the importance of the activity, and their motivation for change on 10-point scales. The importance and motivation ratings can be used to establish treatment priorities for treatment planning. An overall mean score for attainment can be calculated at any given point by dividing the sum of the attainment ratings for all goals by the number of goals set. Change can be examined by subtracting the average goal attainment score at discharge from the average goal attainment score at baseline. The guidelines for use of the BGSI-2 are freely available (see resource section).

Informal Goal Rating within the Multicontext Approach

Within the MC approach, goals can be rated by the client, significant other, and/or clinician using the goal-rating methods described above. Informal goal-rating methods with rating anchors specific to the client's preferences or level of understanding can also be used. For example, a numerical scale can be converted to words such as "Lots of room for improvement," "partially met," "almost met," "goal is met." The use of word descriptors may be easier for some clients (Turner-Stokes, 2009). Goals for functional performance, strategy use, or awareness can be placed into goal-rating formats by defining measurable levels of goal attainment. Table 12.3 illustrates an example of a goal rating scale for a functional goal (cooking dinner 1x/week). It includes both word descriptors and numerical ratings. Appendix D.17 includes additional sample goal rating scales for functional goal performance, specific strategy use, and self-monitoring that could be used with the MC approach, while Appendix C.29 provides a blank goal rating form for clinical use.

Table 12.2 Modified 3-point Goal Attainment Scale for Self-Ratings

Goal Met	Criteria	GAS Rating Scale	Client/Informant Rating Scale
Goal	Achieved	1	3
Goal Not Met	Partially achieved	0	2
Goal Not Met	No Change	-1	1

Table 12.3 Example Goal Rating Scale for the Functional Goal of "Cooking Dinner 1x/Week"

Levels of performance	Achievement	Rating
Cooks dinner 1x/week (100%)	Goal is met	5
Cooks dinner almost weekly, ~3x/month (75%)	Almost met	4
Cooks dinner every other week, ~2x/month (50%)	Partially met	3
Cooks dinner ~1x/month (25%)	Lots of room for improvement	2
Does not cook dinner (0%)	Baseline	1

Clinical Example 12.5 provides an example of how goal rating methods were used by both a client and his wife.

Clinical Example 12.5 Informal Goal Rating

Joe has significant memory problems following resection of a brain tumor. In the initial evaluation, Joe's wife indicated that Joe constantly relied on her and other family members for all information. This increased her level of frustration and stress. Joe was constantly asking questions about the schedule for the day, upcoming events, and general information, instead of using external sources. Joe generally acknowledged that his memory was not what it used to be but seemed to be generally unaware of the frequency with which he asked others for information. He agreed to this as a goal when his wife raised this issue.

Treatment focused on helping Joe identify systems that would help him keep track of information. For example, he agreed to use a digital voice assistant to set reminders. He also agreed to keep a digital journal to record daily conversations or events. Joe's wife was simultaneously coached on methods of guided questioning to help Joe use external sources to obtain information.

The goal of decreasing reliance on others was placed into a goal rating format (Table 12.4). Joe and his wife separately rated this goal at the end of every week during treatment (Table 12.5). Discrepancies in goal ratings were discussed with the therapist.

It is interesting to note that although Joe consistently rated himself as only occasionally asking others for information, his wife noted reductions in this behavior over time such that their ratings converged by the end of treatment. Joe started referring to his digital journal and calendar more frequently. Others in the family also noticed this difference as well. Joe's initial rating and discrepancy with his wife's may have reflected poor awareness, personality variables, resistance to verbally acknowledging problems, or difficulty with coping and accepting limitations. The lack of change in Joe's self-rating illustrates the importance of including both client and significant others in goal rating to ensure change or progress is captured. In this situation, the discrepancy between the Joe and his wife's ratings decreased, which represented an important change.

ASSESSING OUTCOMES

Whereas Chapter 11 discussed methods for tracking changes in awareness, strategy use, and activity performance within and across treatment sessions, this section discusses methods for capturing change before and after the entire course of treatment (i.e., intervention outcomes). Prior to treatment, it is important to identify the indicators of successful intervention and determine how these outcomes will be assessed (Cicerone et al., 2005). Outcome measures may vary depending on the practice setting as well as other factors, such as the stage of recovery that the client is in at the time of intervention and the client's goals. A combination of self and proxy ratings or questionnaires, along with performance-based measures, are recommended to examine change from before to after intervention, whenever possible. A quote from Corrigan and Bogner (2004) highlights the importance of obtaining the person's perspective "to conclude that an outcome is either successful or unsuccessful in the absence of the person's assessment of the situation seems counterintuitive" (p. 447).

Outcome measures, regardless of the setting, need to be consistent with the treatment targets and intervention model. Outcome measures can be conceptualized in terms of distance from the intervention. Proximal outcome measures are those most closely related to the intervention, whereas distal outcome measures represent

Table 12.4 Joe's Goal Rating Scale for the Goal of Decreasing Reliance on Others

Levels of performance	Achievement	Rating
Client does not rely on others for information	Met	5
Client relies on others for information occasionally (< 25%)	Almost met	4
Client relies on others for information about half of the time (50%)	Partially met	3
Client relies on others for information the majority of the time (75%)	Lots of room for improvement	2
Client relies on others for information, all of the time (e.g., schedule, upcoming events, past events, news items)	Baseline	1

Table 12.5 Goal Rating Across Treatment

	Week 1	Week 2	Week 3	Week 4
Client	4	4	4	4
Wife	2	3	3	4

broader areas of function that could be influenced by the intervention and other factors (Whyte, 2006). This is akin to the distinction in the RTSS between treatment theory and enablement theory and their associated outcomes (discussed in Chapter 11). Changes in proximal measures should be observed immediately or shortly after the intervention ends, whereas changes in distal measures may not be observed until months later.

Proximal Outcome Measures

This chapter discussed goal rating methods as a proximal outcome measure. Indicators of increased awareness, such as decreased discrepancy between actual performance, self-ratings, and ratings of others within activities, increased engagement in goal setting, and appropriate goal readjustments can also be used as proximal outcome measures. The sections below provide examples of additional standardized proximal outcome measures that are recommended for use with the MC approach. This list is not exhaustive, and selection of outcome measures depends on a variety of factors. The reader is referred to the resource section at the end of this book and assessment resources on www.multicontext.net for links to the below measures as well as to additional measures.

Awareness

Self-Regulation Skills Interview (SRSI) (Ownsworth, et al., 2000)

The SRSI interview has been used as a measure of outcome for the MC approach (Toglia et al., 2010) and is recommended because unlike other awareness interviews, it includes questions that probe understanding of the conditions under which cognitive difficulties emerge as well as questions on strategies.

Weekly Calendar Planning Activity (WCPA) (Toglia, 2015)

The WCPA is a performance-based measure of functional cognition that includes assessment of awareness. It includes a measure of online awareness or the number of times the person self-recognizes errors. It also includes questions that investigate the person's perceptions of task challenges and their performance as well as self-ratings and estimations of performance that can be compared to actual performance.

Contextual Memory Test-2 (Toglia, 2019).

The Contextual Memory Test (CMT-2) measures awareness within the context of a recall task involving 20 photos that are related to an everyday scene (morning or restaurant). Actual recall is compared to the person's predicted (before task) and estimated (after task) memory scores. Both the direction of discrepancy (under, accurate, or over) and the magnitude of discrepancy are examined. The CMT-2 is web-based and is administered on a computer or iPad.

Strategy Use

Weekly Calendar Planning Activity (WCPA) (Toglia, 2015)

The WCPA also includes direct observation of strategy use within activity performance and measures the frequency, type, and effectiveness of strategies used. Awareness of strategies or task methods used, as well as the ability to generate alternate strategies, are investigated in an after-task interview.

Contextual Memory Test-2 (Toglia, 2019)

Strategy use is measured on the CMT-2 by coding the type or quality of strategies reported in an after-task interview. A total strategy score is calculated, based upon responses.

Compensatory Cognitive Strategies Scale (Becker et al., 2019)

This is a recently developed scale that includes a list of 24 strategies. The person is asked to indicate how frequently they use each strategy in their daily lives on a 5-point scale. The psychometric characteristics of this scale have been tested on people with multiple sclerosis and need to be examined with other populations.

Cognition

Performance-Based Measures of Functional Cognition

Any functional task that is not directly used as a treatment activity can be used as an outcome measure. Some of these measures were described in Chapter 5. The WCPA is most compatible with the MC approach because it examines awareness, strategy use, and performance of an instrumental activities of daily living (IADL) task, and it has alternate versions for repeat testing; however, other performance-based functional cognitive measures are appropriate. For example, Toglia et al. (2010, 2011) also describe use of the Multiple Errand Test (MET) (Knight et al., 2002) and the Executive Function Performance Test (EFPT) Bill Paying subtest (Baum, et al., 2008) as outcome measures in MC case studies. Similar to the WCPA, the MET also has a focus on the process of how a person goes about doing an activity and records types of errors. The Actual Reality Test (AR) (Goverover & DeLuca, 2015) is a functional test that consists of using commercial websites to accomplish three everyday life tasks of purchasing (1) flight tickets, (2) cookies for a birthday present, and (3) two large pizza pies for a party. Both errors and observable cognitive capacities are rated. WCPA and AR performance have been found to be significantly associated (Goverover et al., 2019).

Questionnaires Assessing Functional Cognition

While performance-based functional cognitive assessments provide an objective snapshot of a client's performance in a specific context, questionnaires can provide information on a client's functional cognition in general in their everyday life situations. Although issues such as impaired awareness or depression may limit the reliability or validity of these types of measures, they are important for providing the client and/or caregiver perspective and, as discussed throughout this chapter, can provide insight into a person's level of awareness through comparison of self- and informant ratings.

Daily Living Questionnaire (DLQ) (Rosenblum et al., 2017): The DLQ is available freely on www.multicontext.net. Part 1 of the DLQ examines the person's perceptions regarding cognitive difficulty within IADL such as financial management and household activities, as well as participation in social, community, and work activities. Part 2 focuses on the person's perceptions regarding difficulty in EF and memory skills. Part 3 is optional and involves general questions regarding overall ability to function, perceived changes in roles and responsibilities, and degree of satisfaction with what the person needs and wants to do in their daily lives. The DLQ can be administered to both the client and significant other, and the discrepancy between them can be compared. The psychometric characteristics of the DLQ including comparison of healthy people to those with multiple sclerosis have been reported for Parts 1 and 2, however, research on additional populations is needed.

Activity Measure Post-Acute Care (AM-PAC)-Applied Cognitive Scale (Coster et al., 2004): This measure is a clinician or self-reported measure of cognitive-IADL activities. Different forms are available including a short paper form and an online computer adapted version. Scores are standardized and cluster within five functional levels. The AM-PAC is quick and is well suited for an inpatient setting (see resource section).

Behavior Rating Inventory of Executive Function – Adult Form (BRIEF-A) (Roth et al., 2005): The BRIEF-A measures everyday behaviors associated with the domains of EF and has normative data on 1,136 adults ages 18-90 years. It has been validated across a wide variety of diagnostic categories. The BRIEF-A includes 75 items within nine clinical scales: Inhibit, Self-Monitor, Plan/Organize, Shift, Initiate, Task Monitor, Emotional Control, Working Memory, and Organization of Materials. It provides an overall summary score as well as two indices (Behavioral Regulation and Metacognition). The BRIEF-A includes a client form and an informant form. Toglia (2010, 2011) included the use of the BRIEF-A in MC case studies.

Cognitive Self-Efficacy

Cognitive Self-Efficacy Questionnaire (CSEQ) (Toglia & Johnston, 2017): The CSEQ was designed to assess a person's beliefs regarding their ability to recognize, monitor, and manage cognitive symptoms (e.g., cognitive fatigue, slow processing speed, and difficulty organizing information) and everyday challenging cognitive activities (e.g., coordinating schedules or following a group conversation). In addition, it examines the ability to identify and apply strategies to everyday problem situations that involve cognitive skills. The CSEQ includes beliefs about the ability to recognize and manage cognitive lapses and cognitively demanding tasks as well as the ability to identify and self-generate potential strategies. Normative data has been collected on 200 participants (100 under the age of 60 and 100 people over the age of 60) and provides a foundation for interpretation of clinical populations. The CSEQ is freely available on www.multicontext.net.

DISTAL OUTCOME MEASURES

Distal outcomes include broader areas of function such as frequency of participation in social, productive, and community activities, satisfaction with activity patterns, subjective well-being, quality of life, overall activity level, life space, and measures of caregiver strain. Distal outcome measure selection depends on many factors (Whyte, 2006). Examples of such measures that might be considered include the Participation, Objective, Subjective (POPS) (Brown, 2006) the Patient-Reported Outcomes Measurement Information System (PROMIS) or Quality of Life in Neurological Disorders (NeuroQoL) scales (www.healthmeasures.net), and the Activity Card Sort (ACS) (Baum et al., 2008).

SUMMARY

Client-centeredness begins with facilitating client engagement in goal setting and treatment planning. However, client-centered goal setting is not an all-or-none construct and instead occurs on a continuum. Thus, in the MC approach, goal setting is conceptualized as a dynamic process that varies across treatment and individuals. This chapter discussed the impact of various cognitive impairments on goal setting and offered a range of strategies to support cognitive skills and optimize engagement in goal setting. In addition, it discussed the central role of self-awareness in the process of goal setting. MC treatment supports and facilitates the process of goal adjustment. Treatment within the MC approach is designed to help a person self-discover their new cognitive strengths and limitations so that realistic goals can emerge.

Greater engagement in goal setting and an increased ability to identify realistic goals are positive signs that represent desired treatment outcomes.

There are several ways to monitor and document progress and outcomes consistent with the treatment targets and intervention model of the MC approach. This chapter provided methods for rating goals and specific techniques for supporting goal rating in clients with cognitive impairment. It also discussed methods for measuring change from before to after intervention and presented a selection of proximal and distal outcome measures consistent with the MC approach.

KEY POINTS

- The extent of engagement in goal setting can differ between individuals depending on their cognitive abilities, level of awareness, and individual needs.

- Strategies such as narrowing the focus of questions, repeating the same question in a different way, daily goal reminders, pictorial or visual supports, and sub-goaling can support people with cognitive impairment in goal setting.

- Some individuals may not be ready to set realistic goals as they may have not had the opportunity to try to resume previous roles and activities and may be unaware of their strengths and limitations. Enhancing self-awareness through structured activity experiences using the metacognitive framework and mediated learning may be required before an individual can set realistic goals.

- As self-awareness, self-efficacy, or acceptance increase with treatment, goals may be adjusted or changed entirely. This represents progress in treatment.

- Progress in functional goals, strategy use, and awareness can be monitored and documented using formal (e.g., GAS, BGSI-2) and informal goal rating methods.

- Proximal outcomes of the MC approach include strategy use, awareness, functional cognitive performance, and self-efficacy, whereas distal outcomes are broad and can include participation, occupational performance, quality of life, well-being, etc.

- A variety of standardized outcome measures are available that are consistent with the MC approach. Measure selection depends on client- and setting-specific factors.

Chapter 13

The Multicontext Approach: Putting It All Together

Background information, theoretical concepts, and a comprehensive description of each component of the Multicontext (MC) approach were reviewed in this book. Key MC treatment elements were specified, guidelines to operationalize the elements were described, and tools to support implementation of this approach were provided. In addition, assessments of both therapist delivery and client progress were provided. This chapter summarizes the steps of the MC approach and is designed to help therapists review key information and get started with implementing this approach. Suggestions for self-assessment of knowledge of foundational information as well as for practicing delivery of treatment components are provided. Integration of information for treatment planning, challenges to implementation, and frequently asked questions are discussed. Examples of treatment session activities, outlines, and existing treatment protocols further illustrate treatment implementation.

CONTENTS OF CHAPTER 13

Steps of the Multicontext Approach
Learning and Gaining Proficiency in the Multicontext Approach
    Foundational Knowledge and Skills
    Assessment and Synthesis of Assessment Results as a Foundation for Treatment
    Planning and Implementing the Key Treatment Components
    Assessing Multicontext Treatment Delivery, Treatment Response, and Functional Outcomes
What does a Multicontext Treatment Session Look Like?
    Variation with Consistency
    Sample Treatment Protocols
    Practicing a Multicontext Treatment Session
Challenges in Implementing the Multicontext Approach
    Using Guided Learning
    Focusing on the Process Rather than the Task Outcome
    Selecting Activities at the Optimal Level of Challenge
    Clients with Defensive Denial
    Clients with Aphasia
Typical Frequently Asked Questions
Summary and Key Points

STEPS OF THE MULTICONTEXT APPROACH

The steps involved in using the MC approach that have been reviewed throughout this book are summarized in Exhibit 13.1. These are further described in the section below along with suggested methods to learn and gain proficiency in their implementation.

LEARNING AND GAINING PROFICIENCY IN THE MULTICONTEXT APPROACH

Use of the MC approach requires a shift in thinking and practice. Unlike many contemporary approaches in rehabilitation, the initial design of the MC approach integrated principles of transfer and generalization into intervention structure and techniques. Activities are presented horizontally rather than graded vertically, there is a focus on cognitive strategies to manage cognitive lapses and performance errors rather than on task components or functional task skills, and the process of how someone goes about an activity is emphasized rather than the outcome. In contrast to conventional practice, guided learning methods are used instead of direct cues, feedback, or instruction. Implementation of this approach requires an investment of time and effort to shift perspectives, break treatment habits, and learn, practice, and apply the new methods described.

In addition to this book, there are training workshops for the MC approach posted on the www.multicontext.net website. Increases in the frequency of training workshops are planned in the near future. While attending workshops, reading this book, and trying out structured MC activities with clients is a critical beginning, it is not enough. Repeated practice in using these methods, particularly mediated learning techniques, is needed to gain proficiency in the MC approach. The below outline provides guidance in learning and applying the MC approach with corresponding chapters, tools and resources.

Foundational Knowledge and Skills

Learning the MC approach begins with foundational knowledge of cognition, functional cognition, and the influence of activity and environmental demands on cognitive performance. Since MC treatment involves helping a person recognize, understand, and control cognitive lapses and performance errors, it is important to have a full understanding of the types of cognitive symptoms and errors that can occur within activities, as well as the conditions that increase and decrease symptoms. Similarly, knowledge of the multi-dimensional aspects of metacognition and self-awareness and how they interact with self-efficacy and self-identity provides critical foundational information. The Dynamic Comprehensive Model of Awareness (DCMA) provides a theoretical framework for understanding self-awareness and distinguishes between awareness within and outside the context of specific activities.

Additionally, the Dynamic Interactional Model of cognition provides a broad, overarching model for

---

Exhibit 13.1 Steps of the Multicontext Approach

1. *Assessment:* Based on interviews or questionnaires and performance analysis, identify client concerns, error patterns, awareness and strategy use, treatment targets, and expected outcomes.

2. *Treatment Planning*
    a. Plan cognitive strategy use: Identify the types of strategies that are likely to be most effective given the person's error patterns, awareness, and cognitive abilities.
    b. Plan cognitive functional treatment activities: Determine if structured activities will be used, identify activity themes, brainstorm activities, and establish transfer criteria. If feasible, two structured activities are used within each treatment session.
    c. Plan metacognitive framework and mediated learning methods: Depending on the identified treatment targets, consider when and which guided questions will be asked and whether structured self-evaluation will be used.

3. *Implementation:* Use treatment activities in each session within a structured metacognitive framework that uses mediated learning techniques before, during, and/or after activities. End each treatment session with strategy bridging methods.

4. *Tracking and Documenting Client Progress*: Use methods to document observations and track change in treatment targets within and across treatment activities and sessions and to track change in broader functional goals across treatment.

understanding cognition and explains cognitive symptoms as a mismatch between the person's abilities and activity and environmental demands. Performance can be changed by manipulating activity demands, environmental demands, the person's awareness or strategy use, or a combination of all three. The MC approach is based on the Dynamic Interactional Model, but it focuses more specifically on self-awareness within the context of activities and cognitive strategy use while at the same time adjusting activity and environmental demands to be at the optimal level of challenge. This requires application of activity analysis skills to the components of executive function (EF). This background knowledge, summarized in Exhibit 13.2, provides the foundation for performance analysis and assessment as well as for understanding the MC approach.

Assessment and Synthesis of Assessment Results as a Foundation for Treatment

The combination of information from client and/or caregiver interviews, questionnaires or rating scales, and

---

Exhibit 13.2 Gaining Foundational Knowledge and Skills: Advice for the Therapist

Chapter 1: Cognition, Occupational Performance, and Participation

- Be familiar with the definition and importance of functional cognition. This includes the ability to discuss the difference between standardized assessments of cognitive skills and functional cognitive assessment.
- Recognize and explain how cognition can have an impact on all areas of daily function (IADL, work, leisure), behavior, social interactions, self-identity, coping skills, and overall health.

Chapter 2: Functional Cognition: Understanding How Executive Function and Memory Impairments are Expressed in Everyday Life

- Be familiar with the types of cognitive errors observed in functional activities.
- Complete learning activities for Chapter 2 in Appendix A.1-A.6 and develop a solid understanding of how different types of executive function and memory impairments are expressed in everyday life. This is a foundational skill for interpreting observations of performance and choosing treatment activities that match the person's functional cognitive abilities.

Chapter 3: Self-Awareness, Metacognition, and Self-Efficacy

- Identify, describe, and differentiate between different types of awareness.
- Identify the components of online awareness (Exhibit 3.2).
- Be familiar with denial reactions and guidelines for managing them.
- Describe and explain the general principles of awareness training.
- Analyze case scenarios in Appendix A.7 and identify the type of self-awareness deficit.

Chapter 4: The Dynamic Interactional Model of Cognition and Activity and Environmental Demands

- Be familiar with the Dynamic Interactional Model of cognition and complete Appendix A.14.
- Practice manipulating activity directions and characteristics to place different demands on executive function skills (Appendix A.11) and/or practice using pre-made activities in the MC Activity Schedule Module (separate purchase) with a variety of different clients to observe how the same functional materials can be used to address different cognitive performance problems by varying the activity directions and components. The ability to analyze executive function components of activities and how to adjust them provides a foundational skill for analysis of performance during both assessment and treatment.
- Select an activity that is functionally relevant to your client and complete Appendix A.12- A.13.

Chapter 6: Introduction to the Multicontext Treatment Approach

- Be familiar with the goals and key characteristics of the MC approach.

performance analysis provides a strong foundation for MC treatment planning.

The assessment summary form in Appendix B.10 is used to integrate assessment information from different sources as the first step in treatment planning and includes the following:

- *Client's functional cognitive concerns and limitations, strengths, and goals.*
- *Cognitive performance errors or behaviors that go across different activities and contexts*: This includes the error patterns or symptoms that interfere with performance across a number of different tasks as well as the activity characteristics or conditions under which errors are most likely and least likely to occur.
- *Strategies use and effectiveness*: This involves observing how strategies are used during performance, such as initiation, type, frequency, efficiency, and effectiveness of strategies, as well as the ability to self-generate alternate strategies when appropriate. It also involves identifying potential obstacles to effective strategy use.
- *Self-awareness both outside and inside the context of an activity:* This includes the ability to recognize strengths and limitations, set realistic goals, self-correct performance within an activity, identify task challenges before, during, or after activities, determine strategies or task methods used, and appraise task difficulty compared to actual performance.
- *Potential for change*: This includes responsiveness to probing, questions, or mediation from others. The test-teach-retest dynamic method can be used to make this determination if needed.
- *Initial focus of treatment and treatment targets for change.*

- Chapter 5 reviews several assessment tools that can be used to gather the basic needed information. Tools such as the DIM Performance Analysis Guide and the Weekly Calendar Planning Activity (WCPA) incorporate analysis of strategy use and awareness. Performance analysis also helps the therapist identify cognitive functional activities and activity characteristics that are at the "optimal level of challenge" (not too hard and not too easy), which then guides the selection of treatment activities. Exhibit 13.3 summarizes key assessment tools to practice, learn and use with clients.

Planning and Implementing the Key Treatment Components

An MC treatment planning worksheet is included in Appendix C.2 for therapist's use (completed example Appendix D.12). This form can be helpful in guiding the therapist to synthesize information from assessment and think through each MC treatment component before beginning treatment.

Cognitive Strategy Use

The MC approach focuses on methods to manage cognitive performance errors that are observed across different situations. This requires understanding the client's specific performance problems, characteristics of strategies, and analysis of strategy use.

Although guided learning methods are used in the MC approach to help the client generate their own strategies, the therapist should use their knowledge of strategies to identify or hypothesize about strategies that would be most effective for the observed performance errors across different activities. The types of activity conditions that are most likely to elicit these strategies and the type of strategy

---

Exhibit 13.3 Assessment and Synthesis of Results: Advice for the Therapist

- Use DIM Performance Analysis Guide with a client and a selected relevant activity (Appendix B.3).
- Use DIM Analysis of Task Errors: Identify a task that is relevant to a client. Divide the task into steps and analyze performance (Appendix B.6).
- Use WCPA with a client and analyze results following the WCPA manual (requires separate purchase).
- *Additional:* Contextual Memory Test (CMT-2) (available for free online); cognitive performance observation tool with a selected task (Appendix B.4); Multiple Smart Phone Tasks (B.8); Upper Body Dressing Error Analysis (UBDEA) (B.9).
- Practice synthesizing and summarizing assessment results of a client using the MC Assessment Summary form (Appendix B.10).

training that would be most appropriate (strategy-specific, situational, or flexible) should also be specified.

Identifying effective strategies beforehand can help the therapist structure and guide the strategy generation process if it is needed as described in Chapter 10. For example, if the client chooses an inefficient strategy, the therapist should not intervene but instead should help the client reflect on strategy effectiveness and generate alternate strategies. Questions can be posed in a way that leads the client to the pre-identified effective strategy (e.g., What type of image or picture can you think of to help you use "just right timing"?). The therapist should also identify and plan to address any potential obstacles to effective strategy use (e.g., poor recall, awareness, self-efficacy, lack of initiation). Exhibit 13.4 summarizes ways to apply information on strategies from Chapter 7.

Cognitive Functional Treatment Activities

A series of structured treatment activities that challenge the client's functional cognition and provide the context for gaining awareness of performance and strategy use is recommended for those who are not fully aware of their cognitive performance errors. These treatment activities are structured horizontally in the MC approach so that cognitive demands remain constant while transfer distance and breadth is gradually increased. This requires familiarity with a wide range of functional cognitive activities as well as skill in adjusting and manipulating activity characteristics to promote transfer.

Structured activities provide consistent cognitive demands to elicit similar error patterns that can be managed with the same strategies. This builds awareness and understanding of abilities and limitations by providing repeated opportunities to recognize that the same errors are interfering with performance across situations. It also helps the person recognize that the same strategies are effective in reducing performance errors across different activities.

If the person is fully aware, has identified specific personal goals, and easily perceives connections between activity experiences, structured activities may not be necessary, and a series of self-chosen functional cognitive activities can be used. Alternatively, the MC activity modules (Appendix D.5-D.6) provide pre-made parallel structured activities that can be combined to create horizontal activity transfer continuums for a variety of clients (purchased separately). Exhibit 13.5 outlines the steps in selecting treatment activities and situating them along a horizontal continuum.

Metacognitive Framework and Mediated Learning Methods

The MC approach focuses on online awareness of performance within the context of an activity. Chapter 9 provides general information on metacognitive strategy interventions and guidelines for guided and mediated learning methods. Chapter 10 provides specific guidelines for using a metacognitive framework within MC treatment. This includes the types of guided questions that should be asked and mediated learning techniques (reflection of observations, re-stating, reframing, rephrasing, or interpretation of client statements) that can be used before, during, and immediately after an activity as needed, to help

---

Exhibit 13.4 Observing and Analyzing Strategy Use: Advice for the Therapist

- Analyze the strategies that you use when faced with cognitively challenging activities (Appendix A.5).
- Think about a strategy you are currently using with a client and complete the Worksheet for Analysis of Strategy Attributes (Appendix B.11). Think about how the same strategy might be used differently by changing the attributes.
- Be familiar with the range, variety, and types of cognitive strategies in advance (Chapter 7 and Appendix D.1).

Choose a client, and …

- Think about possible strategies that would help the client control or reduce errors *across* different activities.
- Think about the type of strategy intervention that is most appropriate for the client (task-specific, strategy-specific, situational, or flexible strategy use) (Table 7.3).
- Identify and create a plan to address obstacles to effective strategy use (Table 7.4).
- Consider characteristics that affect the quality of strategy use (Table 7.5) and use this as a guide for observing and analyzing strategy use.
- Practice using the checklists in Appendix B.12 (Therapist Worksheet for Observing Types of Strategies) and Appendix B.13 (Therapist Checklist for Observation and Analysis of Strategy Use).
- Complete the strategy section of the treatment planning worksheet (Appendix C.2).

> **Exhibit 13.5 Creating a Horizontal Treatment Activity Continuum: Advice for the Therapist**
>
> 1. *Ensure that you have access to a wide variety of activities* (see Chapter 8 and Appendix D.3). This may involve creating activity kits or using those that are already developed and organizing activities in your clinic so they can be readily used.
> 2. *Identify the activity theme:* Specify the cognitive demands that remain consistent throughout a series of activities so that the same or similar strategies can be practiced (Appendix D.2).
> 3. *Brainstorm activities:* Identify and describe several different activities that can be used within the activity theme to help the client recognize error patterns in performance and/or practice similar strategies.
>   - Activities should vary in motor demands, type of materials, and contexts.
>   - Cognitive demands (e.g., amount of detail, number of steps) should remain at the same level of difficulty. Activities should be at the optimal level of challenge; for example, the client should be able to complete 70-75% without errors or assistance.
>   - Keep the individual's lifestyle, interests, activity preferences, goals, and personality in mind.
>   - Incorporate physical goals into cognitive activities when feasible (standing, walking, reaching, fine motor activities).
> 4. *Establish transfer criteria:* Specify how the physical (surface) characteristics of the task will be gradually changed without significantly increasing cognitive complexity level. Arrange activities across the transfer continuum (guideline only, not fixed categories): (Appendix C.4)
>   - *Very Similar or Near Transfer:* Alternate forms of the same activities, change 1-2 task parameters.
>   - *Somewhat Similar or Intermediate Transfer:* Looks somewhat different than the
>   - original activity change 3-6 task parameters.
>   - *Different or Far Transfer:* Looks completely different from the original activity, change all or nearly all task parameters.

the person build online awareness, use strategies, and make connections between activity experiences.

First, review and become familiar with the different mediation guidelines (see Table 9.3-9.4 and Appendices D.7-D.8) and the treatment session framework. Consider when guided questions will be asked (before, during, and/or after activities) and identify the questions that might be used. The focus of guided questions should match the identified treatment targets. Determine if structured self-assessments or self-ratings will be used and what strategy bridging methods will be used. The treatment session framework is summarized below:

- *Pre-Activity Discussion:* Focused on analyzing activity demands, making connections to previous activities, anticipating possible challenges, and generating strategies or error prevention methods.
- *During Activity Mediation*: Stop and review questions focused on either error detection or effectiveness and efficiency of task methods or strategies.
- *Post-Activity Discussion:* Focused on either self-recognition of errors or assessment of the effectiveness of task methods or strategies used.
- *End of Session Strategy Bridging:* Focused on relating strategies to previous and future activity experiences. Journaling or strategy worksheets can be used.

Although Chapter 10 provides specific guidelines and resources for using guided learning and the metacognitive framework, reading Chapter 10 is not enough. As mentioned previously, shifting from traditional modes of practice (e.g., direct instruction, cueing) to implementing this approach is challenging and takes practice and self-reflection. It is important for you to notice when and how you question or use prompts. The MC approach avoids use of task-specific questions, whenever possible. The content of questions gradually progresses from a *general* focus to *performance or symptom-specific* or to *task-specific*, if needed (Table 9.4, Differences in Type and Content of Guided Questions). This type of questioning needs to become automatic for the therapist. An investment of time and effort is needed to become proficient in this method. Exhibit 13.6 includes tips from therapists who use the MC approach to help facilitate the transition to using mediated learning methods.

> **Exhibit 13.6 Practicing Mediated Learning Methods: Advice for the Therapist**
>
> - Practice using guided learning methods and the metacognitive framework with a variety of clients. Use the pre- and post- Guided Anticipation and Strategy Generation questions in Appendices C.7-C.8. Be sure the questions flow like a conversation or discussion and not a formal interview.
> - Practice guided questioning with a colleague. Use the role play scenarios in Appendix A.16 or use your own scenarios and have a colleague be the client.
> - Keep a list of the questions or prompts that you use during a session so you can identify what you are doing and what needs more attention. Compare and analyze the questions you used to the guidelines in Chapter 10. Or analyze the type of questions or prompts that you used using Table 9.4 (Differences in Type and Content of Guided Questions).
> - Be aware of common errors and try to avoid them (Exhibit 11.1).
> - Write down a list of helpful guided questions or reframing statements (cheat sheet) and keep them out for reference during initial use of the approach.
> - Make it a habit to pause for 10 seconds before cueing a client. This will help in self-monitoring personal cueing style. It also helps the therapist inhibit their tendency to "jump in" and help.
> - Video or audio record your treatment sessions and review and reflect on your implementation of guided questioning and mediation. Think about if other questions or mediated techniques could have been used (Appendix C.12). Use the MC Treatment Fidelity Tool (Appendix C.13) to guide a structured self-reflection on methods used.

Assessing Multicontext Treatment Delivery, Treatment Response, and Functional Outcomes

MC treatment elements were further specified using the RTSS framework included in Appendix D.10 and described in Chapter 11. Measurement of treatment effectiveness involves ensuring that essential intervention elements are implemented as intended by the therapist (treatment fidelity). It also involves identifying specific treatment targets for improvement that are directly affected by intervention elements. The RTSS was used as a foundation for the development of tools to measure the fidelity of therapist treatment delivery and client treatment response. Specific proximal treatment measures for tracking, monitoring, and documenting client response presented in Chapter 11 were differentiated from broader functional cognitive goals and outcome measures discussed in Chapter 12. While Chapter 11 focused on progress occurring within MC treatment sessions and across treatment activities, Chapter 12 discussed broader goals and outcome measures used to examine change before and after treatment.

Chapter 12 also discussed goal setting in the MC approach as a dynamic process that is adjusted and revised across MC treatment as awareness and acceptance change. Increased engagement in goal setting, increased specificity of goals, goal adjustment, or the addition of new attainable goals are viewed as positive treatment outcomes. The use of goal rating, and goal attainment scaling, are optional components that can be used within the MC approach to track progress and measure functional outcomes.

Exhibit 13.7 summarizes steps in measuring client and treatment effectiveness, therapist fidelity, and outcomes.

WHAT DOES A MULTICONTEXT TREATMENT SESSION LOOK LIKE?

Variation with Consistency

While some intervention programs offer a step-by-step prescribed outline of what to do in each treatment session, the MC approach provides guidelines that are tailored to client needs and treatment settings. The flexibility of the MC approach is an advantage and allows treatment to be adjusted to meet the needs of different clients and settings. This permits wide clinical applications across ages, clinical problems, levels of severity, and contexts. At the same time, this presents challenges in treatment delivery because it increases complexity and demands a higher level of knowledge, skill, and clinical reasoning from the therapist.

MC treatment involves embedding structured or self-chosen activities into a metacognitive framework. There is a consistent focus on optimizing strategy use and self-monitoring skills across different activities and situations; however, the treatment focus, targets, and techniques used differ depending on the needs, abilities, and responsiveness of the client. For example, structured functional cognitive activities are recommended to build an understanding of cognitive performance strengths and limitations, but they are not appropriate for all clients. Some clients benefit

CHAPTER 13   The Multicontext Approach: Putting It All Together   183

> **Exhibit 13.7 Assessing and Documenting Treatment Delivery, Client Progress and Outcomes: Advice for the Therapist**
>
> *Chapter 11: Multicontext Approach: Assessing Treatment Delivery and Client Response*
>
> - Use the MC Treatment Fidelity tool (Appendix C.13) after treatment sessions, role plays, or as you are reviewing video or audio sessions to review and rate your own delivery.
> - Use the MC Treatment Fidelity tool during supervision of others.
> - Identify MC treatment targets for change (Exhibit 11.2) (see RTSS framework – Appendix D.10).
> - After Session: Use the MC Treatment Session Summary Worksheet to document observations and track progress *within* treatment (Appendix C.11).
> - Rate performance on Pre- and Post-activity questions using Rating scales in Appendices B.14-B.16.
> - Use the MC metacognitive framework to structure treatment progress notes of sessions.
>
> *Chapter 12: Goal Setting and Measuring Functional Outcomes*
>
> - Practice techniques for facilitating engagement in goal setting such as narrowing the focus of questions, repeating the same question in a different way, providing choices from a pre-made goal sheet, daily goal reminders, pictorial or visual supports, and sub-goaling (Appendix C.24-C.27).
> - Select a client that has potential for changes in self-awareness. Track goals and goal adjustments or revisions across treatment (Appendix C.28).
> - Practice developing and using a goal rating or attainment scale for a targeted strategy or self-monitoring technique (See sample Appendix D.17, blank form, C.29).
> - Identify measures (post-treatment measures) that could be used to measure outcome of MC treatment.

from activities that gradually differ in physical features (horizontal transfer continuum) because it makes it easier for them to recognize cues necessary to apply cognitive strategies. Other clients spontaneously recognize the application of strategies across a wide range of activities so that treatment activities do not need to be structured horizontally.

Similarly, the metacognitive framework has three phases, but only the post-activity discussion phase is used with all clients. The extent that mediation or pre-activity questioning is used depends on self-awareness and responses to questions. In addition, the type of strategies that are promoted and how they are trained also differ. Therapists must use their understanding of EF and cognitive skills to guide clients in the use of effective strategies, but these strategies are not fixed or prescribed. Also, in some instances, treatment focuses on a single strategy, whereas in other situations strategy training involves use of multiple strategies.

In addition, the MC approach is dynamic and can vary within treatment for an individual client. The emphasis, methods, and techniques used can change across a treatment program. For example, the type, content, focus, and frequency of guided questions often change as awareness or strategy use improves. This is illustrated in a sample outline of MC treatment sessions in Exhibit 13.8. The session outline illustrates that treatment may initially have a focus on improving awareness of performance errors during or after an activity. As this improves, treatment progresses to a focus on anticipating challenges, generating strategies, and assessing strategy effectiveness and efficiency. In the latter phase of treatment, strategy reinforcement, practice, and generalization across activities are emphasized. Although the same post-discussion questions (addressing all areas) are used, the emphasis and time spent on each area can differ across treatment. Similarly, the use of pre-activity guided questions and mediation can vary as clients progress. In some cases, treatment may focus entirely on strategy efficiency across sessions; in other cases, the focus of treatment remains on awareness of performance errors.

Sample Treatment Protocols

Despite its variations, there are consistent elements that go across all MC interventions. As described and illustrated in Chapters 14 and 15, the principles and key elements of the MC approach can be applied in different settings and client populations. A sample generic treatment session outline is presented on the bottom of page 185. Additional protocols that have been implemented in research and clinical practice follow on p.185-186. As you review the treatment protocol outlines, identify the similarities and differences.

Exhibit 13.8 Sample Outline of Multicontext Treatment Sessions

Session Focus	Session Outline
Sessions 1-2 Observe process. Focus on understanding the person's perspectives and building recognition of performance errors after the task.	**Session 1, Activity 1** • *Introduce activity:* Discuss how it relates to client goals. • *Structured activity at optimal challenge level:* Observe activity process, no mediation. • *Post-activity:* Structured self-assessment and guided discussion focusing on challenges encountered (i.e., what went right and what could be improved). **Session 1, Activity 2** • *Pre-activity:* Discussion is eliminated because client did not recognize errors after activity. • *Alternate structured activity at optimal challenge level:* Observe process and mediate within activity because client had difficulty reflecting back on performance. • *Post activity:* Structured self-assessment and guided questions with a focus on things to watch out for (e.g., tendency to miss or skip over information). • **End of Session:** Strategy worksheet, journaling is completed at the end along with guided questions (e.g., What did I learn? What would I do differently next time? What activities are similar?).
Sessions 3-5 Continue building awareness of error patterns after activities. Focus on error prevention and monitoring strategies. Self-monitoring of errors within activities.	**Session 4, Activity 1** • *Introduce activity* • *Pre-activity:* Pre-discussion is used because client vaguely recognizes difficulties after activities in session 3. Questions focus on similarities to previous session activities, identifying possible challenges, and staying a step ahead. Strategy generation questions are asked, but inefficient or inappropriate strategies are not corrected. • *Structured activities continue:* Focus on self-monitoring within the activity, with mediation as needed. • *Post-activity:* Guided discussion on error patterns, things to watch out for, and methods to stay a step ahead. **Session 4, Activity 2** • *Pre-activity:* Guided questions on connection to previous activities are eliminated to see if client spontaneously perceives similarities between activities. Questions focus on identification of challenges and strategy generation. • *Structured activity:* Same focus as above. Therapist and client decide if structured activities should continue or if client would like to self-choose their own activity. • *Post-activity:* Same as above. Structured evaluation methods are eliminated after session 4 because client self-recognizes errors. • **End of Session:** Action plan, strategy worksheet or journaling is completed along with strategy bridging questions.

Exhibit 13.8 Sample Outline of Multicontext Treatment Sessions *(continued)*

Session Focus	Session Outline
Sessions 6-7 Focus on strategy initiation, effectiveness, and efficiency.	**Session 7, Activity 1** • *Introduction* • *Pre activity:* Focus on strategy generation. Identification of challenge questions are eliminated because person identifies challenges and perceives strategy need. • *Self-chosen activities or provide activity choice:* Mediation focuses on adjusting task methods and increasing efficiency of strategies. • *Post-activity:* Guided discussion with a focus on building strategy awareness, assessing effectiveness of strategies used, and generating alternate strategies. **Session 7, Activity 2** • Same as above. • **End of Session:** Action plan or journaling is completed along with strategy bridging questions.
Sessions 8-10 Focus on strategy efficiency and connections to other activities.	**Activity 1** • *Pre-activity:* Discussion is eliminated. • *Self-chosen activity:* No mediation. • *Post-activity:* Guided discussion on awareness of methods used and how or why they worked. Strategy use is reinforced with a greater focus on connections and generalization to previous sessions and everyday life activities. **Activity 2** • Same as above if feasible. • **End of Session:** Strategy bridging questions and development of specific cognitive action plan.

Generic Multicontext Treatment Session Outline

1. *Introduce activity.*
2. *Pre-Activity Discussion*: Skipped in session 1. Guided questions focused on connections with previous experiences (optional), analyzing activity demands, anticipating possible challenges, and generating strategies or error prevention methods (Appendix C.7).
3. *Observe and Analyze Strategy Use During Activity*: Observe the process of how the person goes about the activity. Use observation worksheets to assist in structuring observations (B.4, B.13-14). Mediate if needed (e.g., Stop and review questions focused on either error detection or strategy use).
4. *Post-Activity Discussion*: Structured self-assessment (optional), guided questions directed at identification of challenges, or effectiveness of task methods or strategies used (Appendix C.8).
5. Repeat above steps with a second activity if feasible to observe immediate carryover.
6. *End of Session*: Use strategy bridging methods such as cognitive action plan, journaling, or strategy worksheets (Appendix C.9, C.14-C.18).

Treatment Protocol: Chronic Traumatic Brain Injury (Toglia et al., 2010, 2011)

Participants: 3 years or more post-TBI, aged 27-50 years, able to attend for at least 30 minutes, difficulty in managing multi-step instrumental activities of daily living

(IADL), not currently receiving cognitive rehabilitation or OT services, at least a rating of 5 on the Functional Independence Measure (FIM) Communication scale.

Outcome Measures: Self-Regulation Skills Interview (SSRI) (Ownsworth, et al., 2000), Executive Function Performance Bill Paying subtest (EFPT) (Baum et al., 2008), Multiple Errands Test (MET) (Knight et al., 2002), Behavior Rating Inventory of Executive Function (BRIEF) (Roth et al., 2005), Awareness Questionnaire (AQ) (Sherer, 2004), and the Canadian Occupational Performance Measure (COPM) (Law et al., 2014). (See Chapter 12 for measures.)

1. *Treatment Setting*: Day program
2. *Key Treatment Protocol Features:*
3. *Treatment session duration*: 75 minutes
4. *Frequency of treatment sessions*: 2 times per week
5. *Length of treatment program:* 9 treatment sessions (4-5 weeks)
6. Structured activities for the first four sessions were the same for all participants.
7. All activities involved following complex directions that included specific criteria or rule constraints.
8. All activities had a checklist of questions for self-assessment of performance.
9. *Strategies emphasized:* simplifying, creating a list, breaking information down, or for those unable to create a list, strategies included asking for a simplified list, and using strategies to ensure accuracy in following the list.
10. Strategy-specific training was used for two clients, and flexible strategy use was used for two other clients.
11. After Session 4, clients were asked to choose their own treatment activity. If they had difficulty, they were asked to choose from a pre-made list of activities.
12. *Metacognitive Framework:* Pre and post discussion used in all sessions. Mediation during activity was used with all clients as needed.
13. Journaling was used at the end of all sessions.

Treatment Protocol: Inpatient Acquired Brain Injury (Jaywant et al., 2020; current ongoing trial)

Participants: Stroke, brain tumor, or TBI on an acute inpatient rehabilitation unit, aged 24-76 years, ranged from 4 days to 4 weeks post-injury. All were cognitively independent in self-care activities with FIM Comprehension and Expression score of 4 or greater, impaired performance on at least one screening measure of EF, and able to attend to a cognitive task for at least 10 minutes.

Outcome Measures: SSRI, WCPA (see Chapter 12)

Treatment Setting: Acute Rehabilitation Unit in an academic medical center

Key Treatment Protocol Features

1. *Treatment session duration*: 30-45 minutes, implemented within the context of routine OT sessions.
2. *Frequency of treatment sessions:* Daily
3. *Length of treatment program:* Varied with length of stay but involved a median of seven treatment sessions.
4. All clients received two 10-minute brief activities in each session.
5. All clients received six structured activities for at least the first 3-4 sessions.
6. Level 1 activities from the Schedule, Menu, and Business MC Activity modules were used with the module supplementary activities.
7. Therapists chose Level 1 activities from the pre-made MC Activity modules for the following themes: searching and locating, keeping track, and shifting. The theme and activities chosen depended on client error patterns.
8. Activities incorporated client physical goals (standing, ambulating, reaching, fine motor).
9. All structured activities had self-evaluation samples so participants could check their own work.
10. *Strategies emphasized*: verbal rehearsal, self-talk, self-monitoring, creating external cues to keep track, planning ahead, taking pauses for self-checks.
11. Strategy training focused on either situation-specific or flexible strategy use across clients.
12. Strategy worksheets and journaling were not used due to time constraints.
13. *Metacognitive Framework:* Pre-discussion questions were not used in Session 1.
14. End of session strategy bridging questions were used during the mid-to-end phases of treatment since the initial sessions focused on awareness. Strategy worksheets or journaling was not used due to time constraints.

Treatment Protocol: Parkinson's Disease (Foster et al., 2017, and current ongoing randomized pilot)

Participants: Community-dwelling people with Parkinson's disease without dementia with subjective cognitive concerns.

Outcome Measures: SRSI, CSEQ, WCPA, BGSI-2 (See Chapter 12)

Treatment Setting: Participants' homes

Key Treatment Protocol Features:

1. *Treatment session duration:* 60 minutes
2. *Frequency of treatment sessions:* once per week
3. *Length of treatment program:* 10 sessions (10 weeks)
4. All participants received at least five structured activities for the first three sessions.
5. Therapists selected Level 3 activities from the pre-made MC Activity modules.
6. The main activity theme involved complex questions requiring organization and planning (see example Appendix D.6).
7. All structured activities had self-evaluation samples so participants could check their own work.
8. *Strategies emphasized:* simplifying, breaking down information, planning ahead, self-monitoring
9. *Metacognitive Framework:* Pre discussion not used in Session 1. Post discussion was used in all sessions. Mediation during activity was used with all clients as needed.
10. Strategy bridging questions and cognitive strategy action plans were used at the end of each session.

The MC treatment protocols above illustrate differences in duration, length of treatment sessions, and types of treatment activities. Each protocol was conducted in a different setting with clients who had neurological disorders but differed in age, length of onset, and diagnosis. Despite the differences, all protocols involved use of (a) structured activities in initial sessions, followed by self-chosen or activity choices as treatment progressed, (b) two structured activities in each session, (c) metacognitive framework and mediated learning techniques, (d) a focus on strategies, (e) structured self-assessment, or checking responses against completed activity samples, answers, or checklists, (f) end of session strategy bridging questions, journaling or action plans.

Practicing a Multicontext Treatment Session

MC treatment sessions involve functional cognitive activities embedded within a structured metacognitive framework. If feasible, two brief activities within one treatment session are recommended. A sample treatment session that uses two structured activities from the MC Schedule Module (Toglia, 2017) is included in Appendix C.6. The treatment activities are embedded within guided questions asked before and after each activity. Strategy bridging questions for use at the end of the session are included. The client directions, activity, and guided questions are reproducible and can be copied and trialed with an appropriate client (activity at just-right level of challenge) using MC treatment principles and guidelines.

The sample MC activities require the person to recall items from a list while they search in cabinets and closets to retrieve information that needs to be written on the list. This activity example places cognitive demands on keeping track or holding information in mind while searching and locating information (activity theme). The activities' difficulty can be increased or decreased to meet the level of the client by adjusting the number of items on the list.

Depending on their cognitive abilities and limitations, two people can demonstrate different error patterns or have problems with this activity for varied reasons. For example, one client may miss information on the list or repeatedly re-read information because of a difficulty holding information in mind (working memory) while another person may become easily sidetracked or distracted by irrelevant items as they search in cabinets and may choose incorrect or extraneous items (inhibition). The therapist must carefully observe how the person goes about doing the activity. Specific guidance and mediation for error recognition or strategy generation and use depend on error patterns and behaviors that are observed.

CHALLENGES IN IMPLEMENTING THE MULTICONTEXT APPROACH

As described above and throughout this book, the MC approach is a complex multicomponent intervention that varies with the response and needs of the client. Although there is a consistent framework as illustrated with examples of protocols, the MC approach is highly dependent on the skills and clinical reasoning of the therapist for intervention delivery. The therapist observes, analyzes, interprets, and mediates all at the same time. Based on client responses, the therapist often makes on-the-spot decisions about how to proceed or what to say or do next. Therapist training and fidelity (Chapter 11) is therefore critical for ensuring that the MC approach is carried out as intended (Toglia et al., 2020).

Practitioners have described several specific challenges in implementing the MC approach that are discussed below. The most common challenge involves use of mediated learning methods and shifts in practice.

Using Guided Learning

One therapist indicated that it was difficult for her to avoid the tendency to talk too much or to jump in quickly when someone was having difficulty. It took time for her to feel more comfortable with silence, sitting back to observe the process, and allowing time for a client to struggle and figure out solutions themselves. A common concern that therapists express is *not knowing when to jump in or how much to say* (Toglia, et al., 2020). A general rule is that *the less said, the better* because the aim is to help a person learn to solve problems and generate strategies on their own. At the same time, frustration and negative emotional responses need to be avoided, so there is a balance.

Focusing on the Process Rather than the Task Outcome

As one therapist stated, "It doesn't matter if the task is not finished. It's more about the process... rather than the end product and it took time for me to realize how valuable that was" (Toglia et al., 2020, p. 369). An emphasis on the task process rather than the end product requires a shift in thinking. Therapists have indicated that fitting two activities within a session can be challenging with time constraints. Although task completion may be desired, it is not always necessary to complete both activities. The focus of treatment is on learning from activity experiences. For example, a person might realize that they went about the activity the wrong way because they overfocused on parts of the directions. This is an opportunity to help the person generate alternate strategies for ensuring directions are fully understood and that the overall goal is clear. At this point, rather than continuing with the same activity, it would be appropriate to stop and switch to another similar activity. This provides the opportunity for the person to start fresh and apply what has just been learned.

Two treatment activities within a session allow for repeated practice in identifying challenges and using strategies. It also provides the opportunity to examine carryover of learning. This requires a large assortment of functionally relevant activities and materials as discussed in Chapter 8.

Selecting Activities at the Optimal Level of Challenge

Another challenge that therapists have identified is selecting treatment activities at the optimal level of challenge. Performance in people with cognitive impairments can fluctuate with many factors including fatigue, emotional status, time of day, and the cumulative effects of activities. It is important to get a sense of how the person feels before treatment. If inconsistency in performance has been observed, it is important to investigate factors that might be contributing to variability. A quick rating scale for fatigue, mood, or mental sharpness can help the therapist judge the person's level prior to treatment. There are times, however, that activities may be easier or more difficult than desired. Activity analysis skills that are part of the core of occupational therapy are required to make on-the-spot adjustments when needed.

Clients with Defensive Denial

Finally, therapists have also expressed challenges in using the MC approach in people with defensive denial. People who respond to guided questions with resistance or hostility may not be well suited for this approach. Therapists are encouraged to address the person's physical or other goals first to develop a therapeutic rapport while gently introducing cognitive functional activities. Pre-activity questions often need to be eliminated. A focus is not on identification of challenges but on awareness of methods that contribute to success. This focus can sometimes engage those who might otherwise be hostile and defensive, but if resistance persists, a different approach may be warranted (see Chapter 3).

Clients with Aphasia

Limitations of the MC approach include heavy dependence on communication and language. Therefore, the MC approach is not well suited for people with moderate to severe aphasia. Although methods can be adapted for those with expressive aphasia (e.g., providing choices, simple rating scales, pictorial representations for responses to questions), those with significant comprehension difficulties require an alternate approach.

TYPICAL FREQUENTLY ASKED QUESTIONS

What is the frequency of MC treatment?

This depends on the client and setting and has ranged from daily treatment in an inpatient setting to 1-3 times per week in outpatient settings. Outpatient treatment may need to begin three times a week to obtain carryover between sessions. Gradually frequency can be decreased to once or twice a week.

What is the duration of a treatment session?

The duration of treatment has ranged from 30 to 90 minutes, depending on the setting and clients. In inpatient settings, brief 5- and 10-minute functional cognitive treatment activities have been designed so that MC treatment can be used within a 30-minute session. In outpatient settings, a 45-60 minute session is recommended.

How long is an MC treatment program?

In general, a minimum of a 9-12 session program is recommended; however, more or fewer sessions may be indicated depending on the client and setting. A gradual decrease in the frequency of treatment with continued follow-up is recommended when it is feasible rather than an abrupt stop. This provides the opportunity for the therapist to ensure and probe for maintenance of gains, promotes further generalization, and provides continued support for clients as new or unexpected life challenges arise.

Is awareness required for implementation of the MC approach?

Improved *online self-awareness of performance* is a goal of the MC approach. It is not required for the start of treatment, but there should be potential for gain in this area. By the third or fourth treatment session, some indications of performance changes (changes in strategy use, self-monitoring skills, or error detection skills) should be observed; otherwise, alternate treatment approaches should be considered. Additional intervention methods for individuals with low self-awareness are discussed in Chapter 14. It should be noted as discussed in Chapter 3 that limited online awareness of performance is different from acknowledgment of problems in an interview. Unawareness within an interview does *not* preclude use of the MC approach.

When are activities increased in difficulty? How do you know when to increase difficulty level of activities?

Activities are typically increased in difficulty when the person has demonstrated application of strategy use across near, intermediate, or far transfer activities that are approximately at the same level of difficulty. Some clients immediately see connections between far transfer tasks within the initial 1-2 sessions, while others require a series of tasks that represent near transfer distance (5-7 sessions) before strategy transfer is observed within similar tasks. In the latter case, treatment complexity may not be increased within the treatment time frame. As complexity or difficulty level is increased, a temporary decline in strategy use may be observed. It should be noted that effective strategy use is tied to task difficulty level. The MC approach improves awareness and strategy use in activities and situations that are within optimal levels of challenge. If activities considerably exceed the person's abilities, strategy use may be ineffective. Therefore, it is important to help the person and others understand the conditions in which strategy use is most effective. This is further described in Chapter 7-8.

Why does treatment start with structured activities instead of asking the person to choose activities?

Structured activities are used to build online self-awareness of performance by providing repeated opportunities for the person to recognize and self-assess error patterns across activities. As awareness increases, greater engagement in goal setting and selection of treatment activities occurs and are viewed as indicators of increased awareness or acceptance. It is important to note that structured activities are not used with all clients. If the client has good awareness and specific self-identified goals, structured activities are not used. Structured activities are also a tool that can be used to repeatedly practice generating and using strategies effectively. Since these activities are functionally relevant, most clients have rated high enjoyment and satisfaction with them (Jaywant et al., 2020). However, if the client does not perceive the relevance or value of an activity, it should not be used. Functional cognition can be addressed with nearly any cognitive IADL or daily life activity.

It should be noted that the MC approach always incorporates the client's functional goals (including physical goals), preferences, and experiences into activities. At the start of treatment, however, many clients with cognitive impairments do not have a full understanding of their abilities and limitations. Goals are often vague and overly general. While techniques can be used to help a person break down goals and identify specific activities, this can take multiple sessions and require extensive guidance, rephrasing, and direction from the therapist. These techniques are therefore more commonly used within treatment as awareness begins to emerge (as the result of structured activity experiences) rather than at the very beginning of treatment. Goal setting is viewed as a dynamic process that changes across treatment. Improvements in goal identification, specificity, or revisions are considered positive treatment outcomes as indicated above.

Questions Related to Strategy Use (also see Appendix D.7)

What if the person generates strategies but doesn't use them or uses them ineffectively?

It has been commonly observed that people can generate strategies before they are able to use them effectively. As a person becomes involved in activities, habitual ways of doing things may take over. It can take practice to learn to do things differently or to think in new ways. Strategy learning can require developing new mental habits and this sometimes involves readjusting or inhibiting previous methods that were used to approach activities. Greater opportunities for strategy practice might be needed.

Common difficulties in strategy execution can also be related to difficulty in shifting actions or responses. Assuming that the person is generally aware that things are not going smoothly or efficiently within an activity, the focus of intervention might need to be on recognizing when they are "stuck" within an activity or when the method they are using is not working as well as it could be. The next step is helping the person stop and evaluate the effectiveness of methods within the activity. This involves helping the person understand why their methods or strategies are not working and generating alternate options or plans. An emphasis may be needed on creating a backup plan or generating alternate strategies or task methods before activities.

Alternatively, the cognitive load of activities may be too high. As a person is involved in an activity, cognitive resources and attention are devoted to doing the activity. If the activity is too effortful or challenging, the use of strategies may further inhibit performance because strategy use itself can require additional cognitive resources. In these situations, simplifying or grading the activity complexity downward might be needed.

What if the person does not initiate strategies spontaneously?

Lack of strategy initiation can be related to lack of perceived need (poor ability to assess task challenge in relation to abilities) or to general difficulty in initiation and the ability to get started in activities (see Chapter 2). Lack of strategy initiation can also be related to depression, low self-efficacy, lack of acceptance, resistance to change one's ways of doing things, or an activity that is above the individual's processing capacity. The reason for the lack of spontaneous strategy initiation needs to be sorted out to determine the best approach.

If the lack of strategy use is related to decreased awareness, self-awareness, and anticipation of the need to use strategies should be the initial focus of intervention. If decreased spontaneous strategy use is part of an error pattern observed across activities, the following could be considered:

1. Consider starting treatment with single strategy training.
2. Increase automaticity of the strategy to help the person use the strategy as a mental habit. This requires intense practice and strategy reminders or use of *if-then* statements (implementation intentions; see Chapter 7) to increase automaticity.
3. Increase the saliency of cues for strategy initiation in the environment. For example, alarm messages, timers, text message reminders, pictures or video message reminders. One client that enjoyed music chose specific tunes to help her get started and persist with different activities.
4. Guide the person in identifying things that help cue actions (e.g., things that help me get started, things that would help me remember to make a list).
5. Help the person create an action plan for things that can help them get started or get going.

What if the person does not show carryover of strategies?

This may be related to poor recall and lack of continuity between treatment sessions, or it might be related to other factors including lack of a perceived need to use strategies or belief that strategies will not help. It is important to understand the reasons for lack of carryover or obstacles to strategy use as discussed in Chapter 7, as different obstacles require different methods for addressing them.

If there are issues with recall from session to session, techniques to bridge, trigger, or support recall from session to session may be needed. This can include having the person make a video clip summary of what they just did in a session, the methods they used, and what they plan to do differently next time, keep a digital journal, or take photos of completed activities to cue recall. Text reminders of goals and strategies between sessions may be needed to increase retention. It might be helpful to start each session by showing the person the treatment activity from the previous session to determine if visual representation of the activity triggers recall of what previously occurred.

If a lack of continuity and recall between sessions continues to exist, single strategy training that focuses on practicing and initiating use of one strategy across different activities can be used to increase automaticity and capitalize on procedural memory for strategy learning (see case example in Chapter 15). Alternatively, task-specific strategy training can be used to improve performance in an identified task, rather than across tasks.

SUMMARY

The MC approach is a complex multicomponent approach to cognitive rehabilitation. Although it was initially described in 1991, the complexity and lack of specification of practical intervention guidelines made it difficult to implement consistently across therapists. This book has operationalized the MC approach, clearly identifying the key treatment ingredients so that intervention can be delivered with greater consistency in clinical practice. While the MC approach provides consistent core treatment elements, it does not provide a fixed set of procedures for all clients. Intervention is tailored to the needs of the individual and settings. Therefore, it has wide applications. Examples of broad clinical applications are further illustrated in Chapters 14 and 15. While the flexibility and broad applications of the MC approach are advantages, treatment delivery depends on the skill of the therapist. It is therefore critical for therapists to invest time and practice in learning and using this approach. This chapter presented suggestions for therapists to learn, practice, and gain proficiency in the MC approach. Advice for learning, implementation, and self-assessment were provided along with guidelines, corresponding chapters, tools, and resources. This chapter also discussed some common challenges and frequently asked questions related to implementing MC treatment along with strategies for managing them.

KEY POINTS

- Advantages of the MC approach are that it has wide clinical applications, can be tailored to individual client needs or settings, and directly addresses the areas of function that present major obstacles to rehabilitation in people with cognitive impairments (self-awareness, transfer and generalization).

- Key treatment components of the MC approach are well specified, linked to theoretical concepts, and are evidence-based.

- Challenges in implementing the MC approach include variations in treatment focus and techniques according to client needs and settings, requirements for shifts in clinical practice, procedures and ways of interacting with clients, and dependence on therapist skill and reasoning for treatment delivery.

- Although this book provides detailed guidelines and indications for the MC approach, simply reading it is not enough. The MC approach requires practice in application and self-reflection to gain proficiency. It takes time and commitment to replace old methods with new ones.

- In particular, mediated learning techniques need to be practiced by the therapist, so they become a habitual way of interacting with clients.

- Therapist training and practice using role-play, video review, supervision, and the MC Fidelity Tool are methods therapists can use to gain proficiency.

PART III

CLINICAL APPLICATIONS OF THE MULTICONTEXT APPROACH

Chapter 14

Applying the Multicontext Approach Across Different Clinical Problems or Contexts

This chapter describes considerations for application of the Multicontext (MC) approach across different situations. This includes certain client factors, such as level of awareness, cognitive ability, and spatial neglect, as well as environmental factors, such as the treatment setting. The MC approach is broad, and different aspects of this approach can be emphasized to better fit the client's abilities, needs, and goals as well as any constraints or affordances of the treatment setting.

CONTENTS OF CHAPTER 14

Client-Related Factors
  Low Self-Awareness
  Low Cognitive Functioning
  Self-Identified Cognitive Concerns or Subtle Cognitive Deficits
  Spatial Neglect
Treatment Setting
  The Multicontext Approach in Acute Inpatient Rehabilitation
  The Multicontext Approach Within an Interprofessional Team
  The Multicontext Approach in the Home: Collaborating with Care Partners or Significant Others
  Group Applications of the Multicontext Approach
Summary and Key Points

CLIENT-RELATED FACTORS

The MC approach focuses on helping people gain an understanding of their cognitive performance strengths and weaknesses. The type and extent of guided questions used in the metacognitive framework can vary depending on the client's level of cognitive functioning and awareness. Similarly, the extent to which activities are structured along a horizontal continuum can differ depending on the severity of cognitive symptoms and self-awareness of deficits. Those that are at the low and the high ends of the spectrum require special considerations. This section will first discuss application of the MC approach to clients who have poor self-awareness and lower cognitive functioning and then to those who have self-identified cognitive concerns and subtle cognitive deficits.

Low Self-Awareness

In general, clients with low self-awareness require short parallel-structured activities in the initial stages of treatment to provide the opportunity to recognize repeated error patterns. There is typically a greater emphasis on mediation *during* the activity than on reflection after the activity. Additional methods may be needed to supplement the metacognitive framework. For example, video review of activity performance with guided questioning is recommended if the person shows limited awareness with post-discussion questions (Schmidt, et al., 2013; Schmidt, et al., 2015). Role reversal methods can also be used. No empirical studies, however, have investigated the use of this method. Both methods are described below.

Appendix D.11 provides general guidelines for people who exhibit different levels of awareness (low, partial/vague, high). It is important to recognize that those who have low awareness may also be high functioning while those who have moderate-severe cognitive deficits can be well aware of their limitations. Thus, Appendix D.11 provides broad guidelines based on clinical experiences, but it is over-simplified and does not fit all situations.

Video Review

Video review of activity performance provides the opportunity for self-observation and can be used to self-assess performance. The video of the treatment activity is paused at certain segments and guided questions are used to help the person retrospectively identify and assess performance errors and/or generate alternate task strategies. The combination of structured self-observation and guided questioning can help clients gain a better understanding of their own strengths and weaknesses (Schmidt et al., 2015).

Video review requires selecting or choosing activities that readily lend themselves to observing and detecting errors on the screen. Activities such as setting the table, sorting laundry into piles, making coffee or a smoothie are ideal because it is easy to visually detect errors. In contrast, tasks such as paying bills or computer activities present challenges to the video review method as errors are not easily observed on video.

Video review has the advantage of allowing self-observation of performance and providing objective, concrete, and vivid feedback. It is easier to detect errors during the process of video review because the person is just focusing on observing and is not involved in doing the task. During activity performance, the person is involved in both action or "doing" and self-monitoring, so additional cognitive resources are required compared to watching the video alone. There is some evidence that video review of performance may be more effective in enhancing online awareness than verbal feedback alone in people with moderate-severe acquired brain injury (Fleming, et al., 2019; Schmidt et al., 2013). This is particularly true for those who are unable to recall or reflect on performance.

Role Reversal

Role reversal involves observing someone else perform an activity with cognitive performance errors that the person might typically make. This might be a video of someone performing an activity with errors or it might be the therapist performing the activity in real-time. The client is asked to identify errors and suggest strategies to reduce performance errors. Viewing another person making errors can be less threatening for a client and can assist in building up error detection and strategy generation skills (Toglia, 2018).

It should be noted that if a client has strong denial, the methods described above will likely not be effective. A person with denial already acknowledges errors but makes excuses for them. The problem is not error recognition but one of acceptance and coping. This requires a different approach as described in Chapter 8.

Low Cognitive Functioning

Strategy training for those with moderate-severe cognitive deficits should begin with single strategy training as described in Chapter 7. Additional treatment methods, such as errorless learning, task adaptations, or technology to support performance or strategy use can be considered for single strategy training. Use of task-specific training methods or errorless learning can be used to train *strategy initiation* or create strategy habits such as referring to a list within an activity, setting timers, reviewing "to-do lists," or referring to a digital journal. For example, automated text messages or recurrent reminders can be used to prompt strategy use (e.g., referring to a list or writing in a digital journal). As strategy initiation becomes more habitual, technology prompts can be faded, but other strategies may be needed. For example, once a person consistently refers to a list, other strategies to effectively manage items on the list such as underlining or checking off, might be needed. Guided questions could be used to help a person generate methods for ensuring that all parts of the list are attended to (or that nothing is missed).

In addition to methods to initiate strategy use, technology can be used to prompt self-monitoring habits (e.g., stop and review) or emotional regulation strategies (e.g., "take a deep breath, relax, and stay calm"). Videos of activities can be used to initially support mental imagery or visualization strategies and then faded. The person should be involved in choosing images or making the video. Technology can also be used to help a person monitor a tendency to "get stuck" or to prematurely end an activity. Preset voice messages, vibrating signals, or auditory tones/alarms can be used as prompts for the person to review what they are doing, switch from one activity to the next, or "keep going" during an activity.

If the person has difficulty recalling previous sessions due to memory deficits, memory supports to increase continuity of treatment should be considered. For example, a digital journal or notebook that includes photos or videos of parts of previous treatment sessions, daily automated text messages of goals, or photo reminders of previous treatment activities can help to increase continuity of treatment. Regardless of the technique, the person should be involved in choosing methods to increase continuity of information from day to day or session to session. Frequency of treatment might also need to be increased to obtain carryover until continuity of treatment can be established.

Goal-Focused Methods

Goal-focused methods can be used to increase specific or discrete behaviors. Exhibit 14.1 provides examples of focused goals. Although the goals are focused, they are not task-specific and instead represent behaviors that go across situations.

> **Exhibit 14.1 Examples of Focused Goals**
>
> - Sustain activity for 10 minutes (avoid stopping prematurely).
> - Stay task focused for 10 minutes.
> - Initiate looking at or reviewing task list on the bulletin board during multi-step activities.
> - Follow through tasks to completion such as brushing teeth or dressing.

Goals are presented to the client for discussion, adjustment if needed, and agreement. Goal behaviors are self-rated on a simplified scale during and immediately after activities. The same guidelines for structuring activities are used (similar to dissimilar) and the same metacognitive framework is applied, but the questions are more structured and targeted. Exhibit 14.2 presents examples of pre-discussion questions that could be used within goal-focused methods.

External cues such as a large visible timer, periodic voice messages, or a large salient task list (e.g., on yellow poster board), can be used in initial stages during activities to promote attentional focus. Immediately after the task, the client and therapist can both rate goal performance (staying focused for 10 minutes) using a simplified self-rating scale that focuses on the targeted behavior (Appendix C.21-C.22).

Positive feedback and reinforcement are provided for all attempts toward goal achievement (even if it results in goals that are only partially met). Ratings, scores, charts, or graphs that visually illustrate progress toward the goal (e.g., time spent that is task-focused) can be effective in increasing effort and engagement. In some cases, incentives may also be needed. The post-discussion is similar to that described in Chapter 10 (e.g., What did you do to help yourself stay focused?) and includes identification of other everyday activities where the same behaviors are needed or where the same strategies could apply.

Specific behaviors such as interrupting others, continuous talking, impulsivity, or perseveration can also be targeted for reduction.

Clinical Example: Targeting Specific Behaviors

Clinical Example 14.1 describes a person with low cognitive functioning and awareness. This is followed by a description of how MC intervention can be combined with other techniques to address a targeted behavioral problem.

> **Clinical Example 14.1 Low Awareness and Excessive Talking**
>
> John is a 32-year-old who suffered a traumatic brain injury three weeks ago. He has difficulty controlling verbal output and talks incessantly in a tangential manner during occupational therapy (OT), physical therapy (PT), and speech therapy. This makes it difficult to accomplish anything during treatment. Other patients avoid him because it is difficult to hold a meaningful conversation with him. He vaguely acknowledges that it is sometimes hard to concentrate, but he does not realize how frequently he goes off task or that his talking is a problem.

> **Exhibit 14.2 Pre-Discussion Example: Goal of staying focused on task for 10 minutes**
>
> - Before we begin, what are some of the things that can interfere with ____ (goal, e.g., staying focused)?
> - What are some of the things that can be distracting and cause things to get sidetracked?
> - What can you do to help stay focused on the activity or resist that tendency to get distracted by other things?
> - Let's think of some things that you should do if you notice you are getting sidetracked. If others notice you are getting sidetracked what should they say or do?
> - How would you know that you are getting sidetracked? What can you do if you notice that you are getting distracted? What can you say to yourself? What actions can you take?

Since John did not realize that his constant talking was interfering with task completion, the therapist decided to use video review within the first couple of treatment sessions. During the video review, the therapist asked, "What things are interfering with completing the activity? Let's think about some things that can help you stay on task or resist the tendency to talk during the activity." John agreed that a visual timer set for 5 minutes at a time might help him monitor his talking. He also chose a few pictures/icons including a picture of binoculars (focus) and a person gesturing to keep quiet within sight, as reminders to stay focused.

After each activity, John self-rated his ability to stay on task. The video was then reviewed and discussed with guided questions. Immediately after watching and discussing the video, he was given the option to adjust his self-ratings if desired. The therapist also rated his ability to stay on task. If there were discrepancies, the video was reviewed again and discrepancies were discussed. The therapist kept a tally of the number of minutes John spent on task (including conversations that were related to the task) with the goal to increase time spent on task.

In addition, an automated daily text message was sent to John six times a day that had the message "Stay focused" with a picture of his binoculars and the "keep quiet" picture icon. As John's awareness gradually emerged, video review was faded and replaced by mediation during the task and anticipation questions (e.g., Before we do this task, what are some things that you might need to watch out for or that could interfere with task completion? What can you say to yourself or do if you have thoughts that are not related to the activity?). Initially, John generated the idea of keeping a paper handy to write down irrelevant ideas that popped into his head instead of talking about them and/or asking for a break if he felt he needed to talk about a non-task related topic. Although this interfered with task performance, it helped him initially recognize and monitor off-task behaviors. Eventually, he was able to use mental images and self-cues to help him stay on task and control his verbal output. All team members used the same metacognitive questions and self-ratings within treatment sessions so that John could see how the same pattern of behavior was interfering with performance across different activities and contexts.

The same MC activity progression and metacognitive framework were used; however, treatment was targeted at reducing a specific behavior. Additional external supports and goal-focused methods were used to enhance awareness and performance across treatment sessions.

Self-Identified Cognitive Concerns or Subtle Cognitive Deficits

People who readily self-identify cognitive concerns and are aware of changes in thinking and performance require special considerations. This can include people with multiple sclerosis (Goverover et al., 2019), Parkinson's disease (Foster et al., 2017), lupus (Harrison et al., 2005), mild cognitive deficits following cancer treatment (Fernandes et al., 2019), older adults with subjective cognitive complaints (Rodakowski et al., 2014), or those with mild acquired brain injury (Dikmen et al., 2017). Those who self-identify subtle cognitive concerns are often high-functioning individuals who are engaged in cognitively demanding occupations or who have busy and complex home and social lives.

Although subtle cognitive deficits are described as mild, the impact on a person's life is not mild. They can significantly impact self-esteem, self-efficacy, emotional status, and the ability to function at prior levels in complex work or life tasks (Stenberg et al., 2020). A person that is aware of cognitive difficulties may avoid tasks with cognitive challenges because they might immediately anticipate difficulties and believe they are not going to be successful before they even try. This can lead to decreased participation in activities and social situations that were previously enjoyed. In addition, awareness or anticipation of difficulties without tools to manage or cope with these difficulties results in negative psychological and emotional responses such as performance anxiety, increased stress, depressive symptoms, or frustration.

The person with self-identified cognitive concerns notices cognitive changes in themselves that are not easily visible to others. Families or co-workers may expect the person to function as they did before the illness or injury. Struggles in functioning might be recognized by others but attributed to behavioral or emotional issues such as lack of effort or motivation, which further compounds the negative effects of subtle cognitive deficits (see Chapter 1). In these cases, treatment needs to address cognitive difficulties along with the social and psychological issues that result from having an invisible disability.

Assessment: Subtle Cognitive Deficits

People with self-identified or subtle cognitive deficits may be able to provide specific examples of cognitive performance difficulties; however, these difficulties are not readily observed. For example, the person may be able to complete higher-level cognitive instrumental activities of daily living (IADL) tasks without difficulty in a clinic setting, yet they can provide numerous real-life examples in work and social situations in which they experience cognitive challenges or lapses (e.g., keeping up with group conversations, solving complex problems, learning to use new technology, remembering to do things). Sometimes, subtle cognitive deficits only emerge after sustained cognitive activity or as the cumulative effects of a combination of activities. For these reasons, it can be challenging to identify assessment and treatment tasks that provide an adequate cognitive challenge for those who are higher functioning.

Performance-based assessments may not always reveal limitations in individuals who have subtle cognitive limitations. Higher-level assessments such as the Complex Task Performance Assessment (CTPA) (Wolf, et al., 2017), Actual Reality Test (Goverover & DeLuca, 2018), or the WCPA – level III (Toglia, 2015) can be used, but measures that examine social engagement, participation, and the ability to fulfill roles and work responsibilities should also be incorporated into assessment (Toglia, Askin, et al., 2019). In addition, tools such as the Bangor Goal Setting Interview (Clare et al., 2016), self-ratings of everyday cognitive symptoms, mental fatigue, and a measure of cognitive self-efficacy (CSEQ) (Toglia & Johnston, 2017) are recommended (see Resources).

Treatment: Subtle Cognitive Deficits

Management of stress, emotions, and cognitive fatigue play a key role in the treatment of people with subtle cognitive deficits. Stress, anxiety, depression, or mood changes can significantly magnify subtle cognitive symptoms and increase the frequency of cognitive lapses. Similarly, poor sleep and mental fatigue contribute to inconsistencies in performance. The person may be aware of fluctuating performance errors but may not fully understand when or why they occur. The MC approach helps the person identify the triggers or anticipate, monitor, and manage symptoms that may be influencing the consistency of cognitive performance. Self-ratings of anxiety, stress level, mood, or mental fatigue before, during, and after activities can help a person gain a deeper understanding of how these factors might be affecting performance. Also, daily journals or logs of cognitive lapses (see cognitive log below) can help people identify patterns in performance as well as generate strategies to optimize performance.

Enhancing cognitive self-efficacy is particularly important in treatment with those with self-identified cognitive concerns. Subtle changes in the ability to remember, think on one's feet, or organize information can dramatically impact self-confidence, one's sense of self, and ability to function. Often, the person can identify cognitive problems but believes there is nothing that can be done to improve cognitive performance. If the person recognizes cognitive difficulties but does not have tools to cope with or manage cognitive challenges, self-efficacy is lowered, and activity avoidance can occur. At the same time, mood, mental fatigue, or emotional reactions such as anxiety, stress, or depression can emerge and overshadow performance (Brands, et al., 2019).

The metacognitive framework can help enhance self-efficacy in both situations. For example, often people who anticipate that a task will be very difficult cannot identify which specific aspects of the task will be easy or hard or why they think the task will be hard. This can contribute to a tendency to become quickly overwhelmed and a sense of a lack of control over performance. The metacognitive framework can be used to help a person analyze task demands to identify aspects that might be tricky and generate methods and back-up plans to "stay a step ahead." Development of action or goal plans can be particularly helpful for those who are aware of cognitive lapses or difficulties (Chapter 10 and 13).

If the person demonstrates negative emotional reactions to challenges, treatment involves a focus on emotional regulation strategies as described in Chapter 7. This involves first acknowledging the emotional response and helping the person recognize and monitor emotional triggers that can interfere with performance through mediation during an activity. For example, the therapist might begin by asking "what are the warning signs to watch out for as you do this activity?" If the therapist observes warning signs, the activity can be paused, and mediation can be used to help the person become aware of their emotional reactions. For example, "Let's stop and identify what is happening" or It seems as though you are getting frustrated – I see the *temperature* rising. What part is frustrating? Let's try to work this through and figure out a way to break this activity down" or, "It seems as though the anxiety is rising. Let's think about a way to lower the anxiety and make things less overwhelming."

It is important to help the person understand that negative emotional responses (e.g., anxiety, bad mood, or frustration) impede performance (Champion, 2006). Self-ratings of emotions or mood during activities can help the person see the connection between emotions and performance. An emotional regulation action plan (Appendix C.18) can be utilized to enhance the ability to recognize emotional warning signs and identify strategies. For example, relaxation exercises, mindfulness, meditation, or guided mental imagery can be integrated within action plans to decrease anxiety or stress. Positive self-coaching or the re-framing of problems can be used to manage negative beliefs and emotions (see Chapter 7).

Similarly, mental fatigue requires understanding how fatigue symptoms influence performance, analyzing the conditions that increase or decrease symptoms and evaluating strategies that reduce mental fatigue. For example, some people may find that setting a timer to take frequent and brief mental rest breaks every 20 minutes can reduce mental fatigue, while others might find that mental fatigue can be decreased by short bursts of physical activity within daily routines, re-arranging and balancing complex activities with routine or repetitive activities, avoiding mentally challenging activities at certain times of day, decluttering the environment and workspace, or removing potential interruptions to reduce cognitive load before starting tasks.

The focus of treatment is on providing positive support, managing stress, mental fatigue, or emotions, facilitating emotional regulation, and reframing negative beliefs while simultaneously increasing awareness of methods that can be used to cope with cognitive challenges in complex activities (Cantor et al., 2014). This may include modifying beliefs or helping the person realize that there are techniques they can use to control symptoms, improve performance, and manage cognitive challenges successfully. The MC Activity modules include complex treatment activities for high functioning people with subtle difficulties (see Appendix D.6). Repeated practice in cognitively complex activities provides the opportunity to practice the strategies described above as well as increase self-confidence and build self-efficacy for managing activities with high cognitive demands.

The complete metacognitive framework described in Chapter 10 may not be needed in clients that have self-identified cognitive concerns. It may be that the pre-activity discussion can be skipped, and the focus might be on reflection and assessment of performance. This is particularly true if the person has a good ability to identify challenges and strategies. If the client can already anticipate difficulties and self-recognize performance errors, the therapist may focus on further enhancing self-understanding or monitoring of cognitive performance, guiding the generation and use of effective strategies, increasing the range and breadth of strategy application, and enhancing cognitive self-efficacy.

Cognitive Log

Ongoing daily logs or journals of cognitive lapses and cognitively challenging occupational situations can be powerful in helping clients self-reflect and interpret cognitive performance experiences (Toglia, 2018). The cognitive log is a structured journal of cognitive lapses, including when and where they occurred, the context in which they occurred (including the individual's mood, stress level, fatigue level, emotional reaction, environment, and presence of other people), and reflection about whether anything could have been done differently to prevent the lapse (Exhibit 14.3; blank form in Appendix C.19).

For example, a client can be asked to keep a log of cognitive lapses or cognitive performance errors that occur during daily occupations. The log of problems and their contexts can then be reviewed and analyzed collaboratively in treatment sessions so the client can learn more about themselves as well as the conditions under which difficulties are most likely to emerge. A cognitive log kept over time can reveal patterns in everyday cognitive symptoms and can help a person anticipate situations where difficulties might arise. Cognitive logs can be quite powerful in helping a client gain self-understanding as illustrated in the following quote of a person with subtle cognitive difficulties:

> "When it comes to the point that you cannot do your work or whatever it is that is important to you in your life, that frustration can build up to the point that it paralyzes you. It becomes a real block. The Cog Logs help you take a step back . . . and look at what happened. And when you do that week after week, by the third or fourth week, you just see things a lot clearer. . . . You see patterns that help you understand things in a different way . . . . The Cog Logs were key."

Exhibit 14.3 Sample Cognitive Log

Date and Time of event	Problem: What Happened?	When? Describe the context:	Why do you think this may have occurred?	Methods for Prevention
	Describe troublesome cognitive experience or cognitive lapse or functional problem	Where were you? Were other people involved? What occurred immediately before, how did you feel at the time? (e.g., tired, relaxed, angry)		Strategies? Adaptations?

Cognitive logs can also be used to monitor changes in awareness and strategy use. At the beginning of treatment, descriptions of cognitive lapses and analysis of why the lapse may have occurred are typically vague, and strategies for prevention are often nonexistent. Possible methods of preventing future lapses or performance problems are reviewed during treatment sessions for each daily life situation, practiced in the context of simulated functional activities during treatment, and even assigned as real-life "homework." The person can be encouraged to develop action plans for applying strategies in certain situations or environments to control performance errors and prevent future problems (Appendix C.16) (Toglia, 2018). As treatment progresses and the person has a better understanding of their cognitive lapses, entries into the cognitive logs gradually become more specific, and a variety of strategies and methods for the prevention of cognitive lapses are generated.

Activity Challenges

People with cognitive difficulties gradually begin to avoid cognitively challenging activities. It is important to help a person identify activities that they have avoided or have given up because they were too difficult. An activity challenge log (Exhibit 14.4) requires the client to identify cognitively challenging activities that they would like to do. It provides a structure to encourage the person to choose an activity goal, make a plan for success, try the activity, self-assess, and reflect upon performance. The aim is to increase participation in cognitively challenging activities. See the sample activity challenge log below. Alternatively, the cognitive action plan form (Appendix C.16) can also be used to create a plan that addresses participation in challenging activities.

Clinical Example: Subtle Cognitive Deficits

The following case is an example of using the MC approach in an outpatient setting with a person who had a mild traumatic brain injury (TBI) and who exhibited awareness of cognitive deficits and poor cognitive self-efficacy. Treatment focused on helping the client develop a sense of control over cognitive performance or enhance self-efficacy. Case #3 in Chapter 15 is another example of the MC approach with an individual with mild cognitive deficits.

> **Clinical Example 14.2 Awareness and Low Self-Efficacy**
>
> Deborah readily identified cognitive concerns in the areas of organization and ability to keep track of information in higher-level tasks. She consistently under-estimated performance and became easily overwhelmed with cognitively challenging tasks before she even attempted them. During activities, she easily recognized difficulties and errors but continued to use the same ineffective task methods. This only heightened anxiety because she knew what was wrong but did not know how to correct it. As a result, she often withdrew from tasks or gave up. She constantly made negative self-statements such as "This is too hard for me," "I can't do this," and "My brain isn't working right." For example, in attempting to follow complex directions to an online shopping activity with multiple criteria regarding sizes, prices, and types of items, Deborah highlighted almost all of the directions. As she was highlighting, she appeared overwhelmed and stated, "This isn't helping," but continued to highlight sentences rather than stop and simplify or re-organize the information.

Exhibit 14.4 Activity Challenge Log and Plan

Challenging Activity	Make a Plan for Success — Environment or Context	Self-Evaluate	Self-Reflect	Plan
		What went well? What challenges or obstacles did I run into? What strategies did I use? How well did the strategies work? What parts need more practice?	How did I feel during the activity (e.g., confident, unsure, anxious, tired, frustrated)? Is there anything I could do differently next time? What other strategies could I use?	Would I do this activity again? (If so, when? If not, identify another activity.) What would I do differently?

The initial treatment focus was on helping Deborah to recognize the "warning signs" that signaled she was becoming overwhelmed or anxious within a multi-step activity before it escalated. She identified that visual images such as a "calm ocean" and breathing techniques made her feel less anxious. Treatment also guided her in reframing negative self-statements into positive thinking. For example, instead of saying, "This is too hard. I will never be able to do it," she was encouraged to say, "This is a challenge; I need to stop, stay calm, and split it up." As treatment progressed, she was also able to generate methods to make multi-step complex tasks more manageable by using methods of task simplification and mental imagery or rehearsal before performing an activity. For example, she imagined herself performing the activity (or similar activity) in the past. Rehearsing the activity mentally decreased her anxiety and helped her preplan actions. These strategies were incorporated into her emotional regulation action plan (Appendix C.18). With repeated use of guided questioning before, during, and after cognitively complex activities, she learned to recognize the need to stop and adjust task methods when they were ineffective and create back-up plans in case things did not go as planned. These strategies were summarized into strategy cue sheets that Deborah created for herself and reviewed every morning to start her day.

Spatial Neglect

Although this manual has focused on executive functions, the MC approach has also been described with people with spatial neglect and other visual perceptual disorders (Golisz, 1998; Toglia, 1989; Toglia & Chen, 2020) Limitations in self-awareness are a major obstacle to performance in people with neglect; however, the nature of awareness difficulties is different in people with and without spatial neglect. The person with spatial neglect typically perceives the world or visual scenes in front of them as complete (Chen & Toglia, 2019). They do not realize they are missing information until they are cued to look at the neglected space. Cues such as "look to the left" are not always effective because the person thinks they are already looking toward the left. They may not know where the left side of space is because their brain is not signaling that they are missing information. Strategies that a person with spatial neglect can use to help themselves attend to the left are listed in Exhibit 14.5 (Toglia & Chen, 2020).

Disassociation between awareness outside and inside the context of an activity is also observed in people with spatial neglect (Chen & Toglia, 2019). Clinically, we have observed that people with spatial neglect often show improvements in intellectual awareness or the knowledge that they miss information first, without changes in behavior within the context of an activity (e.g., making sure to scan entire table to find specific items from a list). This might be because other people are constantly telling them that they are missing information, and they remember this, but they do not know when it occurs because they perceive the world as complete.

Assessment: Spatial Neglect

Spatial neglect is not a unitary disorder. There are different subtypes and varying combinations of symptoms that can occur. Spatial neglect can vary across frames of space (e.g., individual object or number string, space within reach, size of a table, room, and large environment). For example, a person may miss the left side of a number or object but have no difficulty negotiating large spaces. The opposite may also be true. The person may bump into doorways and walls but have no difficulty in paper and pencil tasks (Toglia, Golisz, et al., 2018). The conditions that influence the manifestation of neglect such as size of space, density, or number of stimuli within space, and the task instructions (e.g., copying, detecting or organizing

---

Exhibit 14.5 Strategies for Spatial Neglect

- *Intellectual override* – Encouraging a person to initiate double-checking by making an extra effort to feel and see the space around them, and disregard the perception from their brain that is telling them that they have seen everything around them.
- *Self-chosen anchor* – Person chooses a salient object or stimuli to place on the left side.
- *Visual imagery* – With eyes closed, the person describes the space that is in front of them including the left side.
- Finger-pointing during scanning or reading.
- Tapping the left side to provide auditory cues to increase attention to the left side.
- *Stimuli reduction* – The person covers what they see on the right side so that attention can be drawn to the left.
- Tapping the left foot to increase attention to the left side.

information within space) need to be analyzed during performance analysis.

Treatment: Spatial Neglect

The MC approach uses the same metacognitive framework with guided questions before, during, and after functional cognitive activities to help a person with spatial neglect develop awareness within the context of activity performance. The emphasis is on helping the person 1) recognize that they sometimes "miss information," 2) recognize the need to use strategies to ensure that they have seen everything around them, and/or 3) initiate strategies to do so across a variety of activities. The same structured activities using functionally relevant materials across a horizontal transfer continuum can also be used; however, the focus is on attending to and working with objects or information in space (Toglia, 2011). Treatment activities can be generally grouped into those that involve searching and locating information that exists in the environment or those that involve placing and organizing information within different-sized spaces.

Clinical Example: Person with Stroke and Spatial Neglect

Clinical Example 14.3 includes examples of treatment activities using the MC approach for someone with spatial neglect.

> **Clinical Example 14.3 Person with Stroke and Spatial Neglect**
>
> Eva is a 62-year-old female with spatial neglect following a right cerebral hemorrhage five months ago. She ambulates independently without an assistive device and has partial functional use of her left upper extremity (LUE). Visual fields are intact. Eva readily acknowledges missing information on the left side and can provide specific examples. She describes not being able to find objects, not realizing that a pot on the left side is boiling over or that the gas burner is still on, and missing information when reading. During shopping trips to the grocery store, she had so much difficulty finding items that she began to use a cane simply because "people would realize she had a disability and would be more willing to help her." Although Eva appeared to have excellent awareness, she demonstrated significant neglect in activities such as setting a table for six people and finding items on a schedule. Her goal was to "get better" and not make "stupid mistakes." She described embarrassment when others pointed out information she missed that was right in front of her.

Treatment activities for Eva were structured along the horizontal continuum (Chapter 8) and included a variety of activities that initially involved placing items on both sides of space. For example, Eva was asked to place spoons, napkins, and tea bags next to sixteen cups that were spread all over a large conference table. Similarly, other activities involved placing crackers, cheese, or other food items on plates, placing pencils and Post-it® notes next to name cards and placing a cookie in lunch bags spread out on tables or counters. The metacognitive framework and guided questions were used within each session. Initially, Eva did not anticipate any difficulties in these activities and did not perceive the need to use any special strategies. As soon as she moved to the opposite side of the table, she was able to immediately recognize that she had missed information on the left side. At first, she believed there was nothing she could do to change task outcomes. She seemed to believe that missing things "just happened" unpredictably due to her stroke.

An important aspect of treatment involved using the metacognitive framework and guided learning questions to empower her to "plan ahead" and identify situations in which she was more vulnerable to emergence of neglect symptoms (e.g., distracting or new environments, information crowded together or spread across large spaces). In these situations, she was encouraged to use special methods to make sure she "sees everything." She began to generate strategies and self-initiated the use of anchors or choosing an object and placing it to the left before beginning an activity. Activities progressed to those such as dealing cards or chips to four or six people, arranging cookies on a baking sheet, arranging photos on a large poster board, or placing take-out menus on a large bulletin board. When reading a large newspaper, she initiated folding it so it would be narrow. She also started to use stimuli reduction methods.

At this point, specific goals started to emerge. Eva felt she was ready to try making dinner for her family. She worked with her OT to create an action plan that was then reviewed and shared with family members. Some of the strategies within the plan included 1) only one pot on the stove at a time, 2) rotating a baking dish before putting it in the oven to ensure food was distributed evenly, 3) preparing a salad and setting the table several hours beforehand, and 4) checking the table setting by walking around the table and viewing it from different perspectives.

TREATMENT SETTING

The Multicontext Approach in Acute Inpatient Rehabilitation

The acute inpatient rehabilitation setting is challenging because of time constraints and shortened length of inpatient stays. The therapist often has a variety of different types of clients on their caseload, with different diagnoses and needs. Clients have not yet had the opportunity to return home and try many of their daily activities, and the inpatient rehabilitation setting does not challenge cognition in ways similar to real life (i.e., reduced responsibilities, structured environment), so they and their families may be unaware of any cognitive limitations. Because physical impairments are more obvious, the focus during inpatient rehabilitation is often on physical functioning while cognitive limitations are not always detected or adequately addressed in this type of setting.

The importance of identifying and addressing functional cognitive limitations early in the recovery process cannot be understated. A person who leaves inpatient rehabilitation with inadequately understood cognitive difficulties will likely experience difficulty once they attempt to resume life activities. They may have difficulty managing medications or following health instructions and routines, and this can ultimately lead to re-admission (Wolf, 2018). Return to work and social activities may result in unexpected struggles or failures that produce negative psychological and emotional responses or decline in function. This highlights the need for both screening and intervention of cognitive limitations within an inpatient setting.

The Montreal Cognitive Assessment (MoCA) has been typically used as a tool to screen for cognitive impairments. Toglia and colleagues (2017) found that those who score below 20 on the MoCA are likely to have instrumental activities of daily living (IADL) deficits. However, for those who score 20 or more on the MoCA, functional cognition cannot be reliably predicted and should be directly assessed. This underscores the importance of using functional cognitive performance-based tests even for those who score normally on a cognitive screening exam or who do not show obvious cognitive deficits (Toglia et al., 2017).

Feasibility of the Multicontext Approach in an Inpatient Setting

We tested the feasibility, acceptability, and client satisfaction with the MC approach in a case series of eight individuals with acquired brain injury (ABI) in an acute inpatient rehabilitation setting, during the context of routine OT. The median length of stay was 7-8 days. Criteria for inclusion included those with deficits in functional cognition or IADL and who were cognitively independent in self-care activities (Jaywant, et al., 2020).

Pre-made functional cognitive activity kits were designed along a horizontal transfer continuum (see Chapter 8) so that they were brief (10-15 minutes), could easily be adjusted to different cognitive abilities, and could provide repeated opportunity to apply the same strategies across different activities. The activities included functional materials such as menus, schedules, food circulars, business cards, lists as well as cards and written directions. Some of these activities are included in the MC Activity modules (Level 1) and are described in Appendix D.5.

Therapists were trained to position and arrange materials to support the person's physical goals. For example, schedules or menus were placed on a bulletin board, while materials such as lists or cards were placed in different areas of the room. This required holding and keeping track of information while walking from one location to the next. Some activities were presented in the seated position and required reaching, writing, or fine motor skills, while others required standing, bending, reaching, or moving from sitting to standing. The motor requirements addressed the client's goals while at the same time provided the opportunity for the person to experience functionally relevant activities with cognitive demands (Jaywant et al., 2020).

The MC approach was integrated successfully within the context of daily inpatient OT treatment. Treatment sessions of the eight clients were videotaped and assessed for pre/post changes. The majority of clients in the inpatient feasibility study only identified physical goals at the start of treatment. The focus of initial sessions was on increasing awareness of cognitive performance errors. Addressing motor goals while simultaneously placing demands on cognitive skills appeared to facilitate the emergence of self-awareness. Clients began to recognize cognitive challenges and added goals such as "keeping track of directions" or "remembering what I just read" during treatment.

All clients with ABI demonstrated significant changes in pre/post measures assessing executive function, strategy use, and awareness performed by an independent therapist. Client engagement, perceived improvement, and satisfaction with treatment was high. Despite the short length of stay, we demonstrated feasibility and changes in awareness, strategy use, and functional cognition within the time constraints of this setting, however, the absence of a control group limits conclusions that can be made (Jaywant, et al., 2020). An in-depth case example of the application of the MC approach in an inpatient setting is illustrated in Chapter 15 (Case #1).

In an inpatient rehabilitation setting, there is typically

a focus on direct instruction and showing the person and their families what to do and how to do it. This made it particularly challenging for therapists who had caseloads of people with both orthopedic and neurological conditions to shift and use alternate treatment methods. Therefore, we discovered that we underestimated the degree of practice and training that it took for therapists to feel comfortable and achieve competence with the use of guided questioning (Toglia, et al., 2020).

The OTs using this approach began to collaborate with families and other disciplines such as PT and speech to encourage them to use the metacognitive framework and guided questions as well. They realized that the same framework could be used across a range of different activities, and they began to broaden the application beyond that of the pilot study to the interprofessional team. They found that the MC approach works best when an entire team shares a similar philosophy and uses consistent methods of interacting with clients as described below.

The Multicontext Approach within an Interprofessional Team

The MC approach can easily be integrated within an inter-professional team approach. Cognitive performance errors affect performance across all areas of function and are relevant to all disciplines. The same cognitive errors that affect successful completion of a meal preparation task can also be observed during communication or physical activities. Although the goals of team members may be different, the same metacognitive framework, guided learning techniques, and strategies can be used or reinforced by different team members across a wide range of activities. Similar questions (pre, during, and post-activity) can be used by team members for self-care activities, wheelchair transfers, reading, organizing medications, communication activities, group activities, or physical activities such as following directions to a new exercise, learning to use a walker, or ambulating in different environments. For example, a client can be asked to identify things they might need to watch out for before getting up from a wheelchair and transferring to a chair. Questions can ask about things that could possibly go wrong and methods that might be used to ensure success. Afterward, the client could be asked how they went about the wheelchair transfer and the methods that they used.

A unified approach by all team members helps the client practice self-monitoring skills and strategies across different contexts and achieves the best outcomes. Clinical Example 14.4 below illustrates how the same error pattern interfered with performance across all disciplines. The same metacognitive framework and strategies were used by different team members.

> **Clinical Example 14.4 Same Error Pattern Across Situations**
>
> Anne was 43 years old and suffered a stroke two years ago, shortly after giving birth to twins. She previously worked as a marketing director for a large firm. She struggles with mild cognitive difficulties and a tendency to become sidetracked, tangential, disorganized, and lose goal focus. This is reflected in her communication as well as activity performance and ambulation. For example, when creating a birthday invitation for her daughter's party, she became sidetracked with concern about party decorations and began making a list of party supplies, forgetting about the invitation. During conversations, she begins discussing topics that are not relevant to the topic at hand, and during ambulation, she tends to forget to use her cane properly when involved in an activity. As she reflected on her past rehabilitation experiences, she stated, "I had about 12 different goals between OT, PT, and speech, and it was overwhelming. I wondered how I could get better with so many different goals. When I realized that some of the same issues were causing difficulties across different situations and some of the same strategies helped, it felt so much more manageable to me."

In Anne's case, the OT, PT, and speech therapists collaborated and agreed that they would all ask her to (1) think about what she needed to watch out for before beginning any activity (i.e., getting sidetracked) and (2) generate methods she could use to help her stay focused. Initially, her responses were vague such as "I have to concentrate." Team members asked her to identify what they should say or do if they noticed she was straying off task or becoming tangential. For example, should they wait and not say anything or should they say "Stop and review"? Anne indicated that they should wait at least two minutes before saying anything, as she wanted to try to monitor herself. All team members agreed to reinforce self-corrections or any attempts at catching her going off track (even if it was partial). They also agreed on more structured questions to help Anne generate strategies. For example, "What can you do to help make sure the goal of this activity is kept in mind and doesn't slip away? What type of image or picture can you think of to help you stay focused on the goal during this activity?" All team members agreed to leave time at the end of the treatment sessions to discuss the methods or strategies used.

This type of interprofessional collaboration requires a shared understanding and philosophy about guided learning techniques versus direct instructional methods. All team members can benefit from training in guided learning methods. This requires discussion, in-services, and coordination by team members and supervisors. The form illustrated in Exhibit 14.6 may be useful for an interprofessional team and may facilitate discussion on how each discipline can help reinforce similar strategies across treatment activities for a client.

The example in Exhibit 14.6 describes a client who was impulsive and had difficulty pacing his speed of response. Each discipline had different goals. Physical therapy's goal was safe and independent ambulation, speech therapy's goal was the ability to write e-mails accurately and generate appropriate questions for seeking information, and OT's goal was independence in IADL such as meal preparation, following a list of daily errands, and ordering groceries online. Once again, although the end goals were different, the same cognitive performance pattern was interfering with function across disciplines, so all team members worked together to help the client recognize and manage performance errors. A blank interprofessional team worksheet is included in Appendix C.3 for clinical use.

The Multicontext Approach in the Home: Collaborating with Care Partners or Significant Others

The home setting offers many advantages for use of the MC approach. The person's natural environment and everyday activities are easily integrated within treatment. For example, within a person's home, the person can be asked to compare a recipe to ingredients in their kitchen and create a shopping list for missing items. Similarly, they can be asked to identify toiletries in their bathroom that are low or will need to be purchased within the next month and create a shopping list.

Treatment within the home setting also provides an ideal opportunity to collaborate closely with the family, significant others, or care partners to reinforce cognitive strategies or support cognitive functioning. Cognitive difficulties are not always visible, and it can be challenging for others to understand and manage. It can be exhausting to deal with a person that constantly asks the same questions, repeats actions, forgets important information, or fails to follow simple directions. Even mild cognitive difficulties can contribute to caregiver burden and stress among others, particularly if self-awareness is limited (Jones et al., 2017; Kelleher, et al., 2016). Home care intervention can help others gain a better understanding of observed cognitive errors or behaviors as a foundation for learning effective management strategies. The care partner or significant other should be involved in identifying error patterns across activities, collaborating on goals, and generating possible strategies or solutions.

The same metacognitive framework used in the MC approach with clients can be used with family members

---

Exhibit 14.6 Example of How to Use the Multicontext Approach Within an Interprofessional Team

Functional Team Goal: Independent in IADL (preparing meals, paying bills, shopping, planning activities, and communication)

Cognitive Performance Errors Across Situations	Sample Treatment Strategies Used by All Disciplines	OT	Speech	PT
Haphazard, impulsive approach to higher-level functional tasks. Does things without thinking.	Anticipate task challenges before task. Identify things to watch out for before the task. Generate strategies to follow all steps on a list. Generate images to help stay focused and pace speed during activity. Discuss – "How will I know if it is just right timing?" Stops and self-checks within tasks. Self-rates timing immediately after tasks (too slow, just right, a little too quick or too fast).	During meal prep, paying bills, shopping online. Following a list of errands.	Making telephone calls to seek information. Writing e-mails to seek information.	Walking with a walker. Learning a new exercise.

or significant others as a means of guiding problem identification, generation of strategies, and problem-solving. The first step is helping significant others identify concerns and problem areas and guiding them in (1) recognizing error patterns or problem behaviors across situations and (2) identifying the conditions under which the behaviors or errors are most likely to occur. This is followed by a collaborative goal-setting process including developing goals that are specific and measurable.

Once problem areas are identified and goals are established, the care partner is guided in generating strategies or adaptations of tasks and environments. They are also asked to anticipate challenges or obstacles they might encounter in implementing solutions or strategies and developing back-up plans (i.e., coping planning). After implementation, care partners are asked to assess the effectiveness of the methods used. If needed, strategies or adaptations are modified, adjusted, or changed. Care partners are also asked to think broadly about how the same methods might be useful in other situations. This shares similarity with the occupational performance coaching model described in the literature (Belliveau, et al., 2016; Kahjoogh, et al. 2016).

The cognitive log described earlier in this chapter can be modified and completed by the care partner to document everyday functional cognitive challenges or problem situations that have occurred (see Exhibit 14.7). The log can be reviewed during treatment and used as a tool to facilitate collaboration with significant others including the generation of strategies and solutions for management of problem areas. In addition to use during treatment, logs can be used to track the frequency and type of everyday problem situations occurring across treatment.

In addition to the therapist using the metacognitive framework and mediation techniques to guide and coach care partners, care partners or significant others can be taught how to use mediated learning techniques with their loved ones to facilitate strategy use or performance.

The therapist should carefully observe how the significant other provides cues or assistance including tone of voice, timing, type, and content of prompts. Different methods for facilitating performance should be discussed with significant others. It is natural and faster for others to jump in and help rather than to watch someone struggle or help them problem solve. There are some activities where both the client and significant other may agree that direct assistance is most practical. However, there may be other activities where guided learning methods may be most appropriate in helping the person gain independence and a sense of control. This determination requires collaborating with the care partner or significant other to identify and understand everyday problems, set priorities or goals, and generate strategies or methods for dealing with everyday challenges. Alternative methods of managing problems and using guided learning techniques can be practiced and role-played using scenarios or problems identified by the significant other. The role of care partners or significant others in mediating the occupational performance of their family member is important in optimizing performance.

Group Applications of the Multicontext Approach

The MC approach has wide applications to group programs, particularly for populations with hidden or subtle cognitive deficits and subjective cognitive concerns such as those with cancer-related cognitive impairment (CRCI), early Parkinson's disease, concussion, ABI, mild cognitive impairment, multiple sclerosis, and lupus (Harrison et al, 2005, Toglia, 2018). It has also been applied within a middle-school classroom to enhance strategies for organization of lockers and materials (Waldman-Levi & Steinmann Obermeyer, 2018).

Consistent with the MC approach, group programs have a focus on three areas across sessions: (1) strategy use, (2) metacognitive skills, and (3) self-efficacy. Groups use the same guided questioning techniques and bridging methods

Exhibit 14.7 Care Partner Log of Everyday Functional Cognitive Challenges

Date	Problem: What Happened? Describe situation or functional problem	When? Describe the context: Were other people involved? What occurred immediately before (environment, mood)?	Why do you think this may have occurred?	Strategies and Solutions

described in Chapter 10. Participants are provided with a cognitively challenging activity without prior discussion. Immediately following the activity, the group facilitator uses guided questioning to facilitate discussion on methods or strategies used and challenges encountered. Discussion questions proceed from general to more structured in each session as discussed in Chapter 10. For example, questions to facilitate group discussion can include the following: How did you go about doing this activity? What challenges did you run into? What did you do to help yourself stay organized? How was this activity similar to activities that you do in everyday life? Participants are encouraged to share, discuss, and evaluate the effectiveness and efficiency of methods used as well as to generate alternate strategies if needed.

Throughout the program, group participants are asked to keep a cognitive log and complete a strategy worksheet or action plan every week. Each group session begins with a summary of the previous group by a participant and a sharing of cognitive logs (Appendix C.19). Each session ends with completion of the strategy worksheet. The strategy worksheet provides an ongoing tool to help participants learn about which strategies worked best for them and in what situations. A consistent format is used within group sessions and is summarized in Exhibit 14.8.

The activities used within a group program center on activity themes such as keeping track of information or what is read, simplifying complex activities, or coping with multitasking situations (see Appendix D.2 for other examples of activity themes). Typically, two or more brief activities that are similar and require the same underlying skills are completed within one group session so that the same strategies can be practiced repeatedly within a single session.

For high functioning groups, each session can introduce different activities, themes, and strategies that build upon previous groups. Alternatively, the same group framework outlined in Exhibit 14.8 can be used with a series of activities that require practice of the same strategies across different group sessions. Activities from the MC Activity modules can be used within a group program by using the sample eight treatment sessions and activities that are outlined in Appendix D.5 (lower level activities) or D.6 (higher-level activities). For example, Appendix D.5 includes a series of activities, across eight sessions that require basic ability to keep track of a limited amount of information. These activities place consistent demands on working memory across different types of tasks. Therefore, the same strategies (e.g., verbal or mental rehearsal, chunking, or associations) are applicable and can be practiced repeatedly across the group sessions. The group framework outlined in Exhibit 14.8 is applicable; however, tools such as the cognitive log and action plan are most appropriate for higher functioning groups.

Exhibit 14.8 Multicontext Approach: Consistent Group Format

- *Intro and review:* Summary of previous session, discussion of homework or strategy action plan, and review and sharing of the cognitive log.

- *Mental exercise and/or cognitive functional activity experience:* Participants engage in an individual activity without prior discussion.

- *Self-assessment and guided discussion:* Group guided discussion after each activity using principles and similar questions presented in Chapter 10. For example, questions posed to the group may include "Share how you went about doing this activity," "What did you do first, second, etc.?" "What challenges did you run into?" "How did you manage to keep track of everything?" The group leader encourages generation of alternate strategies.

- *Repetition of similar activities:* This provides the opportunity to try and practice strategies that were discussed. Activities include alternate forms of the same activity as well as activities that are physically dissimilar but require the same cognitive skills (Chapter 8).

- *Connecting experiences and strategy bridging:* Group discussion relates activities in the group to each other and to everyday situations. Participants discuss how the same strategies apply to other daily life activities. Participants complete the strategy worksheet, action plan, or journal and identify activities in which they will practice the strategy (see Chapter 10).

- *Summarize main points:* One or two members are also asked to be prepared to summarize the key points of the group session at the start of the next session.

The metacognitive framework used in the MC approach has also been applied to lower functioning clients by focusing on a single strategy such as the ability to follow or create a checklist across a series of activities. For example, a group of 4-5 people with mild dementia might participate in a series of activities, such as making banana pudding, brownies, or fruit salad, that involve following a five- or six-item list of simple steps. Participants can be asked to identify challenges using the list *before* activities, encouraged to help or remind each other to use the list *during* activities, and discuss results *after* the activity. The group checklist method can be used across different group activities as well as individual activities.

Finally, the MC approach principles can also be applied

to group projects that require collaboration in activities with a common goal (Toglia & Golisz, 1990). For example, activities such as putting together a newsletter, designing a web page, interviewing a physician within the facility, or planning and organizing a bake sale require shared planning and organization of multiple steps that go across several sessions or weeks. Group projects can simulate working in a team and require collaboration, negotiation, and interpersonal communication. They require identification of the tasks that need to be done, prioritization, timelines, and decisions about subtasks and division of work. The goals in this type of group include awareness of interpersonal behaviors, social communication, and strategies to effectively manage social situations across different activities. Similar to descriptions of previous groups, a consistent format can be used across different sessions (Toglia, 2018).

SUMMARY

This chapter illustrates how the MC approach can be applied broadly across a range of clinical severity, problems, and settings. Although the type of activities, strategies, and guided questions differ across clients who have different levels of self-awareness and cognitive functioning, the same core concepts are applicable. In addition to the application across ranges of function, the MC approach can be used to address perceptual problems such as spatial neglect. The MC approach is suited for inpatient, outpatient, home care settings, and groups. It can also be extended across an interprofessional team, including collaboration with family and care partners. Integration of the MC approach within a team provides cohesiveness and further reinforces self-monitoring skills and strategies across contexts.

KEY POINTS

- The same core components of the MC approach can be applied across clients with a range of functioning, problems, and settings; however, the treatment focus, types of activities, strategies used, timing, and types of guided questions differ.

    Lower functioning clients:
    - Generally require multiple short parallel (near transfer) activities that follow the transfer continuum.
    - Mediation is often used during the activity (rather than after).
    - Questions are structured and may initially be focused on the task.
    - Single-strategy training
    - Targeting discrete behaviors
    - Video review and technology are often used to promote awareness and carryover of strategies, particularly for those with significant memory impairments.

    Higher functioning clients:
    - Activities are complex, may be self-chosen, and often do not follow the transfer continuum.
    - Multiple flexible strategies are addressed in treatment.
    - There is an emphasis on cognitive self-efficacy.
    - Application of efficient strategies across situations is often an area of emphasis.
    - Mediation is used before and/or after the activity (not during).
    - Guiding questions are broad or general and are not task-focused.
    - Tools such as a cognitive log or diary of cognitive lapses and an activity challenge log to increase engagement in challenging activities are often used.

- The MC approach can be used across different settings, including home care and inpatient rehabilitation.

- All members of an interprofessional team can use the MC approach and guided learning methods to help the client practice self-monitoring and strategies across different contexts and achieve the best outcomes.

- The MC metacognitive framework can be used to facilitate problem identification and strategy generation by care partners or significant others. Mediated learning techniques can also be taught to care partners or significant others as a means of facilitating strategy use or optimizing function.

- The MC approach and metacognitive framework can also be applied in groups to promote awareness, strategy use, and self-efficacy. The same activities used in individual treatment can be completed within a group setting and/or in collaboration with others. Guided questions are used to facilitate sharing of experiences, challenges, or strategies used and to make connections with everyday life activities.

Chapter 15

Case Examples of the Multicontext Approach

This section includes three case examples and applications of the Multicontext (MC) approach with different settings, diagnoses, functional cognitive status, and stages of recovery. Each case includes a summary of assessment, the treatment program (including a table of sample treatment activities), and outcomes. Additionally, comprehensive case descriptions can be found in the following sources: Toglia et al. (2011), Toglia (2018), Steinberg & Zlotnik (2019).

> **CONTENTS OF CHAPTER 15**
> Case 1: Inpatient Setting, Stroke
> Case 2: Outpatient Day Program, Traumatic Brain Injury
> Case 3: In-Home Treatment, Parkinson's Disease
> Summary

CASE 1: INPATIENT SETTING, STROKE

This case discusses application of the MC approach for a person with impulsivity and difficulty inhibiting responses in an inpatient rehabilitation setting. This case was initially presented in Chapter 5 (See Clinical Example 5.1). A sample of the treatment planning worksheet for this case is presented in Appendix D.12. The client, Fred, is unaware of cognitive limitations and is only motivated to address physical deficits. This case illustrates how treatment can begin with the client's physical concerns and gradually increase awareness of cognitive limitations simultaneously. Treatment activities include use of lists as an inherent part of activities that involve gathering information or attending to details, rather than as a strategy.

Overview of Current Functional Status and Occupational History

Fred is 64 years old and had a stroke two weeks ago. He is in an inpatient rehabilitation setting. He actively participates in therapy and is motivated to "get better" so he can return to work and living independently in his apartment. He is independent in all self-care activities. His cognitive screening Montreal Cognitive Assessment (MoCA) score was 20/30, indicating mild cognitive impairment. Fred presently has limited standing tolerance and ambulates approximately 8-10 feet with a walker and close supervision. He has full active range of motion (AROM) in his right upper extremity (RUE), but his strength is 3/5.

Prior to his stroke, Fred lived alone in an urban setting and worked as an inventory control manager for an electronic company. Fred describes himself as an organized person that likes to "get things done." He prepared meals, took care of finances, grocery shopped, and ordered items online such as books, music, electronics, or food. His social life revolved around work, and he typically engaged in leisure activities on his own. Fred enjoyed going out to restaurants and digital photography. He used a tablet and computer (was familiar with Excel and PowerPoint but has not used either since the stroke). He does not have family in the immediate area and plans to temporarily live with his brother and his brother's wife, who live several hours away when he is discharged.

Client's Goals

Fred's goal is to return to living in his apartment, resume driving, and return to work part-time within 3-4 weeks after discharge (unrealistic). He perceives physical deficits as the major obstacle to his function and articulates goals related to walking and increasing strength of his RUE.

Occupational Therapy Evaluation

Initial Assessment Results

The following is a description of Fred's pre-treatment assessment results. Pre- and post-treatment scores are presented and compared in 15.4 Case Example 1.

Self-Regulation Skills Interview

Fred indicated he does not have any cognitive concerns and focused on his physical deficits.

Weekly Calendar Planning Activity – 10-item version

Fred entered 8/10 appointments into the calendar but only 3/8 were correct, resulting in a total of 7 errors. He jumped into the activity without preplanning and did not refer to written instructions and rules during the task. He inconsistently checked off items before they were entered and skipped to different appointments on the list without any apparent order. He broke 4/5 rules and crossed out appointments frequently. Appointments were often missing key details. For example, he wrote down "lunch" instead of "lunch with cousin." As he was doing the task, he began to speak about irrelevant personal experiences that were triggered by some of the appointments. For example, he began talking about the last movie he saw (triggered by "movie with friends") and about his neighborhood dry cleaner that recently raised prices (triggered by the dry-cleaning appointment).

Awareness: During the activity, Fred recognized appointment conflicts and occasional errors after the fact. He broke rules (without awareness that he was doing so) by crossing out. After task completion, Fred indicated that the task was trickier than he thought it would be and acknowledged that he placed a few appointments in the wrong place, but in general, he overestimated his performance.

Strategy Use: During the activity, Fred inconsistently checked off items on the list but no other strategies were observed. He said that next time he would take his time and go more slowly.

Performance Analysis of a Bill-Paying Task

Described in Chapter 5, Clinical example 5.1.

Functional Cognitive Problems

The following issues were observed or reported early in Fred's inpatient stay by his occupational therapist, other members of his care team, or his family.

- Meal Preparation – Prepares routine snacks and a sandwich but unable to accurately follow a list of directions on packages or recipes. Needs close supervision for using appliances or the stove.

- Ordered food from a menu that did not adhere to his dietary restrictions.

- Medication – When asked to place 15 pills into an organizer for a week following directions from 2 different medication bottles, he made 6 errors placing pills in the wrong locations.

- Bill Paying – Fred only paid 2 out of 3 bills. He placed one bill in the wrong envelope and made out a check for the incorrect amount. He also exceeded the amount in his account.

- Safety – Fred has been observed to get up without locking his wheelchair, stand up with incorrect hand placement on the walker before listening to directions, and he almost took a hot pan off the stove without using a potholder.

Treatment Targets

Build awareness and self-monitoring skills across simple IADL:

- Ability to identify task challenges prior to an activity.

- Error recognition and/or correction during an activity.

- Recognize that similar performance errors are occurring across activities.

- Recognizes need for a strategy to manage performance errors across activities.

15.1 Case Example 1 Inpatient Case (Fred): Summary of Assessment

Client Concerns and Goals	• Physical concerns and goals, especially related to walking. • No cognitive concerns or goals.
Functional Cognitive Concerns by Others	• Other team members and family are concerned about impulsivity and safety in activities such as transfers and ambulation.
Functional Cognitive Performance *(activity limitations and/or participation restrictions)*	• Requires close supervision in instrumental activities of daily living (IADL): use of a stove in cooking, placing pills into an organizer or appointments into a calendar, or paying a bill. • Mobility (rushing, unsafe) • Unable to return to independent living, work.
Cognitive performance errors or behaviors that go across activities	• Jumps into tasks without preplanning and rushes without following directions/procedures accurately, attending to details, or adhering to rules and criteria. • Misses or omits details, information, or steps. • Easily sidetracked by irrelevant thoughts or extraneous information.
Activity/environment characteristics that increase likelihood of errors	• Nonroutine activities • Activities that involve following 4 or more step directions • Less familiar or novel activities • Activities with distractions, extraneous materials, interruptions, rules or criteria to adhere to
Awareness *Outside of Task* *Before Task* *During* *After*	• Describes physical deficits (walking) as the main obstacle to function. Did not acknowledge cognitive concerns or limitations. • Poor anticipation – overestimates abilities within a task. • Recognizes errors after the fact. • Acknowledges task errors and is surprised by them. He is not aware that his impulsivity and tendency to become sidetracked are contributing to these errors.
Strategy Use *Generation and initiation* *Type* *Frequency and timing* *Efficiency and effort* *Flexibility* *Consistency* *Effectiveness*	• Does not anticipate or generate strategies before the task. • Occasionally inconsistent but ineffective strategy use observed during a task. • After tasks, occasionally makes general statements (need to pay more attention, take a little more time) but does not identify specific strategies.
Potential for Learning and Change	• Client acknowledges task errors with structured self-assessment and is responsive to guided questions. He recalls information from day to day and attempts to use some strategies spontaneously. He has not yet had the opportunity to try many IADL. With structured experiences and guided questions, there is good potential for increased self-awareness.

Treatment Goals

1. Client will use a 10-item list to gather items and attend to details as a prerequisite to IADL such as bill paying and meal preparation.
2. Client will stand and ambulate 10 feet with a walker in the kitchen independently (without verbal cues) by using strategies to mentally review steps and pace/regulate actions.
3. Client will pay one bill accurately without verbal cues to self-recognize and correct performance errors.
4. Client will make a hot breakfast with only occasional cues.

Summary of Treatment Sessions

Fred was seen daily for individual treatment sessions within an inpatient setting. 15.2 Case Example 1 presents sample activities used across treatment. In sessions 1-3, Fred engaged in activities that involved both physical and cognitive challenges such as standing, reaching for items in cabinets and drawers while simultaneously following a list, and recording information. The activities addressed Fred's motor goals while also requiring attention to relevant details. Initially, Fred made several performance errors that he recognized with structured self-evaluation methods. Post-task questions during these sessions focused on helping Fred think about methods he could use before and during the task to help make sure that the task went smoothly. The therapist reflected on observations and used guided questioning techniques. For example, "I noticed that you jumped right into the task and did it very quickly. What could you do before the task to help make things go more smoothly? What type of image or picture or "saying" can you think of to help you pace your speed and timing so that you don't go too fast?" Since Fred likes music, he thought of an image of a metronome. During the task, however, he acknowledged that he forgot to use the strategy.

By session 4, Fred generally recognized that he needed to slow down his performance and resist the tendency to get sidetracked by extraneous information and thoughts. Following task experiences, Fred began to generate additional strategies, with structured questions. For example, he thought of a slow, calm melody to "play" in his head and sayings such as "plan and review" or "SC" (for Stop and Check). Although he was beginning to identify strategies that he could use, he did not carry out his plans consistently. He often realized this after errors occurred or after task completion. It is important to note that at this point, Fred continued to identify physical goals as his main area of concern. He did not acknowledge any cognitive limitations during a general interview and did not change

15.2 Case Example 1 Inpatient Case (Fred): Sample treatment activities across the horizontal continuum

	Very Similar → Somewhat Similar		Different → Very Different	
Session	Sessions 1-3	Sessions 4-5	Sessions 6-7	Sessions 8-9
Session focus	Promoting awareness of performance: error recognition and need to use different task methods.	Anticipation of "things to watch out for" and initial generation of strategies.	Task difficulty increased. Strategy generation and monitoring strategy use.	**Self-Chosen activities** Monitoring and assessing the effectiveness of strategies.
Sample activities	List of ingredients in kitchen cabinets. Retrieve ingredients and write calories on list (working on standing and reaching). Kitchen supply list provided. Need to take inventory (# of coffee cups, frying pans, etc.).	Two menus on bulletin board and list on table. Needs to find items on the list that are also on the menu and write the price and name of restaurant on the list. Requires walking back and forth. Supply cabinet inventory – write the number of each item (boxes of paper, pens, pencils). *Ambulating 15 ft.*	Ambulate on floor and write location of electronic devices (computers, phones). Find items in gift shop on a list that meet criteria and write down price and item. Cafeteria – identify items for lunch that meet dietary restrictions.	Make breakfast – scrambled eggs, coffee, and toast. Pay bill online.
Outcomes	Awareness of performance errors emerges with structure. Begins to generate general strategies with guidance after the task.	Beginning to self-monitor. Performance shows improvement. Recognizes need to use different methods by session 4, but during the task does not always use them. Only occasional errors in session 4, by session 5, no errors.	Recognizes performance errors. With questioning, acknowledges that he did not use the strategy.	Anticipates possible challenges such as "missing something." Uses strategies.

his goals. At the same time, however, his *awareness of performance* was changing, along with his task outcomes. By the end of session 5, he was successfully self-monitoring performance in activities that involved following a simple list or directions. The physical therapist was reporting that he was consistently following mobility directions and was no longer standing up in an unsafe manner.

At this point, activities were graded up slightly in complexity to include rules, additional criteria, and distractions within task and environment. As complexity increased, Fred's ability to implement his strategies fluctuated and remained inconsistent. In distracting environments, Fred was more likely to act impulsively. For example, at the gift store, he picked up candy (which he was not supposed to have) and started eating it before paying. He immediately realized this was inappropriate when the cashier asked him to pay. By sessions 7 and 8, he began to ask about trying additional activities. For example, he expressed interest in activities such as shopping online for electronics and preparing scrambled eggs, coffee, and toast for breakfast. At the start of the treatment program, he did not think he would have any difficulties with these activities but now he was unsure of himself. Although this was a point that functional cognitive goal planning and goal rating could have been introduced, Fred was discharged to his brother's home, three hours away. The therapist spent time with his brother's wife on the phone reviewing his program and progress and highlighting the need to seek additional occupational therapy treatment.

In general, all treatment activities were at Fred's physical level and involved standing, walking, and reaching. The incorporation of physical activities that were consistent with Fred's goals increased his engagement and motivation in treatment. As his physical capacity and standing tolerance increased, activities involving ambulating were included. Although the activities met Fred's physical goals, they were also simultaneously designed to facilitate self-awareness and strategy use across activities.

Outcome

Change in Treatment Targets within Treatment Sessions

Fred showed changes in treatment targets within treatment sessions (15.3 Case Example 1) as well as across pre/post outcome measures (15.4 Case Example 1). 15.3 Case Example 1 illustrates that within functional cognitive tasks, Fred's ability to identify challenges, generate strategies, monitor and recognize errors, and make connections between activity experiences increased across treatment sessions. Toward the end of treatment, Fred also began to identify new goals and activities as described in sessions 7-8, further providing indications of changes in awareness.

Post-Treatment Assessment Results

Post-treatment outcome measures also demonstrate positive changes compared to initial scores. However, at the same time, they indicate that there is additional room for improvement (see 15.4 Case Example 1).

Self-Regulation Skills Interview (SSRI)

Fred's responses on the SRSI were considerably different from the initial interview. He now stated that sometimes he tends to miss information because he goes too fast, especially if there are a lot of directions, but he could not provide specific examples within the interview. He also stated that he needed to stop and plan, remember to go slowly, and check his work, but he was unable to provide details on how he used these strategies (although they were observed during treatment).

15.3 Case Example 1 Inpatient Case (Fred): Summary of Changes in Treatment Targets

Activity	Identification of Challenges	Strategy Generation	Error Recognition During Performance	Mediation Provided	Recognition of Performance errors	Strategy generation	Connection to other activities
1	None	None	None	No	With self-assessment	None	No
4	Rushing	Go slower	Occasionally	Yes	With self-assessment	Yes	Yes, with prompts
8	Missing something	Stop and check	Yes	No	Initiates self-check	Yes	Yes

15.4 Case Example 1 Inpatient Case (Fred): Summary of Pre-Post Treatment Outcomes

Test	Pre-treatment Score	Post-treatment Score
SRSI		
Awareness (0-20)	20	14
Strategy Behavior (0-30)	28	15
Total (0-50)	48	28
WCPA-10		
Total time	8:09	14:13
Planning time	0	1:30
# Entered appointments (0-10)	8/10	10
# Accurate appointments (0-10)	3/8	6/10
# Missing	2	0
# Total Errors	7	4
# Rules followed	1/5	3/5
Total strategies used	1	3
Activity Measure Post-Acute Care (AM-PAC)- Applied Cognitive scale	-------	38.61 (minor difficulties)
Pill Box Organizer (15 pills)	9/15	14/15

Weekly Calendar Planning Activity (WCPA)

On the WCPA, changes were noted in performance accuracy, rules followed, strategy use, and responses to the after-task interview. Compared to initial performance, Fred entered all appointments; however, he continued to make some errors in location and details (although reduced). He took more time planning and reviewing the list before starting. He consistently checked off each appointment after it was entered and did not randomly jump around on the list as he did initially. At the same time, however, he did not use efficient methods (went down the list in order). This created appointment conflicts. He also continued to miss some details but was observed to be more focused and adhered to more rules. In addition to consistently checking off the list, Fred spontaneously checked and compared the number of appointments entered against the list (although he did not check details) and used the strategy of crossing out the day on the calendar, so that no appointments could be entered. Afterward, he identified challenges and generated additional strategies he could have used (placing fixed appointments first).

Performance of Cognitive Functional Tasks

Similarly, performance on functional tasks such as organizing a pillbox and completing a bill-paying task (dynamic performance analysis) improved; however, occasional errors and a tendency to miss details were noted. For example, on the bill-paying task, Fred paid all bills (initially he omitted one bill); however, he paid the total amount for one of the bills rather than the balance due and this exceeded the balance in the checking account. During the pillbox task, he placed one too many pills in one slot, however, this was a considerable improvement from initial assessment when he made six errors. Physical therapy also no longer reported safety concerns during ambulation. These observations were consistent with his discharge score on the Applied Cognitive Scale of the Activity Measure of Post-Acute care that categorized performance as minor difficulties in cognitive IADL.

Summary

In summary, Fred demonstrated improvements in awareness and self-monitoring skills that corresponded with changes observed in functional cognitive tasks. He was observed to take time for planning and to spontaneously initiate strategies across different activities; however, he continued to have a tendency to miss details in complex activities. Continued outpatient or home-based occupational therapy is recommended to increase the effectiveness of Fred's self-monitoring skills and strategy use and increase the ability to manage novel and complex situations.

CASE 2: OUTPATIENT DAY PROGRAM, TRAUMATIC BRAIN INJURY

This case describes application of the MC approach with a person with chronic traumatic brain injury (TBI) and severe memory deficits in a community day program. The person, Mike, readily acknowledges memory deficits but does not anticipate or recognize memory errors as they occur within an activity. This case illustrates *strategy-specific training*; namely, helping a person use a list as a tool to support memory within an activity as a strategy. It also illustrates integration of other approaches, such as errorless learning and technology, to address other aspects of behavior, while simultaneously enhancing awareness of performance and increasing self-monitoring and effectiveness of use of a single strategy (list).

Overview of Current Functional Status and Occupational History

Mike is a 27-year-old male, three years post-TBI with severe memory problems. Mike attended a community day program daily. He was unemployed and living with his parents at the time of treatment. He reported that his three-year-old son from a former relationship visited him once a week, under the supervision of his parents. Mike did not have any physical disabilities and was independent in self-care activities. He participated in a case study project involving nine intervention sessions and pre and post-testing. Before his injury, Mike worked as an HVAC technician and also at a friend's deli, preparing sandwiches or salads and assisting with cooking. He lived in an apartment with a roommate. Mike expressed an interest in cars, building things, and doing activities with his son.

Client's Goals

Mike was unable to state any goals except to "get better." With specific questioning, he stated that he would like his memory to improve. When asked what he would like to remember better, he stated "everything" and was unable to provide examples.

Occupational Therapy Evaluation

Initial Assessment Results

Self-Regulation Skills Interview

Mike readily acknowledged problems with short-term memory with structured questions, but he could not spontaneously provide examples and stated he doesn't rely on his memory. During the interview, he was unable to hold onto information for more than a few minutes and frequently repeated the same stories without realizing he had already shared them. When asked about strategies, he indicated that his mother writes information that he needs to remember on a whiteboard in the house, but he could not generate anything else that he could do on his own to remember things. He appeared to believe that there was nothing he could do to help his memory and indicated that his brain was messed up from the accident.

Awareness Questionnaire

The Awareness Questionnaire (AQ) is a 17-item scale that is rated on a scale of 1 (much worse than before) to 5 (much better) (Sherer et al., 1998). Discrepancy scores are obtained by subtracting the informant's score from the client's self-rating. Scores range from -68 to +68, with higher positive discrepancy scores indicating greater impairment of self-awareness. A score of >20 indicates clinically significant impairment in self-awareness (Evans et al., 2005). Mike rated himself as generally being either the same or better in most areas since his injury, except memory. The discrepancy between himself and a staff member was 15, indicating good general awareness.

Contextual Memory Test (CMT)

On the CMT Mike recalled 5/20 items and after 15 minutes only recalled 2 items. Before the activity, he predicted he would have difficulty (prediction = 4/20 items). After the activity, he acknowledged he only remembered 2 items.

Multiple Errands Test (MET)

Mike carried out 5 out of 12 errands, but only one errand was completed. He put the list in his pocket and got distracted by items he saw in a nearby vending machine and appeared to forget entirely about the list. He spent most of the time walking around the hospital lobby aimlessly. For example, when he had to pick up an envelope at the security desk, he walked to the desk but then appeared to forget why he had walked to the desk and did not look at the list. The same behavior was observed while walking into the gift shop (he appeared to forget why he was there). At the end of the task, he rated it as easy and appeared to be unaware of his errors.

Executive Function Performance Test - Bill Paying Subtest (EFPT-B)

On the bill-paying task, Mike wrote down incorrect amounts on the ledger and checks and needed multiple direct cues to complete the task, however, he rated himself as "efficient" and was unaware of his errors.

Weekly Calendar Planning Activity (WCPA)

Mike entered 7 appointments into the calendar, however, only 3/7 were correct, resulting in a total of 14 errors. Mike did not check off any items on the list and entered several appointments twice without realizing that he had done so. Half of the appointments he entered were incomplete or only partially correct (right location, wrong time slot). At one point, he appeared to forget that the list existed and began entering his own appointments. He pulled out his daily schedule and began copying the schedule into the calendar. During the after-task interview, he stated the task was easy. With specific probing, he acknowledged that he forgot to look back at the appointment list.

Functional Cognitive Problems

The following issues were observed or reported by Mike's therapists, family, or friends:

- Does not accurately follow 2-3 step directions and loses track of the goal or what step he is up to during activities.
- Unable to follow a recipe, pay bills, go shopping, or perform multiple-step IADL such as cooking.
- Does not recall previous conversations or events from the day before.
- Meal Preparation – prepares routine snacks and a sandwich but is unable to accurately follow a list of directions on packages or recipes. Needs close supervision for using appliances or the stove.
- Received a new phone and is unable to remember how to enter appointments into the calendar.

Treatment Targets

Build awareness and self-monitoring skills related to using a list:

- Recognize repeated error pattern (missing info).
- Identify the need to use a list.
- Anticipates challenges in following a list.
- Self-generates strategies for managing a list.
- Identifies how/why strategies help performance with a task.

Treatment Goals

1. Client will anticipate the need to use a list in a multiple-step cognitive IADL task.
2. Client will consistently refer to a written list of directions or list as a pre-requisite for functional use.
3. Client will use a 6- to 8-step list accurately in completing IADL such as shopping and following a recipe.
4. Client will follow a provided 8-step list with 95% accuracy.

Summary of Treatment Sessions

Mike was seen at his day program for individual sessions twice a week for four weeks. The first four sessions involved two structured activities each, across the horizontal continuum. Mike was asked to self-select or identify treatment activities for sessions 5 and above and initially he was unable to do so. Instead, he self-selected activities from a pre-made list presented by the therapist. Towards the end of treatment (session 8-9), Mike self-identified goals and activities he wanted to work on, and goal planning techniques were used. 15.6 Case Example 2 summarizes the focus of treatment sessions, sample activities, and the observed outcomes. After each session, the therapist guided Mike in summarizing his experiences in a structured activity journal that included the activity, areas for improvement, methods that helped performance, and things to watch out for as well as other observations. Each session began with a review of the journal from the previous session and ended with documentation in the journal.

During the initial treatment sessions, Mike was unable to anticipate any difficulties or generate any strategies, even with prompts and questions. He readily agreed that using a checklist would be helpful during an activity; however, he did not initiate looking at the list or marking the list

15.5 Case Example 2 Outpatient Day Program Case (Mike): Summary of Assessment

Client Concerns and Goals	• I want my memory to get better.
Functional Cognitive Concerns by Others	• Poor memory • Asks the same questions, • Repeats same steps within tasks because he forgets what he just did.
Functional Cognitive Performance *(activity limitations and/or participation restrictions)*	• IADL activities and following any multistep activity. • Unable to pay bills, follow a list of directions, follow a recipe. • Unable to return to independent living, work.
Cognitive performance errors or behaviors that go across activities	• Repetition of task steps and omission of details or steps are the most frequent errors due to a lack of the ability to keep track of information. • Forgets what step he has just completed and what should be done next. • Forgets conversations, previous events, or what was done the day before.
Activity/environment characteristics that increase likelihood of errors	• Nonroutine activities with three or more steps. • Activities that involve following three or more step directions. • Less familiar or novel activities.
Awareness *Outside of Task* *Before Task* *During* *After*	• Readily acknowledges poor memory in an interview but is unable to provide examples (States he is unable to remember anything). • Anticipates and acknowledges difficulties on a memory task but overestimates abilities on functional cognitive tasks. • Poor self-monitoring – Does not recognize errors within a functional cognitive activity or immediately afterwards. • With structured questions, or self-assessment – acknowledges some errors but generally overestimates performance.
Strategy Use *Generation and initiation* *Type* *Frequency and timing* *Efficiency and effort* *Flexibility* *Consistency* *Effectiveness*	• No strategies observed. • Makes multiple errors in multiple step tasks. • Does not consistently refer back to written lists or directions. • Does not initiate use of strategies.
Potential for Learning and Change	• Acknowledges memory deficits but appears to believe there is nothing he can do about his memory deficits (poor memory self-efficacy). • Poor online awareness and self-monitoring. • Has difficulty recalling information from session to session. Will need repetition, practice, and increased self-efficacy to effect change.

unless he was cued to do so. During the first session, Mike frequently lost track of what he had just done within the activity and repeated already completed steps on the checklist. He needed nearly continual cues to refer to the list and when he referred to it, he did not mark off completed steps.

During session 2, he was provided with a vibrating timer. The timer was used as a "cue" to remind him to check the list every 5 minutes within the activity. Initially, when he felt the vibrating signal, he would recognize "I'm supposed to do something" but he did not know what he was supposed to do. Errorless learning techniques such as pointing to the list if Mike appeared not to know what to do when the signal went off were used. The use of the vibrating signal was gradually withdrawn. By the end of session 5, he was checking the list the majority of time on his own without the vibrating timer, so the timer was discontinued.

In addition, to inconsistently referring to the checklist, Mike had difficulty remembering what step he was up to on the list. A focus of treatment was on helping Mike recognize that if he marked the list when he completed a step, it would help him keep track of what had been completed. Changes in awareness relating to use of the list began to emerge. During the first two treatment sessions, Mike did not anticipate any difficulties and could not generate any strategies. As treatment progressed, he anticipated that he may have a little difficulty but could not provide examples. By session 5, he began to anticipate and recognize difficulties using and marking the list. For example, when asked if he anticipated any difficulty or challenges, he states "not if I mark the list; sometimes I forget to mark it." Although he marked each step, he also sometimes missed the details or only followed part of the step. Mike began to self-generate strategies such as circling or underlining keywords in each step on the list. His accuracy in completing activities also significantly increased.

In session 5, Mike was asked to self-select treatment activities but could not identify any activities he wanted to work on. He was presented with a ready-made list and identified activities within his interest, including using an internet site to "build a car" and learning to use the calendar and alarm function for his new cell phone. At this point, he began to self-identify his own goals. For example, at the end of session 7, he stated he wanted to make dinner for his family. A goal-planning worksheet was used to help him identify what he needed to do to prepare (making a shopping list, checking the kitchen for needed supplies and ingredients, shopping, and cooking), as well as to help him anticipate possible challenges and strategies for success. During the shopping trip, he realized he forgot to bring a pen and repeatedly told the therapist, "I need a pen to mark the list." At this point, he was consistently marking the list and self-monitoring his use of the list. Staff reported that when he was presented with a series of directions or confronted with a complex activity, he began to initiate asking staff for a written checklist.

At the end of treatment, Mike began to initiate other goals. For example, he indicated he would like to be able to be more independent from his mother and provided an example of shopping in the mall without his mother next to him in every store. Since Mike was participating in a study, treatment was discontinued after session 9. Recommendations were made to continue OT treatment, but due to the length of time since his injury and insurance restrictions, therapy could not continue; however, the facility agreed to have an OT consultant monitor his progress. The facility and family were provided with recommendations including a plan to increase independence in cooking and shopping.

Outcome

Post-treatment Assessment Results

On immediate post-testing, changes were observed in all measures (15.7 Case Example 2).

Awareness

General awareness as measured by the AQ remained unchanged; however, on the SRSI, Mike was now able to provide examples of memory difficulties and strategies. For example, he was able to describe the list strategy and stated, "If I don't mark the list, things get messed up and I leave things off."

Contextual Memory Test

Mike continued to demonstrate significant memory deficits, but his encoding of information slightly improved. He attempted to use strategies during the memory task; however, they were ineffective and inefficient. For example, he tried to remember items in pairs rather than in larger groups or clusters; though, this was an improvement from initial testing, when he did not initiate any strategies.

Multiple Errands Test

On the MET, Mike actively used the checklist and marked items off on the list; however, he did not attend to all parts of the page and missed a few steps. He rated his performance on the MET as inefficient (as compared to the pre-tests when he rated his performance as efficient).

Executive Function Performance Test – Bill Paying Subtest

On retest, Mike kept track of all three bills. He no longer needed direct verbal cues, but he did need verbal and gestural guidance to complete the task accurately.

Weekly Calendar Planning Activity

During the WCPA, Mike was also observed to refer to the list and marked it off consistently. Although he missed a few items, he made active attempts to underline keywords and self-check responses. His ability to manage the number of items on the list significantly improved as compared to initial assessment; however, he continued to have difficulty accurately holding on to all the information he needed (appointment name, time, location, and day) as he moved from the list to the calendar.

15.6 Case Example 2 Outpatient Day Program Case (Mike): Sample Treatment Activities Across the Horizontal Continuum

Very Similar → Somewhat Similar → Different → Very Different

Session	Sessions 1-2	Sessions 3-4	Sessions 5-7	Sessions 8-9
Session focus	Refer to list during activity Increase recognition of tendency to lose track during the activity and need to look at list.	Refer to list during activity Initial anticipation – What do you need to watch out for? Increase awareness of how/why the list improves performance. Self-assessment	Increase anticipation and initiation of asking for a written list (when provided with verbal directions) Self-generation of list Focus on using list effectively – attend to all parts of the instruction.	Self-generation of list Focus on using list effectively – attend to all parts of the instruction.
Sample activities	*Structured activities* Follow a list of directions to make a fruit salad, slice and bake cookies, decorate cookies and enter items into a weekly menu.	*Structured activities* Follow a list to enter items into a TV schedule. Follow a list to create a series of e-vites on the computer.	*Self-selected from a list* Follow a list to take photos and save them in a folder on a computer. Follow a list of directions to "Build a Honda car" from a website. Follow a list of directions to set appointments in phone.	*Self-Selected activities* Making dinner for family. Checking kitchen for supplies and ingredients, making shopping list of needed items, shopping at supermarket and following directions.
Techniques	Vibrating timed device introduced in session 2 as a reminder to look at list every 3-5 minutes. *Questioning* – Why is it important to look at the list? What does the list help you do?	Vibrating device gradually faded within sessions.	Vibrating timer was discontinued after session 5.	Use of Goal Planning worksheet.
Session	Sessions 1-2	Sessions 3-4	Sessions 5-7	Sessions 8-9
Outcomes	Lost track of what was completed within the activity and re-did already completed tasks on the checklist. Needed frequent reminders to use list.	Over-estimated performance; did not identify. Used list consistently with external vibrating signal.	By the end of session 5, was checking the list the majority of time on his own. Anticipated before tasks that he might forget to "check and mark the list," and began reminding himself to check the list within activities (self-talk). When confronted with a complex activity began to initiate asking for a list. Self-identified goals emerge	Consistently anticipates possible challenges such as "forgetting to mark the list. Marking the list consistently, skipping a step or missing something the majority of time of the time.

15.7 Case Example 2 Outpatient Day Program Case (Mike): Summary of Pre-Post Treatment Outcomes

Test	Pre-treatment Score	Post-treatment Score
Awareness Questionnaire Discrepancy (-68 to +68)	15	14
SRSI		
Awareness (0-20)	20	13
Strategy Behavior (0-30)	25	15
Total (0-50)	45	28
CMT		
Immediate recall (0-20)	5/20	8/20
Delayed Recall (0-20)	2/20	3/20
Strategy (0-12)	none	Minimal association
Awareness Discrepancy	-1	-3
WCPA-17		
Total time		
Planning time	0	30 seconds
# Entered appointments (0-17)	7	15
# Accurate appointments (0-17)	3	8
# Missing	10	2
Total # Errors	14	9
# Rules followed (0-5)	1	2
Total strategies used	0	3 Checked off list, underlined keywords, self-checked
MET (12 tasks to carry out)	11 errors	6 errors
Marked list	0	6x
EFPT - Bill Paying subtask (0-25)	11	6

Observed Changes in Functional Cognition

Although Mike continued to demonstrate difficulties within functional tasks, a trend toward improvement across all measures was observed. There was also evidence of increased self-efficacy. Initially, Mike didn't seem to believe there was anything he could do to help his memory and was unable to identify specific goals except to "get better and improve his memory." Toward the end of treatment, Mike began to identify specific goals and was initiating strategies, including asking others to provide him with a list, if directions were too long to remember. The gains that were observed were maintained upon retesting four weeks later. In addition, after four weeks, staff continued to report that Mike asked for lists if multiple-step directions were provided and consistently checked it off.

Six-Month Follow-Up

An informal video interview at six months post-intervention indicated that Mike recalled activities that were done during treatment such as making dinner for his family and a digital photography task. Given the extent of his memory impairment, it was surprising that he was able to recall these activities. Both of these activities, however, were meaningful and enjoyable to him and also had a procedural component. Mike was also able to continue to articulate that use of a list helps to make sure he doesn't forget things. He reported engaging in more activities and using lists that his mother created for household errands and activities. For example, he reported cooking for his family about once a week with a list.

CASE 3: IN-HOME TREATMENT, PARKINSON'S DISEASE

This case discusses application of the MC approach for a person with mild cognitive deficits in their home environment. It took place as a part of a research study on the use of the MC approach with community-dwelling adults with Parkinson's disease (PD) without dementia. The person, Sue, was aware of and could describe some emerging cognitive difficulties and trouble completing complex tasks, and she expressed frustration, feeling overwhelmed, and reduced self-efficacy as a result. The case illustrates how structured activities and discussion can foster a deeper understanding of cognitive performance and strategies to control it; the use of a cognitive log, homework, and action planning to promote generalization of strategies to everyday life; and improved self-efficacy through the use of strategies to cope with cognitive challenges.

Overview of Current Functional Status and Occupational History

Sue is a 74-year-old woman who has been diagnosed with PD for 7 years. She is Hoehn and Yahr stage II, indicating generally mild bilateral motor symptoms with intact balance. She has been diagnosed with probable mild cognitive impairment (PD-MCI) based on a MoCA score of 24/30, an in-depth clinical interview (Clinical Dementia Rating Scale), and a comprehensive neuropsychological assessment.

Sue is a retired teacher who lives in a ranch-style home with her husband, who is also retired. She is independent in all self-care and instrumental ADL at home and in the community. Her husband handles the household finances. She spends her days running errands, performing home duties (e.g., cleaning, cooking, laundry), exercising (4-5x/week), and in quiet leisure. She and her husband attend church every Sunday morning and afterward teach Sunday school to 3 year old's, and they participate in a Bible study discussion group most weeks. They have an active social life and have two children and four grandchildren who live nearby that they see regularly.

Client's Goals

Sue enrolled in the study because she noticed thinking and memory problems in her everyday life, and she wanted to learn ways to address or overcome them. Treatment-related goals were established collaboratively with the therapist after an in-depth evaluation of her functional cognition (see below under Treatment Goals).

Occupational Therapy Evaluation

Initial Assessment Results

Self-Regulation Skills Interview

Sue stated that her main area of difficulty was "organization" and provided examples such as not having all of the items needed for a recipe, misplacing items around her home, and having difficulty following her lesson plans while teaching Sunday school. She noticed that these difficulties mainly occur when there are more people around and more things going on (e.g., company in the kitchen while she's trying to cook). When asked about strategies she could use or is using to cope, she said that she's been trying to get rid of unnecessary items around her home and cooking in bigger batches so she has leftovers and does not need to cook as often.

Weekly Calendar Planning Activity

Sue entered 8/17 appointments within 25 minutes, at which point she was frustrated and gave up with the task. Of the eight appointments entered, only three were accurate, despite using a variety of strategies (e.g., circling key words, rearranging materials, talking aloud). She attempted to plan the calendar out in writing first; however, she tried to organize the appointments by day and could not handle conflicts when they arose. She was also bothered and distracted by the Saturday-Sunday reversal and how the time increments were displayed on the calendar.

During the activity, Sue was generally aware that she was having difficulty and indicated she was feeling overwhelmed and confused, but she did not appear to recognize why she was having difficulty and did not adjust her approach even though it was not effective. After the activity, she could verbalize her difficulty and confusion and identify the flexible appointments as problematic. She stated that writing in the fixed appointments first, then going back and filling in the flexible appointments would be a helpful strategy; however, she continued to state that she would go day by day (which was an ineffective strategy).

Behavioral Rating Inventory of Executive Function – Adult Form

Sue self-reported increased problems with Inhibition, Shifting, Emotional Control, Working Memory, Planning and Organization, and Task Monitoring compared to age-appropriate normative data. Her Behavioral Regulation Index, Metacognition Index, and Global Executive Composite scores were also elevated. Using the informant-report version of this questionnaire, her husband rated her everyday cognitive and emotional regulation as typical.

Cognitive Self-Efficacy Questionnaire

Sue reported relatively low confidence (≤ 5 on a scale of 1-10) in her ability to self-recognize cognitive lapses and implement strategies to cope with mentally challenging tasks. Her confidence in her ability to perform everyday cognitive tasks was higher for some activities (e.g., remember at least five items in the refrigerator without looking, mentally keep track of two different medications, understand a 10-minute lecture) but low to moderate on most others (e.g., plan and organize a party with 25 people, follow written directions to a new location that involves 7-8 steps).

Functional Cognitive Problems

Sue completed a cognitive log for one week between the pre-treatment assessment and the goal-setting discussion in which she documented "troublesome cognitive experiences or cognitive lapses" that occurred in her daily life. The following is a summary of the issues she noted:

- Forgetting to buy items at the grocery store.
- Trouble listening to sermon and taking notes at the same time (for discussion group).
- Difficulty/problems doing laundry and cooking because distracted by the TV and phone ringing.
- Misplacing items around the home.
- Not having all information at hand when beginning tasks (e.g., insurance card and calendar while trying to schedule a doctor's appointment on the phone; ingredients for recipes).
- Losing place in recipes.
- Not being able to finish activities due to frustration/anxiety/stress.
- Difficulty staying on track and following the lesson plan while teaching Sunday school.

Treatment Targets

Build awareness, self-monitoring skills, and strategy use across IADL:

- Online awareness of performance errors
- Anticipation of task challenges prior to an activity
- Independent initiation of strategies to avoid or prevent performance errors
- Application of self-monitoring skills and strategies across everyday activities

Treatment Goals

After reviewing her pre-treatment assessment results, cognitive log, and completing a brief occupational profile focusing on functional cognition, Sue listed several functional cognitive problem areas to address during treatment. She then rated them on 10-point scales for Performance and Satisfaction with Performance (using the scales from the Canadian Occupational Performance Measure, COPM; higher scores indicate better perceived Performance and Satisfaction) (15.9 Case Example 3). Sue's Performance ratings ranged from 3-6, and her Satisfaction ratings ranged from 2-6.

Summary of Treatment Sessions

Sue was seen weekly at her home for six sessions. 15.10 Case Example 3 presents sample activities used across treatment. Sessions consisted of simulated treatment activities and discussion to promote awareness, strategy generation, strategy use, connection to everyday situations, and self-efficacy. In addition, between sessions, Sue continued her cognitive log and created homework action plans to monitor her daily functional cognitive performance and to implement strategies that were generated during treatment sessions in her everyday life.

In sessions 1-2, treatment activities and discussions focused on promoting Sue's awareness of cognitive performance errors that go across activities or situations and the initial generation of strategies to control them. Initially, in structured activities, Sue made errors during the self-checking portion of the activities. With therapist prompting and questioning, she identified her errors and determined that difficulty keeping track while shifting back and forth was the source. She was able to generate several strategies to help her keep track with

15.8 Case Example 3 Home Setting (Sue): Summary of Assessment

Client Concerns and Goals	• Multitasking • Organization • Managing frustration • Dealing with distractions and interruptions
Functional Cognitive Concerns by Others	• Husband agrees with everything discussed by client and additionally adds digressing during conversations as an issue that he has noticed
Functional Cognitive Performance *(activity limitations and/or participation restrictions)*	• Preparing meals – specifically those that require coordinating multiple dishes and/or new recipes • Housework • Shopping • Church – following sermons and discussion groups • Teaching Sunday school
Cognitive performance errors or behaviors that go across activities	• Difficulty inhibiting irrelevant information • Difficulty with flexibility – shifting attention between different sets of information, trying new approaches to solving problems if one way isn't working • Organization of materials, personal space, and information • Working memory – keeping track of where she is in a task; following group conversations • Difficulty returning to a task once interrupted • Difficulty managing emotions/frustration/anxiety
Activity/environment characteristics that increase likelihood of errors	• Time pressure • Lots of stimuli, distractions, disorganization, interruptions • Multitasking
Awareness *Outside of Task* *Before Task* *During* *After*	• Able to describe difficulties after experiencing them • Able to connect difficulties in activity performance (e.g., cooking, shopping) to cognitive errors or behaviors (e.g., getting distracted or frustrated) and activity/environment characteristics (e.g., multitasking, interruptions) • Lack of anticipation or planning ahead to avoid difficulties
Strategy Use **Generation and initiation** *Type* *Frequency and timing* *Efficiency and effort* *Flexibility* *Consistency* *Effectiveness*	• Generates a number of appropriate and potentially useful strategies for problems in discussion but has not implemented any of them
Potential for Learning and Change	• High, motivated

15.9 Case Example 3 Home Setting (Sue): Canadian Occupational Performance Measure Initial Scores

Problem Area	Performance	Satisfaction
Cooking (coordinating meals, new recipes)	6	3
Teaching Sunday school	6	3
Multitasking	5	2
Dealing with distractions and interruptions	4	6
Managing frustrations	3	3
Organizing *(this goal was refined over the course of treatment to be more specific – See 15.11 Case Example 3 below under Outcomes)*	5	4
Digressing during conversation	4	2

therapist guidance including using her finger, marking off, and double-checking. On subsequent attempts, she implemented her strategies but inconsistently unless prompted by the therapist (at which point she was successful). Discussions and homework focused on the application of these strategies to her everyday life, including checking off ingredients and recipe steps while cooking and checking grocery items off the list as she placed them in her cart. Additionally, it was determined that problems multitasking could also be prevented by taking steps to avoid doing multiple things at once. For example, instead of trying to take notes while listening to the sermon in real time, she realized that she could simply listen to the sermon while in church and then access the church's recording (available online) afterward for note-taking and deeper thought.

15.10 Case Example 3 Home Setting (Sue): Sample treatment activities across the horizontal continuum

	Very Similar → Somewhat Similar → Different → Very Different		
Session	**Sessions 1-2**	**Sessions 3-4**	**Sessions 5-6**
Session focus	Promoting awareness of cognitive performance errors across situations and initial generation of strategies.	Anticipation of challenges and consistent use of strategies. Task difficulty increases.	Consistent use of strategies. Application and monitoring effectiveness of strategies in real-life situations.
Sample activities	Use different colored pens to mark $2, $3, and $4 coupons off on a page. Transfer answers to a chart and check own work against an answer key. Use different-colored pens to mark different types of activities on a calendar. Check work against an answer key.	Transfer different types of films (Comedy, Drama, Documentary) from a list to separate calendars. Check work against answer keys. Review two recipes and the items in your kitchen, and make a shopping list for a party.	Created action plans to apply strategies to real-world activities: Shopping for and preparing a meal for family. Teaching Sunday school.
Outcomes	Awareness of performance errors and generation of strategies to control performance with therapist questioning and guidance. Some independent use of strategies; successful use when prompted.	Carryover and use of previously generated strategies. Fewer performance errors. Increased task difficulty prompted the generation of additional strategies.	Independent use of a variety of strategies in everyday life in relation to self-identified goals.

In sessions 3-4, treatment focused on anticipation of challenges and independent and consistent use of strategies. Sue successfully used her strategies for keeping track to control performance errors, so the structured treatment activities increased in difficulty (e.g., more complex instructions, more information to sort through, higher shifting demands) and incorporated her own objects and environment. As task difficulty increased, she gained additional awareness (with therapist guidance) of the need to break down or simplify more complex activities or instructions so they are not overwhelming, and "pre-planning" before beginning activities. Through discussion, she realized that these strategies might help her to avoid becoming frustrated, as well as ensure she has everything she needs before beginning an activity. Sessions 5-6 focused on consistent application and monitoring of strategies across real-world situations.

Discussions during sessions 3-6 helped make explicit connections between Sue's strategies for keeping track, pre-planning, avoiding doing two things at once, and her goals. For example, that making lists and checking things off as she goes can support her cooking, Sunday school teaching, dealing with distractions or interruptions, and multitasking. In addition, pre-planning in terms of making lists and gathering all materials before beginning a task can also help with complex activities. Strategies for pre-planning and keeping track can also reduce her frustration, which is caused by difficulty managing interruptions and feeling overwhelmed, and help her feel more in control and confident. Homework involved continued application of strategies for keeping track while cooking, shopping, and teaching Sunday school; taking the time to pre-plan before making a phone call or cooking to ensure she has everything she needs and to plan strategy use, and further ways to reduce multitasking and distractions (e.g., turn the phone and TV off while cooking, making some dishes of a multi-course meal a day ahead of time).

Improvements in self-efficacy were evident in the reflections completed by Sue at the end of each treatment session, illustrated by the following quotes:

- Session 1: "I'm normal!" "I can get help – I can adapt."
- Session 2: "Multitasking is most difficult for me – I do have new strategies for that. [I learned that] I can still do things I enjoy with some new strategies."
- Session 4: "Going back several times to check my work HELPS!"
- Session 6: "I like that I feel more successful and have great ideas that are working for me."

Outcome

Post-Treatment Assessment Results

A comparison of pre and post treatment results, using standardized outcome measures is presented in 15.11, Case Example 3.

Self-Regulation Skills Interview

Regarding her stated difficulty with "organization" from her pre-treatment assessment, Sue additionally noted that this problem occurs when there are distractions (she has a hard time getting back on track) and time pressure. She listed a number of strategies that work well to help keep her organized and on track including using lists and checking off completed items, checking her pantry and fridge against recipes before going to the store, writing information down, avoiding multitasking, and giving herself more time.

Weekly Calendar Planning Activity

Sue entered 4/17 appointments and then became frustrated and quit at around 13 minutes. After entering the first appointment rather quickly, she reported getting "confused almost immediately" and not knowing "where to start." She attempted to enter the fixed appointments first and organize the appointments by day – starting at the top of the list with Thursday – but was overwhelmed by the amount of information and got stuck.

Behavior Rating Inventory of Executive Function – Adult Form

Sue continued to report increased problems with Shifting, Working Memory, Planning and Organization, and Task Monitoring, which resulted in elevated Metacognition Index and Global Executive Composite scores. However, now her Inhibition, Emotional Control, and Behavior Regulation Index scores were in the normal range. Similar to pre-treatment, her husband rated her everyday cognitive and emotional regulation as typical.

Cognitive Self-Efficacy Questionnaire

Sue's confidence in her ability to self-recognize cognitive lapses and implement strategies to cope with mentally challenging tasks was slightly higher but still in the low-moderate range. Her confidence in her ability to perform everyday cognitive tasks remained stable and in the moderate range overall.

15.11 Case Example 3 Home Setting (Sue): Summary of Pre-Post Treatment Outcomes

Test	Pre-treatment Score	Post-treatment Score
SRSI (average scores)		
Awareness	5	4.5
Strategy Behavior	6	3
WCPA		
Total time	Quit task at 26 minutes	Quit task at 13 minutes
Planning time	15 minutes	1 minute
# Entered appointments	8	4
# Accurate appointments	3	2
# Errors	5 (1 self-recognized)	2
# Missing	9	13
# Rules followed	3	NA
Total strategies used	7	4
BRIEF Self-rating (T-scores)		
Behavioral Regulation Index	71	61
Metacognition Index	71	75
General Executive Composite	71	70
CSEQ		
Part 1, Recognize lapses	3.8	4.8
Part 2, Implement strategies	3.9	5
Part 4, Perform daily cognitive tasks	4.6	4.5
COPM average ratings		
Performance	4	7
Satisfaction with Performance	3.3	8.4

Treatment Goals

Sue's performance ratings now ranged from 4-9, and her Satisfaction ratings ranged from 7-10 (see 15.12). Although her problem of "digressing during conversation" was never addressed during treatment, Sue's satisfaction rating improved dramatically (from 2 to 8). This may be due to the increased self-efficacy or generally more positive attitude Sue demonstrated after having gone through the intervention.

Client's Reflection and Report

After treatment, Sue reported consistent use of strategies to reduce multitasking, keep herself on track, and pre-plan. She knows she needs to continue using them so they become habits. She noted still feeling frustration and wanting to deal with it better, but also that she is better at accepting her problems and using strategies to work around them, make things easier, and avoid mistakes. She said the intervention "validated to me where I am" and that

15.12 Case Example 3 Home Setting (Sue): Canadian Occupational Performance measure: Post-Treatment Results

Problem Area	Performance	Satisfaction
Cooking (coordinating meals, new recipes)	8	10
Teaching Sunday school	8	8
Multitasking	7	8
Dealing with distractions and interruptions	8	9
Managing frustrations	4	7
Organizing/gathering needed materials and information before beginning a task (i.e., "pre-planning").	9	9
Digressing during conversation	5	8

"it's difficult to lose cognitive ability but it helps to know there are ways to cope."

Summary

After six treatment sessions, Sue demonstrated improved ability to anticipate performance problems, plan, and use effective strategies in the context of functional activities, and her perceived performance and satisfaction with her real-world functional cognitive problems/goals improved. Results from the other standardized assessments indicate slight improvements in awareness, self-rated everyday cognition, and cognitive self-efficacy. However, her WCPA performance was worse in that she got frustrated and gave up sooner. This may have stemmed from her prior negative experience with the task, as she remembered having difficulty with it at pre-assessment, so this negative reaction may have interfered with her performance. This finding indicates that Sue still needs support in simplifying complex tasks and managing her emotional reactions to cognitively challenging or overwhelming tasks. While Sue is now able to use a variety of strategies to address her self-identified problem areas, it is unclear if she could self-initiate and independently use the process of problem-solving and generating strategies to address any new cognitive challenges that might arise. Although Sue is moving in the right direction, she would likely benefit from more treatment sessions (10-12 total).

SUMMARY

This chapter described application of the MC approach across different settings, clinical problems, and client populations. It demonstrated how similar assessments and treatment structure can be used in inpatient, outpatient, and home-based settings, how assessment results can be summarized and synthesized to guide treatment (including the use of the Assessment Summary table, Appendix B.10) and measure outcomes, and how treatment activities and focus progress across treatment sessions. It illustrated how the MC treatment components of cognitive strategies, horizontally structured treatment activities, the metacognitive framework and mediation can be used to improve self-awareness, self-monitoring, and strategy use in clients with mild, moderate, and severe cognitive impairment. In clients with severe cognitive impairment, treatment might focus on optimizing the use of a specific strategy (e.g., Case 2: Mike); whereas in clients with subtle cognitive deficits, treatment might focus more on anticipation of challenges and flexible, independent initiation of strategy use across daily life activities (e.g., Case 3: Sue). In some clients, treatment may need to focus on raising awareness of cognitive performance problems before addressing strategy use (e.g., Case 1: Fred). Regardless, the focus is always on using functional activity experiences to help the person self-discover their performance challenges and generate their own strategies to control them. Ultimately, this leads to improved self-efficacy and functional cognitive performance.

Resources

Chapter 2

Videos of EF and EF symptoms: www.multicontext.net; navigate to Resources, Video Resources of Cognitive Perceptual Symptoms

Chapter 5

Weekly Calendar Planning Activity (WCPA): American Occupational Therapy Association (AOTA) Press https://myaota.aota.org/shop_aota/index.aspx or Amazon. Additional resources on https://multicontext.net/weekly-calendar-planning-activity

Contextual Memory Test 2 (CMT-2): https://cmt.multicontext.net/

Other Performance-Based Assessments: www.multicontext.net, navigate to Resources, Adult IADL assessments.

Chapter 7

Goal Plan Do Review Worksheet: http://tres.hcpss.org/sites/default/files/Goal_Plan_Do_Review.pdf

GoalPlanDo App (by NYSARC, INC): https://apps.apple.com/us/app/goalplando/id961194974

Chapter 8

MC Functional Activity Kits: www.multicontext.net, navigate to Products

Chapter 10

swapmymood – App that guides the user through problem solving or emotional regulation (www.livewellrerc.org/swapmymood).

Chapter 11

Rehabilitation Treatment Specification: Moss Rehabilitation Institute

https://mrri.org/mrri-develops-rehab-treatment-specification-system/

Chapter 12: Outcome Measures

Activity Measure Post Acute Care (AM-PAC): Pearson Assessments, www.pearsonassessments.com

Activity Card Sort – 2nd Edition – American Occupational Therapy Association (AOTA) Press https://myaota.aota.org/shop_aota/index.aspx or Amazon.

Bangor Goal Setting Interview and Manual, version 2, University of Exeter, REACH: The Centre for Research in Ageing and Cognitive Health, Freely available. http://medicine.exeter.ac.uk/reach/publications/

Behavior Rating inventory of Executive Function (Adult Form) – Psychological Assessment Resources (PAR). www.parinc.com

Canadian Occupational Performance Measure (COPM): http://www.thecopm.ca/

Cognitive Self-Efficacy Questionnaire (CSEQ): www.multicontext.net, Free download; go to Resources, Assessment Tools, Questionnaires. or https://multicontext.net/assessments-questionnaires

Daily Living Questionnaire (DLQ): www.multicontext.net; Free download, go to Resources, Assessment Tools, Questionnaires or https://multicontext.net/assessments-questionnaires

Goal Attainment Scaling (GAS) in Rehabilitation, Kings College of London: GAS Engagement Scales - Client and Family Engagement in Goal Setting; Freely available resources on www.kcl.ac.uk/cicelysaunders/resources/tools/gas.

Life Interests and Values Cards (LiV): UNC School of Medicine, Division of Speech and Hearing Sciences, Center for Aphasia and Related Disorders www.med.unc.edu/ahs/sphs/card/resources/liv-cards.

Patient-Reported Outcomes Measurement Information System (PROMIS): www.healthmeasures.net

Quality of Life in Neurological Disorders (Neuro-QoL): www.neuroqol.org.

For digital download of Appendices: https://multicontext.net/book-appendix **Passcode: Mcappendix4**

References

Abreu, B., Seale, G., Scheibel, R. S., Huddleston, N., Zhang, L., and Ottenbacher, K. J. (2001). Levels of self-awareness after acute brain injury: How patients' and rehabilitation specialists' perceptions compare. *Arch Phys Med Rehabil, 82*(1), 49-56. doi:10.1053/apmr.2001.9167

Abreu, B., and Toglia, J. (1987). Cognitive rehabilitation: A model for occupational therapy. *The American Journal of Occupational Therapy, 41*(7), 439-448. doi:10.5014/ajot.41.7.439

Allan, J., McMinn, D., and Daly, M. (2016). A bidirectional relationship between executive function and health behavior: Evidence, implications, and future directions. *Frontiers in Neuroscience, 10* doi:10.3389/fnins.2016.00386

Allen, C. K., Earhart, C. A., and Blue, T. (1992). *Occupational therapy treatment goals for the physically and cognitively disabled*. AOTA Press.

Altgassen, M., Rendell, P. G., Bernhard, A., Henry, J. D., Bailey, P. E., Phillips, L. H., and Kliegel, M. (2015). Future thinking improves prospective memory performance and plan enactment in older adults. *Quarterly Journal of Experimental Psychology, 68*(1), 192-204. doi:10.1080/17470218.2014.956127

American Occupational Therapy Association. (2018). Guidelines for documentation of occupational therapy. *American Journal of Occupational Therapy, 72*(Suppl. 2), 7212410010. doi:10.5014/ajot.2018.72S203

Anderson, F. T., McDaniel, M. A., and Einstein, G. O. (2017). Remembering to remember: An examination of the cognitive processes underlying prospective memory. *Learning and Memory: A Comprehensive Reference E, 2*, 451-463.

Anderson, R. E., and Birge, S. J. (2016). Cognitive dysfunction, medication management, and the risk of readmission in hospital inpatients. *Journal of the American Geriatrics Society*, doi:10.1111/jgs.14200

Aurah, C. M. (2013). The effects of self-efficacy beliefs and metacognition on academic performance: A mixed method study. *American Journal of Educational Research, 1*(8), 334-343. doi:10.12691/education-1-8-11

Baddeley, A. (2012). Working memory: Theories, models, and controversies. *Annual Review of Psychology, 63*, 1-29. doi:10.1146/annurev-psych-120710-100422

Baddeley, A., Eyesench, M. W., and Anderson, M. C. (2015). *Memory* (2nd ed.). Psychology Press.

Baddeley, A., and Hitch, G. (1974). Working memory. In G. H. Bower (Ed.), *Psychology of learning and motivation* (Vol. 8 ed., pp. 47-89), Academic Press.

Bailey, H., Dunlosky, J., and Hertzog, C. (2010). Metacognitive training at home: Does it improve older adults' learning? *Gerontology, 56*(4), 414-420. doi:10.1159/000266030

Bandura, A. (1982). Self-efficacy mechanism in human agency. *American Psychologist, 37*(2), 122-147. doi:10.1037/0003-066X.37.2.122

Bandura, A. (1995). *Self-efficacy in changing societies*. Cambridge University Press.

Bandura, A. (1997). *Self-efficacy: The exercise of control*. W.H. Freeman and Company.

Barco, P. P., Crosson, B., Bolesta, M. M., Wets, D., and Stout, R. (1991). Training awareness and compensation in postacute head injury rehabilitation. In J. S. Kreutzer, and P. H. Wehman (Eds.), *Cognitive rehabilitation for persons with traumatic brain injury: A functional approach* (pp. 129-146). Paul H. Brookes Publishing Co.

Bar-Haim Erez, A., and Katz, N. (2018). Cognitive functional evaluation. In N. Katz, and J. Toglia (Eds.), *Cognition, occupation, and participation across the lifespan* (4th ed., pp. 69-85). AOTA Press. doi:10.7139/2017.978-1-56900-479-1

Barnett, S. M., and Ceci, S. J. (2002). When and where do we apply what we learn?: A taxonomy for far transfer. *Psychological Bulletin, 128*(4), 612-637. doi:10.1037/0033-2909.128.4.612

Baum, C. M., Connor, L. T., Morrison, T., Hahn, M., Dromerick, A. W., and Edwards, D. F. (2008). Reliability, validity, and clinical utility of the executive function performance test: A measure of executive function in a sample of people with stroke. *American Journal of Occupational Therapy, 62*(4), 446-455. doi:10.5014/ajot.62.4.446

Baum, C. M., and Edwards, D. (2008). *Activity card sort* (2nd ed.). AOTA Press.

Beadle, E. J., Ownsworth, T., Fleming, J., and Shum, D. (2016). The impact of traumatic brain injury on self-identity: A systematic review of the evidence for self-concept changes. *The Journal of Head Trauma Rehabilitation, 31*(2), E12-E25. doi:10.1097/HTR.0000000000000158

Beadle, E. J., Ownsworth, T., Fleming, J., and Shum, D. H. (2018). Personality characteristics and cognitive appraisals associated with self-discrepancy after severe traumatic brain injury. *Neuropsychological Rehabilitation*, 1-19. doi.org/10.1080/09602011.2018.1469416

Becker, H., Stuifbergen, A. K., Henneghan, A., Morrison, J., Seo, E. J., and Zhang, W. (2017). An initial investigation of the reliability and validity of the compensatory cognitive strategies scale. *Neuropsychological Rehabilitation, 29*(5), 739-753. doi:10.1080/09602011.2017.1329154

Belliveau, D., Belliveau, I., Camire-Raymond, A., Kessler, D., and Egan, M. (2016). Use of occupational performance coaching for stroke survivors (OPC-stroke) in late rehabilitation: A descriptive case study. *The Open Journal of Occupational Therapy, 4*(2), 7. doi:10.15453/2168-6408.1219

Besnard, J., Allain, P., Aubin, G., Chauvire, V., Etcharry-Bouyx, F., and Le Gall, D. (2011). A contribution to the study of environmental dependency phenomena: The social hypothesis. *Neuropsychologia, 49*(12), 3279-3294. doi:10.1016/j.neuropsychologia.2011.08.001

Best, J., Miller, P., and Jones, L. (2009). Executive functions after age 5: Changes and correlates. *Developmental Review, 29*(3), 180-200. doi:10.1016/j.dr.2009.05.002

Bier, N., Brambati, S., Macoir, J., Paquette, G., Schmitz, X., Belleville, S., . . . Joubert, S. (2015). Relying on procedural memory to enhance independence in daily living activities: Smartphone use in a case of semantic dementia. *Neuropsychological Rehabilitation, 25*(6), 913-935. doi:10.1080/09602011.2014.997745

Bier, N., and Macoir, J. (2010). How to make a spaghetti sauce with a dozen small things I cannot name: A review of the impact of semantic-memory deficits on everyday actions. *Journal of Clinical and Experimental Neuropsychology, 32*(2), 201-211. doi:10.1080/13803390902927885

Bjork, R. A., and Richardson-Klavehn, A. (1989). On the puzzling relationship between environmental context and human memory. In C. Izawa (Ed.), *Current issues in cognitive processes: The tulane flowerree symposium on cognition* (pp. 313-344). Lawrence Erlbaum Associates, Inc.

Bjorklund, D., and Causey, K. (2017). *Children's thinking: Cognitive development and individual differences* (6th ed.). SAGE Publications.

Blair, C., McKinnon, R., and Family Life Project Investigators. (2016). Moderating effects of executive functions and the teacher–child relationship on the development of mathematics ability in kindergarten. *Learning and Instruction, 41*, 85-93. doi:10.1016/j.learninstruc.2015.10.001

Blair, C., and Raver, C. (2016). Poverty, stress, and brain development: New directions for prevention and intervention. *Academic Pediatrics, 16*(3), S30-S36. doi:10.1016/j.acap.2016.01.010

Bol, Y., Duits, A. A., Hupperts, R. M., Verlinden, I., and Verhey, F. R. (2010). The impact of fatigue on cognitive functioning in patients with multiple sclerosis. *Clinical Rehabilitation, 24*(9), 854-862. doi:10.1177/0269215510367540

Bortolato, B., Miskowiak, K. W., Köhler, C. A., Maes, M., Fernandes, B. S., Berk, M., and Carvalho, A. F. (2016). Cognitive remission: A novel objective for the treatment of major depression? *BMC Medicine, 14*(1), 9. doi:10.1186/s12916-016-0560-3

Bottari, C. L., Shun, P. L., Le Dorze, G., Gosselin, N., and Dawson, D. (2014). Self-generated strategic behavior in an ecological shopping task. *The American Journal of Occupational Therapy, 68*(1), 67-76. doi:10.5014/ajot.2014.008987

Bottiroli, S., Cavallini, E., Dunlosky, J., Vecchi, T., and Hertzog, C. (2017). Self-guided strategy-adaption training for older adults: Transfer effects to everyday tasks. *Archives of Gerontology and Geriatrics, 72*, 91-98. doi:10.1016/j.archger.2017.05.015.

Brands, I., Kohler, S., Stapert, S., Wade, D., and van Heugten, C. (2014). How flexible is coping after acquired brain injury? A 1-year prospective study investigating coping patterns and influence of self-efficacy, executive functioning and self-awareness. *Journal of Rehabilitation Medicine, 46*(9), 869-875. doi:10.2340/16501977-1849

Brands, I., Stapert, S., Köhler, S., Wade, D., and van Heugten, C. (2015). Life goal attainment in the adaptation process after acquired brain injury: The influence of self-efficacy and of flexibility and tenacity in goal pursuit. *Clinical Rehabilitation, 29*(6), 611-622. doi:10.1177/0269215514549484

Brands, I., Verlinden, I., and Ribbers, G. M. (2019). A study of the influence of cognitive complaints, cognitive performance and symptoms of anxiety and depression on self-efficacy in patients with acquired brain injury. *Clinical Rehabilitation, 33*(2), 327-334. doi:10.1177/0269215518795249

Bransford, J. D., and Stein, B. S. (1993). *The IDEAL problem solver: A guide for improving thinking, learning, and creativity* (2nd ed.). W.H. Freeman.

Bransford, J., Brown, A. L., and Cocking, R. R. (2000). *How people learn: Brain, mind, experience, and school*. National Academy of Sciences Press. doi:10.17226/9853

Bransford, J. D., Sherwood, R. D., and Sturdevant, T. (1987). Teaching thinking and problem-solving. In J. Baron, and R. Sternberg (Eds.), *Teaching thinking skills: Theory and practice* (pp. 162-181). W.H. Freeman/Times Books/Henry Holt and Co.

Bray, N. W., Huffman, L. F., and Fletcher, K. L. (1999). Developmental and intellectual differences in self-report and strategy use. *Developmental Psychology, 35*(5), 1223-1236. doi:10.1037/0012-1649.35.5.1223

Brom, S. S., and Kliegel, M. (2014). Improving everyday prospective memory performance in older adults: Comparing cognitive process and strategy training. *Psychology and Aging, 29*(3), 744-755. doi:10.1037/a0037181

Brown, A. L., and Ferrara, R. A. (1985). Diagnosing zones of proximal development. In J. Wertsch (Ed.), *Culture, communication and cognition: Vygotskian perspectives* (pp. 272-305). Cambridge University Press.

Brown, C., Rempfer, M., and Hamera, E. (2009). *The test of grocery shopping skills* AOTA Press.

Brown, M. (2006). Participation objective, participation subjective. *The Center for Outcome Measurement in Brain Injury.* http://www.tbims.org/combi/pops (accessed June 23, 2020).

Brum, P. S., Yassuda, M. S., and Forlenza, O. V. (2013). Subjective memory and strategy use in mild cognitive impairment and healthy aging. *Psychology and Neuroscience, 6*(1), 89-94. doi:10.3922/j.psns.2013.1.13

Budson, A. E., and Price, B. H. (2005a). Memory dysfunction. *New England Journal of Medicine, 352*(7), 692-699. doi:10.1056/NEJMra041071

Budson, A. E., and Price, B. H. (2005b). Memory: Clinical disorders. *Encyclopedia of Life Sciences,* doi:10.1038/npg.els.0004052

Burgess, P. W. (2015). Serial versus concurrent multitasking: From lab to life. In M. F. Fawcett, E. F. Risko and A.

Kingstone (Eds.), *The handbook of attention* (pp. 443-462), MIT Press.

Burgess, P. W., Alderman, N., Forbes, C., Costello, A., Coates, L., Dawson, D. R., . . . Channon, S. (2006). The case for the development and use of "ecologically valid" measures of executive function in experimental and clinical neuropsychology. *Journal of the International Neuropsychological Society, 12*(2), 194-209. doi:10.1017/S1355617706060310

Burgess, P. W., Quayle, A., and Frith, C. D. (2001). Brain regions involved in prospective memory as determined by positron emission tomography. *Neuropsychologia, 39*(6), 545-555. doi:10.1016/S0028-3932(00)00149-4

Burke, L. A., and Hutchins, H. M. (2007). Training transfer: An integrative literature review. *Human Resource Development Review, 6*(3), 263-296. doi:10.1177/1534484307303035

Buslovich, S., and Kennedy, G. J. (2012). Potential effect of screening for subtle cognitive deficits on hospital readmission. *Journal of the American Geriatrics Society, 60*(10), 1980-1981. doi:10.1111/j.1532-5415.2012.04135.x

Butler, A. C., Black-Maier, A. C., Raley, N. D., and Marsh, E. J. (2017). Retrieving and applying knowledge to different examples promotes transfer of learning. *Journal of Experimental Psychology: Applied, 23*(4), 433-446. doi:10.1037/xap0000142

Cahn, D. A., Sullivan, E. V., Shear, P. K., Pfefferbaum, A., Heit, G., and Silverberg, G. (1998). Differential contributions of cognitive and motor component processes to physical and instrumental activities of daily living in parkinson's disease. *Archives of Clinical Neuropsychology, 13*(7), 575-583. doi:10.1093/arclin/13.7.575

Campione, J. C., and Brown, A. L. (1990). Guided learning and transfer: Implications for approaches to assessment. In N. Frederiksen, and R. Glaser (Eds.), *Diagnostic monitoring of skill and knowledge acquisition* (pp. 141-172). Lawrence Erlbaum Associations.

Cantor, J., Ashman, T., Dams-O'Connor, K., Dijkers, M. P., Gordon, W., Spielman, L., . . . Oswald, J. (2014). Evaluation of the short-term executive plus intervention for executive dysfunction after traumatic brain injury: A randomized controlled trial with minimization. *Archives of Physical Medicine and Rehabilitation, 95*(1), 1-9. doi:10.1016/j.apmr.2013.08.005

Caplan, B., Bogner, J., Brenner, L., Twamley, E. W., Thomas, K. R., Gregory, A. M., . . . Lohr, J. B. (2015). CogSMART compensatory cognitive training for traumatic brain injury: Effects over 1 year. *Journal of Head Trauma Rehabilitation, 30*(6), 391-401. doi:10.1097/HTR.0000000000000076

Carretti, B., Borella, E., Zavagnin, M., and De Beni, R. (2010). Impact of metacognition and motivation on the efficacy of strategic memory training in older adults: Analysis of specific, transfer and maintenance effects. *Archives of Gerontology and Geriatrics*, doi:10.1016/j.archger.2010.11.004

Cella, M., Reeder, C., and Wykes, T. (2015). Lessons learnt? the importance of metacognition and its implications for cognitive remediation in schizophrenia. *Frontiers in Psychology, 6*, 1259. doi:10.3389/fpsyg.2015.01259

Cermak, S. A. (2018). Cognitive rehabilitation of individuals with attention deficit hyperactivity disorder. In Katz, N. and Toglia, J. (Ed.), *Cognition, occupation, and participation across the lifespan* (4th ed., pp. 189-217). AOTA Press. doi:10.7139/2017.978-1-56900-479-1

Cermak, S. A., and Toglia, J. (2018). Cognitive development across the lifespan: Development of cognition and executive functioning in children and adolescents. In N. Katz, and J. Toglia (Eds.), *Cognition, occupation, and participation across the lifespan* (4th ed., pp. 9-27). AOTA Press. doi:10.7139/2017.978-1-56900-479-1

Chai, W. J., Abd Hamid, A. I., and Abdullah, J. M. (2018). Working memory from the psychological and neurosciences perspectives: A review. *Frontiers in Psychology, 9*, 401. doi:10.3389/fpsyg.2018.00401

Champion, A. J. (2006). *Neuropsychological rehabilitation: A resource for group-based education and intervention*. John Wiley and Sons.

Chan, R. C., Shum, D., Toulopoulou, T., and Chen, E. Y. (2008). Assessment of executive functions: Review of instruments and identification of critical issues. *Archives of Clinical Neuropsychology, 23*(2), 201-216. doi:10.1016/j.acn.2007.08.010

Chaytor, N., Schmitter-Edgecombe, M., and Burr, R. (2006). Improving the ecological validity of executive functioning assessment. *Archives of Clinical Neuropsychology, 21*(3), 217-227. doi:10.1016/j.acn.2005.12.002

Chen, P., and Toglia, J. (2019). Online and offline awareness deficits: Anosognosia for spatial neglect. *Rehabilitation Psychology, 64*(1), 50-64. doi:10.1037/rep0000207

Cicerone, K. D. (2005). Evidence-based practice and the limits of rational rehabilitation. *Archives of Physical Medicine and Rehabilitation, 86*(6), 1073-1074. doi:10.1016/j.apmr.2005.01.003

Cicerone, K. D. (2012). Facts, theories, values: Shaping the course of neurorehabilitation. The 60th John Stanley Coulter Memorial Lecture. *Archives of Physical Medicine and Rehabilitation, 93*(2), 188-191. doi:10.1016/j.apmr.2011.12.003

Cicerone, K. D., and Azulay, J. (2007). Perceived self-efficacy and life satisfaction after traumatic brain injury. *The Journal of Head Trauma Rehabilitation, 22*(5), 257-266. doi:10.1097/01.HTR.0000290970.56130.81

Cicerone, K. D., Goldin, Y., Ganci, K., Rosenbaum, A., Wethe, J. V., Langenbahn, D. M., . . . Nagele, D. (2019). Evidence-based cognitive rehabilitation: Systematic review of the literature from 2009 through 2014. *Archives of Physical Medicine and Rehabilitation, 100*(8), 1515-1533. doi:10.1016/j.apmr.2019.02.011

Cicerone, K. D., Mott, T., Azulay, J., Sharlow-Galella, M. A., Ellmo, W. J., Paradise, S., and Friel, J. C. (2008). A randomized controlled trial of holistic neuropsychologic rehabilitation after traumatic brain injury. *Archives of Physical Medicine and Rehabilitation, 89*(12), 2239-2249. doi:10.1016/j.apmr.2008.06.017

Cizman Staba, U., Vrhovac, S., Mlinaric Lesnik, V., and Novakovic-Agopian, T. (2020). Goal-oriented attentional self-regulation training in individuals with acquired brain injury in a subacute phase: A pilot feasibility study. *International Journal of Rehabilitation Research, 43*(1), 28-36. doi:10.1097/MRR.0000000000000380

Clare, L., Nelis, S. M., and Kudlicka, A. (2016). *Bangor Goal-Setting interview manual*.

Clerc, J., Miller, P. H., and Cosnefroy, L. (2014). Young children's transfer of strategies: Utilization deficiencies, executive function, and metacognition. *Developmental Review, 34*(4), 378-393. doi:10.1016/j.dr.2014.10.002

Cockburn, P. H. J. (1998). Concurrent performance of cognitive and motor tasks in neurological rehabilitation. *Neuropsychological Rehabilitation, 8*(2), 155-170. doi:10.1080/713755565

Corrigan, J. D., and Bogner, J. (2004). Latent factors in measures of rehabilitation outcomes after traumatic brain injury. *The Journal of Head Trauma Rehabilitation, 19*(6), 445-458.

Coster, W. J., Haley, S. M., Ludlow, L. H., Andres, P. L., and Ni, P. S. (2004). Development of an applied cognition scale to measure rehabilitation outcomes. *Archives of Physical Medicine and Rehabilitation, 85*(12), 2030-2035. doi:10.1016/j.apmr.2004.05.002

Craik, F. I., and Lockhart, R. S. (1972). Levels of processing: A framework for memory research. *Journal of Verbal Learning and Verbal Behavior, 11*(6), 671-684. doi:10.1016/S0022-5371(72)80001-X

Cramm, H., Krupa, T., Missiuna, C., Lysaght, R., and Parker, K. (2016). The expanding relevance of executive functioning in occupational therapy: Is it on your radar? *Australian Occupational Therapy Journal, 63*(3), 214-217. doi:10.1111/1440-1630.12244

Culley, C., and Evans, J. J. (2010). SMS text messaging as a means of increasing recall of therapy goals in brain injury rehabilitation: A single-blind within-subjects trial. *Neuropsychological Rehabilitation, 20*(1), 103-119. doi:10.1080/09602010902906926

Dahlberg, C. A., Cusick, C. P., Hawley, L. A., Newman, J. K., Morey, C. E., Harrison-Felix, C. L., and Whiteneck, G. G. (2007). Treatment efficacy of social communication skills training after traumatic brain injury: A randomized treatment and deferred treatment controlled trial. *Archives of Physical Medicine and Rehabilitation, 88*(12), 1561-1573. doi:10.1016/j.apmr.2007.07.033

Dawson, D., Binns, M. A., Hunt, A., Lemsky, C., and Polatajko, H. J. (2013). Occupation-based strategy training for adults with traumatic brain injury: A pilot study. *Archives of Physical Medicine and Rehabilitation, 94*(10), 1959-1963. doi:10.1016/j.apmr.2013.05.021

Dawson, D., Gaya, A., Hunt, A., Levine, B., Lemsky, C., and Polatajko, H. J. (2009). Using the cognitive orientation to occupational performance (CO-OP) with adults with executive dysfunction following traumatic brain injury. *Canadian Journal of Occupational Therapy, 76*(2), 115-127. doi:10.1177/000841740907600209

Dawson, D., Richardson, J., Troyer, A., Binns, M., Clark, A., Polatajko, H., . . . Bar, Y. (2013). An occupation-based strategy training approach to managing age-related executive changes: A pilot randomized controlled trial. *Clinical Rehabilitation*, 1-10. doi:10.1177/0269215513492541

Diamond, A. (2013). Executive functions. *Annual Review of Psychology, 64*, 135-168. doi:10.1146/annurev-psych-113011-143750

Diamond, A., and Ling, D. S. (2016). Conclusions about interventions, programs, and approaches for improving executive functions that appear justified and those that, despite much hype, do not. *Developmental Cognitive Neuroscience, 18*, 34-48. doi:10.1016/j.dcn.2015.11.005

Dikmen, S., Machamer, J., and Temkin, N. (2017). Mild traumatic brain injury: Longitudinal study of cognition, functional status, and post-traumatic symptoms. *Journal of Neurotrauma, 34*(8), 1524-1530. doi:10.1089/neu.2016.4618

Dockree, P. M., Tarleton, Y. M., Carton, S., and FitzGerald, M. C. (2015). Connecting self-awareness and error-awareness in patients with traumatic brain injury. *Journal of the International Neuropsychological Society*, 1-10. doi:S1355617715000594

Doig, E., Fleming, J., and Lin, B. (2017). Comparison of online awareness and error behaviour during occupational performance by two individuals with traumatic brain injury and matched controls. *Neurorehabilitation, 40*(4), 519-529. doi:10.3233/NRE-171439

Doig, E., Fleming, J., Ownsworth, T., and Fletcher, S. (2017). An occupation-based, metacognitive approach to assessing error performance and online awareness. *Australian Occupational Therapy Journal, 64*(2), 137-148. doi:10.1111/1440-1630.12322

Duval, J., Coyette, F., and Seron, X. (2008). Rehabilitation of the central executive component of working memory: A re-organisation approach applied to a single case. *Neuropsychological Rehabilitation, 18*(4), 430-460. doi:10.1080/09602010701573950

Ellis, S. J., and Small, M. (1993). Denial of illness in stroke. *Stroke, 24*(5), 757-759. doi:10.1161/01.STR.24.5.757

Engel, L., Chui, A., Goverover, Y., and Dawson, D. R. (2017). Optimising activity and participation outcomes for people with self-awareness impairments related to acquired brain injury: An interventions systematic review. *Neuropsychological Rehabilitation, 29*(2), 163-198. doi:10.1080/09602011.2017.1292923

Engle, R. A., Lam, D. P., Meyer, X. S., and Nix, S. E. (2012). How does expansive framing promote transfer? several proposed explanations and a research agenda for investigating them. *Educational Psychologist, 47*(3), 215-231. doi:10.1080/00461520.2012.695678

Ernst, A., Blanc, F., De Seze, J., and Manning, L. (2015). Using mental visual imagery to improve autobiographical memory and episodic future thinking in relapsing-remitting multiple sclerosis patients: A randomised-controlled trial study. *Restorative Neurology and Neuroscience,* doi:10.3233/RNN-140461

Eslinger, P. J., and Grattan, L. M. (1993). Frontal lobe and frontal-striatal substrates for different forms of human cognitive flexibility. *Neuropsychologia, 31*(1), 17-28. doi:10.1016/0028-3932(93)90077-D

Evans, C. C., Sherer, M., Nick, T. G., Nakase-Richardson, R., and Yablon, S. A. (2005). Early impaired self-awareness, depression, and subjective well-being following traumatic brain injury. *Journal of Head Trauma Rehabilitation, 20*(6), 488-500.

Evans, J. J. (2012). Goal setting during rehabilitation early and late after acquired brain injury. *Current Opinion in Neurology, 25*(6), 651-655. doi:10.1097/WCO.0b013e3283598f75

Fasoli, S. E., Ferraro, M. K., and Lin, S. H. (2019). Occupational therapy can benefit from an interprofessional rehabilitation treatment specification system. *American Journal of Occupational Therapy, 73*(2), 7302347010p1-7302347010p6. doi:10.5014/ajot.2019.030189

Fernandes, H. A., Richard, N. M., and Edelstein, K. (2019). Cognitive rehabilitation for cancer-related cognitive dysfunction: A systematic review. *Supportive Care in Cancer, 27*(9), 3253-3279. doi:10.1007/s00520-019-04866-2

Ferreira, F., and Monteiro, L. (2018). Ecological assessment of executive dysfunction in anxiety. *Clinical and Biomedical Research, 38*(1), 22-29. doi:10.4322/2357-9730.76288

Feuerstein, R., Falik, L., and Feuerstein, R. S. (2015). *Changing minds and brains—The legacy of Reuven Feuerstein: Higher thinking and cognition through mediated learning.* Teachers College Press.

Fish, J., Evans, J. J., Nimmo, M., Martin, E., Kersel, D., Bateman, A., . . . Manlya, T. (2007). Rehabilitation of executive dysfunction following brain injury: "Content-free" cueing improves everyday prospective memory performance. *Neuropsychologia, 45*(6), 1318-1330. doi:10.1016/j.neuropsychologia.2006.09.015

Fisher, A. G., and Bray Jones, K. (2012). *Assessment of motor and process skills: Vol. 1 - development, standardization, and administration manual* (7th ed.). Three Star Press, Inc.

Flavell, J., Miller, P., and Miller, S. (2002). *Cognitive development* (4th ed.). Prentice-Hall Inc.

Fleming, J., Braithwaite, H., Gustafsson, L., Griffin, J., Collier, A. M., and Fletcher, S. (2011). Participation in leisure activities during brain injury rehabilitation. *Brain Injury, 25*(9), 806-818. doi:10.3109/02699052.2011.585508

Fleming, J., Goh, A., Lannin, N., Ownsworth, T., and Schmidt, J. (2019). An exploratory study of verbal feedback on occupational performance for improving self-awareness in people with traumatic brain injury. *Australian Occupational Therapy Journal,* doi:10.1111/1440-1630.12632

Fleming, J., Lucas, S. E., and Lightbody, S. (2006). Using occupation to facilitate self-awareness in people who have acquired brain injury: A pilot study. *Canadian Journal of Occupational Therapy, 73*(1), 44-55. doi:10.2182/cjot.05.0005

Fleming, J., and Strong, J. (1999). A longitudinal study of self-awareness: Functional deficits underestimated by persons with brain injury. *The Occupational Therapy Journal of Research, 19*(1), 3-17. doi:10.1177/153944929901900101

Foster, E. R., and Hershey, T. (2011). Everyday executive function is associated with activity participation in Parkinson's disease without dementia. *OTJR: Occupation, Participation and Health, 31*(1), 16-22. doi:10.3928/15394492-20101108-04

Foster, E. R., Spence, D., and Toglia, J. (2017). Feasibility of a cognitive strategy training intervention for people with Parkinson's disease. *Disability and Rehabilitation, 40*(10), 1127-1134. doi:10.1080/09638288.2017.1288275

Frey, N., and Fisher, D. (2010). Identifying instructional moves during guided learning. *The Reading Teacher, 64*(2), 84-95. doi:10.1598/RT.64.2.1

Fride, Y., Adamit, T., Maeir, A., Ben Assayag, E., Bornstein, N. M., Korczyn, A. D., and Katz, N. (2015). What are the correlates of cognition and participation to return to work after first ever mild stroke? *Topics in Stroke Rehabilitation, 22*(5), 317-325. doi:10.1179/1074935714Z.0000000013

Gage, M., and Polatajko, H. (1994). Enhancing occupational performance through an understanding of perceived self-efficacy. *The American Journal of Occupational Therapy, 48*(5), 452-461. doi:10.5014/ajot.48.5.452

Geary, E. K., Kraus, M. F., Rubin, L. H., Pliskin, N. H., and Little, D. M. (2011). Verbal learning strategy following mild traumatic brain injury. *Journal of the International Neuropsychological Society, 17*(4), 709-719. doi:10.1017/S1355617711000646

Gick, M. L., and Holyoak, K. J. (1983). Schema induction and analogical transfer. *Cognitive Psychology, 15*(1), 1-38. doi:10.1016/0010-0285(83)90002-6

Gick, M. L., and Holyoak, K. J. (1987). Transfer of learning: Contemporary research and applications. In S. M. Cormier, and J. D. Hagman (Eds.), *The cognitive basis of knowledge transfer* (pp. 9-42). Academic Press.

Giles, G. M. (2018). Neurofunctional approach to rehabilitation after brain injury. In N. Katz, and J. Toglia (Eds.), *Cognition, occupation and participation across the life span: Neuroscience, neurorehabilitation and models of intervention in occupational therapy* (4th ed., pp. 419-442). AOTA Press. doi:10.7139/2017.978-1-56900-479-1

Giles, G. M., Edwards, D. F., Baum, C., Furniss, J., Skidmore, E., Wolf, T., and Leland, N. E. (2020). Making functional cognition a professional priority. *American Journal of Occupational Therapy, 74*(1), 7401090010p1-7401090010p6. doi:10.5014/ajot.2020.741002

Giles, G. M., Edwards, D. F., Morrison, M. T., Baum, C., and Wolf, T. J. (2017). Screening for functional cognition in post-acute care and the improving Medicare post-acute care transformation (IMPACT) act of 2014. *American Journal of Occupational Therapy, 71*(5), 7105090010p1-7105090010p6. doi:10.5014/ajot.2017.715001

Ginns, P. (2005). Imagining instructions: Mental practice in highly cognitive domains. *Australian Journal of Education, 49*(2), 128-140. doi:10.1177/000494410504900202

Goldstein, G. (1990). Contributions of Kurt Goldstein to neuropsychology. *Clinical Neuropsychologist, 4*(1), 3-17. doi:10.1080/13854049008401492

Golisz, K. M. (1998). Dynamic assessment and multicontext treatment of unilateral neglect. *Topics in Stroke Rehabilitation, 5*(2), 11-28. doi:10.1310/C5EU-A605-L7UQ-1QXB

Golisz, K., Waldman-Levi, A., Swierat, R. P., and Toglia, J. (2018). Adults with intellectual disabilities: Case studies using everyday technology to support daily living skills.

British Journal of Occupational Therapy, 81(9), 514-524. doi:10.1177/0308022618764781

Gollwitzer, P. M. (1999). Implementation intentions: Strong effects of simple plans. *American Psychologist, 54*(7), 493-503. doi:10.1037/0003-066X.54.7.493

Goode, M. K., Geraci, L., and Roediger, H. L. (2008). Superiority of variable to repeated practice in transfer on anagram solution. *Psychonomic Bulletin and Review, 15*(3), 662-666. doi:10.3758/PBR.15.3.662

Gould, F., McGuire, L. S., Durand, D., Sabbag, S., Larrauri, C., Patterson, T. L., . . . Harvey, P. D. (2015). Self-assessment in schizophrenia: Accuracy of evaluation of cognition and everyday functioning. *Neuropsychology, 29*(5), 675-682. doi:10.1037/neu0000175

Goverover, Y. (2018). Cognitive rehabilitation: Evidence-based interventions. In N. Katz, and J. Toglia (Eds.), *Cognition, occupation, and participation across the lifespan* (4th ed., pp. 51-68). AOTA Press. doi:10.7139/2017.978-1-56900-479-1

Goverover, Y., Arango-Lasprilla, J. C., Hillary, F. G., Chiaravalloti, N., and DeLuca, J. (2009). Application of the spacing effect to improve learning and memory for functional tasks in traumatic brain injury: A pilot study. *American Journal of Occupational Therapy, 63*(5), 543-548. doi:10.5014/ajot.63.5.543

Goverover, Y., Chiaravalloti, N., and DeLuca, J. (2010). Pilot study to examine the use of self-generation to improve learning and memory in people with traumatic brain injury. *American Journal of Occupational Therapy, 64*(4), 540-546. doi:10.5014/ajot.2010.09020.

Goverover, Y., Chiaravalloti, N., Genova, H., and DeLuca, J. (2017). A randomized controlled trial to treat impaired learning and memory in multiple sclerosis: The self-GEN trial. *Multiple Sclerosis Journal, 24*(8), 1096-1104. doi:10.1177/ 1352458517709955

Goverover, Y., and DeLuca, J. (2015). Actual reality: Using the internet to assess everyday functioning after traumatic brain injury. *Brain Injury, 29*(6), 715-721. doi:10.3109/02699052.2015.1004744

Goverover, Y., and DeLuca, J. (2018). Assessing everyday life functional activity using actual reality in persons with MS. *Rehabilitation Psychology, 63*(2), 276-285. doi:10.1037/rep0000212

Goverover, Y., Genova, H., Hali, G., Chiaravalloti, N., and DeLuca, J. (2014). Metacognitive knowledge and online awareness in persons with multiple sclerosis. *Neurorehabilitation*, doi:10.3233/NRE-141113

Goverover, Y., Johnston, M. V., Toglia, J., and Deluca, J. (2007). Treatment to improve self-awareness in persons with acquired brain injury. *Brain Injury, 21*(9), 913-923. doi:10.1080/02699050701553205

Goverover, Y., O'Brien, A. R., Moore, N. B., and DeLuca, J. (2010). Actual reality: A new approach to functional assessment in persons with multiple sclerosis. *Archives of Physical Medicine and Rehabilitation, 91*(2), 252-260. doi:10.1016/j.apmr.2009.09.022

Goverover, Y., Toglia, J., and DeLuca, J. (2019). The weekly calendar planning activity in multiple sclerosis: A top-down assessment of executive functions. *Neuropsychological Rehabilitation*, 1-16. doi:10.1080/09602011.2019.1584573.

Graham-Scott (2007). *30 days to a more powerful memory*. AMACOM Books.

Green, C. R. (2012). *Total memory workout: 8 easy steps to maximum memory fitness*. Bantam Publishers.

Gustafsson, H., Nordström, P., Stråhle, S., and Nordström, A. (2015). Parkinson's disease: A population-based investigation of life satisfaction and employment. *Journal of Rehabilitation Medicine, 47*(1), 45-51. doi:10.2340/16501977-1884

Gutierrez, A. P., and Price, A. F. (2017). Calibration between undergraduate students' prediction of and actual performance: The role of gender and performance attributions. *The Journal of Experimental Education, 85*(3), 486-500. doi:10.1080/00220973.2016.1180278

Hagger, M. S., and Luszczynska, A. (2014). Implementation intention and action planning interventions in health contexts: State of the research and proposals for the way forward. *Applied Psychology: Health and Well-Being, 6*(1), 1-47. doi:10.1111/aphw.12017

Haley, K. L., Womack, J., Helm-Estabrooks, N., Lovette, B., and Goff, R. (2013). Supporting autonomy for people with aphasia: Use of the life interests and values (LIV) cards. *Topics in Stroke Rehabilitation, 20*(1), 22-35. doi:10.1310/tsr2001-22

Han, K., Chapman, S. B., and Krawczyk, D. C. (2018). Neuroplasticity of cognitive control networks following cognitive training for chronic traumatic brain injury. *NeuroImage: Clinical, 18*, 262-278. doi: 10.1016/j.nicl.2018.01.030

Han, K., Davis, R. A., Chapman, S. B., and Krawczyk, D. C. (2017). Strategy-based reasoning training modulates cortical thickness and resting-state functional connectivity in adults with chronic traumatic brain injury. *Brain and Behavior, 7*(5), e00687. doi:10.1002/brb3.687

Harris, K. R., Alexander, P., and Graham, S. (2008). Michael Pressley's contributions to the history and future of strategies research. *Educational Psychologist, 43*(2), 86-96. doi:10.1080/00461520801942300

Harris, K. R., and Pressley, M. (1991). The nature of cognitive strategy instruction: Interactive strategy construction. *Exceptional Children, 57*(5), 392-404. doi:10.1177/001440299105700503

Harris, M. T., and Rempfer, M. V. (2020). Profiles of self-evaluation as a metacognitive skill: An indicator of rehabilitation potential among people with schizophrenia. *Psychiatric Rehabilitation Journal*, doi:10.1037/prj0000412

Harrison, M. J., Morris, K. A., Horton, R., Toglia, J., Barsky, J., Chait, S., . . . Robbins, L. (2005). Results of intervention for lupus patients with self-perceived cognitive difficulties. *Neurology, 65*(8), 1325-1327. doi:10.1212/01.wnl.0000180938.69146.5e

Harrison, S. L., Laver, K. E., Ninnis, K., Rowett, C., Lannin, N. A., and Crotty, M. (2019). Effectiveness of external cues to facilitate task performance in people with neurological disorders: A systematic review and meta-analysis. *Disability and Rehabilitation, 41*(16), 1874-1881. doi:10.1080/09638288.2018.1448465

Hart, T., Dijkers, M. P., Whyte, J., Turkstra, L. S., Zanca, J. M., Packel, A., . . . Chen, C. (2019). A theory-driven system for the specification of rehabilitation treatments. *Archives of Physical Medicine and Rehabilitation, 100*(1), 172-180. doi:10.1016/j.apmr.2018.09.109

Hart, T., and Vaccaro, M. J. (2017). Goal intention reminding in traumatic brain injury: A feasibility study using implementation intentions and text messaging. *Brain Injury, 31*(3), 297-303. doi:10.1080/02699052.2016.1251612

Hart, T., Vaccaro, M., Collier, G., Chervoneva, I., and Fann, J. R. (2019). Promoting mental health in traumatic brain injury using single-session behavioural activation and SMS messaging: A randomized controlled trial. *Neuropsychological Rehabilitation, 29*, 1-20. doi:10.1080/09602011.2019.1592761

Hart, T., Whyte, J., Djikers, M., Packel, A., Turkstra, L., Zanca, J., Ferraro M., Chen C.,Van Stan, J. (2019). *Manual for rehabilitation treatment specification* (v6.2).

Hartman-Maeir, A., Harel, H., and Katz, N. (2009). Kettle test--a brief measure of cognitive functional performance: Reliability and validity in stroke rehabilitation. *American Journal of Occupational Therapy, 63*(5), 592-599. doi:10.5014/ajot.63.5.592

Haskell, R. E. (2001). *A vol. in the educational psychology series. Transfer of learning: Cognition, instruction and reasoning.* Academic Press.

Haskins, E. C., Cicerone, K. D., and Trexler, L. E. (2012). *Cognitive rehabilitation manual: Translating evidence-based recommendations into practice.* ACRM Publishing.

Herrmann, D. J. (1991). *Super memory: A quick-action program for memory improvement* Rodale Press.

Hewitt, J., Evans, J. J., and Dritschel, B. (2006). Theory driven rehabilitation of executive functioning: Improving planning skills in people with traumatic brain injury through the use of an autobiographical episodic memory cueing procedure. *Neuropsychologia, 44*(8), 1468-74. doi:10.1016/j.neuropsychologia.2005.11.016

Hock, M., and Mellard, D. (2005). Reading comprehension strategies for adult literacy outcomes. *Journal of Adolescent and Adult Literacy, 49*(3), 192-200. doi:10.1598/JAAL.49.3.3

Hoerold, D., Pender, N. P., and Robertson, I. H. (2012). Metacognitive and online error awareness deficits after prefrontal cortex lesions. *Neuropsychologia, 5*(3), 385-391. doi:10.1016/j.neuropsychologia.2012.11.019

Holm, M. B., and Rogers, J. (2008). The performance assessment of self-care skills (PASS). In B. Hemphill-Pearson (Ed.), *Assessments in occupational therapy mental health* (2nd ed., pp. 101-110). Slack Inc.

Hotz, G., and Helm-Estabrooks, N. (1995). Perseveration. part II: A study of perseveration in closed-head injury. *Brain Injury, 9*(2), 161-172. doi:10.3109/02699059509008189

Hurst, F. G., Ownsworth, T., Beadle, E., Shum, D. H. K., and Fleming, J. (2020). Domain-specific deficits in self-awareness and relationship to psychosocial outcomes after severe traumatic brain injury. *Disability and Rehabilitation, 42*(5), 651-659. doi:10.1080/09638288.2018.1504993

Ihle, A., Albiński, R., Gurynowicz, K., Kliegel, M., and Albiński, R. (2018). Four-week strategy-based training to enhance prospective memory in older adults: Targeting intention retention is more beneficial than targeting intention formation. *Gerontology, 64*(3), 257-265. doi:10.1159/000485796

Ishii, A., Tanaka, M., and Watanabe, Y. (2014). Neural mechanisms of mental fatigue. *Reviews in the Neurosciences, 25*(4), 469-479. doi:10.1515/revneuro-2014-0028

Issurin, V. B. (2013). Training transfer: Scientific background and insights for practical application. *Sports Medicine, 43*(8), 675-694. doi:10.1007/s40279-013-0049-6

Jaywant, A., Steinberg, C., Lee, A., and Toglia, J. (2020). Feasibility and acceptability of the multicontext approach for individuals with acquired brain injury in acute inpatient rehabilitation: A single case series. *Neuropsychological Rehabilitation.* DOI: 10.1080/09602011.2020.1810710.

Job, J. M., and Klassen, R. M. (2012). Predicting performance on academic and non-academic tasks: A comparison of adolescents with and without learning disabilities. *Contemporary Educational Psychology, 37*(2), 162-169. doi:10.1016/j.cedpsych.2011.05.001

Johansson, B., Berglund, P., and Ronnback, L. (2009). Mental fatigue and impaired information processing after mild and moderate traumatic brain injury. *Brain Injury, 23*(13-14), 1027-1040. doi:10.3109/02699050903421099

Johansson, B., and Ronnback, L. (2014). Evaluation of the mental fatigue scale and its relation to cognitive and emotional functioning after traumatic brain injury or stroke. *Int J Phys Med Rehabil, 2*(1) doi:10.4172/2329-9096.1000182

Jonasson, A., Levin, C., Renfors, M., Strandberg, S., and Johansson, B. (2018). Mental fatigue and impaired cognitive function after an acquired brain injury. *Brain and Behavior, 8*(8), e01056. doi:0.1002/brb3.1056

Jones, A. J., Kuijer, R. G., Livingston, L., Myall, D., Horne, K., MacAskill, M., . . . Dalrymple-Alford, J. C. (2017). Caregiver burden is increased in Parkinson's disease with mild cognitive impairment (PD-MCI). *Translational Neurodegeneration, 6*(1), 17. doi:10.1186/s40035-017-0085-5

Josman, N., and Regev, S. (2018). Dynamic interactional model in severe mental illness: Metacognitive and strategy-based intervention. In N. Katz, and J. Toglia (Eds.), *Cognition, occupation, and participation across the lifespan* (4th ed., pp. 387-403). Bethesda, MD: American Occupational Therapy Association, Inc. doi:10.7139/2017.978-1-56900-479-1

Just, M. A., and Buchweitz, A. (2016). What brain imaging reveals about the nature of multitasking. In S. Chipman (Ed.), *The Oxford Handbook of Cognitive Science.* Oxford University Press.

Kable, J. A., Taddeo, E., Strickland, D., and Coles, C. D. (2016). Improving FASD children's self-regulation: Piloting phase 1 of the GoFAR intervention. *Child and Family Behavior Therapy, 38*(2), 124-141. doi:10.1080/07317107.2016.1172880

Kahjoogh, M. A., Rassafiani, M., Dunn, W., Hosseini, S. A., and Akbarfahimi, N. (2016). Occupational performance coaching: A descriptive review of literature. *New Zealand Journal of Occupational Therapy, 63*(2), 45-49. ISSN: 1171-0462.

Kaizerman-Dinerman, A., Josman, N., and Roe, D. (2019). The use of cognitive strategies among people with schizophrenia: A randomized comparative study. *The Open Journal of Occupational Therapy, 7*(3), 1-12. doi:10.15453/2168-6408.1621

Kaizerman-Dinerman, A., Roe, D., and Josman, N. (2018). An efficacy study of a metacognitive group intervention for people with schizophrenia. *Psychiatry Research, 270*, 1150-1156. doi:10.1016/j.psychres.2018.10.037

Kannan, S., Chandramohan, V., and Kannan, S. R. (2017). Efficacy of cognitive intervention using CogSMART in the management of cognitive problems in mild traumatic brain injury. *Indian Journal of Health and Wellbeing, 8*(9), 1008-1011. Retrieved from http://www.iahrw.com/index.php/home/journal_detail/19#list

Karr, J. E., Areshenkoff, C. N., Rast, P., Hofer, S. M., Iverson, G. L., & Garcia-Barrera, M. A. (2018). The unity and diversity of executive functions: A systematic review and re-analysis of latent variable studies. *Psychological bulletin, 144*(11), 1147.

Kavaliunas, A., Danylaite Karrenbauer, V., Gyllensten, H., Manouchehrinia, A., Glaser, A., Olsson, T., . . . Hillert, J. (2017). Cognitive function is a major determinant of income among multiple sclerosis patients in Sweden acting independently from physical disability. *Multiple Sclerosis Journal*, 1-9. doi:10.1177/1352458517740212

Kegel, J., Dux, M., and Macko, R. (2014). Executive function and coping in stroke survivors. *Neurorehabilitation, 34*(1), 55-63. doi:10.3233/NRE-131010

Kelleher, M., Tolea, M. I., and Galvin, J. E. (2016). Anosognosia increases caregiver burden in mild cognitive impairment. *International Journal of Geriatric Psychiatry, 31*(7), 799-808. doi:10.1002/gps.4394

Kennedy, M. R., and Coelho, C. (2005). Self-regulation after traumatic brain injury: A framework for intervention of memory and problem-solving. *Seminars in Speech and Language, 26*(4), 242-255. doi:10.1055/s-2005-922103

Kircher, T., and David, A. (2003). *The self in neuroscience and psychiatry.* Cambridge University Press.

Kiresuk, T. J., and Sherman, R. E. (1968). Goal attainment scaling: A general method for evaluating comprehensive community mental health programs. *Community Mental Health Journal, 4*(6), 443-453. doi:10.1007/BF01530764

Knight, C., Alderman, N., and Burgess, P. W. (2002). Development of a simplified version of the multiple errands test for use in hospital settings. *Neuropsychological Rehabilitation, 12*(3), 231-255. doi:10.1080/09602010244000039

Kompier, M. A. (2006). New systems of work organization and workers' health. *Scandinavian Journal of Work, Environment and Health, 32*(6), 421-430. Retrieved from www.jstor.org/stable/40967595

Kortte, K. B., and Wegener, S. T. (2004). Denial of illness in medical rehabilitation populations: Theory, research, and definition. *Rehabilitation Psychology, 49*(3), 187-199. doi:10.1037/0090-5550.49.3.187

Krasny-Pacini, A., Chevignard, M., and Evans, J. (2014). Goal management training for rehabilitation of executive functions: A systematic review of effectiveness in patients with acquired brain injury. *Disability and Rehabilitation, 36*(2), 105-116. doi:10.3109/09638288.2013.777807

Krasny-Pacini, A., Evans, J., Sohlberg, M. M., and Chevignard, M. (2016). Proposed criteria for appraising goal attainment scales used as outcome measures in rehabilitation research. *Archives of Physical Medicine and Rehabilitation, 97*(1), 157-170. doi:10.1016/j.apmr.2015.08.424

Laakso, H., Hietanen, M., Melkas, S., Sibolt, G., Curtze, S., Virta, M., . . . Erkinjuntti, T. (2019). Executive function subdomains are associated with post-stroke functional outcome and permanent institutionalization. *European Journal of Neurology, 26*(3), 546-552. doi:10.1111/ene.13854

Landa-Gonzalez, B. (2001). Multicontextual occupational therapy intervention: A case study of traumatic brain injury. *Occupational Therapy International, 8*(1), 49-62. doi:10.1002/oti.131

Lane-Brown, A., and Tate, R. L. (2010). Evaluation of an intervention for apathy after traumatic brain injury: A multiple-baseline, single-case experimental design. *Journal of Head Trauma Rehabilitation, 25*(6), 459-469. doi:10.1097/HTR.0b013e3181d98e1d

Lane-Brown, A., and Tate, R. L. (2011). Apathy after traumatic brain injury: An overview of the current state of play. *Brain Impairment, 12*(1), 43-53. doi:10.1375/brim.12.1.43

Law, M., Baptiste, S., Carswell, A., McColl, M. A., Polatajko, H. J., and Pollock, N. (2014). *Canadian Occupational Performance Measure* (5th ed.). CAOT publications.

Lengenfelder, J., Chiaravalloti, N. D., and DeLuca, J. (2007). The efficacy of the generation effect in improving new learning in persons with traumatic brain injury. *Rehabilitation Psychology, 52*(3), 290-296. doi:10.1037/0090-5550.52.3.290

Lepping, R. J., Brooks, W. M., Kirchhoff, B. A., Martin, L. E., Kurylo, M., Ladesich, L., . . . Savage, C. (2015). Effectiveness of semantic encoding strategy training after traumatic brain injury is correlated with frontal brain activation change. *Int.J.Phys.Med.Rehabil, 3*(1) doi:10.4172/2329-9096.1000254

Levine, B., Robertson, I. H., Clare, L., Carter, G., Hong, J., Wilson, B. A., . . . Stuss, D. T. (2000). Rehabilitation of executive functioning: An experimental–clinical validation of goal management training. *Journal of the International Neuropsychological Society, 6*(3), 299-312. doi:10.1017/S1355617700633052

Levine, B., Schweizer, T. A., O'Connor, C., Turner, G., Gillingham, S., Stuss, D. T., . . . Robertson, I. H. (2011). Rehabilitation of executive functioning in patients with frontal lobe brain damage with goal management training. *Frontiers in Human Neuroscience, 5*, 9. doi:10.3389/fnhum.2011.00009

Levy, L. L. (2018). Cognitive information-processing memory. In N. Katz, and J. Toglia (Eds.), *Cognition, occupation, and participation across the lifespan* (4th ed., pp. 105-127). Bethesda, MD: American Occupational Therapy Association, Inc. doi:10.7139/2017.978-1-56900-479-1

Lezak, M., Howieson, D. B., Bigler, E. D., and Tranel, D. (2012). *Neuropsychological assessment* (5th ed.). Oxford University Press.

Lidz, C. S. (2002). Mediated learning experience (MLE) as a basis for an alternative approach to assessment. *School Psychology International, 23*, 68-84. doi:10.1177/0143034302023001731

Lipskaya-Velikovsky, L., Zeilig, G., Weingarden, H., Rozental-Iluz, C., and Rand, D. (2019). Executive functioning and daily living of indivduals with chronic stroke: Measurement and implications. *International Journal of Rehabilitation Research, 41*(2), 122-127. doi:10.1097/MRR.0000000000000272

Liu-Ambrose, T., Pang, M. Y., and Eng, J. J. (2007). Executive function is independently associated with performances of balance and mobility in community-dwelling older adults after mild stroke: Implications for falls prevention. *Cerebrovascular Diseases, 23*(2-3), 203-210. doi:10.1159/000097642

Liu, K. P., Chan, C. C., Lee, T. M., and Hui-Chan, C. W. (2004). Mental imagery for promoting relearning for people after stroke: A randomized controlled trial. *Archives of Physical Medicine and Rehabilitation, 85*(9), 1403-1408. doi:10.1016/j.apmr.2003.12.035

Liu, K. P., Chan, C. C., Wong, R. S., Kwan, I. W., Yau, C. S., Li, L. S., and Lee, T. M. (2009). A randomized controlled trial of mental imagery augment generalization of learning in acute post-stroke patients. *Stroke, 40*(6), 2222-2225. doi:10.1161/STROKEAHA.108.540997

Lobato, J., Rhodehamel, B., and Hohensee, C. (2012). "Noticing" as an alternative transfer of learning process. *Journal of the Learning Sciences, 21*(3), 433-482. doi:10.1080/10508406.2012.682189

Loya, F., Novakovic-Agopian, T., Binder, D., Rossi, A., Rome, S., Murphy, M., and Chen, A. J. (2017). Long-term use and perceived benefits of goal-oriented attentional self-regulation training in chronic brain injury. *Rehabilitation Research and Practice, 2017* doi:10.1155/2017/8379347

Lussier, A., Doherty, M., and Toglia, J. (2019). Weekly calendar planning activity. In T. J. Wolf, D. F. Edwards and G. M. Giles (Eds.), *Functional cognition and occupational therapy: A practical approach to treating individuals with cognitive loss* (1st ed., pp. 75-89). AOTA Press.

Maddox, G. B., and Balota, D. A. (2015). Retrieval practice and spacing effects in young and older adults: An examination of the benefits of desirable difficulty. *Memory and Cognition, 43*(5), 760-774. doi:10.3758/s13421-014-0499-6

Maeir, A., Traub Bar-Ilan, R., Kastner, L., Fisher, O., Levanon-Erez, N., and Hahn-Markowitz, J. (2018). An integrative cognitive-functional (cog-fun) intervention model for children, adolescents, and adults with ADHD. In N. Katz, and J. Toglia (Eds.), *Cognition, occupation, and participation across the lifespan* (4th ed., pp. 335-351). AOTA Press. doi:10.7139/2017.978-1-56900-479-1

Majd, M. A., Asgharpour, S., and Ghiasvand, M. (2017). Effectiveness of educating problem-solving and decision making skills on mental health and resilience of female university students. *International Journal of Applied Behavioral Sciences, 3*(3), 9-14. doi:10.22037/ijabs.v3i3.15495

Mansbach, W. E., and Mace, R. A. (2018). Predicting functional dependence in mild cognitive impairment: Differential contributions of memory and executive functions. *The Gerontologist,* doi:10.1093/geront/gny097

Man, D. W., Soong, W. Y., Tam, S. F., and Hui-Chan, C. W. (2006). Self-efficacy outcomes of people with brain injury in cognitive skill training using different types of trainer-trainee interaction. *Brain Injury : [BI], 20*(9), 959-970. doi:10.1080/02699050600909789

McCraith, D. B., and Earhart, C. A. (2018). Cognitive disabilities model: Creating fit between functional cognitive abilities and cognitive activity demands. In N. Katz, and J. Toglia (Eds.), *Cognition, occupation, and participation across the lifespan* (4th ed., pp. 469-497). AOTA Press. doi:10.7139/2017.978-1-56900-479-1

McDaniel, M. A., and Einstein, G. O. (2007). *Prospective memory: An overview and synthesis of an emerging field.* SAGE Publications.

McDonald, S. (2013). Impairments in social cognition following severe traumatic brain injury. *Journal of the International Neuropsychological Society, 19*(3), 231-246. doi:10.1017/S1355617712001506

McDonald, S., Code, C., and Togher, L. (2016). *Communication disorders following traumatic brain injury,* Psychology press.

McDonald, S., Gowland, A., Randall, R., Fisher, A., Osborne-Crowley, K., and Honan, C. (2014). Cognitive factors underpinning poor expressive communication skills after traumatic brain injury: Theory of mind or executive function? *Neuropsychology, 28*(5), 801-811. doi:10.1037/neu0000089

McEwen, S. E., Mandich, A., and Polatajko, H. J. (2018). CO-OP Approach™: A cognitive-based intervention for children and adults. In Katz, N. and Toglia, J. (Ed.), *Cognition, occupation, and participation across the lifespan* (4th ed., pp. 315-334). AOTA Press. doi:10.7139/2017.978-1-56900-479-1

McGlynn, S. M., and Schacter, D. L. (1989). Unawareness of deficits of neuropsychological syndromes. *Journal of Clinical and Experimental Neuropsychology, 11*, 143-205. doi:10.1080/01688638908400882

McKeough, A., Lupart, J. L., and Marini, A. (2013). *Teaching for transfer: Fostering generalization in learning.* Routledge.

Medley, A. R., and Powell, T. (2010). Motivational interviewing to promote self-awareness and engagement in rehabilitation following acquired brain injury: A conceptual review. *Neuropsychological Rehabilitation,* 1-28. doi:10.1080/09602010903529610

Meichenbaum, D. (1975). A self-instructional approach to stress management: A proposal for stress inoculation training. *Stress and Anxiety, 1*, 237-263.

Meichenbaum, D. (1977). Cognitive behaviour modification. *Cognitive Behaviour Therapy, 6*(4), 185-192. doi:10.1080/16506073.1977.9626708

Meichenbaum, D., and Goodman, J. (1971). Training impulsive children to talk to themselves: A means of developing self-control. *Journal of Abnormal Psychology, 77*(2), 115-126. doi:10.1037/h0030773

Mentis, M., Dunn-Bernstein, M. J., and Mentis, M. (2008). *Mediated learning: Teaching, tasks, and tools to unlock cognitive potential.* Corwin Press.

Mestre, J. (2002). Transfer of learning: Issues and research agenda. Paper presented at the *National Science Foundation*, Arlington, VA.

Miller, P. H. (1990). The development of strategies of selective attention. In D. F. Bjorklund (Ed.), *Children's strategies: Contemporary views of cognitive development* (pp. 157-184). Lawrence Erlbaum Associates.

Miyake, A., and Friedman, N. (2012). The nature and organization of individual differences in executive functions: Four general conclusions. *Current Directions in Psychological Science, 21*(1), 8-14. doi:10.1177/0963721411429458

Mlinac, M. E., and Feng, M. C. (2016). Assessment of activities of daily living, self-care, and independence. *Archives of Clinical Neuropsychology, 31*(6), 506-516. doi:10.1093/arclin/acw049

Morin, A. (2009). Self-awareness deficits following loss of inner speech: Dr. jill bolte Taylor's case study. *Consciousness and Cognition, 18*(2), 524-529. doi:10.1016/j.concog.2008.09.008

Morris, P. E., and Gruneberg, M. (1992). Prospective memory: Remembering to do things. In M. Gruneberg, and P. E. Morris (Eds.), *Aspects of memory: The practical aspects.* (2nd ed., pp. 196-222). Routledge.

Murphy, R., Tubridy, N., Kevelighan, H., and O'Riordan, S. (2013). Parkinson's disease: How is employment affected? *Irish Journal of Medical Science, 182*(3), 415-419. doi:10.1007/s11845-013-0902-5

Njomboro, P. (2017). Social cognition deficits: Current position and future directions for neuropsychological interventions in cerebrovascular disease. *Behavioural Neurology, 2017* doi:10.1155/2017/2627487

O'Brien, A., Chiaravalloti, N., Arango-Lasprilla, J. C., Lengenfelder, J., and DeLuca, J. (2007). An investigation of the differential effect of self-generation to improve learning and memory in multiple sclerosis and traumatic brain injury. *Neuropsychological Rehabilitation, 17*(3), 273-292. doi:10.1080/09602010600751160

O'Brien, A. N., and Wolf, T. J. (2010). Determining work outcomes in mild to moderate stroke survivors. *Work, 36*(4), 441-447. doi:10.3233/WOR-2010-1047

Oddy, M., Worthington, A., and Francis, E. (2009). Motivational disorders following brain injury. In M. Oddy, and A. Worthington (Eds.), *The rehabilitation of executive disorders: A guide to theory and practice* (pp. 37-56). Oxford University Press.

O'Keeffe, F., Dockree, P., Moloney, P., Carton, S., and Robertson, I. H. (2007). Awareness of deficits in traumatic brain injury: A multidimensional approach to assessing metacognitive knowledge and online-awareness. *Journal of the International Neuropsychological Society, 13*(1), 38-49. doi:10.1017/S1355617707070075

Ownsworth, T. (2005). The impact of defensive denial upon adjustment following traumatic brain injury. *Neuropsychoanalysis, 7*(1), 83-94. doi:10.1080/15294145.2005.10773476

Ownsworth, T., and Clare, L. (2006). The association between awareness deficits and rehabilitation outcome following acquired brain injury. *Clinical Psychology Review, 26*(6), 783-95. doi:10.1016/j.cpr.2006.05.003

Ownsworth, T., Desbois, J., Grant, E., Fleming, J., and Strong, J. (2006). The associations among self-awareness, emotional well-being, and employment outcome following acquired brain injury: A 12-month longitudinal study. *Rehabilitation Psychology, 51*(1), 50. doi:10.1037/0090-5550.51.1.50

Ownsworth, T., Fleming, J., Desbois, J., Strong, J., and Kuipers, P. (2006). A metacognitive contextual intervention to enhance error awareness and functional outcome following traumatic brain injury: A single-case experimental design. *Journal of the International Neuropsychological Society, 12*, 54-63. doi:10.1017/S135561770606005X

Ownsworth, T., Fleming, J., Tate, R., Beadle, E., Griffin, J., Kendall, M., . . . Shum, D. (2017). Do people with severe traumatic brain injury benefit from making errors? A randomized controlled trial of error-based and errorless learning. *Neurorehabilitation and Neural Repair, 31*(12), 1072-1082. doi:10.1177/1545968317740635

Ownsworth, T., McFarland, K. M., and Young, R. M. (2000). Development and standardization of the self-regulation skills interview (SRSI): A new clinical assessment tool for acquired brain injury. *The Clinical Neuropsychologist, 14*(1), 76-92. doi:10.1076/1385-4046(200002)14:1;1-8;FT076

Ownsworth, T., and Shum, D. (2008). Relationship between executive functions and productivity outcomes following stroke. *Disability and Rehabilitation, 30*(7), 531-540. doi:10.1080/09638280701355694

Palermo, L., Cinelli, M. C., Piccardi, L., De Felice, S., Ciurli, P., Incoccia, C., . . . Guariglia, C. (2018). Cognitive functions underlying prospective memory deficits: A study on traumatic brain injury. *Applied Neuropsychology: Adult, 27*(2), 158-172. doi:10.1080/23279095.2018.1501374

Palm, S., Rönnbäck, L., and Johansson, B. (2017). Long-term mental fatigue after traumatic brain injury and impact on employment status. *Journal of Rehabilitation Medicine, 49*(3), 228-233. doi:10.2340/16501977-2190

Pearson, D., Deeprose, C., Wallace-Hadrill, S. M., Heyes, S. B., and Holmes, E. A. (2013). Assessing mental imagery in clinical psychology: A review of imagery measures and a guiding framework. *Clinical Psychology Review, 33*(1), 1-23. doi:10.1016/j.cpr.2012.09.001

Pearson, J., Naselaris, T., Holmes, E. A., and Kosslyn, S. M. (2015). Mental imagery: Functional mechanisms and clinical applications. *Trends in Cognitive Sciences, 19*(10), 590-602. doi:10.1016/j.tics.2015.08.003

Perez, F. M., Tunkel, R. S., Lachmann, E. A., and Nagler, W. (1996). Balint's syndrome arising from bilateral posterior cortical atrophy or infarction: Rehabilitation strategies and their limitation. *Disability and Rehabilitation, 18*(6), 300-304. doi:10.3109/09638289609165884

Perkins, D. N., and Salomon, G. (1992). Transfer of learning. *International encyclopedia of education* (2nd ed., pp. 6452-6457). Pergamon Press.

Perkins, D. N., and Salomon, G. (2012). Knowledge to go: A motivational and dispositional view of transfer. *Educational Psychologist, 47*(3), 248-258. doi:10.1080/00461520.2012.693354

Plant, S. E., Tyson, S. F., Kirk, S., and Parsons, J. (2016). What are the barriers and facilitators to goal-setting during rehabilitation for stroke and other acquired brain injuries? A systematic review and meta-synthesis. *Clinical Rehabilitation, 30*(9), 921-930. doi:10.1177/0269215516655856

Polatajko, H. J., and Mandich, A. (2004). *Enabling occupation in children: The cognitive orientation to daily occupational performance*. CAOT Publications.

Prescott, S., Fleming, J., and Doig, E. (2018). Rehabilitation goal setting with community dwelling adults with acquired brain injury: A theoretical framework derived from clinicians' reflections on practice. *Disability and Rehabilitation, 40*(20), 2388-2399. doi:10.1080/09638288.2017.1336644

Pressley, M., Borkowski, J. G., and Schneider, W. (2010). Cognitive strategies: Good strategy users coordinate metacognition and knowledge. *Annals of Child Development, 4*, 89-129.

Pressley, M., and Harris, K. R. (2009). Cognitive strategies instruction: From basic research to classroom instruction. *Journal of Education, 189*(1-2), 77-94. doi:10.1177/0022057409189001-206

Pressley, M., Woloshyn, V., Lysynchuk, L. M., Martin, V., Wood, E., and Willoughby, T. (1990). A primer of research on cognitive strategy instruction: The important issues and how to address them. *Educational Psychology Review, 2*(1), 1-58. doi:10.1007/BF01323528

Prigatano, G. (2008). Neuropsychological rehabilitation and psychodynamic psychotherapy. In J. E. Morgan, and J. H. Ricker (Eds.), *Textbook of clinical neuropsychology* (pp. 985-995). Taylor and Francis Group.

Prigatano, G., and Klonoff, P. S. (1998). A clinician's rating scale for evaluating impaired. self-awareness and denial of disability after brain injury. *The Clinical Neuropsychologist, 12*(1), 56-67. doi:10.1076/clin.12.1.56.1721

Radomski, M. V., Anheluk, M., Bartzen, P., and Zola, J. (2016). Effectiveness of interventions to address cognitive impairments and improve occupational performance after traumatic brain injury: A systematic review. *American Journal of Occupational Therapy, 70*(3), 7003180050p1-7003180050p9. doi:10.5014/ajot.2016.020776

Radomski, M. V., Giles, G., Finkelstein, M., Owens, J., Showers, M., and Zola, J. (2018). Implementation intentions for self-selected occupational therapy goals: Two case reports. *The American Journal of Occupational Therapy, 72*(3), 7203345030p1-7203345030p6. doi:10.5014/ajot.2018.023135

Raphael-Greenfield, E., Toglia, J., and Hartman, A. (2020). The contextual memory test. In B. J. Hemphill-Pearson, and C. K. Urish (Eds.), *Assessments in occupational therapy mental health: An integrative approach* (4th ed., pp 223-237). Slack Inc.

Raskin, S. A., Smith, M. P., Mills, G., Pedro, C., and Zamroziewicz, M. (2019). Prospective memory intervention using visual imagery in individuals with brain injury. *Neuropsychological Rehabilitation, 29*(2), 289-304. doi:10.1080/09602011.2017.1294082

Raskin, S. A., Williams, J., and Aiken, E. M. (2018). A review of prospective memory in indvdiuals with acquired brain injury. *Clinical Neuropsychologist*, doi:10.1080/13854046.2018.1455898

Rath, J., Hradil, A. L., Litke, D. R., and Diller, L. (2011). Clinical applications of problem-solving research in neuropsychological rehabilitation: Addressing the subjective experience of cognitive deficits in outpatients with acquired brain injury. *Rehabilitation Psychology, 56*(4), 320-328. doi:10.1037/a0025817

Rath, J., Simon, D., Langenbahn, D. M., Sherr, R. L., and Diller, L. (2003). Group treatment of problem-solving deficits in outpatients with traumatic brain injury: A randomised outcome study. *Neuropsychological Rehabilitation, 13*(4), 461-488. doi:10.1080/09602010343000039

Rende, B. (2000). Cognitive flexibility: Theory, assessment, and treatment. *Seminars in Speech and Language, 21*(2) 121-133. doi:10.1055/s-2000-7560

Richardson, C., McKay, A., and Ponsford, J. L. (2015). Factors influencing self-awareness following traumatic brain injury. *Journal of Head Trauma Rehabilitation, 30*(2), E43-E54. doi:10.1097/HTR.0000000000000048

Robertson, K., and Schmitter-Edgecombe, M. (2015). Self-awareness and traumatic brain injury outcome. *Brain Injury, 29*(7-8), 848-858. doi:10.3109/02699052.2015.1005135

Rochat, L., Beni, C., Billieux, J., Azouvi, P., Annoni, J., and Van der Linden, M. (2010). Assessment of impulsivity after moderate to severe traumatic brain injury. *Neuropsychological Rehabilitation, 20*(5), 778-797. doi:10.1080/09602011.2010.495245

Rodakowski, J., Skidmore, E. R., Reynolds, C. F., Dew, M. A., Butters, M. A., Holm, M. B., . . . Rogers, J. C. (2014). Can performance on daily activities discriminate between older adults with normal cognitive function and those with mild cognitive impairment? *Journal of the American Geriatrics Society, 62*(7), 1347-1352. doi:10.1111/jgs.12878

Rosenblum, S., Josman, N., and Toglia, J. (2017). Development of the daily living questionnaire (DLQ): A factor analysis study. *The Open Journal of Occupational Therapy, 5*(4), 4. doi:10.15453/2168-6408.1326

Rotenberg-Shpigelman, S., Rosen-Shilo, L., and Maeir, A. (2014). Online awareness of functional tasks following ABI: The effect of task experience and associations with underlying mechanisms. *Neurorehabilitation, 35*(1), 47-56. doi:10.3233/NRE-141101

Roth, R., Isquith, P. K., and Gioia, G. A. (2005). *Behavior rating inventory of executive function - adult version*. Psychological Assessment Resources Inc.

Royall, D. R., Lauterbach, E. C., Kaufer, D., Malloy, P., Coburn, K. L., and Black, K. J. (2007). The cognitive correlates of functional status: A review from the committee on research of the American Neuropsychiatric Association. *The Journal of Neuropsychiatry and Clinical Neurosciences, 19*(3), 249-265. doi:10.1176/jnp.2007.19.3.249

Rummel, J., and McDaniel, M. A. (Eds.) (2019). *Prospective memory*. Routledge.

Sala, G., Aksayli, N. D., Tatlidil, K. S., Tatsumi, T., Gondo, Y., and Gobet, F. (2019). Near and far transfer in cognitive training: A second-order meta-analysis. *Collabra: Psychology, 5*(1).

Salas, C. E., Gross, J. J., & Turnbull, O. H. (2019). Using the process model to understand emotion regulation changes after brain injury. *Psychology & Neuroscience, 12*(4), 430.

Salas, C., Vaughan, F., Shanker, S., & Turnbull, O. (2013). Stuck in a moment: Concreteness and psychotherapy after acquired brain injury. *Neuro-disability and Psychotherapy, 1*(1), 1-38.

Salazar-Villanea, M., Liebmann, E., Garnier-Villarreal, M., Montenegro-Montenegro, E., and Johnson, D. K. (2015). Depressive symptoms affect working memory in healthy older adult Hispanics. *Journal of Depression and Anxiety, 4*(4) doi:10.4172/2167-1044.1000204

Salomon, G., and Perkins, D. (1988). Teaching for transfer. *Educational Leadership, 46*(1), 22-32.

Sandson, J., and Albert, M. L. (1984). Varieties of perseveration. *Neuropsychologia, 22*(6), 715-732. doi:10.1016/0028-3932(84)90098-8

Schmidt, J., Fleming, J., Ownsworth, T., and Lannin, N. A. (2013). Video feedback on functional task performance improves self-awareness after traumatic brain injury: A randomized controlled trial. *Neurorehabilitation and Neural Repair, 27*(4), 316-324. doi:10.1177/1545968312469838

Schmidt, J., Fleming, J., Ownsworth, T., and Lannin, N. A. (2015). An occupation-based video feedback intervention for improving self-awareness: Protocol and rationale. *Canadian Journal of Occupational Therapy., 82*(1), 54-63. doi:10.1177/0008417414550999

Selwood, A., Bennett, J., Conway, M. A., Loveday, C., and Kuchelmeister, V. (2020). Mnemoscape: Supporting older adults' event memory using wearable camera photographs on an immersive interface. *Gerontology,* 1-11. doi:10.1159/000505848

Shallice, T., and Burgess, P. W. (1991). Deficits in strategy application following frontal lobe damage in man. *Brain, 114*(2), 727-741. doi:10.1093/brain/114.2.727

Shea-Shumsky, N. B., Schoeneberger, S., and Grigsby, J. (2019). Executive functioning as a predictor of stroke rehabilitation outcomes. *The Clinical Neuropsychologist, 33*(5), 854-872. doi:10.1080/13854046.2018.1546905

Sherer, M., Boake, C., Levin, E., Silver, B. V., Ringholz, G., and High, W. M. (1998). Characteristics of impaired awareness after traumatic brain injury. *Journal of the International Neuropsychological Society, 4*(4), 380-387.

Sherer, M. (2004). The Awareness Questionnaire. *The Center for Outcome Measurement in Brain Injury.* http://www.tbims.org/combi/aq (accessed July 26, 2020)

Skidmore, E. R. (2017). Functional cognition: Implications for practice, policy, and research. *The American Journal of Geriatric Psychiatry, 25*(1), 483-484. doi:10.1016/j.jagp.2016.12.020

Skidmore, E. R., Butters, M., Whyte, E., Grattan, E., Shen, J., and Terhorst, L. (2017). Guided training relative to direct skill training for individuals with cognitive impairments after stroke: a pilot randomized trial. *Archives of physical medicine and rehabilitation, 98*(4), 673-680.

Skidmore, E. R., Whyte, E. M., Butters, M. A., Terhorst, L., and Reynolds, C. F. (2015). Strategy training during inpatient rehabilitation may prevent apathy symptoms after acute stroke. *PM and R: The Journal of Injury, Function, and Rehabilitation, 7*(6), 562-570. doi:10.1016/j.pmrj.2014.12.010

Skidmore, E. R., Whyte, E. M., Holm, M. B., Becker, J. T., Butters, M. A., Dew, M. A., . . . Lenze, E. J. (2010). Cognitive and affective predictors of rehabilitation participation after stroke. *Archives of Physical Medicine and Rehabilitation, 91*(2), 203-207. doi:10.1016/j.apmr.2009.10.026

Sohlberg, M., and Turkstra, L. (2011). *Optimizing cognitive rehabilitation: Effective instructional methods.* Guilford Press.

Spiess, M. A., Meier, B., and Roebers, C. M. (2016). Development and longitudinal relationships between children's executive functions, prospective memory, and metacognition. *Cognitive Development, 38,* 99-113. doi:10.1016/j.cogdev.2016.02.003

Spikman, J. M., Timmerman, M. E., Milders, M. V., Veenstra, W. S., and van der Naalt, J. (2012). Social cognition impairments in relation to general cognitive deficits, injury severity, and prefrontal lesions in traumatic brain injury patients. *Journal of Neurotrauma, 29*(1), 101-111. doi:10.1089/neu.2011.2084

Stamenova, V., and Levine, B. (2019). Effectiveness of goal management training® in improving executive functions: A meta-analysis. *Neuropsychological Rehabilitation, 29*(10), 1569-1599. doi:10.1080/09602011.2018.1438294

Steinberg, C. J., and Zlotnick, S. (2019). The multicontext approach. In T. J. Wolf, D. F. Edwards and G. M. Giles (Eds.), *Functional cognition and occupational therapy: A practical approach to treating individuals with cognitive loss* (1st ed., pp. 219-237). AOTA Press.

Stokes, P. D., Lai, B., Holtz, D., Rigsbee, E., and Cherrick, D. (2008). Effects of practice on variability, effects of variability on transfer. *Journal of Experimental Psychology: Human Perception and Performance, 34*(3), 640-659. doi:10.1037/0096-1523.34.3.640

Stuss, D. T., Picton, T. W., and Alexander, M. P. (2001). Consciousness, self-awareness, and the frontal lobes. In S. P. Salloway, P. F. Malloy and J. D. Duffy (Eds.), *The frontal lobes and neuropsychiatric illness* (pp. 101-109). American Psychiatric Publishing, Inc.

Suchy, Y. (2016). *Executive functioning: A comprehensive guide for clinical practice.* Oxford University Press.

Sumowski, J. F., Wood, H. G., Chiaravalloti, N., Wylie, G. R., Lengenfelder, J., and DeLuca, J. (2010). Retrieval practice: A simple strategy for improving memory after traumatic brain injury. *Journal of the International Neuropsychological Society : JINS, 16*(6), 1147-1150. doi:10.1017/S1355617710001128

Swanson, H. L., Lussier, C. M., and Orosco, M. J. (2015). Cognitive strategies, working memory, and growth in word-problem solving in children with math difficulties. *Journal of Learning Disabilities, 48*(4), 339-358. doi:10.1177/0022219413498771

Swanson, H. L., and Sachse-Lee, C. (2000). A meta-analysis of single-subject-design intervention research for students with LD. *J Learn Disabil, 33*(2), 114-36. doi:10.1177/002221940003300201

Tailby, R., and Haslam, C. (2003). An investigation of errorless learning in memory-impaired patients: Improving the technique and clarifying theory. *Neuropsychologia, 41*(9), 1230-1240. doi:10.1016/S0028-3932(03)00036-8

Tamir, R., Dickstein, R., and Huberman, M. (2007). Integration of motor imagery and physical practice in group treatment applied to subjects with Parkinson's disease. *Neurorehabilitation and Neural Repair, 21*(1), 68-75. doi:10.1177/1545968306292608

Tate, R., Kennedy, M., Ponsford, J., Douglas, J., Velikonja, D., Bayley, M., and Stergiou-Kita, M. (2014). INCOG recommendations for management of cognition following traumatic brain injury, part III: Executive function and self-awareness. *The Journal of Head Trauma Rehabilitation, 29*(4), 338-352. doi:10.1097/HTR.0000000000000068

Toglia, J. (1989). Visual perception of objects: A model for assessment and intervention. *American Journal of Occupational Therapy, 44*, 587-595. doi:10.5014/ajot.43.9.587

Toglia, J. (1991). Generalization of treatment: A multicontext approach to cognitive perceptual impairment in adults with brain injury. *The American Journal of Occupational Therapy, 45*(6), 505-516. doi:10.5014/ajot.45.6.505

Toglia, J. (1992). A dynamic interactional approach to cognitive rehabilitation. In N. Katz (Ed.), *Cognitive rehabilitation: Models for intervention in occupational therapy* (pp. 104-143). Andover Medical Publishing.

Toglia, J. (1993a). *Contextual memory test*. The Psychological Corporation.

Toglia, J. (1993b). Lesson 4: Attention and memory. *AOTA self-study series: Cognitive rehabilitation* (pp. 4-27). AOTA Press.

Toglia, J. (1998). A dynamic interactional model to cognitive rehabilitation. In N. Katz (Ed.), *Cognition and occupation in rehabilitation* (pp. 5-50). AOTA Press.

Toglia, J. (2011). The dynamic interactional model of cognition in cognitive rehabilitation. In N. Katz, and J. Toglia (Eds.), *Cognition, occupation and participation across the life span: Neuroscience, neurorehabilitation and models of intervention in occupational therapy* (4th ed., pp. 161-201). AOTA Press. doi:10.7139/2017.978-1-56900-479-1

Toglia, J. (2015). *The weekly calendar planning activity (WCPA): A performance test of executive function*. AOTA Press.

Toglia, J. (2017). *Schedule activity module: Functional cognitive rehabilitation activities and strategy based intervention*. MC CogRehab Resources, LLC.

Toglia, J. (2018). The dynamic interactional model and the multicontext approach. In N. Katz, and J. Toglia (Eds.), *Cognition, occupation, and participation across the lifespan* (4th ed., pp. 355-385). AOTA Press. doi:10.7139/2017.978-1-56900-479-1

Toglia, J. (2019). Contextual memory test 2 (CMT-2): Assess recall, memory awareness, and strategy use in children or adults. Retrieved from cmt.multicontext.net

Toglia, J., Askin, G., Gerber, L. M., Jaywant, A., and O'Dell, M. W. (2019). Participation in younger and older adults post-stroke: Frequency, importance and desirability of engagement in activities. *Frontiers in Neurology, 10*, 1108. doi:10.3389/fneur.2019.01108

Toglia, J., Askin, G., Gerber, L., Taub, M., Mastrogiovanni, A., and O'Dell, M. (2017). Association between two measures of cognitive instrumental activities of daily living and their relationship to the Montreal Cognitive Assessment in persons with stroke. *Archives of Physical Medicine and Rehabilitation*, doi:10.1016/j.apmr.2017.04.007

Toglia, J., and Berg, C. (2013). Performance-based measure of executive function: Comparison of community and at-risk youth. *The American Journal of Occupational Therapy, 67*(5), 515-523. doi:10.5014/ajot.2013.008482

Toglia, J., and Chen, P. (2020). Spatial exploration strategy training for spatial neglect: A pilot study. *Neuropsychological Rehabilitation*, 1-22. doi.org/10.1080/09602011.2020.1790394

Toglia, J., and Golisz, K. (2012). Therapy for activities of daily living: Theoretical and practical perspectives. In N. D. Zasler, D. Katz and R. Zafonte (Eds.), *Brain injury* (2nd ed), Demos Medical Publishing.

Toglia, J., and Golisz, K. (2017). Traumatic brain injury (TBI) and the impact on daily life. In N. Chiaravalloti, and Y. Goverover (Eds.), *Changes in the brain* (1st ed., pp. 117-143). Springer. doi:10.1007/978-0-387-98188-8_6

Toglia, J., and Golisz, K. M. (1990). *Cognitive rehabilitation: Group games and activities*. Communication Skill Builders/Therapy Skill Builders.

Toglia, J., Golisz, K., and Goverover, Y. (2018). Evaluation and intervention for cognitive perceptual impairments. In B. A. Boyt Schell, and G. Gillen (Eds.), *Willard and Spackman's occupational therapy* (13th ed., pp. 901-941). Lippincott Williams and Wilkins.

Toglia, J., Goverover, Y., Johnston, M. V., and Dain, B. (2011). Application of the multicontextual approach in promoting learning and transfer of strategy use in an individual with TBI and executive dysfunction. *OTJR: Occupation, Participation and Health, 31*(1), S53-S60. doi:10.3928/15394492-20101108-09

Toglia, J., and Johnston, M. V. (2017). Cognitive Self-Efficacy Questionnaire. Retrieved from https://multicontext.net/assessments-questionnaires

Toglia, J., Johnston, M. V., Goverover, Y., and Dain, B. (2010). A multicontext approach to promoting transfer of strategy use and self-regulation after brain injury: An exploratory study. *Brain Injury, 24*(4), 664-677. doi:10.3109/02699051003610474

Toglia, J., and Katz, N. (2018). Executive functioning: Prevention and health promotion for at-risk populations and those with chronic disease. In N. Katz, and J. Toglia (Eds.), *Cognition, occupation, and participation across the lifespan* (4th ed., pp. 129-140). AOTA Press. doi:10.7139/2017.978-1-56900-479-1

Toglia, J., and Kirk, U. (2000). Understanding awareness deficits following brain injury. *Neurorehabilitation, 15*(1), 57-70. doi:10.3233/NRE-2000-15104

Toglia, J., Lee, A., Steinberg, C., and Waldman-Levi, A. (2020). Establishing and measuring treatment fidelity of a complex cognitive rehabilitation intervention: The multicontext approach. *British Journal of Occupational Therapy*, 1-12. doi:10.1177/0308022619898091

Toglia, J., and Maeir, A. (2018). Self-awareness and metacognition: Effect on occupational performance and outcome across the lifespan. In N. Katz, and J. Toglia (Eds.), *Cognition, occupation, and participation across the lifespan* (4th ed., pp.

143-163). Bethesda, MD: American Occupational Therapy Association, Inc. doi:10.7139/2017.978-1-56900-479-1

Toglia, J., Rodger, S. A., and Polatajko, H. J. (2012). Anatomy of cognitive strategies: A therapist's primer for enabling occupational performance. *Canadian Journal of Occupational Therapy, 79*(4), 225-236. doi:10.2182/cjot.2012.79.4.4

Toglia, J., and White, S. (2020). The weekly calendar planning activity. In B. J. Hemphill-Pearson, and C. K. Urish (Eds.), *Assessments in occupational therapy mental health: An integrative approach* (4th ed., pp 239-259). Slack Inc.

Tornås, S., Lovstad, M., Solbakk, A. K., Evans, J., Endestad, T., Hol, P. K., . . . Stubberud, J. (2016). Rehabilitation of executive functions in patients with chronic acquired brain injury with goal management training, external cuing, and emotional regulation: A randomized controlled trial. *Journal of the International Neuropsychological Society : JINS, 22*(4), 436-452. doi:1017/S1355617715001344

Tsai, N., Eccles, J. S., & Jaeggi, S. M. (2019). Stress and executive control: mechanisms, moderators, and malleability. *Brain and Cognition, 133,* 54-59.

Turner, B. J., Ownsworth, T., Turpin, M., Fleming, J., and Griffin, J. (2008). Self-identified goals and the ability to set realistic goals following acquired brain injury: A classification framework. *Australian Occupational Therapy Journal, 55*(2), 96-107. doi:10.1111/j.1440-1630.2007.00660.x

Turner-Stokes, L. (2009). Goal attainment scaling (GAS) in rehabilitation: A practical guide. *Clinical Rehabilitation, 23*(4), 362-370. doi:10.1177/0269215508101742

Turner-Stokes, L., Rose, H., Ashford, S., and Singer, B. (2015). Patient engagement and satisfaction with goal planning: Impact on outcome from rehabilitation. *International Journal of Therapy and Rehabilitation, 22*(5), 210-216.

Ubukata, S., Tanemura, R., Yoshizumi, M., Sugihara, G., Murai, T., and Ueda, K. (2014). Social cognition and its relationship to functional outcomes in patients with sustained acquired brain injury. *Neuropsychiatric Disease and Treatment, 10,* 2061-2068. doi:10.2147/NDT.S68156

Ucok, A., Cakir, S., Duman, Z. C., Discigil, A., Kandemir, P., and Atli, H. (2006). Cognitive predictors of skill acquisition on social problem-solving in patients with schizophrenia. *European Archives of Psychiatry and Clinical Neuroscience, 256*(6), 388-394. doi:10.1007/s00406-006-0651-9

Umanath, S., Toglia, J., and McDaniel, M. A. (2016). Training prospective memory for transfer. In T. Strobach, and J. Karbach (Eds.), *Cognitive training: An overview of features and applications* (pp. 81-91) Springer International Publishing.

Vakil, E., and Heled, E. (2016). The effect of constant versus varied training on transfer in a cognitive skill learning task: The case of the tower of hanoi puzzle. *Learning and Individual Differences, 47,* 207-214. doi:10.1016/j.lindif.2016.02.009

Van Bost, G., Van Damme, S., and Crombez, G. (2019). Goal reengagement is related to mental well-being, life satisfaction and acceptance in people with an acquired brain injury. *Neuropsychological Rehabilitation,* 1-15. doi:10.1080/09602011.2019.1608265

Van der Kemp, J., Kruithof, W. J., Nijboer, T. C., van Bennekom, C. A., van Heugten, C., and Visser-Meily, J. M. (2019). Return to work after mild-to-moderate stroke: Work satisfaction and predictive factors. *Neuropsychological Rehabilitation, 29*(4), 638-653. doi:10.1080/09602011.2017.1313746

van Moorselaar, D., & Slagter, H. A. (2020). Inhibition in selective attention. *Annals of the New York Academy of Sciences, 1464*(1), 204.

Van Stan, J. H., Dijkers, M. P., Whyte, J., Hart, T., Turkstra, L. S., Zanca, J. M., and Chen, C. (2019). The rehabilitation treatment specification system: Implications for improvements in research design, reporting, replication, and synthesis. *Archives of Physical Medicine and Rehabilitation, 100*(1), 146-155. doi:10.1016/j.apmr.2018.09.112

Vaughan, L., and Giovanello, K. (2010). Executive function in daily life: Age-related influences of executive processes on instrumental activities of daily living. *Psychology and Aging, 25*(2), 343-355. doi:10.1037/a0017729

Villalobos, D., Bilbao, Á., López-Muñoz, F., and Pacios, J. (2019). Improving self-awareness after acquired brain injury leads to enhancements in patients' daily living functionality. *Brain Impairment, 20*(3), 268-275. doi:10.1017/BrImp.2019.10

Vygotsky, L. S. (1962). In Hanfmann E., Vakar G. (Eds.), *Thought and language.* MIT Press.

Vygotsky, L. S. (1978). *Mind in society: The development of higher psychological processes.* Harvard University Press.

Waldman-Levi, A., and Steinmann Obermeyer, I. (2018). Addressing executive function in schools. In N. Katz, and J. Toglia (Eds.), *Cognition, occupation, and participation across the lifespan* (4th ed., pp. 259-271). AOTA Press. doi:10.7139/2017.978-1-56900-479-1

Waldum, E. R., Dufault, C. L., and McDaniel, M. A. (2016). Prospective memory training: Outlining a new approach. *Journal of Applied Gerontology, 35*(11), 1211-1234. doi:10.1177/0733464814559418

Waters, H. S., and Kunnmann, T. W. (2010). Metacognition and strategy discovery in early childhood. In H. S. Waters, and W. Schneider (Eds.), *Metacognition, strategy use, and instruction.* (pp. 3-22). Guilford Press. Retrieved from http://search.ebscohost.com/login.aspx?direct=trueanddb=psyhandAN=2009-18875-001andsite=ehost-live

Waters, H. S., and Schneider, W. (2010). In Waters H. S., Schneider W. (Eds.), *Metacognition, strategy use, and instruction.* Guilford Press.

Wesson, J., Clemson, L., Brodaty, H., and Reppermund, S. (2016). Estimating functional cognition in older adults using observational assessments of task performance in complex everyday activities: A systematic review and evaluation of measurement properties. *Neuroscience and Biobehavioral Reviews, 68,* 335-360. doi:10.1016/j.neubiorev.2016.05.024

Wesson, J., and Giles, G. M. (2019). Understanding functional cognition. In T. J. Wolf, D. F. Edwards and G. M. Giles (Eds.), *Functional cognition and occupational therapy: A practical approach to treating individuals with cognitive loss* (pp. 7-20). AOTA Press.

West, R. L., Bagwell, D. K., and Dark-Freudeman, A. (2008). Self-efficacy and memory aging: The impact of a memory intervention based on self-efficacy. *Aging,*

Neuropsychology, and Cognition, 15(3), 302-329. doi:10.1080/13825580701440510

Whiting, D. L., Deane, F. P., Ciarrochi, J., McLeod, H. J., and Simpson, G. K. (2015). Validating measures of psychological flexibility in a population with acquired brain injury. *Psychological Assessment, 27*(2), 415-423. doi:10.1037/pas0000050

Whyte, J. (2006). Using treatment theories to refine the designs of brain injury rehabilitation treatment effectiveness studies. *The Journal of Head Trauma Rehabilitation, 21*(2), 99-106.

Whyte, J., Dijkers, M. P., Hart, T., Van Stan, J. H., Packel, A., Turkstra, L. S., . . . Ferraro, M. (2019). The importance of voluntary behavior in rehabilitation treatment and outcomes. *Archives of Physical Medicine and Rehabilitation, 100*(1), 156-163. doi:10.1016/j.apmr.2018.09.111

Whyte, J., Dijkers, M. P., Van Stan, J. H., and Hart, T. (2018). Specifying what we study and implement in rehabilitation: Comments on the reporting of clinical research. *Archives of Physical Medicine and Rehabilitation, 99*(7), 1433-1435. doi:10.1016/j.apmr.2018.03.008

Wieber, F., Thürmer, J. L., and Gollwitzer, P. M. (2015). Promoting the translation of intentions into action by implementation intentions: Behavioral effects and physiological correlates. *Frontiers in Human Neuroscience, 9*, 395. doi:10.3389/fnhum.2015.00395

Wilson, B. A. (2009). *Memory rehabilitation: Integrating theory and practice* Guilford Press.

Wilson, B. A. (2013). Memory deficits. In M. P. Barnes, and D. C. Good (Eds.), *Handbook of clinical neurology* (Vol. 110 ed., pp. 357-363). Netherlands: Elsevier. doi:10.1016/B978-0-444-52901-5.00030-7

Winkens, I., Van Heugten, C. M., Wade, D. T., and Fasotti, L. (2009). Training patients in time pressure management, a cognitive strategy for mental slowness. *Clinical Rehabilitation, 23*(1), 79-90. doi:10.1177/0269215508097855

Wolf, T. J. (2018). Occupational therapy's role in identifying functional cognitive changes in the acute care setting. In N. Katz, and J. Toglia (Eds.), *Cognition, occupation, and participation across the lifespan* (4th ed., pp. 165-171). AOTA Press. doi:10.7139/2017.978-1-56900-479-1

Wolf, T. J., Baum, C., and Connor, L. T. (2009). Changing face of stroke: Implications for occupational therapy practice. *American Journal of Occupational Therapy, 63*(5), 621-625. doi:10.5014/ajot.63.5.621

Wolf, T. J., Dahl, A., Auen, C., and Doherty, M. (2017). The reliability and validity of the complex task performance assessment: A performance-based assessment of executive function. *Neuropsychological Rehabilitation, 27*(5), 707-721. doi:10.1080/09602011.2015.1037771

Wolf, T. J., Doherty, M., Kallogjeri, D., Coalson, R. S., Nicklaus, J., Ma, C. X., . . . Piccirillo, J. (2016). The feasibility of using metacognitive strategy training to improve cognitive performance and neural connectivity in women with chemotherapy-induced cognitive impairment. *Oncology, 91*(3), 143-152. doi:10.1159/000447744

Wong, A. W., Chen, C., Baum, M. C., Heaton, R. K., Goodman, B., and Heinemann, A. W. (2019). Cognitive, emotional, and physical functioning as predictors of paid employment in people with stroke, traumatic brain injury, and spinal cord injury. *American Journal of Occupational Therapy, 73*(2), 7302205010p1-7302205010p15. doi:10.5014/ajot.2019.031203

Ybarra, O., and Winkielman, P. (2012). On-line social interactions and executive functions. *Frontiers in Human Neuroscience, 6*, 75. doi:10.3389/fnhum.2012.00075

Yeates, K. O., Swift, E., Taylor, H. G., Wade, S. L., Drotar, D., Stancin, T., and Minich, N. (2004). Short- and long-term social outcomes following pediatric traumatic brain injury. *Journal of the International Neuropsychological Society, 10*(3), 412-426. doi:10.1017/S1355617704103093

Ylvisaker, M., Szekeres, S. F., and Feeney, T. J. (1998). Cognitive rehabilitation: Executive functions. In M. Ylvisaker (Ed.), *Traumatic brain injury rehabilitation: Children and adolescents*, (pp. 221-269). Butterworth-Heinemann.

Ylvisaker, M., Turkstra, L. S., and Coelho, C. (2005). Behavioral and social interventions for individuals with traumatic brain injury: A summary of the research with clinical implications. Paper presented at the *Seminars in Speech and Language, 26*(04) 256-267. doi:10.1055/s-2005-922104

Zebdi, R., Goyet, L., Pinabiaux, C., and Guellaï, B. (2016). Psychological disorders and ecological factors affect the development of executive functions: Some perspectives. *Frontiers in Psychiatry, 7* doi:10.3389/fpsyt.2016.00195

Zelazo, P., and Carlson, S. M. (2012). Hot and cool executive function in childhood and adolescence: Development and plasticity. *Child Development Perspectives, 6*(4), 354-360. doi:10.1111/j.1750-8606.2012.00246.x

Zepeda, C. D., Richey, J. E., Ronevich, P., and Nokes-Malach, T. J. (2015). Direct instruction of metacognition benefits adolescent science learning, transfer, and motivation: An in vivo study. *Journal of Educational Psychology, 107*(4), 954-970. doi:10.1037/edu0000022

Zlotnik, S., Sachs, D., Rosenblum, S., Shpasser, R., and Josman, N. (2009). Use of the dynamic interactional model in selfcare and motor intervention after traumatic brain injury: Explanatory case studies. *American Journal of Occupational Therapy, 63*, 549-558. doi:10.5014/ajot.63.5.549

Zogg, J. B., Woods, S. P., Sauceda, J. A., Wiebe, J. S., and Simoni, J. M. (2012). The role of prospective memory in medication adherence: A review of an emerging literature. *Journal of Behavioral Medicine, 35*(1), 47-62. doi:10.1007/s10865-011-9341-9

PART IV

TOOLS, RESOURCES, AND SUPPLEMENTARY MATERIAL

APPENDICES

- Appendix A: Learning Activities for Therapists
- Appendix B: Assessment and Observational Tools
- Appendix C: Treatment Forms
- Appendix D: Supplementary Material

A passcode to access the following website can be used solely *by the purchaser* of this book to download the appendices.

https://multicontext.net/book-appendix   **Passcode**: Mcappendix4

These materials are intended for use only by qualified professionals. Application of these materials in a particular situation is the professional responsibility of the practitioner.

Limited Photocopy License for Appendices: The authors grant non-assignable limited permission to individual purchasers of this book to reproduce all materials in the Appendices for personal use or clinical use with individual clients. This license does not grant the right to reproduce these materials for resale or redistribution, or in other publications, websites, file-sharing sites, internet, handouts or slides for lectures, workshops, or webinars. Permission to reproduce these materials for these purposes must be obtained in writing from the authors. Duplication of this material for commercial purposes is prohibited.

APPENDIX A: Learning Activities for Therapists

APPENDIX A.1	Analyzing Negative Behaviors from the Perspective of Executive Function (Chapters 1-2)
APPENDIX A.2	Social Skills and Sample Underlying Cognitive Components (Chapters 1-2)
APPENDIX A.3	Executive Function Skills Exercise 1 (Chapter 2)
APPENDIX A.4	Executive Function Skills Exercise 2: Medication Schedule (Chapter 2)
APPENDIX A.5	Reflections on Strategy Use for Executive Function Exercises (Chapter 2)
APPENDIX A.6	Functional Cognitive Examples of Executive Function and Memory Deficits (Chapter 2)
APPENDIX A.7	Awareness Clinical Scenario and Strategy Use (Chapter 3)
APPENDIX A.8	Worksheet: Brainstorm Activities and Variations in Directions (Chapter 4)
APPENDIX A.9	Characteristics of Simple and Complex Problem-Solving Tasks (Chapter 4)
APPENDIX A.10	Functional Cognitive Problem-Solving Scenarios (Chapter 4)
APPENDIX A.11	Executive Function Analysis Worksheet (Chapter 4)
APPENDIX A.12	Variations in Activity Demands (Chapter 4)
APPENDIX A.13	Variations in Activity Demands 2 (Chapter 4)
APPENDIX A.14.1 and A.14.2	General Case Analysis using the Dynamic Interactional Model Framework Dynamic Interactional Model Case Analysis Form (Chapter 4)
APPENDIX A.15	Cue Analysis: Picture Yourself in the Situation – What would you say or do? (Chapter 10, 11)
APPENDIX A.16	Treatment Role Play: Metacognitive Questions and Guided Learning (Chapters 10,11,14)
ANSWERS	Answers for Appendices A.1, A.2, A.3, A.4, A.6, A.7, A.8, A.10, A.14, A.15

Appendix A.1. Analyzing Negative Behaviors from the Perspective of Executive Function

Observed Negative Behaviors	Possible Underlying Cognitive Problems
• Careless • Lack of effort, lazy • Unmotivated	
• Repeats same mistakes	
• Doesn't follow directions	
• Lack of follow-through • Unreliable • Irresponsible • Not trustworthy	
• Self-centered • Reduced empathy	
• Rude • Interrupts others	
• Stubborn, rigid • Argumentative	
• Inconsistent work • Unpredictable	
• Emotional outbursts • Low frustration tolerance	

Toglia & Foster: The Multicontext Approach to Cognitive Rehabilitation.

Appendix A.2. Social Skills and Sample Underlying Cognitive Components

Social Skills	Cognitive Components
• Eye contact	
• Keep conversations focused on the topic	
• Keep track of what was already stated	
• Sustain a meaningful conversation	
• Shift with changes in topic, speakers	
• Wait for turn before speaking and self-monitor one's reactions	
• Start conversations and keep the conversation going	
• Recall and maintain continuity between previous conversations and interactions	
• Attend to others' reactions, verbal and nonverbal signs	
• Simultaneously attend to the content of conversation and context	
• Express thoughts in an organized way	
• Understand different perspectives	
• Make inferences about the intentions, beliefs, feelings or emotional state of others	
• Anticipate and recognize consequences of saying something that might evoke unpleasant reactions from others	
• Show empathy	
• Awareness of tone of voice, nonverbal cues, facial expressions, emotional cues or basic emotions of self and others. Use tone and emotions that fit the situation.	
• Ability to interpret sarcastic remarks and humor	

Toglia & Foster: The Multicontext Approach to Cognitive Rehabilitation.

Appendix A.3. Executive Function Skills Exercise 1

Try the below activities:

1) Cooking Competition

Mary loves to cook and would like to enter a recipe into a cooking competition.

Write numbers in the blanks to sequence the steps that she needs to complete in order. There is one rule to follow: You should try not to erase or cross out a number once you have written it as points are subtracted for this. Mark the time down when you start and finish.

____ Buy fresh ingredients for the competition

____ Make the practice recipes

____ Receive confirmation that application has been accepted and find out assigned day/time

____ Choose a couple of recipes to practice with

____ Choose the final recipe to make for the judges

____ Complete and submit the application for the competition before the deadline

____ Prepare the dish for the judges

____ Receive feedback from friends on the practice recipe

____ Find out the rules and eligibility for the competition

____ Buy ingredients for the practice recipes

2) Fixing a Flat Tire

Below is a list of steps to fix a flat tire, but the steps are out of order. In addition, some of the steps may not belong. Write a number next to each step relevant to fixing a flat tire to indicate the sequence or order in which the steps need to be completed.

There is one rule to follow: You should try not to erase or cross out a number once you have written it as points are subtracted for this. Mark the time down when you start and finish.

____ Lower car to ground

____ Use tire iron to loosen tire lug nuts

____ Adjust the rear-view mirror

____ Remove flat tire

____ Get out the jack, crank, tire iron

____ Use tire iron to tighten lug nuts

____ Jack up car

____ Completely loosen lug nuts and remove from threaded wheel studs

____ Place spare tire on

____ Insert the key in the ignition

____ Put flat tire in trunk

____ Insert lug nuts onto the threaded wheel studs

____ Get out spare tire

Toglia & Foster: The Multicontext Approach to Cognitive Rehabilitation.

3) Planning

a. You are planning a surprise retirement party for a colleague. Write down everything you need to consider or do.

b. You have a friend visiting you from out of town that has never been to this area before. List all the things you could do over the next day with your visitor.

c. You know someone that is planning to move into their first apartment. Make a list of all of the essential things they will need to buy.

Appendix A.4. Executive Function Skills Exercise 2: Medication Schedule

Assume that you eat breakfast, lunch, and dinner at the times on the attached schedule. Please indicate what times you should take each medication and how many pills you need to take. Also, indicate when you should drink water and eat any snacks. Try not to erase or cross out. Note the time that you begin and end this task.

Antibiotics: Take 1 blue pill three times a day, at least 30 minutes before meals
Aspirin: Take 2 white tablets every 4 hours with a snack
Blood Pressure Meds: Take 1 yellow pill in the morning and evening, after meals
Anti-Inflammatory meds: Take 1 brown pill an hour after dinner
Water: Drink a full glass of water every 2 hours

Medication Schedule

7:30 a.m.	
8:00 a.m.	
8:30 a.m.	Breakfast
9:00 a.m.	
9:30 a.m.	
10:00 a.m.	
10:30 a.m.	
11:00 a.m.	
11:30 a.m.	
12:00 noon	
12:30 p.m.	Lunch
1:00 p.m.	
1:30 p.m.	
2:00 p.m.	
2:30 p.m.	
3:00 p.m.	
3:30 p.m.	
4:00 p.m.	
4:30 p.m.	
5:00 p.m.	
5:30 p.m.	
6:00 p.m.	Dinner
6:30 p.m.	
7:00 p.m.	
7:30 p.m.	
8:00 p.m.	

Toglia & Foster: The Multicontext Approach to Cognitive Rehabilitation.

Appendix A.5. Reflections on Strategy Use for Executive Function Exercise (A.3, A.4)

1. Identify the activity:

2. What aspects of this activity were most challenging and why?

3. Think about how you went about this activity. What method or approach did you use? *For example:* How did you decide where to start and how did you proceed? Did you use any special methods to help you keep track or generate ideas? Or to keep everything in order? Complete the table below.

Describe Strategy or Method	When was it used? (Before writing any numbers; initial part of activity, middle, end, after, or throughout)	How or why did it help? Or indicate if it hindered performance

4. Describe the executive function skills required in this activity.

Toglia & Foster: The Multicontext Approach to Cognitive Rehabilitation.

Appendix A.6. Functional Cognitive Examples of Executive Function and Memory Deficits

Read the below scenarios and identify the type of executive function and/or memory symptoms that appear to be interfering with performance. Note there may be several possible answers. See sample analysis at the end of Appendix A.

1. Fred is independent in self-care activities. He was asked to pay bills that were on the table; however, before the therapist had finished her instructions, Fred began writing out a check (before he even looked at the bills). The physical therapist also reported that Fred tried to get up and start walking before she finished giving him directions on how to use the walker.

2. Victor can recall events and conversations from the day before without difficulty but states that he has difficulty remembering appointments and errands. For example, he forgets to return phone calls, feed his dog, and pay his bill by the due date.

3. Mark was provided with a simulated scenario and was asked to enter a list of classes and activities into the calendar at specific days and times. He put himself in the situation and entered the classes and activities on the list that he preferred instead of adhering to those on the list. He also added other activities he likes to do, that were not on the list.

4. John spoke for 10 minutes with his daughter. Upon hanging up the phone, he immediately relayed the conversation to his wife. Three hours later, he called his daughter, completely unaware he had spoken to her earlier. When she provided cues and told him what they had spoken about, he still had no recollection of the conversation.

5. During a bill-paying task, Sam read the bill, put it in an envelope, and then had to take it out again to look at the amount. He took the bill in and out of the envelope several times because he failed to get all the information he needed when initially looking at the bill (balance due, address, check payable to, etc.). He was frustrated that it took so long to pay his bills and states that he cannot understand why simple activities now take him so long to complete.

6. Marie was given a list of things to pack in an overnight bag. As she was looking for items, she became sidetracked with other items and stopped looking at the list. She ended up packing several items that she did not need and forgot to include key items, such as her eyeglasses and medication.

Toglia & Foster: The Multicontext Approach to Cognitive Rehabilitation.

7. As Mary was looking over a restaurant menu, she read "hamburger" aloud but realized she had forgotten what a "hamburger" was.

8. Sara is independent in routine self-care activities; however, she does not do any household tasks unless cued and appears content watching TV all day. For example, the sink was filled with dirty dishes, but she did not load the dishwasher. She no longer calls friends and does not pursue previous interests such as exercise, swimming, or socializing with others. Depression has been ruled out. Her family indicates that this is a dramatic change.

9. In an interview, Karen said, "I lose my train of thought. I get some food out of the pantry and then, three seconds later, I head back to the pantry to get something out to eat, not realizing I had just done that seconds ago."

10. Sue was instructed to make anything she wanted for lunch from items that were already in the kitchen. After receiving the instructions, she sat at the kitchen table for several minutes before being cued to look in the refrigerator. As she looked in the refrigerator, she said she didn't know what to make.

11. Kevin can recall how to set the alarm on his cell phone but does not remember when he learned it or who taught it to him. When he was provided with cues, he was then able to recall that his son showed him how to set the alarm and he remembered the room he was in.

12. Mary was asked to put 3 pills in a pillbox organizer: one each in the morning, noon, and night sections. She verbally repeated the directions correctly, but she put all 3 pills in the morning section. When paying 2 bills, she completed paying the first bill and stated, "This bill is paid;" however, she continued to read the first bill, instead of moving on to pay the second bill. When she was asked what she needed to do, she correctly stated she needed to pay the next bill but continued to read the first bill.

13. Dave remembered to turn off his cell phone as soon as he walked into a meeting, but he completely forgot to call his colleague at 2:15 p.m. as he had promised.

Toglia & Foster: The Multicontext Approach to Cognitive Rehabilitation.

14. In a task involving making a cake, Kathy retrieved eggs from the refrigerator but lost track of how many eggs she had put into the bowl. She thought she put 4 eggs into the bowl, but she had only put 3. She searched twice for sugar, unaware that she had previously retrieved it. She put a 1/2 cup of water into the mix twice as she did not realize she had already added water and omitted the tablespoon of oil. She did not understand why the cake looked funny and did not taste right.

15. John was asked to walk to the table, pick up the blue book, bring it to his room, and call a pharmacy to find out what time it closed. He only called the pharmacy to find out the closing time. He did not recall any other directions. Two hours later, he recalled that he had called the pharmacy.

16. Jim was asked to make a schedule for visitors from out of town. He was given a list of possible sightseeing items and things to do as well as criteria. He quickly became anxious and overwhelmed by the amount of information and withdrew from the activity, saying he did not know where to begin.

17. Jose forgot how to operate the microwave oven and did not know what to do, even though he has used the same microwave oven on a regular basis for years.

18. Rosa was asked to write down a list of all the meals she could make for dinner during the week. She wrote down "pasta," but could not think of anything else.

19. Carlos went into a supermarket to purchase a few items. As he walked down the aisle to find a specific brand of cereal, he felt overwhelmed. Everything on the shelves looked the same. He couldn't find what he was looking for. Between the noise, the lights, and the people, he couldn't focus. He left the store without purchasing what he needed.

20. Victoria is unable to recall conversations or events from the day before. However, when she is provided with cues such as the context, who she was with, the general topic of conversation, or type of event, she can then recall many of the details.

Toglia & Foster: The Multicontext Approach to Cognitive Rehabilitation.

Appendix A.7. Awareness Clinical Scenario and Strategy Use

The following clients all have difficulty accurately completing a multiple-step online shopping activity; however, their performance differs in other aspects.

Review each scenario and identify (1) the type of awareness described and (2) the implications for strategy training.

Client 1: In an interview, Mike acknowledged that his thinking skills had changed and said he sometimes had difficulty concentrating. He was unable to provide specific examples. Mike was presented with a list of items to purchase online. He was also given a budget. Mike anticipated the online shopping activity would be easy. During the activity, Mike needed multiple cues to refer to the shopping list as he was easily distracted by other items on the web pages. He did not cross off items on the list once he had located them. He lost track of which items he had found. When he was cued to refer to the list and check off items on the list he had found, he had no difficulty. With cues, he was able to complete the task without errors. Afterward, Mike said the activity was easy.

Client 2: In an interview, John did not acknowledge any changes in his thinking skills. John was presented with a list of items to purchase online. He was also given a budget. John anticipated that the online shopping activity might be challenging but could not identify what would be challenging. John self-initiated referring to and using a list during the task; however, he often missed key details on the list or only remembered part of a step. For example, the list indicated he needed to find a blue shirt, size L. He found the shirt but chose the wrong size. He checked off the list consistently, but on several occasions, he checked off items before he located them, causing him to think he had already located the items when he had not. He self-recognized things were not going well by making comments such as, "This should not be so difficult." After the task, he self-recognized specific errors with an answer sheet. He stated that the activity was very challenging.

Client 3: In an interview, Susan did not acknowledge any changes in her thinking skills. When Susan was presented with the online shopping activity, she repeated the directions correctly but immediately began the activity without re-reviewing the list of items that needed to be purchased or without pre-planning. She became distracted by other stores and extraneous items. She located 8 out of the 10 items but they did not consistently adhere to the criteria or budget. During the activity, Susan never looked back at the directions or the list. When the directions were reviewed, Susan realized that her items did not match those on the list and that she exceeded the budget. Initially, she seemed surprised and was overheard mumbling, "I don't know what happened." She then stated that she decided to purchase things that she liked and decided not to follow the list exactly because it wasn't relevant to her. She also said the budget wasn't accurate because she could use her credit card and had a high credit card limit. She indicated that the activity was easy and did not identify anything else she would do differently next time.

Toglia & Foster: The Multicontext Approach to Cognitive Rehabilitation.

Appendix A.8. Worksheet: Brainstorm Activities and Variations in Directions

Review the items below and identify the key executive function (EF) component based on the activity characteristics.

Directions Key Materials: Menu(s)	Key EF Component(s)
Here is a list and a menu. Let's try to figure how many items from the list are on the menu. Try to look back at the list as few times as possible.	
Out of three menus, which menu has the most dinner items below $18.00? The most vegetarian options?	
You have two friends coming from out of town. One likes steak, while the other is vegetarian and does not eat meat or fish. She will eat salads and pasta dishes. You are looking for a restaurant within 15 minutes of this location that has an average entrée price below $25.00. Review the menus on the table and choose the best options.	
Circle the items on the menu that are $15.00 and below and place a checkmark next to the items that are above $15.00.	
You need to take three business acquaintances to dinner. Choose a restaurant and see if reservations are available.	

EF Demand	Activity Characteristics that Increase EF Demands
Initiation	Vague, ambiguous directions, requires information seeking, asking questions, generating plans, ideas; unstructured, open-ended, identify goals/choices.
Inhibition	Rule constraints or criteria for selection; contains extra information, extraneous materials, or increased amount of irrelevant stimuli, interruptions, distractions, competition.
Working Memory (keeping track)	Increased number of items, steps, or information to hold onto; decreased external cues, tasks requiring mental tracking, updating, or manipulation.
Shifting/Flexibility	Tasks requiring alternating, switching actions, or attention back and forth between several different sources of information. Changing rules or circumstances. Has more than one solution. Requires generating alternative ideas, methods, or solutions.
Planning/ Organization	Anticipate future events; create a plan, develop or decide the order of steps; identify, select, gather and arrange materials or information, grasp main ideas; prioritize, group, summarize or condense information; create an organizational system; decide how much time should be allotted.

Toglia & Foster: The Multicontext Approach to Cognitive Rehabilitation.

Appendix A.9. Characteristics of Simple and Complex Problem-Solving Tasks: Use with Appendix A.10

	Simple	Complex	Demands with Increased Complexity	Sample Complex Treatment Tasks
Identify the Problem	Immediate problem is clear and readily apparent. Examples: Shampoo bottle is empty; toaster is unplugged.	Requires sorting out information to determine where the real problem exists. Anticipating possible consequences.	Places greater demand on initiation, exploration, attention to the environment and the ability to predict ahead and establish goals.	Emphasis on problem recognition or selection of goals (e.g., recognize that a bill entry is missing in a checkbook activity).
Define the Problem precisely	All the necessary information is presented. A small amount of information relevant to the problem is presented.	Requires searching for additional information needed to solve the problem. A large amount of information, both relevant and irrelevant, is included.	Greater demands on selective attention strategies, choosing priorities, simultaneously attending to details and keeping the whole situation in mind. Requires processing of multiple information and strategies for keeping track of a large number of factors.	Emphasis on discriminating between relevant and irrelevant information (e.g., identifying relevant information in a travel advertisement, or "Find the two least expensive restaurants that deliver lunch in the area.").
Explore possible strategies	Limited choices and solutions. The problem may be approached only in one or two ways. Can be solved with trial and error.	Many different possibilities.	Requires ability to generate, plan, test and reject different hypotheses and formulate alternative solutions. Greater demands on flexibility and abstract thinking.	Requires generation of ideas and alternatives (e.g., You are going to visit a friend in another state for four weeks. List everything you will need to do before you leave.)
Act	One to three steps. Minimal to no demands on multi-tasking.	Multiple steps – requires multi-tasking, keeping track of multiple pieces of information while investigating and completing the task	Greater demands on self-regulation and self-monitoring of behaviors and time.	Emphasis on carrying out a task that requires multitasking (e.g., choosing from two options for a vacation and looking through flyers, brochures and internet sites while keeping track of budget, preferences, criteria for location.)
Look at the effects	Incorrect solution is readily apparent and prevents success.	Incorrect solution is not readily apparent. Requires actively comparing solution with original problem.	Requires greater self-monitoring strategies.	Have client fill out a structured self-evaluation rating form or checklist. Gradually reduce the structure of the rating form.

Toglia & Foster: The Multicontext Approach to Cognitive Rehabilitation.

Appendix A.10. Functional Cognitive Problem-Solving Scenarios

There are 3-4 simulated scenarios within each section below (Organizing Your Day and Planning). Complete each scenario as quickly as you can. Think about the differences and similarities between these scenarios. Look at Appendix A.9 on Characteristics of Problem Solving and determine how it applies. After each section, answer the reflection questions at the end of the next page.

1. ORGANIZING YOUR DAY

a. You have a busy day ahead. You have a doctor's appointment. You must also go to the liquor store to buy wine for a party, fill up the car with gas, go to the post office to mail an important package, go to the bank to get enough money to pay the doctor's fee (he demands cash on visits), order and pick up a special ice cream cake for your friend's birthday, bring your prescription to the drug store, and meet a friend for lunch. The post office, bakery, drugstore, and liquor store all close at 5:00 p.m. The bank closes at 3:00 p.m. It is 10:00 a.m. now. Your doctor's appointment is at 2:00 p.m. At what time should you leave the house? Where will you go first, second, third, etc.?

b. It is 90° out today and you have several errands to do. You need to buy a birthday card and postage stamps since your mother's birthday is only a few days away. The bank closes at 3:00 p.m. and you are out of cash, so you plan to stop there. You have to fill up the car with gas and buy milk, eggs, and chicken for tonight's dinner. You also need to register for a yoga class because yoga is one of your favorite leisure activities. Registration times are between 2:00 and 4:00 p.m. You plan to drop off your phone for repair. You dropped the phone accidentally and the screen cracked. It will take 3 hours for repair and you will have to pay by cash only. Your friends are coming over tonight for dinner at 7:30 p.m. and you cannot wait to show them the pictures you took with your phone while you were on vacation. You must pick up your favorite blue dress at the dry cleaner before it closes at 5:00 p.m. Your haircut appointment is at 2:30 p.m. and it usually takes an hour. You have to remember to stop at a department store to buy a present for your mother and be home by 6:15 p.m. at the latest. It is 1:45 p.m. now.

    Make a list of the errands and places that you have to go to during the day. Indicate which place/errand you would go first, second, and so on.

c. It is a very hot summer day and you have several errands to do. You have to get your hair cut at 2:00 p.m., buy bread, milk, and eggs for tonight's dinner, fill the car with gas (it is almost empty), and go to the department store to buy yourself a new dress. It is 1:30 p.m. now.

    Make a list of the errands and places that you have to go to during the day. Indicate which place/errand you would go first, second, and so on.

Toglia & Foster: The Multicontext Approach to Cognitive Rehabilitation.

PLANNING

a. You are organizing a breakfast meeting for 16 people. You plan to offer a continental breakfast with an assortment to choose from. You would like to keep costs low. Investigate three options in the local area.

b. You are organizing a breakfast meeting for 16 people. You plan to offer coffee, tea, and a tray of fruit as well as an assortment of bagels or croissants, muffins, and danishes. Find three options in the local area that can provide delivery (if feasible).

c. You are organizing a breakfast meeting for 16 people. Coffee is $1.50 each, tea is $.75 each, bagels are $1.25 each, doughnuts are $1.10 each, muffins are $1.75 each, and danishes are $2.00 each. You would like to order an assortment. You need to stay under $40.00. Identify two different options.

d. You are organizing a breakfast meeting for 10 people. Coffee is $.75 each and bagels are $.85 each. How much money do you need to order coffee and bagels for all 10 people?

Reflection Questions

Think about how you went about doing these activities.

- Where did you begin and how did you proceed?

- How did the differences between these scenarios influence the skills needed and the strategies or methods used to complete these activities?

- Which scenario was easiest? Which scenario was most challenging? Why? What were the activity characteristics that contributed to increased or decreased complexity?

Toglia & Foster: The Multicontext Approach to Cognitive Rehabilitation.

Appendix A.11. Executive Function Analysis Worksheet

Activity and Directions: _____

	Initiation	Inhibition	Working Memory	Flexibility or Shifting
Task components that place demands on this skill				
Level of cognitive demand *(low, med, high)*				
Methods to decrease demands *(adaptations)*				
Methods to increase demands *(change directions, rules, items, arrangement, distractions, etc.)*				
Task Errors that might be observed				
Context or Environment				

Toglia & Foster: The Multicontext Approach to Cognitive Rehabilitation.

Appendix A.12. Variations in Activity Demands

For Appendix A.12 and A.13, choose a functional or motor activity. Some examples are provided, but any activity can be chosen. Identify how the directions or activity demands of the selected activity can be changed to place more or less demands on different executive function skills.

Executive Function Skills	A Functional Activity (e.g., setting a table, making a sandwich, writing activity, writing an e-mail, making a phone call, using a vending machine, going to the cafeteria) Activity:	A Motor Activity (adding cognitive components) (fine motor activity such as picking up coins, obstacle course, ambulating, following directions to exercise). Activity:
Initiation (Seeking info)		
Working Memory (Keeping track)		
Inhibition (add rules or criteria)		
Flexibility		

Executive Function Skills or Components

- **Initiation** (*seeking information*): Begin activity without procrastination; seek and search for information; generate ideas or plans, persist, complete all parts of activity.
- **Working Memory** (*keeping track*): Hold information in mind for purpose of completing a task; keep track of all items or information; update and manipulate information in one's mind.
- **Inhibition:** Control impulses, automatic tendencies; stop behavior, think before acting, pace actions; follow or select according to rules or criteria; manage extraneous distractions, irrelevant information or interference; delay responses.
- **Flexibility/Shift:** Mentally shift ideas, thoughts and tasks; move freely from one step, activity/situation to another; go back and forth between stimuli/steps; transition and view situations from different perspectives; revise plans, adapt; shift back and forth among changing stimuli or rules.

Toglia & Foster: The Multicontext Approach to Cognitive Rehabilitation.

Appendix A.13. Variations in Activity Demands 2

Selected Activity _____

EF Skills	Activity Characteristics	Activity Directions — Identify directions that place greater demands on the targeted executive function skill
Initiation (Seeking information)	Ambiguous directions	
Working Memory (Keeping track)	Increased number of items and steps.	
Inhibition	Rule constraints, cluttered environment with multiple choices, interruptions.	
Flexibility	Alternating responses, changing rules or obstacles.	
Prospective Memory	Carry out actions or intentions at certain times or with cues.	
Plan/ Organize	Develop a plan, identify, sequence, or arrange steps, gather needed materials or information, and group or consolidate as needed.	

Executive Function Skills or Components (Depending on activity, not all skills may be relevant)

- **Initiation** (*seeking information*): Begin activity without procrastination; seek and search for information; generate ideas or plans, persist, complete all parts of activity.
- **Working Memory** (*keeping track*): Hold information in mind for purpose of completing a task; keep track of all items or information; update and manipulate information in one's mind.
- **Inhibition:** Control impulses, automatic tendencies; stop behavior, think before acting, pace actions; follow or select according to rules or criteria; manage extraneous distractions, irrelevant information or interference; delay responses.
- **Flexibility/Shift:** Mentally shift ideas, thoughts and tasks; move freely from one step, activity/situation to another; go back and forth between stimuli/steps; transition and view situations from different perspectives; revise plans, adapt; shift back and forth among changing stimuli or rules.
- **Prospective Memory (PM):** Time monitoring, time estimation, time planning or organization, carrying out intentions. Time-based PM – remember to carry out intention at a certain time; Event-based PM – remember to carry out intention with a cue; Activity-based PM – completion of activity serves as cue.
- **Plan/Organize:** Anticipate future events; set goals; develop steps; identify and gather materials; grasp main ideas; prioritize, reduce, or cluster information; rearrange materials or information; think ahead or plan action steps.

Toglia & Foster: The Multicontext Approach to Cognitive Rehabilitation.

Appendix A.14.1 General Case Analysis using the Dynamic Interactional Model Framework

Rhonda is a 32-year-old female who sustained a TBI 2 months ago. Prior to the injury, she lived alone and worked for a public relations firm, coordinating events and projects. Presently, she is living with her parents, who are very supportive. She is independent in ambulation and basic self-care activities. In a quiet environment, with structured tasks or step by step directions, she functions well. In an interview, she expressed difficulty concentrating. She also indicated that it takes her a long time to complete daily activities, but she could not explain why. She is aware that she is not ready to return to work but is unable to provide examples of tasks she might have difficulty with. She expressed motivation to get better and get back to work.

Rhonda demonstrates difficulty staying on task in multiple-step or non-routine activities and is easily distracted by extraneous information. Task performance is inefficient and includes extra actions or unnecessary steps. For example, while making lunch, she saw a book on the table that belonged in the bedroom. She brought it into the bedroom, saw her phone, and began texting her friend. She then started hanging clothes and organizing her closet. Then she remembered she was in the middle of making lunch. As she was making lunch, she took extra items out of the refrigerator that were not needed. Similarly, while shopping online for a birthday gift for her 7-year-old niece, she began looking at jewelry, books, and accessories. She received a phone call and when she returned to the task, she had lost track of what she had completed and thought she had already identified a birthday gift. Immediately after the activity, she rated the tasks as easy. No strategies or self-monitoring skills were observed during activities.

Rhonda is able to stay on topic during conversations with one person (e.g., interview) without difficulty. During group conversations, she is often tangential and jumps from one topic to the next without recognizing social cues. Friends have gradually stopped calling her and she is becoming increasingly isolated.

Rhonda previously enjoyed traveling, shopping, and going out with friends or social activities. Now she finds noisy environments or places with lots of people confusing, overwhelming, and anxiety provoking. She avoids crowded places such as a supermarket, mall, train station, restaurant, or theatre.

Case Analysis: Analyze the case information above within the framework of the Dynamic International Model of Cognition by identifying person, activity, and environmental facilitators and inhibitors of performance that are influencing functional cognitive performance using the Dynamic Interactional Model case analysis form in Appendix 14.2.

Toglia & Foster: The Multicontext Approach to Cognitive Rehabilitation.

Appendix A.14.2. Dynamic Interactional Model Case Analysis Form

Dynamic Interactional Model of Cognition: Analysis of Case		
Person Factors	**Activity Demands**	**Environment**
Facilitators	*Facilitators*	*Facilitators*
Inhibitors	*Inhibitors*	*Inhibitors*

Functional Cognitive Performance

Cognitive Behaviors and Performance Errors:

Functional Limitations:

Toglia & Foster: The Multicontext Approach to Cognitive Rehabilitation.

Appendix A.15. Cue Analysis: Picture Yourself in the Situation – What would you say or do?

1. Susan is given a list of five errands that need to be completed (deliver mail, make a phone call, etc.). After completing the first errand, she gets sidetracked and jumps ahead, missing at least three errands on the list. As you observe this, what would you say or do?

2. Tom is given a list of 15 items that need to be retrieved from the kitchen. You notice that he is retrieving several extraneous items that are not on the list.

    a. What could be the underlying reasons for this?

    b. What would you say or do?

3. During an activity involving decorating cookies, Erica reads the directions correctly aloud: "Put chocolate sprinkles on two cookies and icing on three cookies." She puts icing on all the cookies, unaware of her error.

    a. What could be the underlying reason for this?

    b. What would you say or do to facilitate error recognition?

4. Mike, age 11, is working on a multiple-step craft activity. One step of directions states "Cut out the square." Mike cuts out only three sides of the square and checks off the step, thinking he has completed this step. As you observe this, what would you say or do?

5. S. is following a list of directions that need to be completed for a new recipe. You observe that after she reads a step, she immediately checks it off. As she continues, she begins to lose track and skips over steps, thinking the step has been completed (due to the checkmark). She does not realize she is skipping over steps.

    a. What could be the underlying reasons for this?

    b. What would you say or do?

Toglia & Foster: The Multicontext Approach to Cognitive Rehabilitation.

Appendix A.16. Treatment Role Play: Metacognitive Questions and Guided Learning

2 or 3 people required

Materials: Multi-step functional activity (e.g., calling to order flowers for delivery for a special occasion, ordering airline tickets or pizza on the internet, putting appointments into your phone, and searching for information on the internet).

Optional: Video recording (by third person or on tripod).

Therapist Fidelity Tool: For self-assessment and reflection. Completed and discussed with others after the activity (Appendix C.13).

Therapist: Provides activity and uses the metacognitive framework and mediation methods to facilitate performance.

Client: The person playing the client should act out one of the below symptoms but should NOT tell anyone which of the below symptoms are being acted out.

1. **Impulsive/decreased inhibition:** For example, goes quickly before fully reading entire instruction, jumps right into the task; adds extraneous steps, skips over the steps, or jumps ahead and then tries to go back. May get sidetracked or distracted by irrelevant stimuli (e.g., comments on irrelevant details during or after task, information triggers a past story or thought, or the person uses trial and error).

2. **Working memory:** You tend to lose track of what you just did, or what step you just completed. You often only recall part of the directions. You frequently refer back to the directions and re-read the same item (after you look away, you lose track of what you just read and have to go back and re-read).

3. **Decreased Flexibility:** Multiple errors of repetition; repeats the same step (you can easily recall the step out loud but when carrying out the task, you get "stuck." Sometimes you say the right step out loud but do the previous step; may have difficulty moving from one step to the next. Tends to get overfocused on parts or pieces; gets stuck and has difficulty generating alternatives. When you read, you often overfocus on the first part of the directions only or you only recall specific words/pieces of the directions and this causes misinterpretation or inability to accurately complete steps.

4. **Goal neglect:** You tend to get sidetracked and lose sight of the task goal. When distractors are present, you have difficulty inhibiting irrelevant information and tend to show goal neglect. For example, you wander away from the goal and begin doing other tasks. You are unaware of task errors as they are occurring.

Toglia & Foster: The Multicontext Approach to Cognitive Rehabilitation.

SELECTED APPENDIX A ANSWERS

A.1, A.2, A.3, A.4, A.6, A.7, A.8, A.10, A.14, A.15

Answers for Appendix A.1. Analyzing Negative Behaviors from the Perspective of Executive Function. (Chapter 1)

Observed Negative Behaviors	Possible Underlying Cognitive Problems
• Careless • Lack of effort, lazy • Unmotivated	*Decreased initiation:* In unstructured situations, does not know how or where to begin. Difficulty sustaining focus and concentration over time. Quickly becomes overwhelmed or experiences cognitive overload and withdraws from tasks.
• Repeats same mistakes	*Reduced cognitive flexibility:* Does not learn from experiences. Poor episodic memory, but good procedural or implicit memory (error remains in implicit memory).
• Doesn't follow directions	*Limited working memory:* May only recall the first or last part of instructions. Has difficulty keeping track of all steps or directions. *Misinterpretations:* Over-focuses on parts of directions and misses the overall goal. Difficulty shifting from one step to the next. Unable to translate directions into actions or intentions.
• Lack of follow-through • Unreliable • Irresponsible • Not trustworthy	*Sustained attention:* Leaves tasks unfinished due to difficulty focusing on or persisting with a task due to decreased attention span or low mental energy. *Goal neglect:* Tendency to get sidetracked, failure to inhibit distractions, or lose track of the goal.
• Self-centered • Reduced empathy	*Concrete thinking:* Inability to think beyond one's self and understand perspectives or feelings of others. Unable to put oneself in another person's shoes. Focuses on immediate needs or "here and now."
• Rude • Interrupts others	*Disinhibited:* Impulsive, says or does things without thinking. Difficulty regulating actions, speech, volume or tone of voice, or emotions.
• Stubborn, rigid • Argumentative	*Reduced cognitive flexibility:* Perceives situations in one way. Resistant to changing ways, understanding other viewpoints, or imagining other possibilities.
• Inconsistent work • Unpredictable	Performance varies with *mental fatigue or difficulty sustaining focus.* *Impaired executive function:* Subtle changes in level of structure or the ways directions are provided, familiarity, unexpected situations, or novelty affects consistency of performance.
• Emotional outbursts • Low frustration tolerance	*Poor emotional regulation:* Emotional outbursts that are out of proportion to the situation. Lack of self-monitoring and ability to inhibit emotions, control anger, tone or volume of voice.

Toglia & Foster: The Multicontext Approach to Cognitive Rehabilitation.

Answers for Appendix A.2. Social Skills and Sample Underlying Cognitive Components. (Chapter 1)

Social Skills	Cognitive Components
• Eye contact	Sustained attention
• Keep conversations focused on the topic	Attention, concentration, inhibit extraneous thoughts or distractions.
• Keep track of what was already stated	Working memory
• Sustain a meaningful conversation	Sustained attention, persistence, initiates question asking.
• Shift with changes in topic, speakers	Cognitive flexibility, shifting attention
• Wait for turn before speaking and self-monitor one's reactions	Ability to restrain impulses, inhibit actions or speech, think before acting.
• Start conversations and keep the conversation going	Initiate questions and conversations; attentive, shows interest in the other person.
• Recall and maintain continuity between previous conversations and interactions	Episodic memory, ability to retain information from previous interactions.
• Attend to others' reactions, verbal and nonverbal signs	Dual tasking – attend to content of conversation and nonverbal cues at the same time.
• Simultaneously attend to the content of conversation and context	Able to attend to both the broader situation or context of the social situation as well as the specifics.
• Express thoughts in an organized way	Inhibit extraneous thoughts, select the main idea, stay focused on topic; does not go off on tangents.
• Understand different perspectives	Cognitive flexibility – Put oneself in another person's shoes, ability to see another point of view.
• Make inferences about the intentions, beliefs, feelings or emotional state of others	Ability to make inferences, abstract meaning, read between the lines, or pick up on hidden meanings.
• Anticipate and recognize consequences of saying something that might evoke unpleasant reactions from others	Recognize cause and effect, think ahead, beyond the here and now (abstract thinking), reason.
• Show empathy	Cognitive flexibility, abstract thinking; ability to put oneself in another person's shoes.
• Awareness of tone of voice, nonverbal cues, facial expressions, emotional cues or basic emotions of self and others. Use tone and emotions that fit the situation.	Attention and awareness of others; awareness of overall context; ability to process and recognize auditory or visual cues while attending to conversation content and context.
• Ability to interpret sarcastic remarks and humor	Abstract thinking, inference (infer hidden meaning).

Toglia & Foster: The Multicontext Approach to Cognitive Rehabilitation.

Answers for Appendix A.3. Executive Function Skills Exercises 1. (Chapter 2)

1) Cooking Competition – The below represents a common way of sequencing these steps, but depending on the person's experiences, more than one way of sequencing the steps is possible.

9	Buy fresh ingredients for the competition
6	Make the practice recipes
3	Receive confirmation that application has been accepted and find out assigned day/time
4	Choose a couple of recipes to practice with
8	Choose the final recipe to make for the judges
2	Complete and submit the application for the competition before the deadline
10	Prepare the dish for the judges
7	Receive feedback from friends on the practice recipe
1	Find out the rules and eligibility for the competition
5	Buy ingredients for the practice recipes

Time started and finished is included; no crossing out or erasures (requires planning ahead and inhibition of responses, discourages trial and error)

Sample Analysis: Although most people have not entered a cooking competition, previous knowledge and experience of the general sequence of cooking and competitions (e.g., choose recipe before buying ingredients; find out rules before applying) is used to order steps. A common strategy is picturing oneself or visualizing another person they know going through the steps.

This task involves integration of all executive function components. It requires initiating, previewing or reading all steps to get a sense of all the subtasks before trying to sequence or organize the steps. Some people initiate an organizational system. For example, they immediately break up, code, or group the steps into chunks (preparation, practice versus competition, or beginning steps versus later steps), prior to assigning the order of steps. This can make the amount of information more manageable. Working memory is required to keep track of what steps have been done and what steps need to come next as the person is doing the task. Inhibition is required to pace speed and resist the tendency to do this task too quickly, without taking the time to consider all possibilities. Once a step has been completed, the person has to shift thinking to the next step. Flexibility of thinking including possible anticipation of consequences (e.g., If I do this . . . , this could result in . . .) is required. In addition, the ability to adopt a simulated or *what if* perspective and think flexibly beyond the here and now or beyond one's own direct experience is also needed.

2) Fixing a Flat Tire – The order below is not completely fixed. *The first two steps are interchangeable.* The spare tire could be removed first or second or third (or before the car is jacked up). Two of the items (N/A) are irrelevant to the task. Time started and finished should be included. No crossing out or erasures (requires planning ahead and inhibition of responses; discourages trial and error).

10	Lower car to ground
3	Use tire iron to loosen tire lug nuts
N/A	Adjust the rear-view mirror
6	Remove flat tire
1	Get out the jack, crank, tire iron *
9	Use tire iron to tighten lug nuts
4	Jack up car
5	Lug nuts are completely loosened and removed
7	Place spare tire on
N/A	Insert the key in the ignition
11	Put flat tire in trunk
8	Insert lug nuts onto the tire studs
2	Get out spare tire *

* interchangeable items

Time started and finished is included; no crossing out or erasures (requires planning ahead and inhibition of responses, discourages trial and error)

Toglia & Foster: The Multicontext Approach to Cognitive Rehabilitation.

Sample Analysis: Most people use their knowledge or experience to guide ordering of the steps. Thinking back to a specific experience such as the last time that you changed a tire or watched someone else change a tire, has been referred to as episodic cueing. Visualization of a past experience such as going through the steps that were taken or what was done first, second, etc. can facilitate completion of this task.

This task involves integration of all executive function components. It requires initiating and previewing or reading all steps to get a sense of all the subtasks before trying to sequence or organize the steps. Some people initiate an organizational system. For example, they immediately break up, code, or group the steps into chunks (steps involved in taking flat tire off the car, steps involved in putting spare tire on the car, or beginning steps versus later steps), prior to assigning the order of steps. This can make the amount of information more manageable. Working memory is required to keep track of what steps have been done and what steps need to come next as the person is doing the task. Inhibition is required to pace speed and resist the tendency to do this task too quickly without taking the time to consider all possibilities. Once a step has been completed, the person has to shift thinking to the next step. Flexibility of thinking, including possible anticipation of consequences (e.g., If I do this…, this could result in…), is required. In addition, the ability to adopt a simulated or *what if* perspective and think flexibly beyond the here and now is also needed.

3) *Planning* – While questions 1 and 2 provided all the information needed to complete the tasks, question 3 presented open-ended ambiguous directions that required brainstorming and generating ideas or steps. There are no right answers. Instead, there are multiple possibilities. Brainstorming ideas is an inherent component of planning and problem solving and is an important daily life skill. For example, identifying possible meals to make for the week or identifying all the things that need to be done to prepare for a holiday dinner require brainstorming as a first step. It is important to analyze the process that you went through in responding to unstructured or open-ended directions. Below are examples of the brainstorming process.

- A person might initially write down whatever comes to mind or use free association. After immediately generating the first 5-10 items automatically, the person may reach a "mind blank" and will need to switch strategies to generate additional possibilities. This can involve thinking of associations or groups as described below, self-questioning, or use of the below methods.

- A person might visualize themselves in a situation or context, think of a previous similar experience, or imagine themselves performing the activity. For example, in thinking of steps involved in planning a party, a person might visualize themselves going through the steps or they might think of a specific time that they planned a party and the order of steps that they went through.

- A person might first generate broad categories or create an outline before identifying specifics. For example, in thinking about planning a party, a person might first think of a framework such as where? when? who? what?, before thinking of specifics. Similarly, in generating a list of things to buy for a first apartment, a person might first think of each room (bedroom, kitchen, bathroom, living room) to structure the process.

Brainstorming requires initiation, flexible thinking, identification of alternatives, ability to switch between broad goals or categories and specifics, and the ability to adjust strategies as needed. Ability to think beyond the here and now or abstract thinking ("what if") is also needed.

Once a list of items or steps is generated, the next step is reviewing the list, eliminating redundancies, and re-organizing the list by identifying similarities or associations among items so that the items can be grouped, clustered, or categorized. Grouping items helps to reduce and simplify information. Planning and problem solving often proceeds from brainstorming lists to categorizing or grouping items on the list to ordering or examining relationships between items.

Lists, therefore, can be a tool for solving problems and can help in identifying relationships and solutions.

Toglia & Foster: The Multicontext Approach to Cognitive Rehabilitation.

Answers for Appendix A.4. Executive Function Exercise 2: Medication Schedule. (Chapter 2)

Antibiotics: Take 1 blue pill three times a day, at least 30 minutes before meals; **Aspirin:** Take 2 white tablets every 4 hours with a snack; **Blood Pressure Meds:** Take 1 yellow pill in the morning and evening, after meals. **Anti-Inflammatory meds:** Take 1 brown pill an hour after dinner; **Water:** Drink a full glass of water every 2 hours. **Time** started and ended should be included.

Sample Medication Schedule

7:30 a.m.	2 white tablets with snack (Aspirin); Drink 1 full glass of water
8:00 a.m.	1 blue pill (Antibiotics)
8:30 a.m.	Breakfast
9:00 a.m.	1 yellow pill (BP)
9:30 a.m.	Drink 1 full glass of water
10:00 a.m.	
10:30 a.m.	
11:00 a.m.	
11:30 a.m.	2 white tablets with snack (Aspirin); Drink 1 full glass of water
12:00 noon	1 blue pill (Antibiotics)
12:30 p.m.	Lunch
1:00 p.m.	
1:30 p.m.	Drink 1 full glass of water
2:00 p.m.	
2:30 p.m.	
3:00 p.m.	
3:30 p.m.	2 white tablets with snack (Aspirin); Drink 1 full glass of water
4:00 p.m.	
4:30 p.m.	
5:00 p.m.	
5:30 p.m.	1 blue pill (Antibiotics); Drink 1 full glass of water
6:00 p.m.	Dinner
6:30 p.m.	1 yellow pill (BP)
7:00 p.m.	1 brown pill (Anti-Inflammatory)
7:30 p.m.	2 white tablets with snack (Aspirin); Drink 1 full glass of water
8:00 p.m.	

Toglia & Foster: The Multicontext Approach to Cognitive Rehabilitation.

> **Answers for Appendix A.6. Functional Cognitive Examples of Executive Function and Memory Dysfunction. (Chapter 2)**

Below are possible interpretations of functional cognitive errors.

1. Fred jumped into the activity before fully listening to the instructions. This is an example of impulsivity or disinhibition. Actions are driven by stimuli, without top-down control. Fred sees a check and begins randomly writing it out, without a goal and without stopping to plan ahead.

2. Victor is having difficulty remembering intentions or things that he needs to do (prospective memory). This is likely related to executive function skills because he is not having difficulty with retrospective memory or recalling things that already occurred.

3. Mark appears to be exhibiting inflexible and/or concrete thinking. He is only able to look at the situation from one way (based on his experience) and cannot adopt an "as if" attitude or consider the situation from different perspectives.

4. This is an example of episodic short-term memory deficits or "rapid forgetting" over time. Since John did not respond to cues, his difficulties may be related to an inability to store or hold onto new information over time.

5. Sam appears to be having difficulty keeping track of what he just saw or did. This appears to be causing unnecessary repetitions. He may have also jumped into the activity without anticipating what was needed or planning ahead. He recognizes that something is wrong but is unaware of his performance inefficiencies.

6. Marie became sidetracked by other items. The goal of the activity seems to have faded away. This has been termed "goal neglect" in the executive functioning literature. Marie may have been unable to inhibit distractions or extraneous information. She also may have had difficulty keeping the goal in mind as she became involved in the activity (limited working memory).

7. This is an example of a semantic memory deficit (declarative memory). Mary can read the word, but she is unable to associate or retrieve the meaning.

8. Sara is demonstrating adynamia. Although she initiates routine self-care activities that are more habitual or automatic, she is unable to self-start or initiate household activities, leisure interests, or socialization.

9. This quote describes difficulty holding and keeping track of information (working memory) within the context of a task.

10. Sue appears to have difficulty initiating with unstructured or ambiguous directions. She did not actively search for items or seek information (ask questions). When she was cued to look in the refrigerator, she was unable to initiate or generate plans for lunch.

11. Procedural memory is intact, but Kevin is experiencing difficulty in declarative memory (short-term event-based or episodic memory). His ability to respond to recall information with cues suggests that new information is being stored but he might be having difficulty accessing or retrieving it.

12. Mary repeated the directions correctly (adequate working memory). She says the correct things but is unable to execute what she verbally states. There is a disassociation between what she says and what she does. Mary appears to have difficulty shifting actions from one step to another (flexibility) and repeated the same action (putting pills in morning slot) rather than switching to noon or evening slots.

13. Dave was able to complete an event-based prospective memory task but had difficulty with time-based prospective memory.

14. Kathy appears to have difficulty keeping track of what she just did (working memory). This is contributing to omissions as well as repetitions. She repeated some steps and left out other steps. She was not aware of her performance errors. Alternatively, she might also have difficulty shifting from one step to the next.

15. John may have only remembered the last item because he was unable to hold all of the information needed in his working memory. Although the information he encoded was limited, he was able to hold onto this information over time.

16. Jim may be having difficulty selecting key information or inhibiting irrelevant information. Emotional responses can flood cognitive processes and result in a brain "shut down." As a result, he appears to be unable to organize or break down the task. Alternatively, he may have difficulty initiating or generating a plan.

Toglia & Foster: The Multicontext Approach to Cognitive Rehabilitation.

17. This is an example of non-declarative memory deficit or procedural memory problem because Jose forgot the procedure or *how to* operate a familiar appliance.

18. Rosa may have difficulty initiating ideas (brainstorming), particularly with unstructured directions. Alternatively, Rosa may have gotten stuck or perseverated on her first response and may have been unable to generate different alternatives.

19. Carlos may have difficulty inhibiting or filtering our extraneous information (attentional inhibition) and as a result is experiencing "brain flooding or information overload". He is unable to select or attend to relevant information and becomes overwhelmed by extraneous stimuli.

20. Victoria has difficulty in short term episodic memory (declarative). Her ability to retrieve information with cues suggests that she was able to encode information and store it over time, but she had difficulty accessing or retrieving this information on her own.

Answers for Appendix A.7. Awareness Clinical Scenario and Strategy Use. (Chapter 3)

The three scenarios illustrate different types of deficits in self-awareness deficits.

Client 1: Mike appears to have *good general awareness*, but it is vague and incomplete. *Online awareness* of performance is poor.

Mike acknowledges that his thinking and concentration have changed, but he is unable to clearly identify what has changed or provide examples of when, where, or what type of symptoms, or problems he is experiencing. He is unable to use his *general awareness* to help him anticipate or monitor performance during activities. With cues, he had no difficulty using strategies and completing the task, but he did not initiate using strategies himself. This is likely because he didn't recognize the need to alter task methods or use strategies. Afterward, he perceived the task as easy. This might be because he ultimately completed the task successfully and may not have recognized how the therapist cues helped his performance.

Treatment Implications: Online awareness of performance should be the focus of treatment. Mike's strengths in his general knowledge and awareness should be used to gradually build anticipation of potential challenges and recognition of the need to use strategies. Direct cues and assistance during the activity should be avoided so that Mike has the opportunity to discover and correct errors himself.

Client 2: Unlike Client 1, John demonstrated *poor general awareness* and at least *partial online awareness.*

Although John did not verbally acknowledge limitations in an interview, he anticipated possible difficulties and spontaneously initiated strategy use within the context of an activity. It might be that John's responses in an interview were overshadowed by personality characteristics, ego, or a tendency to be overconfident. John readily used strategies, suggesting that he recognized the need to do so; however, strategies were ineffective or inefficient. As a result, he made multiple errors. He vaguely recognized difficulties within the context of the activity. Afterward, John acknowledged challenges and identified specific errors with the assistance of a structured self-checking system.

Treatment Implications: The focus of treatment should be on facilitating anticipation and specific identification of challenges as well as detection and monitoring of errors within the context of an activity. General awareness is not addressed directly. With increases in online awareness of performance, across different activities, general awareness may eventually improve as a by-product.

Client 3: Susan exhibits a *denial* reaction and does not acknowledge deficits.

Susan's behavior suggests that she did not anticipate difficulties or recognize the need to use strategies within the activity. She appeared to be unaware of her distractibility or errors during the task. Although she recognized and acknowledged errors after the task, she made excuses and rationalized her errors. Susan acknowledges errors but appears to have difficulty accepting them. Susan might also have difficulty adopting a simulated perspective due to concrete thinking.

Treatment Implications: The experience and value that Susan places on *online shopping* should be considered. Tasks that are familiar and highly valued (e.g., part of work tasks) may elicit more defensiveness than a different task. Performance on tasks that Susan self-chooses should be observed, prior to making conclusions. Treatment should focus on generating the most efficient or effective methods to complete the task, rather than on error recognition. The guidelines in Exhibit 3.6 provides additional information for those who exhibit denial.

Answers for Appendix A.8. Worksheet: Brainstorm Activities and Variations in Directions. (Chapter 4)

The answers below represent <u>the key EF component</u>, *required throughout the activity, based on the activity characteristics in the table below. Please note – all components of EF are involved in each of these scenarios and different clients can have difficulty for entirely different reasons.*

Directions Key Materials: Menu(s)	Key EF Component(s)
Here is a list and a menu. Let's try to figure how many items from the list are on the menu. Try to look back at the list as few times as possible.	Keeping Track – **working memory** Requires the ability to hold onto items from the list while searching the menu. Looking at the list as few times as possible places additional demands on working memory.
Out of three menus, which menu has the most dinner items below $18.00? The most vegetarian options?	**Flexibility/shifting** – has more than one solution.
You have two friends coming from out of town. One likes steak, while the other is vegetarian and does not eat meat or fish. She will eat salads and pasta dishes. You are looking for a restaurant within 15 minutes of this location that has an average entrée price below $25.00. Review the menus on the table and choose the best options.	**Inhibition** – increased rules and criteria with extraneous information place the most demands on inhibition.
Circle the items on the menu that are $15.00 and below and place a checkmark next to the items that are above $15.00.	**Flexibility/shifting** – Requires alternating and switching rules.
You need to take three business acquaintances to dinner. Choose a restaurant and see if reservations are available.	**Initiation** – this is ambiguous and requires asking questions or seeking additional information.

EF Demand	Activity Characteristics that Increase EF Demands
Initiation	Vague, ambiguous directions, requires information seeking, asking questions, generating plans, ideas; unstructured, open-ended, identify goals/choices.
Inhibition	Rule constraints or criteria for selection; contains extra information, extraneous materials, or increased amount of irrelevant stimuli, interruptions, distractions, competition.
Working Memory (keeping track)	Increased number of items, steps, or information to hold onto; decreased external cues, tasks requiring mental tracking, updating, or manipulation.
Shifting/Flexibility	Tasks requiring alternating, switching actions, or attention back and forth between several different sources of information. Changing rules or circumstances. Has more than one solution. Requires generating alternative ideas, methods, or solutions.
Planning/Organization	Anticipate future events; create a plan, develop or decide the order of steps; identify, select, gather and arrange materials or information, grasp main ideas; prioritize, group, summarize or condense information; create an organizational system; decide how much time should be allotted.

Answers for Appendix A.10. Functional Cognitive Problem-Solving Scenarios (Chapter 4)

Scenarios are interpreted within the context of Appendix A.9, Characteristics of Simple and Complex Problem-Solving Tasks.

Scenario 1 situations involve sequencing errands in order. Some information requires thinking ahead or anticipating consequences *(problem identification)*. The scenarios differ in the number of errands, amount of details, and information provided *(problem definition)*. None of the scenarios provide information on the distance or time required to travel from one place to another; however, this information is not essential.

Scenario 1a involves nine errands and requires recognizing that some of these errands (italicized) must be done before the doctor's appointment (bold) and one errand (underlined) must be done last (picking up ice cream cake so it doesn't melt). "Fill up the car with gas" also implies that it is near empty so it should be filled up first. These are all implied and require anticipation, thinking ahead of consequences, or what if. Below is one sample sequence of errands. The items that

Toglia & Foster: The Multicontext Approach to Cognitive Rehabilitation.

are not italicized are flexible and could be switched. Although some items need to be done before and after the doctor's office, the exact order can vary and there are multiple solutions.

Fill up the car with gas	*10:00 a.m.*
Go to bank – before MD office	*10:20 – 10:45 a.m.*
Order ice cream cake	*10:45-11:00 a.m.*
Bring prescription to drugstore	11:00-11:20 a.m.
Buy wine	Flexible
Meet friend for lunch	*12:00 or 12:30 p.m.*
Doctor Appointment	**2:00 p.m.**
Go to post office	Before 3:00 p.m.
Pick up ice cream cake	Must be done last

Scenario 1b involves 12 errands. It requires recognizing that it is a hot day so that groceries should be purchased last and that the bank should be visited before picking up the phone and going to the hair appointment because the hair appointment will be finished after the bank is closed. The phone needs to be dropped off by 2:30 p.m. (or before haircut) and picked up at or after 5:30 p.m. because it takes 3 hours, the person needs to be home by 6:10 p.m., and as in 1a, the gas tank should be filled up first. There is more irrelevant or extraneous information in 1b compared to 1a, so there are more demands on the ability to filter out extraneous information and identify what is most relevant (*problem definition*).

Fill up car with gas	*First errand or 1:45 p.m.*
The bank closes at 3:00 – get cash (before phone)	*Before 2:30 p.m.*
Drop off your phone for repair (3 hours needed)	*Before 2:30 p.m.*
Haircut appointment	2:30 p.m.
Register for a yoga class (before or immediately after haircut)	Between 2:00 and 4:00 p.m.
Pick up dress at the dry cleaner	Before 5:00 p.m.
Buy postage stamps	Flexible
Buy a birthday card	Flexible
Buy birthday present for mother at department store	Flexible
Pick up phone (depending on drop off time)	At or after 5:15-5:30 p.m.
Buy milk, eggs, and chicken for tonight's dinner (last errand, need to be refrigerated, need to be home by 6:10 p.m.)	
Friend's dinner	7:30 p.m.

Scenario 1c has fewer errands, and less information and details than 1a or 1b and generally meets the criteria for a *Simple Problem-Solving Task*. The limited amount of information makes it easier to identify and attend to relevant information and recognize and define the problems (fill car up with gas first because the car is on empty and buy groceries last since it is a hot day). There is only one correct order (below) so there are minimal demands on the exploration of alternate solutions or the ordering of errands. An incorrect solution, however, may not be readily apparent, particularly if the person did not anticipate consequences or attend to all details.

1. Fill the car with gas (now)
2. Hair appointment – 2:00 p.m.
3. Department store to buy new dress
4. Grocery store - Buy bread, milk and eggs

Scenario 2 problems involve planning for a meeting. Compared to Scenario 1, less information is provided; however, as described in 2a, this is not necessarily less difficult than Scenario 1 (it depends on the nature of the person's difficulties). Using the problem-solving characteristics, Scenario 2 places greater demands on *exploration of possible strategies;* whereas Scenario 1 places greater demands on *problem identification and definition*.

Scenario 2a requires generating steps or ideas. Unlike Scenario 1, less information is presented but there are high demands on information seeking and initiation. Scenario 1 situations included all of the details and information needed but it did not require initiation of a plan. Scenario 2 problems are open-ended, unstructured, and require active investigation, planning, and generation of ideas, steps, and options to *explore possible solutions*. Compared to Scenario 1, there are fewer demands on inhibition or selective attention, but greater demands on initiation and flexibility of thinking.

Toglia & Foster: The Multicontext Approach to Cognitive Rehabilitation.

Scenario 2b provides greater structure than 2a because it identifies the items that need to be ordered for the meeting. This provides more constraints, as the person has to adhere to and keep track of the designated items. Similar to 2a, the person needs to actively investigate different options; however, the information provided narrows down choices.

Scenario 2c provides specific items and prices so the person does not have to seek additional information. Instead, the person needs to use the information provided to generate two different options (*explore possible solutions*). This requires cognitive flexibility, attending to details, staying within rule constraints (budget), and keeping track of the amount spent; however, the demands on initiation or information seeking are minimal.

Scenario 2d is more structured and has less information and details and is easier compared to the other problems. The person only has to figure out the amount of money needed from the information provided. The problem is clear and there is only one correct answer (simple problem-solving task).

All of the tasks above require self-monitoring strategies as an incorrect solution is not readily apparent without close inspection or self-checking.

Answers for Appendix A.14.1 General Case Analysis using the Dynamic Interactional Model Framework (chapter 4)

Dynamic Interactional Model of Cognition: Analysis of Case

Person Factors	Activity Demands	Environment
Facilitators Previous high level of functioning; worked in a public relations firm, several interests e.g. social activities. Motivated General vague awareness *Inhibitors* Poor online awareness, decreased awareness of social cues, Easily sidetracked (see below), Anxious or overwhelmed in some situations. No strategies or self-monitoring skills during activities.	*Facilitators* Routine, familiar tasks Structured tasks, step by step directions. *Inhibitors* Non-routine tasks Unstructured tasks Multiple steps Increased amount of information	*Facilitators* Quiet environment, no distractions One to one conversation Supportive parents *Inhibitors* Distractors in environment Crowded, noisy environments with increased visual stimuli or people. Group conversations with 2 or more people

Functional Cognitive Performance

Cognitive Behaviors and Performance Errors:

Extra steps, extraneous actions that are irrelevant to the task, sidetracked away from the goal by irrelevant stimuli, jumps from one task or topic to another (tangential). This contributes to task inefficiencies and increased time for task completion.

Functional Limitations: Difficulty in complex IADL, social, and community participation. Social isolation. Unable to return to work.

Answers for Appendix A.15. Sample Cue Analysis for Picture Yourself in the Situation – What would you say or do? (Chapter 10)

1. *Susan is given a list of five errands that need to be completed (deliver mail, make a phone call, etc.). After completing the first errand, she gets sidetracked and jumps ahead, missing at least three errands on the list. As you observe this, what would you say or do?*
   - Let's stop and check …. Tell me how you are going about following the list.
   - What can you do to be sure that you have completed each errand on the list?
   - What can you do to make sure you are sticking to the list?
   - What can you do to manage that tendency to wander off track or become distracted by other things?

2. *Tom is given a list of 15 items that need to be retrieved from the kitchen. You notice that he is retrieving several extraneous items that are not on the list.*

Toglia & Foster: The Multicontext Approach to Cognitive Rehabilitation.

a. *What could be the underlying reasons for this?*

Tom may have forgotten about the list and the goal. He may have had difficulty adopting a simulated perspective and as a result, he retrieves food items that he likes. He might be impulsive (acting before attending) and therefore fails to attend to details (decreased inhibitory control).

b. *What would you say or do?*

Same mediation above applies.

- Let's stop and check …. Tell me how you are going about following the list.
- How can you be sure that you only retrieve the items from the list?
- What can you do to help make sure that you have all of the correct items?
- What can you do to make sure you are only taking out the items that are on the list?
- *If impulsive*: What can you do to pace your speed or slow down so that you don't have to return the extra items?
- *If it is working memory*: What can you do to help keep track of the item as you are looking for it?

3. During an activity involving decorating cookies, Erica reads the directions correctly aloud "put chocolate sprinkles on 2 cookies and icing on 3 cookies." She puts icing on all of the cookies, unaware of her error.

   a. *What could be the underlying reason for this?*

   May have lost track of directions, difficulty shifting, or poor inhibitory control.

   b. *What would you say or do to facilitate error recognition?*

   - Let's stop and check … . Tell me how you are going about following the directions.
   - How can you be sure that you are following the directions correctly?
   - What can you do to double check yourself?
   - These directions are a little tricky – they involve rules and changing how you are decorating the cookies. What could you do to make it easier to follow directions that are tricky?

4. *Mike, age 11, is working on a multiple-step craft activity. One step of directions states "cut out the square." Mike cuts out only 3 sides of the square and checks off the step, thinking he has completed this step. As you observe this… What would you say or do?*

   - Before you move on … how can you be sure that everything has been completed?
   - Let's make sure that all sides were cut out. Show me how you can be absolutely sure.
   - More structured: Let's check each side to make sure it is completely cut out. Let's check the bottom … now the two sides; now the top.
   - Once errors are discovered: Why do you think that happened (side was missed)? What can you do to help remember to slow down and double-check yourself?

5. *S. is following a list of directions that need to be completed for a new recipe. You observe that after she reads a step, she immediately checks it off. As she continues, she begins to lose track and skips over steps, thinking the step has been completed (due to the check mark). She does not realize she is skipping over steps, but she realizes that something is not quite right and appears to be getting frustrated.*

   a. *What could be the underlying reasons for this?*

   S. might have difficulty inhibiting responses (checking off list before item is done) or has poor working memory and does not realize she has to use extra care to help keep track of what she has just done.

   b. *What would you say or do?*

   - Let's stop and review. Tell me how you are going about this.
   - What can you do to make sure that each step has been completed before you move onto the next step? What can you do after you complete a step?
   - I am noticing some frustration. Let's try to figure out if there is a different way to go about this.

Toglia & Foster: The Multicontext Approach to Cognitive Rehabilitation.

APPENDIX B: Assessment and Observational Tools

APPENDIX B.1	Personality Characteristic Checklist (client) (Chapter 1)
APPENDIX B.2	Personality Characteristic Checklist (other) (Chapter 1)
APPENDIX B.3	Dynamic Interactional Model: Performance Analysis Guide (Chapter 5)
APPENDIX B.4	Cognitive Performance Observation Tool (Chapter 5)
APPENDIX B.5.1 and B.5.2	Directions for Pizza Phone Delivery Task and Pizza Phone Delivery Task: Analysis of Task Errors (Chapter 5)
APPENDIX B.6	Performance Analysis of Task Errors (Chapter 5)
APPENDIX B.7	Multi-step Activity Error Analysis (Chapter 5)
APPENDIX B.8.1 and B.8.2	Smartphone: Multiple Tasks Smartphone: Multiple Tasks Scoresheet (Chapter 5)
APPENDIX B.9	Upper Body Dressing Error Analysis (UBDEA) (Chapter 5)
APPENDIX B.10	Assessment Summary (Chapter 5)
APPENDIX B.11	Worksheet for Analysis of Strategy Attributes (Chapter 7)
APPENDIX B.12	Therapist Worksheet for Observing Types of Strategies (Chapter 7)
APPENDIX B.13	Therapist Checklist for Observation and Analysis of Strategy Use (Chapter 7)
APPENDIX B.14.1 and B.14.2	Guidelines for Challenge Identification Questions and Rating Scale. Challenge Identification Rating Scale (Chapter 11)
APPENDIX B.15.1 and B.15.2	Guidelines for Strategy Generation Questions and Rating Scale Strategy Generation Rating Scale (Chapter 11)
APPENDIX B.16	Strategy Awareness Questions and Rating Scale (Chapter 11)

Appendix B.1. Personality Characteristic Checklist (client)

Name: _____ Date: _____

We would like you to describe yourself <u>before</u> your injury or illness by rating the personal characteristics listed below on a 1 to 3 scale:

1 = Most like me
2 = Somewhat like me
3 = Least like me

_____ Cheerful	_____ Quick	_____ Serious
_____ Outspoken	_____ Easily adaptable	_____ Risk-taker
_____ Dependable	_____ Anxious	_____ Popular
_____ Good sense of humor	_____ Energetic	_____ Somewhat disorganized
_____ Impatient	_____ Leader	_____ Imaginative
_____ Conscientious	_____ An observer	_____ Friendly, outgoing
_____ Good listener	_____ Practical, matter-of-fact	_____ Waits and studies a situation
_____ Quiet and reserved	_____ Decisive	_____ Meticulous
_____ Very organized	_____ Goal-oriented	_____ Thinks quickly on his/her feet
_____ Detail-oriented	_____ Jumps right into things	_____ Holds in feelings
_____ Perfectionist	_____ People-oriented	_____ Efficient work style
_____ Private person	_____ Easily takes charge	_____ Gives direction well to others
_____ Skeptical	_____ Laid back	_____ Open to advice from others
_____ Prefers to be alone	_____ Moody	_____ Works well in groups/teams
_____ Patient	_____ A doer	_____ Takes time to get things right
_____ Empathic	_____ Very friendly	_____ Follows directions carefully
_____ Easy, relaxed style (low key)	_____ Creative	_____ Good at 'being in charge'
_____ A follower	_____ Readily admits mistakes	_____ Persistence and perseverance
_____ Always has lots of ideas	_____ Set in own ways	_____ Argumentative
_____ Even-tempered	_____ Passive	_____ Assertive
_____ Optimistic	_____ Opinionated	_____ Flexible
_____ Easily compromises and collaborates	_____ Easily expresses thoughts, feelings	_____ Avoids Challenges

To what extent has your personality changed since the injury/illness?

_____ Not at all   _____ A little   _____ A lot

Place an asterisk (*) next to any characteristics that you feel have changed since the injury or illness.

Toglia & Foster: The Multicontext Approach to Cognitive Rehabilitation.

Appendix B.2. Personality Characteristic Checklist (other)

Name: _____   Date: _____

We would like you to describe your relative's personal traits before the injury or illness by rating the characteristics listed below on a 1 to 3 scale:

1 = Most like your relative before the injury
2 = Somewhat like your relative
3 = Least like your relative

____ Cheerful	____ Quick	____ Serious
____ Outspoken	____ Easily adaptable	____ Risk-taker
____ Dependable	____ Anxious	____ Popular
____ Good sense of humor	____ Energetic	____ Somewhat disorganized
____ Impatient	____ Leader	____ Imaginative
____ Conscientious	____ An observer	____ Friendly, outgoing
____ Good listener	____ Practical, matter-of-fact	____ Waits and studies a situation
____ Quiet and reserved	____ Decisive	____ Meticulous
____ Very organized	____ Goal-oriented	____ Thinks quickly on his/her feet
____ Detail-oriented	____ Jumps right into things	____ Holds in feelings
____ Perfectionist	____ People-oriented	____ Efficient work style
____ Private person	____ Easily takes charge	____ Gives direction well to others
____ Skeptical	____ Laid back	____ Open to advice from others
____ Prefers to be alone	____ Moody	____ Works well in groups/teams
____ Patient	____ A doer	____ Takes time to get things right
____ Empathic	____ Very friendly	____ Follows directions carefully
____ Easy, relaxed style (low key)	____ Creative	____ Good at 'being in charge'
____ A follower	____ Readily admits mistakes	____ Persistence and perseverance
____ Always has lots of ideas	____ Set in own ways	____ Argumentative
____ Even-tempered	____ Passive	____ Assertive
____ Optimistic	____ Opinionated	____ Flexible
____ Easily compromises and collaborates	____ Easily expresses thoughts, feelings	____ Avoids Challenges

To what extent has your relative's personality changed since the injury/ illness?

_____ Not at all   _____ A little   _____ A lot

Place an asterisk (*) next to any personality characteristics that have changed since the injury or illness. If you feel that your relative's personality has changed a lot, please fill out another rating form that describes your relative now.

Toglia & Foster: The Multicontext Approach to Cognitive Rehabilitation.

Appendix B.3. Dynamic Interactional Model: Performance Analysis Guide

1. **Personal Context, Environment, and Activity Demands**
   Personal context:

   Activity:

   Context:

   Specify activity/environmental demands:

2. **Performance: Observation of Process and Outcome**
   a. *Performance outcome*:

   b. *What are the cognitive performance error(s) or behaviors? Why do you think the errors occurred?*

   c. *Strategies: What task methods or strategies does the person use during performance?*

3. **Self-Perceptions and Awareness:** *What is the client's perspective before and after the task?*
   a. *Before task: Anticipate possible challenges? Generate strategies?*

   b. *During task: Recognize challenges? Detect and/or correct performance errors?*

   c. *After task: Aware of performance, task challenges, task methods that were successful versus unsuccessful? Able to generate alternate strategies?*

4. **Functional Implications**
   a. *Describe the activity demands and environmental conditions under which the performance error(s) or cognitive behaviors are least likely and most likely to emerge.*

   b. *Error patterns: If applicable, identify other activities or situations that the same cognitive behaviors or performance errors have been observed.*

   c. *How or to what extent do the observed performance error(s) or cognitive behaviors impact overall functional performance?*

5. **Treatment Implications**

Toglia & Foster: The Multicontext Approach to Cognitive Rehabilitation.

Appendix B.4. Cognitive Performance Observation Tool

Activity: _____   Date: _____

| **Attends to all Aspects of Task or Directions** |
| (Does not over-focus on parts, pieces, or areas of space; does not miss or omit steps, materials, or info) |

Specific Observations: Task errors/difficulties	*Specific Observations: Strengths/Strategies used*
1.	1.
2.	2.
3.	3.

| **Emotional Regulation and Management: Manages Emotions effectively during an Activity** |
| (Does client become overwhelmed, frustrated, and stop in face of challenge?) |

Specific Observations: Task errors/difficulties	*Specific Observations: Strengths/Strategies used*
1.	1.
2.	2.
3.	3.

| **Generates Alternate Methods, Strategies, Solutions, Ideas when Needed** |
| (When faced with obstacles, switches methods or strategies, brainstorms other possible solutions or ideas) |

Specific Observations: Task errors/difficulties	*Specific Observations: Strengths/Strategies used*
1.	1.
2.	2.
3.	3.

| **Goal-Directed: Stays Focused on Task/Goal** |
| (Resists distractions or irrelevant info; does not become sidetracked) |

Specific Observations: Task errors/difficulties	*Specific Observations: Strengths/Strategies used*
1.	1.
2.	2.
3.	3.

| **Keeps Track of Information/Directions during an Activity** |
| (Does not excessively re-read directions, keeps track of previous responses, steps, or information needed) |

Specific Observations: Task errors/difficulties	*Specific Observations: Strengths/Strategies used*
1.	1.
2.	2.
3.	3.

| **Organized Task Method or Approach** |
| (Gathers needed materials/information; organized search; maintains organization of materials; groups related information, plans ahead) |

Specific Observations: Task errors/difficulties	*Specific Observations: Strengths/Strategies used*
1.	1.
2.	2.
3.	3.

Toglia & Foster: The Multicontext Approach to Cognitive Rehabilitation.

<td colspan="2" align="center">**Paces Timing** (Thinks before acting; regulates timing and speed of actions (does not rush or is not excessively slow))</td>
Specific Observations: Task errors/difficulties 1. 2. 3.	*Specific Observations: Strengths/Strategies used* 1. 2. 3.
<td colspan="2" align="center">**Searches or Seeks Information when Needed** (Asks questions for clarification on directions; initiates searching for additional information when needed)</td>
Specific Observations: Task errors/difficulties 1. 2. 3.	*Specific Observations: Strengths/Strategies used* 1. 2. 3.
<td colspan="2" align="center">**Self-Monitors Performance** (Recognizes errors, obstacles, or potential problems)</td>
Specific Observations: Task errors/difficulties 1. 2. 3.	*Specific Observations: Strengths Strategies used* 1. 2. 3.
<td colspan="2" align="center">**Sequences and Shifts: Moves from one item, step, or activity to the next efficiently** (In order, without redundant actions or extraneous steps)</td>
Specific Observations: Task errors/difficulties 1. 2. 3.	*Specific Observations: Strengths/Strategies used* 1. 2. 3.
<td colspan="2" align="center">**Strategies or Task Methods are Efficient and Effective**</td>
Specific Observations: Task errors/difficulties 1. 2. 3.	*Specific Observations: Strengths/Strategies used* 1. 2. 3.
OTHER:	**OTHER:**

Toglia & Foster: The Multicontext Approach to Cognitive Rehabilitation.

Appendix B.5.1. Directions for Pizza Phone Delivery Task

The calling for pizza task requires the person to use a smartphone with internet connection or a computer/tablet and phone. The person is required to locate a local pizza place that can deliver to the person's current location or vicinity. The therapist role plays the call with the client and provides all of the information needed below during the role-pay (prices, delivery charge, supplies provided, time for order, total charge, closing time)

Task Directions: The therapist presents the below written directions (fold page in half to present directions). The directions are reviewed verbally to ensure client understanding. The written directions can be left out on the table so the client can refer to them during the task. Although directions are presented, no pencil or pen is provided as the person needs to recognize the need and ask for it.

Directions:

Find and call a local pizza place that will deliver to your current location. How you go about doing this is up to you. You need to find out the price of three large plain pies and one large bottle of soda, whether there is a delivery charge, if they can supply plates and napkins, approximate time order will take, total charge for the order, and the closing time on weekends and weekdays.

Write the name, phone number, address of the restaurant, and total charge for the order on the front of this paper and write all the other information you obtain on the back of this paper. Write the time that you begin and end this task on the upper right corner of this page.

Toglia & Foster: The Multicontext Approach to Cognitive Rehabilitation.

Appendix B.5.2. Pizza Phone Delivery Task: Analysis of Task Errors (NO cues or assistance provided)

Steps	√, I, P, X	Task Error or Inefficiency (see options below)	*Error Awareness	Interpretation Why do you think error occurred?
1. Initiates searching on phone or electronic device				
2. Uses appropriate search terms, narrows search appropriately.				
3. *Correctly* ___ identifies local Pizza place ___ phone number				
4. Makes phone call and dials number correctly				
5. *Asks about* ___ price of 3 pies, large soda ___ delivery fee ___ plates & napkins ___ closing time - weekday ___ closing time - weekend				
6. *1st Page - Writes* ___ name, phone number, address ___ total charge ___ start and end time				
7. *2nd paper – Writes* ___ price of 3 pies, large soda ___ delivery fee ___ closing time – weekday ___ closing time – weekend ___ approximate time for order				
% Accurate steps completed _____	Total % inefficient steps _____		Total % partial steps _____	
Time Required: _____	% SR _____ (SR/total errors)	% SR-P _____	% Error corrections _____	

Step Completion: √ = completed accurately, I = inefficient, P = partially accurate, X = inaccurate
Error Awareness: SR = self-recognition of errors, SR-P = self-recognized error after obstacle/problem, EC = error correction

Type of Task Errors

- *Omission*: Leaves out information or misses an action, details, or item. Fails to perform a step.
- *Inaccuracy*: Steps, actions or information are incorrect or do not match directions (eg. writes wrong phone number or identifies a pizza place outside of local area).
- *Incomplete*: Steps, actions, or information is partial or incomplete.
- *Addition*: Extra steps, objects, actions, or information (goal-related).
- *Inefficiency*: Task component could be completed in fewer steps, less time or effort.
- *Repetition*: Repeats a step or item.
- *Sequencing error*: Performs a step in the wrong order.
- *Extraneous actions*: Off-task actions, behaviors, or steps or attends to irrelevant stimuli, materials, items, or information that is unrelated to the goal.
- *Stops prematurely*: Stops before a step is completed.
- *Misinterpretation of instructions*
- *Misplacement*: Items or information placed in the wrong location or arranged incorrectly.

Toglia & Foster: The Multicontext Approach to Cognitive Rehabilitation.

Appendix B.6. Performance Analysis of Task Errors (NO cues or assistance provided)

Activity: _____   Date: _____

Steps	√, I, P, X	Task Error or Inefficiency (see options below)	*Error Awareness	Interpretation Why do you think error occurred?

% Accurate steps completed _____   Total % inefficient steps _____   Total % partial steps _____

Time Required: _____   % SR _____ (SR/total errors)   % SR-P _____   % Error corrections _____

Step Completion: √ = completed accurately, I = inefficient, P = partially accurate, X = inaccurate
Error Awareness: SR = self-recognition of errors, SR-P = self-recognized error after obstacle/problem, EC = error correction

Type of Task Errors

- *Omission:* Leaves out information or misses an action, details, or item. Fails to perform a step.
- *Inaccuracy:* Steps, actions or information are incorrect or do not match directions (eg. writes wrong phone number or identifies a pizza place outside of local area).
- *Incomplete:* Steps, actions, or information is partial or incomplete.
- *Addition:* Extra steps, objects, actions, or information (goal-related).
- *Inefficiency:* Task component could be completed in fewer steps, less time or effort.
- *Repetition:* Repeats a step or item.
- *Sequencing error:* Performs a step in the wrong order.
- *Extraneous actions:* Off-task actions, behaviors, or steps or attends to irrelevant stimuli, materials, items, or information that is unrelated to the goal.
- *Stops prematurely:* Stops before a step is completed.
- *Misinterpretation of instructions*
- *Misplacement:* Items or information placed in the wrong location or arranged incorrectly.

Toglia & Foster: The Multicontext Approach to Cognitive Rehabilitation.

Appendix B.7 DIM: Multi-Step Activity Management

Specify TASK:	Task Errors / Observations	Inefficiency	Omits	Inacc	Seq	Irrelev Actions	Strategies Observed
1. Task Preparation Phase	After initial directions, client initiates actions, takes time to review directions and plan ahead, re-clarifies directions or checks understanding if needed, gathers, organizes or re-organizes relevant tools, materials, directions, lists or information						
2. Task Implementation Phase: *carrying out the task. Identify Main Steps*							
A.							
B.							
C.							
D.							
E.							
F.							
G.							
H.							
3. Task Completion and Self-Check	Persists until task completion, does not stop prematurely; knows when finished (e.g., puts down the items, doesn't continue aimlessly) self-checks work or compares product to initial directions or goal.						
TOTAL							

Recall of directions: _____ Adequate _____ Inadequate
Persistence: _____ Good _____ Needs encouragement to persist _____ Gives up easily
Spontaneous Error Recognition: _____ No error recognition _____ Slight error recognition (misses majority)
_____ Partial error recognition _____ Full error recognition
Pace/Speed: _____ Adequate _____ Too fast (impulsive) _____ Too slow _____ Fluctuates too fast & too slow

Inefficiency: Task could be completed in fewer steps, less time or effort. *Omission:* Misses or omits information, details, items or sub-steps. *Inaccurate -* Selects, or uses incorrect materials, items or information or does not perform the step correctly. *Sequencing error:* Performs a step in the wrong order. *Irrelevant Actions:* Off-task behaviors, actions, or steps unrelated to the goal or attends to irrelevant stimuli, materials, items, or information that is non goal related.

Toglia & Foster: The Multicontext Approach to Cognitive Rehabilitation.

Appendix B.8.1 Smartphone: Multiple Tasks

Using your smartphone, complete all of these tasks as quickly and efficiently as you can. The tasks can be done in any order.

After three minutes into the task, circle the step that you are up to on the list, and write how much time you think you will need to complete the remaining tasks. At 6 minutes, cross out the last step you completed and once again indicate how much longer it will take you to complete all tasks. Do not turn the page over more than once. Tell me when you have completed all tasks.

- Enter a doctor's appointment for _____ 20th at 2:30 p.m. in your calendar.

- Look up the weekend weather forecast in Boston, MA.

- Set an alarm reminder for the doctor's appointment one week before and one day before.

- Send a text message to yourself as a reminder to pick up your bag from the coat check.

- Locate the *Amazon* app and full description. Write the app rating on the back of this page.

- Take a picture of something in the room and e-mail it to yourself.

- Find a hotel in the _____ area and write the address on the back of this page.

- Multiply 164378 by 436 and write the answer in the upper right corner of this page.

- Find today's news headlines and write it on the back of the page.

- Call this phone number _____ and leave a voice mail to confirm your next appointment.

Toglia & Foster: The Multicontext Approach to Cognitive Rehabilitation.

Appendix B.8.2. Smartphone: Multiple Tasks Score Sheet (Chapter 5)

Date: _____   Pt. Initials: _____   Therapist Initials: _____

How familiar are you using your phone to set alarms, text, take and retrieve photos, e-mail, and look up info on the internet?

_____ Not Familiar   _____ Slightly Familiar   _____ Familiar   _____ Very Familiar Task

Start Time: _____   Finish Time _____

Appointments	Order	Completes Task √, X or P (partial)	Accurate √, X, or P	Inefficient	Does not attempt	Task Errors (Write in)	* Error Awareness SR; SR-P; EC
1. Enter doctor's appt. (20th, 2:30) in calendar							
2. Looks up weekend weather in Boston, MA							
3a. Alarm 1 week before							
3b. Alarm 1 day before							
4. Correct text message sent							
5a. Searches and locates Amazon app description							
5b. Writes App rating on back of page.							
6a. Locates hotel							
6b. Writes hotel address on back							
7a. Take a picture							
7b. E-mails photo to self							
8. Multiply 164378 by 436. = 71,668,808							
9a. Locates today's news headlines							
9b. Writes headlines on the back of the page							
10a. Calls phone number							
10b. Leaves voice mail							
Totals							
Total Time: _____							

Completion: √ = task completed, even if inaccurate; P= Partially completed ; X = not done or omitted.
Accuracy: √ = accurate; P = partially accurate; X = inaccurate
Inefficient: Task may be accurate but takes extra time, effort, or includes extra actions or steps or trial and error.
Error Awareness: SR = spontaneously self-recognizes error; SR-P = error recognized after obstacle/problem; EC = error self-corrected
Score – Percentage of steps accurately completed out of 16 (max), and % accurate out of those completed.

Toglia & Foster: The Multicontext Approach to Cognitive Rehabilitation.

After Task: Participant Rating

1. How well did you do this task?

   1 ——— 2 ——— 3 ——— 4 ——— 5
   Extremely Well   Not Well

2. How was your performance on this activity compared to how you would have performed prior to the _____ (illness, injury)

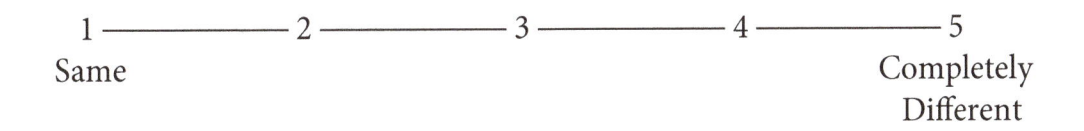

   1 ——— 2 ——— 3 ——— 4 ——— 5
   Same   Completely
                                     Different

3. On a scale of 1 to 5, how challenging was this activity?

   1 ——— 2 ——— 3 ——— 4 ——— 5
   Easy   Very
   Not Challenging   Challenging

4. How efficient would you say you were with completing everything you needed to do?

   1 ——— 2 ——— 3 ——— 4 ——— 5
   Very   Very
   Efficient   Inefficient

5. Tell me how you went about doing this activity. How did you decide what order to do the tasks in?

6. What challenges did you encounter as you were doing this activity?

Toglia & Foster: The Multicontext Approach to Cognitive Rehabilitation.

Clinician Rating

1. How often did the participant look at the clock to monitor time?

    ___ never   ___ occasionally (1-2 times)   ___ frequently (3-6 times)   ___ excessive (7 or more)

2. How often did the participant look at the list/directions?

    ___ never   ___ occasionally (1-2 times)   ___ frequently (3-6 times)   ___ excessive (7 or more)

Rule Following:

___ At 3 minutes: Circles the step on the list ___

   Writes how much time is needed to complete remaining tasks ___

___ At 6 minutes: Crosses out the last step completed ___

   Indicates time needed to complete all tasks ___

___ Follows rule: Do not turn the page over more than once

___ States when all tasks are completed

Additional Observations and Comments:

Toglia & Foster: The Multicontext Approach to Cognitive Rehabilitation.

Appendix B.9. Upper Body Dressing Error Analysis (UBDEA)

This observational assessment is designed to analyze the frequency and type of errors that may occur during upper body dressing (donning an overhead shirt and button-down shirt or sweater) in persons with neurological conditions and cognitive-perceptual impairments. It also examines error recognition, correction, and the ability to recognize need for help or ask for assistance.

Materials: Stopwatch for timing; use a t-shirt *and* a sweater, button-down shirt, or jacket

Context: Record the location of the evaluation, position of the client, and the time of day. For example, indicate if the client is sitting on the edge of a bed, mat, chair, or standing. Also, indicate if the evaluation is taking place in the client's room or the clinic as well as the time of day. For example, note if the evaluation is taking place during the client's normal dressing morning routine (a.m. routine) or if it is taking place at another time in the morning (a.m.) or afternoon (p.m.).

Set up: Garments are presented inside out, upside down.

The person is asked to put on a t-shirt, followed by a button-down shirt, sweater, or jacket (over the t-shirt) as both types of garments are used outside of the hospital setting.

Directions (for each garment):

"**I would like you to put on this shirt by yourself** " (First t-shirt and then repeat with second garment). "**If you need any help, please let me know what type of help you need.**"

<u>Do not verbal cue or offer encouragement</u> unless it is absolutely needed. In other words, if the person is stuck, cannot progress, or is getting nowhere, cues may be provided as per below guidelines for error recognition or error correction.

Completing the Rating/Observational Form during dressing:

Observe and indicate the order of steps that the person takes as each garment is donned by placing the appropriate number next to the corresponding step. Time and record the number of minutes and seconds it takes to put on each garment. Observe task errors carefully and follow the guidelines below.

There are seven columns on the recording form:

1. *Accuracy:* Place a √ if this step was completely accurate; place an X if it was not completely accurate.
2. *Task Errors:* Record any specific errors observed. Examples of errors are listed. Please check off any of the errors that are observed and/or place the error # next to the step that the error occurs if possible.
3. *Error Recognition*:
   a. Client readily recognizes errors: Record **Y** for yes.
   b. Client recognizes some errors but not others: Record **P** for partial recognition.
   c. Client does not appear to recognize errors: Record errors but then cue for error recognition. For example, say, "**Let's stop. Let's look at what is happening. Is everything going the way you want it to be? Is everything going smoothly? Is anything wrong or not quite right? What is wrong?**

      "**I am noticing some things that are not quite right. Do you agree with that?**" *(Only used if the client indicates No to all of the above.)*

      See if the client can identify the error or problem. If the client can now identify the errors, the therapist would record both **Y or P** for full or partial error recognition, but the **Y or P** for error recognition should be **circled** (indicating that error recognition required cues). In addition, **V** = verbal cues should be recorded under the assist column. Comments should describe or specify that error recognition required cues.
4. *Error Correction*:
   a. Client readily corrects errors: If a task error is observed but the client corrects the error themselves, Record Y for yes.
   b. Client corrects some errors but not others: Record P for partial correction.
   c. Unable to correct errors: If the client is unable to recognize errors (#1 above), then it is assumed he or she is unable to correct them and N is recorded.

Toglia & Foster: The Multicontext Approach to Cognitive Rehabilitation.

In some cases, however, the client may recognize that something is wrong but persists with the same incorrect method. An example is presented below along with guided prompts that can be used to facilitate alternative methods and error correction.

Example: Patient with a stroke and minimal movement in their affected arm, puts on shirt, with good arm in sleeve first. Patient recognizes that the affected UE is not in the sleeve but does not know how to correct it and says he needs help.

"Can you think of a different method to make it easier?" or **"Let's stop. Think of a different way to go about doing this?"** or **"Try going about this differently. What else can you try?"**

"If we started again…. What could you do differently?"

"Can you think of a different way to put on the shirt? What arm should go in the sleeve first? Why?"

If the client was able to correct the errors after cues, a Y is recorded but it is **circled**.

5. *Requests assistance:* The client recognizes difficulties and requests help. If client asks for assistance, see if client understands why he needs assistance. e.g., **"How would you like me to help you? What kind of help do you need? Why do you think you are stuck?"**

   If client asks for assistance but needs encouragement or reassurance instead (to continue to persist due to lack of confidence, etc.), encouragement should be provided and recorded as **E** (encouragement only) but comments explaining this should be included and/or the assistance would be labeled as *not* necessary.

6. *Assist is provided:* Assistance is generally not provided unless the person asks for help appropriately or unless the task cannot proceed without assistance. If assistance is provided, indicate whether the assistance is **E** = encouragement or reassurance only; **P** = physical; **V** = verbal; **PV** = combination of physical and verbal assistance provided, or **T** = therapist completes this step for the client.

7. *Inefficient but no assist:* Repetition of steps, correction of multiple errors; extra effort is observed.

Additional Guidelines:

1. If client is unfamiliar with one-handed dressing techniques, do not jump in and provide instruction. Observe how client goes about the task and how they problem solve. Only jump in if absolutely needed. Record that they are unfamiliar with one-handed dressing techniques.

2. If client is going too quickly or is distracted, becomes distracted, etc., do not cue or intervene (unless needed for safety). Observe errors that occur and a person's ability to manage the errors.

3. Indicate cognitive symptoms that appeared to be primarily interfering with dressing under the comment section.

Toglia & Foster: The Multicontext Approach to Cognitive Rehabilitation.

APPENDIX B: Assessment and Observational Tools

T-Shirt (overhead)

Pt. # _____ Age _____ Dx _____

Therapist _____ Date _____

Sitting: ___ Bed   ___ Mat   ___ Chair/WC   ___ Standing   ___ Room   ___ Clinic   ___ a.m. routine

___ a.m.   ___ p.m.

Task Components (place # to indicate order of steps)	√, I or x	2nd try	Task Errors/Problems (specifically describe error or identify errors by number below)	Error Recognition *4,3,2,1	Error Correction ^5,4,3,2,1	Requests assist (Y/N)	Comments or Observations (indicate if error is partially recognized or corrected)
___ Re-orientation of shirt							
___ Affected arm in sleeve							
___ Pulls sleeve up past elbow to shoulder							
___ Good UE in sleeve							
___ Pulls shirt over head							
___ Pulls shirt down in back							

√ = independent; I = inefficient or trial and error but NO cues, encouragement or assistance; X = needs cues/assistance to complete step

*Error Recognition: 4 = Self recognizes error; 3 = Recognizes with general questions; 2 = Recognizes with specific questions/ cues; 1 = Does not recognize error (therapist points out error)

^Error Correction: 5 = Self-corrects; 4 = Self-corrects with general questions; 3 = Self-corrects with specific questions; 2 = Direct cues or tell person what to do; 1 = Physical assistance

Time required _____ minutes   _____ Unfamiliar with one-handed technique

*Able to Generate Alternate Methods: ❏ Y   ❏ N   Assist requested is necessary: ❏ Y   ❏ N

Sample Upper Body Dressing Errors

____ 1. Cannot get started (fails to begin task)
____ 2. Dresses the nonparetic arm first
____ 3. Attempts to put hand through wrong opening of sleeve
____ 4. Stops prematurely or in the middle of task
____ 5. Does not pull shirt down in back
____ 6. Putting garment on backward
____ 7. Chooses wrong garment/ item
____ 8. Repeats same action or step
____ 9. Disorganized approach (example: _____)
____ 10. Puts garment on inside out
____ 11. Neglects to cover the paretic (left) shoulder
____ 12. Does not dress or attend to the affected side
____ 13. Fails to put the paretic hand through the correct hole
____ 14. Fails to push the sleeve high enough over the paretic elbow
____ 15. Puts head through bottom or wrong hole
____ 16. Goal Neglect—strays away from task
____ 17. Extraneous, unrelated task actions
____ 18. Unable to figure out how to position/orient garment correctly
____ 19. Tries to use button-down method for overhead shirt
____ 20. _____ (specify)

Comments/Observations:

___ *Decreased Initiation*   ___ *Impulsive*   ___ *Perseverative*   ___ *Loses Track*   ___ *Neglect*   ___ *Apraxia*

_____

_____

Toglia & Foster: The Multicontext Approach to Cognitive Rehabilitation.

Sweater/Jacket/Button-down shirt

Pt. # _____ Age _____ Dx _____

Therapist _____ Date _____

Sitting: ___ Bed   ___ Mat   ___ Chair/WC   ___ Standing   ___ Room   ___ Clinic   ___ a.m. routine

___ a.m.   ___ p.m.

Task Components (place # to indicate order of steps)	√, I or x	2nd try	Task Errors/Problems (specifically describe error or identify errors by number below)	Error Recognition *4,3,2,1	Error Correction ^5,4,3,2,1	Requests assist (Y/N)	Comments or Observations (indicate if error is partially recognized or corrected)
___ Re-orientation of shirt							
___ Affected arm in sleeve							
___ Pulls sleeve up past elbow to shoulder							
___ Pulls shirt around back							
___ Good Arm in Sleeve							
___ Buttoning							

√ = independent; I = inefficient or trial and error but NO cues, encouragement or assistance; X = needs cues/assistance to complete step

*Error Recognition: 4 = Self recognizes error; 3 = Recognizes with general questions; 2 = Recognizes with specific questions/ cues; 1 = Does not recognize error (therapist points out error)

^Error Correction: 5 = Self-corrects; 4 = Self-corrects with general questions; 3 = Self-corrects with specific questions; 2 = Direct cues or tell person what to do; 1 = Physical assistance

Time required _____ minutes   _____ Unfamiliar with one-handed technique
*Able to Generate Alternate Methods: ❑ Y ❑ N   Assist requested is necessary: ❑ Y ❑ N

Sample Upper Body Dressing Errors (prior to any cues)

Sample Upper Body Dressing Errors

___ 1. Cannot get started (fails to begin task)
___ 2. Dresses the nonparetic arm first
___ 3. Attempts to put hand through wrong opening of sleeve
___ 4. Stops prematurely or in the middle of task
___ 5. Does not pull shirt down in back
___ 6. Putting garment on backward
___ 7. Chooses wrong garment/ item
___ 8. Repeats same action or step
___ 9. Disorganized approach (example: _____)
___ 10. Puts garment on inside out
___ 11. Neglects to cover the paretic (left) shoulder
___ 12. Does not dress or attend to the affected side
___ 13. Fails to put the paretic hand through the correct hole
___ 14. Fails to push the sleeve high enough over the paretic elbow
___ 15. Tries to use overhead method for button-down shirt
___ 16. Goal Neglect - strays away from task
___ 17. Extraneous, unrelated task actions
___ 18. Unable to figure out how to position/orient garment correctly
___ 19. Misaligns buttons
___ 20. _____ (specify)

Comments / Observations:

___ *Decreased Initiation*   ___ *Impulsive*   ___ *Perseverative*   ___ *Loses Track*   ___ *Neglect*   ___ *Apraxia*

_____

_____

Toglia & Foster: The Multicontext Approach to Cognitive Rehabilitation.

Appendix B.10. Assessment Summary

Summary of Assessment Results	
Client Concerns and Goals	
Functional Cognitive Concerns by Others	
Functional Cognitive Performance *(activity limitations and/or participation restrictions)*	
Cognitive performance errors or behaviors that go across activities	
Activity/environment characteristics that increase likelihood of performance errors	
Awareness *Outside of Task* *Before Task* *During* *After*	
Strategy Use *Generation & initiation* *Type* *Frequency & timing* *Efficiency & effort* *Flexibility* *Consistency* *Effectiveness*	
Potential for Learning and change	

Toglia & Foster: The Multicontext Approach to Cognitive Rehabilitation.

Appendix B.11. Worksheet for Analysis of Strategy Attributes

Performance problem	
Desired Outcome	
Strategy	
Strategy Purpose (performance, learning or information processing, self-regulation or monitoring)	
Range of application (task-specific, domain-specific or task category, general)	
Timing of Use (performance phase) Before, during, and/or after activity	
Visibility (overt or covert)	
Permanence (temporary or permanent)	
Strategy target (task, environment, or person's behavior, abilities)	

From: Toglia, J., Rodger, S. A., & Polatajko, H. J. (2012). Anatomy of cognitive strategies: A therapist's primer for enabling occupational performance. *Canadian Journal of Occupational Therapy, 79*(4), 225-236. doi:10.2182/cjot.2012.79.4.4

Toglia & Foster: The Multicontext Approach to Cognitive Rehabilitation.

Appendix B.12. Therapist Worksheet for Observing Types of Strategies

Observable Strategies Not observed, partial/inconsistent use, consistent use	Frequency (Count)	Comments: spontaneous, generated with prompts, used consistently when needed, inconsistent, effective, efficient
Information Seeking/Following Directions ___ Restating instructions or keywords (periodic summaries) ___ Asks questions or clarification ___ Asks for repetition or re-reads directions ___ Reviews all instructions – looks over the entire task ___ Writes down instructions		
Planning Ahead, Organized Methods ___ Pre-gathers all needed items first ___ Organizes/rearranges materials ___ Talks aloud plan or makes a written plan (writes steps) ___ Uses color coding/other methods to group information ___ Uses generic planning outline /questions ___ Rehearses plan		
Attention to Key Features ___ Underlines, circles, or highlights keywords or features		
Searching/ Locating/ Discrimination ___ Finger Pointing or Finger Tracing ___ Systematic search ___ Look from different perspectives (change position) ___ Use of high contrast ___ Get a sense of the "whole" first/look for context cues		
Lists (External Cue) ___ Uses written list/steps ___ Crosses off /check each item as it is completed ___ Creates list (list/ checklist) or writes down		
Uses External Cues ___ Cue card, posted reminders, calendar, clock etc. ___ Visual Cues (e.g., Pictures, symbols) ___ Electronic (alarm, beepers, text message)		
Self-Verbalization Strategies ___ Verbal rehearsal of keywords, directions or steps ___ Self-questions ___ Self-cues ___ Sub-vocalization or talks through problems or solutions		
Stimuli Reduction ___ Removes irrelevant items ___ Screens/covers/blocks part of information		
Paces: ___ Stops and checks; Periodic checking ___ Uses an "alert" strategy and/or requests breaks ___ Counts/taps to ___ ; waits for signal before responding		
Monitoring ___ Recognizes problem—asks for assistance ___ Double checks actions ___ Checks work		
Internal Strategies ___ *Mental Practice* (review or picture what you need to do in your mind, imagine self-performing activity) ___ *"Picture it First"* Visualize what it should look like at the end - picture the goal or end product first.		

Toglia & Foster: The Multicontext Approach to Cognitive Rehabilitation.

Appendix B.13. Therapist Checklist for Observation and Analysis of Strategy Use

Activity _____ Tx Session # _____

	Agree	Disagree	Not Observed or Comments
1. Strategies are **self-generated** prior to the activity			
2. Strategies are **initiated** spontaneously within the activity			
3. **Type of Strategies** used are appropriate and match the performance problem. *List types of strategies observed/reported:*			
4. **Frequency** of strategy use is appropriate for the task (not over or under-used)			
5. **Degree of effort** required to use strategy is manageable			
6. **Timing** of strategies is appropriate (not too early and not too late)			
7. **Strategies adjusted** when needed (does not persist with ineffective task methods)			
8. **Overall #** of strategies used within the task is appropriate or optimal (not too little and not too many)			
9. **Strategies are effective** in contributing to successful/improved performance			
10. **Aware** of effective or ineffective task methods			
Total			

Level of Activity Challenge (circle) (see activity challenge definitions at the end of Appendix C.13)

Not challenging   Somewhat challenging   Challenging   Very challenging

Toglia & Foster: The Multicontext Approach to Cognitive Rehabilitation.

Appendix B.14.1 Guidelines for Challenge Identification Questions and Rating Scale

The therapist rates the client's independent responses to the pre and post-activity questions below by placing a ☒ next to the appropriate level on the Challenge Identification Scale. If mediation is provided, the mediated response can also be indicated on the scale (in addition to the independent response) by an **M** and further specified with below mediation codes, if desired.

___ **PRE-ACTIVITY General Question:** Let's take a look at this activity. What types of challenges (difficulties, roadblocks, or obstacles) do you think you might run into as you do this activity?

___ **POST-ACTIVITY General Question:** What types of challenges (obstacles or roadblocks) did you experience (or run into) as you did this activity?

___ *Elaboration (E) permitted*: Tell me more about that. What exactly about that? Can you give me some examples? *If general responses are provided, ask,* Why? Why would that be (was that) challenging? What kinds of things do you (did you) need to watch out for?

MEDIATION (M): *Should not exceed 3 questions (check type of mediation provided)*

___ *Specific Question (S):* Let's look closely at this task. What parts (aspects) of this activity might be (were) harder than other parts? *or* What parts might be (were) easy and what parts might be (were) tricky/ hard? Why? *or* What types of things do you need to pay special attention to as you do this activity? *or* What did you need to pay special attention to?

___ *Therapist Partially Identifies Challenge (TC):*
Pre-Activity: Let's think about the last time you did an activity similar to this where there was a lot of information. What parts were most challenging? *or* There is a lot of information (details) to keep track of. *or* There are a lot of different papers that needed to be managed. How will this be challenging?
Post-Activity: There were a lot of details. How did all of this information/details present challenges?

___ *Task-Specific Challenges Partially Identified by Therapist (TS)*
Pre-Activity: There are 5 different things to buy within a budget. How will this present challenges?
Post-Activity: The budget was only $75.00 and there were 4 different things to buy. How did this present challenges? *or* The schedule and the information sheet both had different details needed to answer the question. How did this present challenges?

Note: If a client <u>spontaneously</u> identifies strategies they would use/used rather than identifying challenges (e.g., I need to remember to check off the list), it implies that the client is aware of challenges and is thinking ahead (or thought) of solutions. The therapist should ask for elaboration (e.g., Why would that be? Why would that method be needed? Why did you decide to use that method?). If the client can provide an explanation, it is considered good challenge identification (1 or 2). If they cannot explain, it is considered partial challenge identification (3 or 4). If the client was not asked for elaboration, challenge identification cannot be rated.

Toglia & Foster: The Multicontext Approach to Cognitive Rehabilitation.

Appendix B.14.2. Challenge Identification Rating Scale

*Place a ✓ next to the level of independent challenge identification. The levels below are based on independent responses. Optional: Place an **M** next to the level of challenge identification obtained with mediation and code type of mediation (**S, TC, TS**) as defined below, if desired to compare independent and mediated responses. For example, **M-TS** indicates that task-specific mediation was used.*

Optional Rating with Mediation: As an option, code type of mediation (S, TC, TS)
- E = Elaboration questions do not count as mediation and can be coded as E if desired.
- S = Specific questions were provided
- TC = Therapist partially identifies cognitive challenge
- TS = Therapist specifies task components that were challenging

Good Ability to Identify Challenges *(Score = 1)*

1.1. Cognitive Challenges Anticipated with Explanation Provided
____ Client states cognitive challenges (concentration, staying focused, number of items, categorizing, details) *and* can explain why it will be or was challenging.
Examples: miss details or forget instructions because there is (was) a lot of information; misunderstand or misunderstood the instructions because of the amount of information, making it difficult to focus; gloss over things and miss information because the noise outside is hard to filter out and I may get distracted.

1.2. Task-Specific or Environmental Challenges Anticipated with Explanation
____ Client acknowledges key specific task challenges *and* provides specific examples that explain the challenge.
PRE-ACTIVITY examples: I need to stay within $75.00 and make sure that I don't go over the budget; I need to make sure I keep track of the size of the items and the costs (while shopping); identifies task characteristics (e.g., It will be tricky to go back and forth between schedule and the information sheet because the noise outside is hard to filter out).
POST-ACTIVITY examples: I went over $25.00 because I didn't pay attention to the details; I didn't schedule 2 events on Thursday because I lost track and I didn't check off each item; identifies task characteristics (e.g., It was tricky to go back and forth between these 2 pages and I missed a couple of details).

Emerging/Partial Ability to Identify Challenges *(Score = 2)*

2.1. Cognitive Challenges Identified without Explanation
____ Client states cognitive challenges (poor memory, distracted easily, trouble concentrating) but cannot provide specific examples or explain why, or provides several examples that are not key challenges.

2.2. Less Relevant Task or Environmental Challenges Identified or without Explanation
____ Client indicates one specific task challenge without an explanation, identifies task challenges that are less relevant or do not represent the most significant challenges or identifies vague task challenges (e.g., the instructions are long, sorting will be (was) challenging, getting the instructions right) without explaining why it will be challenging *(if directions are just re-stated – see below)*. Environmental challenges may include noise or crowded areas without an explanation.

Limited Ability to Identify Challenges *(Score = 3)*

3.1. Vague Acknowledgement of Mental Challenges without Explanation
____ Client only acknowledges vague challenges with a general question (e.g., mind doesn't work right, brain is messed up) but is unable to provide any examples.

3.2 States Vague Task Challenges but Unable to Identify or Explain
____ Client indicates task will be or was challenging but cannot identify what the challenge will be/was or why. For example, re-states task directions or a list of task steps without specifying any particular challenge.

Toglia & Foster: The Multicontext Approach to Cognitive Rehabilitation.

3.3 Only Physical Challenges or Irrelevant Task Aspects Identified
___ Client only identifies physical task challenges (e.g., hard to open medication, hard to write).

Or

Client identifies aspects of the task that are irrelevant, unimportant, or should not affect performance (e.g., capitalization of words, dough is sticky, the calendar is weekly instead of monthly).

Unable to Identify Challenges *(Score = 4)*

4.1 Uncertain of Challenges
___ Client is unsure or uncertain of challenges. Says it might be (or might have been) challenging. Is uncertain and is not sure what would be (was) challenging.

4.2 Does Not Identify Any Challenges BUT Experienced Difficulties
___ Client does not identify any errors, challenges, or difficulties with the task. Perceives task as easy but is not hostile or defensive when provided with an answer sheet or structured self-evaluation.

4.3 Denial: Identifies or recognizes errors but blames external sources *(post-activity only)*
___ Same as above but is defensive or hostile with questioning. May acknowledge specific errors but blames all errors on other reasons (e.g., faulty directions, memory was never good).

Magnitude of Discrepancy Judged by Therapist
___ (0) Generally a realistic appraisal or underestimates (0)

___ (1) Overestimates abilities: ___ a little   ___ somewhat   ___ a lot

Scoring: The identification of challenges scale can be scored on a scale of 1 to 4 representing 4 levels of awareness or ability to independently identify challenges. Alternatively, items within each level (1.1, 1.2) provide further descriptive categories that were designed to be ordinal (but have not been validated).

NOTE: *If the person does not experience any difficulties and performs task efficiently, quickly, without trial and error with 100% accuracy, awareness of performance errors cannot be assessed or rated.* If the person does not identify challenges, an alternative is the below rating.

___ **1. Does Not Identify Any Challenges and has NO Difficulties**
___ **2. Does Not Identify Any Challenges and has Slight Difficulties** (inefficient, trial and error, increased time, minor errors are recognized and corrected)
___ **3. Does Not Identify Any Challenges and has Some Difficulties** (a few uncorrected errors)
___ **4. Does Not Identify Any Challenges and has a lot of Difficulties** (multiple uncorrected errors)

Toglia & Foster: The Multicontext Approach to Cognitive Rehabilitation.

> **Appendix B.15.1 Guidelines for Strategy Generation Questions and Rating Scale**

The therapist rates the client's independent responses to the pre- and post-activity strategy generation question below by placing a ☒ next to the appropriate level on the Strategy Generation Scale. If mediation is provided, the mediated response can also be indicated on the scale (in addition to the independent response) by an **M** and further specified with below mediation codes, if desired. Independent and mediated responses can be documented and compared.

Strategy generation question:

____ **PRE-ACTIVITY:** Before we start, let's think of the best way to go about doing this. Can you think of some strategies (tricks, methods, special approaches) that you could use to help you complete everything you need to do?

____ **POST-ACTIVITY:** What would you do differently next time? What special methods (tricks, approaches) or strategies could you use the next time you do this activity (to be more efficient, help things go more smoothly)?

____ *Elaboration (E):* Tell me more about that. How will you go about doing this activity? Tell me your plan or plan of action.

MEDIATION (M): *(check type of mediation provided. Use 1 question within each category)*

____ *Symptom-Specific Mediation (SS):* Questions are related to general cognitive symptoms; therapist chooses symptoms based on client. For example,

- This task involves a lot of different steps. Is there anything you can use/do to remind you of which step is next? Locate everything?
- Is there anything you can do that would help you (e.g., pay attention to all of the details, keep track of what you have already completed) as you do this task?

If clarification is needed: Think about things that you could do that might help you (e.g., stay focused, etc.).

____ *Task-Specific Mediation (TS):* Questions specifically related to task components; therapist chooses statements depending on task. For example,

- What can you do can do to help *(insert task component)*? (e.g., remember which items on the list you have already completed or which bills you have already paid, which appointments you have just entered, when to take food out of the oven)

____ *Therapist Provides Strategy Suggestion or Choice (T):* For example, "There may be some methods that can help…"

- Do you think it would be better to write a list or keep track of things in your head?
- It might be helpful to think of an image or picture that will help you to slow down. What picture comes to mind when you think of "slowing down"?
- Look at these pictures – how can a picture help remind you to "slow down"?

Note: *If a person perceives a task as easy, strategies are not considered necessary. If a task is easy or well within the person's abilities, strategies or special methods are not needed. Strategy generation needs to be assessed within a challenging task.*

Toglia & Foster: The Multicontext Approach to Cognitive Rehabilitation.

Appendix B.15.2. Strategy Generation Rating Scale

Place a ✓ next to the level of independent strategy generation. The levels below are based on independent response. <u>Optional</u>: Place an **M** next to the level of strategy generation obtained with mediation and code type of mediation (**SS, TS, T**) as defined below to compare independent and mediated responses. For example, **M-SS** indicates mediation that was symptom specific was used.

Optional Rating with Mediation: As an option, code type of mediation (S, TC, TS)

- E = Elaboration questions do not count as mediation and can be coded as E, if desired.
- S = Specific questions were provided
- TC = Therapist partially identifies cognitive challenge
- TS = Therapist specifies task components that were challenging

Good Strategy Generation (likely to facilitate performance) *(Score = 1)*
___ 1.1 Generates two or more strategies that are appropriate, specific, efficient for the task.
___ 1.2 Generates a key/main strategy that is mostly appropriate, specific, and efficient for task (other strategies not needed).

Note: *If the person identifies the order or the sequence of the steps they will perform and it reflects pre-planning and is* <u>not just repeat of instructions</u>, *it can be considered a strategy.*

Partial Strategy Generation (likely to partially help performance) *(Score = 2)*
___ 2.1 Generates at least one good strategy that is appropriate but other strategies are also needed or would likely be more effective/efficient.
___ 2.2 Identifies key and relevant aspects of the task or instructions that they need to pay special attention to or keep in mind during the task (task specification).
___ 2.3 Generates several strategies that are good but they are either overly general or task-specific or may not be complete or optimal for the task.

Limited Strategy Generation (would be minimally effective or ineffective) *(Score = 3)*
___ 3.1 Describes one aspect of the instructions or a task component to keep in mind or remember, or mentions parts of the task to pay attention that is not important or highly relevant.
___ 3.2 Generates only general or inefficient strategies.
___ 3.3 Generates a task-specific strategy but other strategies are needed.
___ 3.4 Generates strategies that would be likely ineffective, not appropriate for the task, or unrelated to anticipated challenges.

Lack of Strategy Generation (does not help performance) *(Score = 4)*
___ 4.1 Restates task steps or instructions rather than identifying a strategy.
___ 4.2 Generates vague responses that are not strategies (e.g., pay attention, concentrate, use my brain).
___ 4.3 Not sure or unable to think of a strategy but agrees a strategy might be helpful.
___ 4.4 Chooses strategies presented by therapist (agrees it will be helpful).
___ 4.5 Rejects Strategies: Does not believe a strategy or special method is needed or rejects choices.

Scoring: The Strategy Generation scale is scored on a scale of 1 to 4 representing 4 levels of independent strategy generation. Alternatively, items within each level (1.1, 1.2) provide further descriptive categories that were designed to be ordinal (but have not been validated).

Toglia & Foster: The Multicontext Approach to Cognitive Rehabilitation.

Appendix B.16. Strategy Awareness Questions and Rating Scale

The therapist rates the client's independent responses to the post-activity strategy awareness question below after the task by placing a ✓ next to the appropriate level on the Strategy Awareness Scale. If mediation is provided, the mediated response can also be indicated on the scale (in addition to the independent response) by an **M** and further specified with below mediation codes, if desired.

Post-activity strategy awareness question: Tell me how you went about doing this activity. What was your method (plan, strategies or approach)?
____ *Elaboration (E):* Tell me more about that. Where did you begin and how did you proceed?

MEDIATION (M): *(Check type of mediation provided. Limit to 1 question in each category)*
____ *Symptom-Specific (SS):* How did you manage to *(insert cognitive symptom)* (e.g., keep track of everything, stay organized, stay focused, locate or find everything)?
____ *Task-Specific (TS):* Tell me how you managed to *(insert task component)* (e.g., keep track of which bill was already paid)?
____ *Therapist Identifies Strategy Observed (T):* I noticed that you *(insert observed strategy)* (e.g., underlined, used your finger, wrote a list, talked to yourself). Tell me more about that.

Strategy Awareness Rating Scale

Place a ✓ next to the level of independent strategy awareness. The levels below are based on independent responses. <u>Optional:</u> *Place an **M** next to the level of strategy awareness obtained with mediation and code type of mediation (SS, TS, T) as described above, to compare independent and mediated responses. For example, **M-TS** indicates mediation that was task-specific was used.*

Good Strategy Awareness *(Score = 1)*
____ Accurately describes specific strategies used and task methods independently.
____ Recognizes methods that were effective or ineffective.
____ Identifies methods that contributed to success or able to explain why strategy worked.

Partial Strategy Awareness *(Score = 2)*
____ Vaguely or partially describes task methods.
____ Identifies strategies but cannot identify or explain how or why they helped.
____ Identifies methods used but unable to identify if they were effective or ineffective.

Lack of Strategy Awareness *(Score = 3)*
____ Restates tasks steps or directions or what they did rather than strategies used.
____ Does not report using any strategies or special methods, even though they were observed.
____ Therapist shares observations on strategies and client then elaborates.

No Strategies Reported *(Score = 4)*
Scoring: The Strategy Awareness scale is scored on a scale of 1 to 4 representing 4 levels of strategy awareness. Items within each level describe examples of behaviors related to the strategy awareness level.

Toglia & Foster: The Multicontext Approach to Cognitive Rehabilitation.

APPENDIX C: Treatment Forms

APPENDIX C.1	*Dynamic Interactional Model (DIM): Treatment Planning (Chapter 5)
APPENDIX C.2	*Multicontext Treatment Planning Worksheet (Chapter 13; completed sample, D.12)
APPENDIX C.3	*A Team Approach: Multicontext Treatment Planning Worksheet (Chapter 14)
APPENDIX C.4	*Multicontext Activity Worksheet: Increasing Transfer Distance (Chapter 8)
APPENDIX C.5	Sample List of Treatment Activities for Client to Choose From (Chapter 8)
APPENDIX C.6	Sample Structured Multicontext Activity Treatment Session (Chapter 13)
APPENDIX C.7	Pre-Activity Questions: Guided Anticipation & Strategy Generation (Chapter 10)
APPENDIX C.8	Post Activity: End of Session Self-Assessment (Chapter 10)
APPENDIX C.9	End of Session Strategy Bridging Questions or Structured Journal for Client (Chapter 10)
APPENDIX C.10	*Treatment Activity: Therapist Observation Checklist (Chapter 10)
APPENDIX C.11	*Treatment Session: Therapist Summary Worksheet (Chapter 11)
APPENDIX C.12	*Therapist Self-Reflection and Analysis of Mediated Learning Methods (Chapter 11, 13)
APPENDIX C.13.1 And 13.2	13.1 *Multicontext Treatment Fidelity Tool (Chapter 11) 13.2 *Multicontext Fidelity Tool Rating Criteria and Clarifications
APPENDIX C.14	Structured Journal Formats (Chapter 10)
APPENDIX C.15	Client Strategy Worksheet (Chapter 10)
APPENDIX C.16	Cognitive Strategy Action Plan (Chapter 10)
APPENDIX C.17	My Action Plan For Keeping Track (Chapter 7,10)
APPENDIX C.18	Emotional Regulation Action Plan (Chapter 7)
APPENDIX C.19	Cognitive Log (Chapter 14)
APPENDIX C.20	Generic Self-Evaluation (Chapter 10)
APPENDIX C.21	Simplified Self-Ratings (Chapter 10)
APPENDIX C.22	Simplified Self-Monitoring Ratings (Chapter 10)
APPENDIX C.23	Strategy Self-Rating Scale (Chapter 10)
APPENDIX C.24	Pre-Made Goal Examples for Clients (Chapter 12)
APPENDIX C.25	Sample Goal Book (Chapter 12)
APPENDIX C.26	Subgoaling Worksheet (Chapter 12) (see completed samples D.18-D.19)
APPENDIX C.27	Goal Plan (Chapter 12) (see completed sample D.20)
APPENDIX C.28	Goal Setting and Tracking (Chapter 12)
APPENDIX C.29	Blank Goal Rating Form (Chapter 12; see completed sample D.22)

Forms that are used only by therapists for treatment planning, observing, or summarizing. All other forms can be used with clients, either during interviews (C.7-C.8) or as worksheets/forms.

Appendix C.1. Dynamic Interactional Model (DIM): Treatment Planning

Person Factors: *(interests, motivation, experiences, psychosocial, occupations, goals)*
Error patterns across tasks:
Awareness:
Strategy use:

Activity/ Environment conditions that increase/ decrease symptoms:

Functional Problem(s)	Activity Demands Identify any modifications, adaptations, technology	Environment/Context (e.g., environmental cue signs or signals, adaptations, technologies, cues by others)	Person — Strategies Across Situations	Person — Awareness and Self-Monitoring

Toglia & Foster: The Multicontext Approach to Cognitive Rehabilitation.

Appendix C.2. Multicontext Treatment Planning Worksheet

Client Interests/Occupations:

Activity Limitations and/or Participation Restrictions	Task Errors/Symptoms that go Across Activities	Strengths

1. **Client Goals**

2. **Client Perspective, Self-Awareness, and Metacognitive skills** (outside and inside the context of activities)

3. **Intervention Plan:**
   a. What will be the initial focus of treatment? What are the targets for change?

   b. *Considerations and Reasoning:* What will be the initial emphasis? How will treatment proceed?

4. **Building Awareness/Self-Monitoring or Regulation of Symptoms:** How and when will awareness and self-monitoring skills be addressed (before, during, after activities)? Are structured self-assessments needed? Do other techniques need to be considered (video review, role reversal)?

Toglia & Foster: The Multicontext Approach to Cognitive Rehabilitation.

5. **Strategies:**
    a. *Type of Strategy Training:* (strategy specific, situational, flexible)
    b. *Identify possible strategies* that would help the person control or reduce errors across different activities. (Appendix D.1)

Identifying effective strategies beforehand can help the therapist structure the strategy generation process if needed.

Identify Possible Strategies Internal or external strategy or a combination of both	Sample Structured Guiding questions (if needed) for strategy generation:

   c. *Identify potential obstacles to strategy use and plans to address them:*

6. **Training for Generalization:** Think of activities that would require repeated practice in controlling key task errors or symptoms. Consider the starting point and the activity/environment characteristics that increase the likelihood of errors. Activities should be at an optimal level of challenge – not too easy and not too hard. Consider MC Activity Modules, if appropriate.
    a. *Brainstorm sample activities* that can be used to help the client recognize error patterns in performance or practice generating and using similar strategies. Consider goals, interests, experiences, roles, or responsibilities as well as any physical considerations.
    b. *After brainstorming activities, arrange activities on a horizontal continuum* (or use transfer distance worksheet, Appendix C.4)

Activity Theme: What activity demands will remain consistent across activities?

Very Similar:	Somewhat Similar:	Different:
1. *Initial activity:*	1.	1.
2.	2.	2.

7. **Will goal rating, subgoals, or focused goal-setting be used?** (Chapter 12)

8. **Identify the techniques that will be used for "strategy bridging" and reinforcement** (e.g., journaling, strategy worksheet, cognitive action plan).

9. **How will you collaborate with others to support intervention methods or goals?** (care partners, other professionals) (see Appendix C.3)

10. **Other Intervention Considerations:** e.g., Technology to support performance, adaptations, task-specific training for key tasks. (Also see DIM Treatment Planning Worksheet, Appendix C.1)

Toglia & Foster: The Multicontext Approach to Cognitive Rehabilitation.

Appendix C.3. A Team Approach: Multicontext Treatment Planning Worksheet

Client: _____ Date: _____

1. *Functional Team Goal*: Overall rehabilitation program outcome goal.
2. *Identify cognitive error patterns* interfering with performance across all disciplines (e.g., over-attends to details, loses track of directions or steps, impulsive, easily sidetracked).
3. *Identify common treatment strategies* that can be used or reinforced across disciplines.
4. *Identify treatment activities* within each discipline (OT, PT, SLP) that will be used to practice strategies.

Note: The same cognitive strategies can be used to accomplish different goals. Goals for each discipline should be distinct, although methods for addressing cognitive symptoms may be similar.

Functional Team Goal:

Cognitive Performance Errors Across Situations	Treatment Strategies used by All Disciplines	OT	PT	Speech

Toglia & Foster: The Multicontext Approach to Cognitive Rehabilitation.

Appendix C.4. Multicontext Activity Worksheet: Increasing Transfer Distance

Activity Theme (characteristics that stay constant):

Error Patterns:

Processing Strategy/Behavior to Control Errors:

Initial Activity	Very Similar	Somewhat Similar	Different	Very Different

Characteristics that may vary across activities:

Task context				
Type of stimuli				
Directions or rules				
Movement requirements				
Environment				
Other				

Treatment along a horizontal continuum: Number of items and cognitive complexity should remain approximately the same while task characteristics are gradually changed.

Toglia & Foster: The Multicontext Approach to Cognitive Rehabilitation.

Appendix C.5. Sample List of Treatment Activities for Client to Choose From

Directions

- Follow diagram/directions to replace battery in smoke detector.
- Follow directions to assemble a toy.
- Figure out directions to a new card game or new board game and show others how to play.
- Learn a new card game or magic trick to show others. (youtube video)
- Watch video or YouTube demonstrations of "how to"
- Figure out how to use a new APP, electronic device or applicance.

Organize and Planning

- Organize a picture album/scrapbook.
- Create a new organizational system for medications.
- Organize a bookshelf.
- Gardening: Design a window box, garden, or planter; plan, identify materials needed.
- Plan a project (e.g., painting a room, furniture refinishing).
- Plan and make dinner, lunch, dessert, etc. (e.g., No-Bake Pie)
- Schedule/Coordinate: Figure out work shifts based on availability of employees or requests. For example, figure out available appointments in an office, automotive garage, available time slots to book a band, etc.
- Look at bus schedules within the county and plan different routes.
- Theme Collage (e.g., music, fashion, sports, cars).

Investigate

- Identify a new recipe. Identify materials or ingredients needed and try out the recipe.
- Investigate things to do over the weekend and/or with friends, kids, visitors, etc.
- Investigate and locate a book on a certain topic.
- Investigate and compare prices on different products online (or using catalogs) and create a summary table.
- Create a list of things to do with kids (events, outings, activities)

Reading and Writing

- Read an article and summarize it.
- Write letters or an email regarding a problem situation.
- Practice completing different types of applications or forms (e.g., job applications, applications for membership to an organization, library card application, subscription to magazine, health insurance claim form, tax form).

Activities Involving the Computer or Tablet:

- Enter information (eg. balances on bills, invoices, expenses, receipts, calorie information on food packages) into a spreadsheet and create a chart, graph, etc.
- Enter appointments and schedule into Google Calendar.
- Create a PowerPoint slide show on a topic of interest (or life narrative, career, etc.).
- Create a slide show or PowerPoint with photos; create a photo collage.
- Create your own online or printable crossword puzzle and/or word search puzzle (search "create word searches for printing, puzzle maker, create your own crossword puzzles").

Toglia & Foster: The Multicontext Approach to Cognitive Rehabilitation.

- Create signs or invitations on the computer for an event.
- Create/design your own t-shirt online. (design your own coffee mug, jewelry, bookmark)
- Create folders and organize files into folders on computer.
- Create an online survey (e.g., SurveyMonkey).
- Design or set up an e-vite.
- Build your own webpage (investigate sites).
- Make your own online book or journal (e.g., life history, family tree, journal, photo book, comics).
- Make a printable greeting card or bookmark.
- Make business cards, invitations, or a brochure using online templates
- Take digital photos and make a digital jigsaw puzzle (search for "create your own photo puzzles").
- Download pictures from digital camera or phone onto computer and edit, crop, or rotate. Make a picture collage using online templates or Apps
- Follow criteria to create your own jewelry, car, sneakers, etc. online (search for "create/design your own jewelry or sneakers, etc.").
- Learn a new program or new features on a software program (e.g., Excel, PowerPoint, MS Word). For example, how to do a mail merge or how to create a budget sheet in Excel. Locate a video tutorial on the selected topic and follow instructions.
- Follow a YouTube video on "how to" (e.g., prepare a smoothie, learn a magic trick, or learn how to do the basics in Excel).
- Download or organize music on your phone.
- Follow directions to use a new app or online calendar.
- Explore new ways to use your smartphone or iPad (set alarms, reminders, put in appointments, etc.).
- Explore careers and requirements.
- Online shopping and comparison (e.g., shop at a drugstore, virtual supermarket, compare prices of appliances or cars).
- Find a take-out restaurant or meal delivery service; order a take-out meal for delivery.
- Search for different take-out menus in your area and plan meals.
- Investigate information on different websites (e.g., investments, prices, stocks) and create a table that summarizes the information).
- Investigate continuing education or certification courses in your area.
- Investigate and choose a reminder or organizer app. Identify desirable features, make a plan for learning and trialing it.
- Investigate different support groups/online groups, local community services, and resources.
- Investigate exercise classes, courses, workshops, etc. and costs.
- Use online library catalog to find a book, or investigate e-books available on a certain topic.
- Job search and complete a job application.
- Find information on a movie or sports website.
- Investigate and find a concert or play to go to within the next month.
- Download and learn a new App or software program.
- Investigate new computer games and brain teaser puzzles.
- Practice writing e-mails and requesting info.

Toglia & Foster: The Multicontext Approach to Cognitive Rehabilitation.

> **Appendix C.6. Sample Structured Multicontext Activity Treatment Session**

Two sample treatment activities are included: (1) kitchen food list activity (2) travel/toiletry list, with directions, before and after task questions for each activity, and an end of session strategy worksheet. These activities are sample MC supplementary activities from the Schedule Activity Module (S1.1). Directions can be presented in written form or verbally.

List of Kitchen Food Items

Activity Directions (can be written or stated verbally):

1. This is a list of items that can be found in a kitchen or pantry. Study the list and try to remember as many items as you can at one time.

2. Leave the list on the kitchen table and find and retrieve the calorie amount from the items and write them on the list. (If there is more than one of the same item, just choose one).

3. If the item is not in the kitchen, write the name on a separate shopping list.

4. When you are ready, repeat the above (look back at the list and study the next group of items and find the calorie amount).

5. Try to minimize the number of times you look at the list. Keep track of the number of times you look back at the list.

Pre-Activity Questions

1. How is this activity like other activities we have done?

2. What do you think might be challenging about this task? What parts of the task will you have to pay extra close attention to?

3. Think of the best way to go about doing this. What are some special tricks, methods, or strategies you could use to help you complete everything you need to do? Remember the items on the list?

Toglia & Foster: The Multicontext Approach to Cognitive Rehabilitation.

Kitchen List 1

Vegetable or Olive oil

Ketchup

Balsamic Vinegar

Milk

Can of soup

Breadcrumbs

Mayonnaise

Pasta

Salad Dressing

Peanut Butter

Cereal or Oatmeal

Jam/Jelly

Fruit Juice

Mustard

Tomato/Spaghetti Sauce

Butter or Margarine

Canned Tuna

times looked at list _____

Toglia & Foster: The Multicontext Approach to Cognitive Rehabilitation.

After Task Questions:

1. How did you go about doing this activity? What strategies or approaches did you use? How did you manage to ___ (keep track, stay organized)?

2. What types of challenges (obstacles or roadblocks) did you experience (or run into) as you did this activity? What parts were easy and what parts were most challenging?

3. If you did this activity again, what would you do differently next time?

List of Travel/ Toiletry Items

(Sample MC Supplementary Activity from Schedule Activity Module (S1.4))

Activity Directions (can be written or stated verbally):
1. This is a list of items that are needed before packing for a trip.
2. Your task is to see which items you already have and retrieve the size or volume (g, mg, ml) and write it down on the list, next to the item.
3. You will need to check rooms in your apartment or house, including your bedroom and bathroom.
4. Study the list and try to remember as many items as you can at one time before you search. Leave the list on this table.
5. Search for all the items on the list. If you don't have the item, write it on a separate shopping list.
6. Try to minimize the number of times you look at the list. Keep track of the number of times you look back at the list.

Pre-Activity Questions can be skipped to assess spontaneous transfer and strategy use OR 1-2 questions below can be asked (depends on client responses to previous activity).

Pre-Activity Questions
1. How is this activity like the kitchen activity we just completed?

2. What do you think might be challenging about this task? What parts of the task will be most challenging (or require special attention)?

3. Think of the best way to go about doing this. What are some special methods, or strategies you could use to help you complete everything you need to do? Remember the items on the list?

Travel List 1

Shampoo

Mouthwash

Liquid Hand Soap

Cough Syrup

Shaving cream

Vaseline

Powder

Lotion

Body Wash

Hand sanitizer

Tylenol, Aspirin, or other pain reliever (Capsule Amount)

Toothpaste

Hairspray

Face Wash

Deodorant

Sunscreen

Hair Conditioner

times looked at list _____

Toglia & Foster: The Multicontext Approach to Cognitive Rehabilitation.

After Task Questions:

1. How did you go about doing this activity? What strategies or approaches did you use? How did you manage to ___ (keep track, stay organized)?

2. What types of challenges (obstacles or roadblocks) did you experience (or run into) as you did this activity? What parts were easy and what parts were most challenging?

3. If you did this activity again, what would you do differently next time?

4. How do the activities we did today remind you of other activities you might do in everyday life?

5. Think about the strategies or methods you used with these activities. How could these methods help with other tasks?

Complete Strategy Worksheet on next page (or journaling/cognitive strategy action plan (Appendix C.9 or C.14)

Repeat with another horizontal activity. Repeat with list of kitchen supplies (inventory), list of office supplies (inventory), list of menu items (price). The Schedule Activity Module includes other supplemental lists.

Toglia & Foster: The Multicontext Approach to Cognitive Rehabilitation.

Strategy Worksheet:

Identify a strategy (or strategies) reviewed today that you felt was most helpful.

How or why did the strategy help?

Identify specific activities and situations where you could practice this strategy over the next week	When (Date)	Result and Self-Assessment
		Was strategy useful? (circle one) 1 = No 2= A little 3 = Somewhat 4 = A Lot How did it help? or Why didn't it help? What would you do differently next time?
		Was strategy useful? (circle one) 1 = No 2= A little 3 = Somewhat 4 = A Lot How did it help? or Why didn't it help? What would you do differently next time?

Additional Comments:

Toglia & Foster: The Multicontext Approach to Cognitive Rehabilitation.

Appendix C.7. Pre-Activity Questions: Guided Anticipation & Strategy Generation

Name _____   Date _____   Activity _____

Place a checkmark next to the number of all questions that are asked

____ 1. **Let's take a look at this activity. How is this activity similar to other activities we have done?**

____ 2. Anticipation of Challenges: **What types of challenges do you think you might possibly run into as you do this activity?** (or What types of things do you need to pay special attention to as you do this activity? What parts look easy and what parts might be tricky?) **Can you give me some examples?**

Question #2 Probes (optional)

____ 2a. **Let's think about the last time you did an activity similar to this when** _____ (there was a lot of information or details to keep track of). What did you need to pay special attention to? Or What parts were challenging?

____ 3. Strategy Generation: **Before we start, let's think of the best way to go about doing this. Can you think of some strategies (tricks, methods, special approaches) that you could use to help you complete everything you need to do?** *(Optional Probe Questions 3a-3c)*

Question #3 Optional Probes (if needed, identify activity challenges, e.g., there is a lot of information to keep track of)

____ 3a. **Symptom Mediation**: What methods can you use/do to _____ *(insert main symptom, e.g., Remind you of which step is next? Locate everything? Keep track of everything you need to do, etc.)* as you do this task?

____ 3b. **Task Mediation**: What can you do to help _____ *(insert task component, e.g., remember which items on the list you have already completed)?*

____ 3c. **Provide strategy suggestion or choice**: For example, "There may be some methods that can help. Do you think it would be better to _____ (e.g., write a list or keep track of things in your head)?"

Toglia & Foster: The Multicontext Approach to Cognitive Rehabilitation.

Appendix C.8. Post Activity: End of Session Self-Assessment

Name _____ Date _____ Activity _____

___ 1. <u>Strategy Awareness:</u> **Tell me how you went about doing this activity.** What was your method (plan, strategies, or approach)? Where did you begin and how did you proceed? (Reflect on strategy observations if needed.)

Question #1 Probes (if needed)

___ 1a. **Symptom Specific:** How did you manage to _____ *(insert main symptom, e.g., keep track of everything, stay organized, stay focused, or locate or find everything?)*

___ 1b. **Task-Specific:** Tell me how you managed to _____ *(choose task component, e.g., keep track of which bill was already paid)*

___ 2. <u>Identification of Challenges:</u> **What types of challenges (obstacles or roadblocks) did you experience (or run into) as you did this activity?** What did you need to pay special attention to? What parts were hard? Easy?

___ 3. <u>Strategy Generation:</u> **What would you do differently next time?** What special methods (tricks, approaches) or strategies could you use the next time you do this activity (to be more efficient, help things go more smoothly)?

Question 3 Probes (if needed)

___ 3a. **Symptom Mediation:** What methods can you use/do to _____ *(insert main symptoms)*?

___ 3b. **Task Mediation:** What can you can do to help you _____ *(insert main task components)*?

___ 3c. **Provide strategy suggestion or choice**

Toglia & Foster: The Multicontext Approach to Cognitive Rehabilitation.

Appendix C.9. End of Session: Strategy Bridging Questions or Structured Journal for Client

1. What did I do during this session?

2. What did I learn from this experience?

3. What might I do differently next time?

4. Think about the activities in this session. Identify activities that you do (or would like to do) that are similar.

5. How can the strategies or methods used in this session be helpful in your other everyday activities?

Toglia & Foster: The Multicontext Approach to Cognitive Rehabilitation.

Appendix C.10. Treatment Activity: Therapist Observation Checklist

Activity _____

Instructions

Y / N   Pt. confused about instructions. Needs additional clarifications/prompts to **begin** task.
Y / N   Client asks questions or seeks clarification **before** task.
Y / N   Client asks questions, seeks clarification or reassurance, etc. **during** task.

Strategies Observed	Errors/Symptoms Observed
Attention to Key Features	**Before Task**
____ Circles underlines or highlights keywords	____ Does not know how to begin
____ Uses finger to aid in reading or searching	____ Does not read directions carefully
Methods to Keep Track	____ Jumps in without reviewing materials or planning
____ Verbal rehearsal of keywords/criteria	**During Task**
____ Checkmarks, crossing out	____ Appears overwhelmed
____ Lists keywords/criteria to keep track of	____ Misses details
Stimuli Reduction	____ Loses track of key information/criteria
____ Screens/covers/removes part of information	____ Loses track of what they are doing/what step
Planning Ahead	____ Recalls only parts of item or instruction
____ Looks over material before beginning	____ Repeats steps/items (Looks for same item twice)
____ Rearranges materials before beginning	____ Appears to over-focus on pieces of information
Organized Methods	____ Gets sidetracked by thoughts or irrelevant information
____ Uses orderly or systematic approach	____ Does not go back and re-read questions/directions
____ Uses color coding, sorting, etc. to group information	____ Jumps around, haphazard order
____ Sub-vocalization or talks aloud plan	____ Disorganized (no apparent method)
____ Makes a written organized list or plan	____ Difficulty adopting a simulated perspective
____ Simplifies task – breaks apart steps	____ Limited search (searches too quickly, does not persist)
Self-Monitoring	____ Persists with same method, even if it is ineffective
____ Self-checking	**Self-Monitoring**
Other Strategies:	____ No self-checking observed during activity
Strategy use	____ Inconsistent self-checking during activity
Y / N Spontaneous, self-initiated	____ Does not recognize errors during performance
Y / N Frequency appropriate	____ Excessive self-checking
Y / N Timing appropriate	**Other Errors/Symptoms:**
Y / N Number appropriate	Y / N **Self-Recognition of Errors**
Y / N Degree of effort required to use manageable	Y / N **Therapist mediation/prompts provided**
Y / N Adjusted when needed	*Task Accuracy: poor fair good excellent
Y / N Effective	Time (can be estimated): _____
Comments:	

Toglia & Foster: The Multicontext Approach to Cognitive Rehabilitation.

Appendix C.11. Multicontext Treatment Session: Therapist Summary Worksheet

Client _____ Date _____ Session # _____

	Activity 1:	Activity 2:
Before Task		
Recognizes similarities to previous tasks/ sessions/experiences (check one)	❏ Yes ❏ No	❏ Yes ❏ No
Task challenges acknowledged? (check one)	❏ Yes ❏ Partially ❏ No ❏ Therapist identifies chall.	❏ Yes ❏ No ❏ No ❏ Therapist identifies chall.
Prompting used? (check one)	❏ Yes ❏ No	❏ Yes ❏ No
What task challenges were identified? (describe)		
Questions used for strategy generation (check all that apply)	❏ General ❏ Symptom-Specific ❏ Task-Specific ❏ Multiple Choice	❏ General ❏ Symptom-Specific ❏ Task-Specific ❏ Multiple Choice
Probing required to expand on answer? (check one)	❏ Yes ❏ No	❏ Yes ❏ No
Best client strategy generation (describe)		
What are all the strategies generated? (describe)		
During Task		
Strategies utilized (execution) *Effective?* (describe)	❏ Yes ❏ Partially ❏ No	❏ Yes ❏ Partially ❏ No
Error recognition/correction *Stop and review used?*	❏ Yes ❏ No ❏ Yes ❏ No	❏ Yes ❏ No ❏ Yes ❏ No
After Task		
Self-recognition of errors or difficulties (check all that apply)	❏ Spontaneously ❏ During Self-Eval ❏ With guidance ❏ General ❏ Symptom-Specific ❏ Task-Specific ❏ No Recognition	❏ Spontaneously ❏ During Self-Eval ❏ With guidance ❏ General ❏ Symptom-Specific ❏ Task-Specific ❏ No Recognition
Identifies strategies/ methods used If yes, specify:	❏ Yes ❏ No Describe:	❏ Yes ❏ No Describe:
Generates alternate strategies If yes, specify:	❏ Yes ❏ No Describe:	❏ Yes ❏ No Describe:
Identifies other activities where strategies could be applied. If yes, describe:	❏ Yes ❏ No Describe:	❏ Yes ❏ No Describe:

Did Awareness change across activities: ❏ No ❏ Slightly/unsure ❏ Yes
If yes, provide example:

Did Strategy Use change across activities: ❏ No ❏ Slightly/unsure ❏ Yes
If yes, provide example:

Other Observations/Comments:

Toglia & Foster: The Multicontext Approach to Cognitive Rehabilitation.

Appendix C.12. Therapist Self-Reflection and Analysis of Mediated Learning Methods

Describe Question, Probes, or Mediation (What happened?)	Your Analysis	Alternatives: How else could I have phrased this or handled this?

Toglia & Foster: The Multicontext Approach to Cognitive Rehabilitation.

Appendix C.13.1. Multicontext Treatment Fidelity Tool

Therapist/Client _____   Activity _____

Length of Activity/Session _____

Adherence Rating (A) – **bolded questions only, marked as A** – *Provide only 1 overall rating for each numbered question.* Involves rating whether the main treatment component was present or absent. If the treatment component is present, then proficiency for this treatment component is also assessed (see below). If the treatment component is absent, a 0 is assigned for proficiency. Bolded and Numbered Questions are rated for Treatment Adherence.

> A rating scale: 1 = Treatment component was absent although there was opportunity to implement; 2 = Treatment component was fully implemented; 9 = No Opportunity to demonstrate treatment component or component is appropriately missing (guidelines followed or adhered to)

Proficiency Rating – **lettered questions, marked as P**

Proficiency Definitions – This involves rating quality or the extent to which the treatment component follows the guidelines. The lettered questions provide examples of the treatment guidelines, but they are not exhaustive and not all of the lettered questions are appropriate for each client or session.

> P rating scale: 0 = No evidence as treatment component was absent; 1 = Little evidence of proficiency; 2 = Emerging/Adequate proficiency; 3 = Proficient or skilled implementation. P- Cannot be scored if A is scored as 9. 9 = No Opportunity because client spontaneously answers question.

I. Metacognitive Section

	Pre-Activity Discussion Phase	A Rating (1-2; 9)	P Rating (0-3; 9)
1. Orientation to Session	**1. Orientation to the session activities is provided (A)**		
2. Anticipation (not used if person is already aware – 9a)	**2. Discussion related to potential challenges, or task difficulty level (self-ratings of difficulty areas)** ____ yes ____ no **(A)** *Note:* Questions may be skipped before task if person is unaware or it is the first or second session or at end of tx if person is aware (9a). **Guided questions to identify challenges or task difficulty level are used** (Below are sample criteria (C)) Questions proceed from general to more specific: ____ yes ____ no *Probing questions used- if responses were vague, incomplete, unclear or task-specific* (e.g. tell me more about that) ____ yes ____ no		
3. Strategy Generation If strategy is provided with <u>no</u> guiding attempts, this component is absent.	**3. Questions related to strategy generation or task methods (A)** *Note:* May be skipped *If perceives task as easy and it is 1ˢᵗ-2ⁿᵈ session or it is the end of treatment (last sessions) and spontaneous strategy use is expected 9a.* **The Process of Strategy Generation is Guided** ____ yes ____ no **(P)** (e.g., Tell me how you would go about this, what is your plan, what methods, etc.) **Sample criteria (C)** a). Probing questions are used if responses are vague, unclear, incomplete or inefficient strategies are mentioned? ____ yes ____ no ____ No Opportunity b) If the client has difficulty generating strategies, before proceeding to activity, therapist (check all that apply) ____ Focuses strategy question on specific symptoms or task components. ____ Reminds client of strategies used in previous activities ____ Provides choice of strategies or strategy suggestion (as last option)		

Toglia & Foster: The Multicontext Approach to Cognitive Rehabilitation.

	During Activity-Mediated Learning	A (1-2; 9)	P (0-3; 9)
4. Mediation "Stop and Check" Periods Mediated Learning (If no task errors, mediation is not needed)	4. Mediation is used during the activity *if* the person has difficulty (A) ____ yes ____ no ____ No opportunity (no problems) *Frequency of mediation:* ____ 1-2x ____ 2-3x ____ 4-5x ____ > 5x ____ (specify if possible) (F) **Mediation is directed at the task process: (below is sample criteria (P)** a) *The majority of Mediation uses* How/ why, describe or "tell me" questions (open-ended / allow elaboration ____ yes ____ no ____ No Opportunity *Versus* ____ <u>Avoids</u> Direct Cues or Direct feedback (pointing out errors) *If direct cues are used, do they follow attempts at mediation or general questioning?* ____ yes ____ no ____ No opportunity c) Client is asked to explain or describe task methods: ____ yes ____ no d) Questions or cues directed at helping the client (check all that apply) ____ Self-recognize or discover errors ____ Figure out what is wrong/ correct errors ____ Self-monitor cognitive symptoms ____ Generate alternative methods or strategies ____ Task directed questions or questions focused on the task itself (last option) ____ Provide strategy choice, suggestion, only if other attempts fail. *Generally Avoids:* ____ yes/no questions the majority of time (otherwise emerging if above applies) **Overall,** the content of mediation or type of cues are appropriate for the client: ____ yes ____ no *Other Considerations* e) *If client is unaware of errors, therapist* helps client discover errors themselves through questions ____ yes ____ no ____ No Opportunity f) *Therapist repeats or rephrases what the client says or reflects on observations e.g. "It seems as though it is hard to keep track of everything"* ____ yes ____ no ____ No Opportunity h) Awareness of performance errors are increased before strategy mediation? ____ Yes ____ No ____ No Opportunity ____ Missed Opportunity j) Positive feedback on strategy use? ____ yes ____ no ____ No Opportunity h) **Other Observations:**		
	Post Activity Discussion	A (1-2; 9)	P (0-3; 9)
5. Self Assessment	5. Person is asked to reflect on task challenges, difficulty level or self-evaluate performance (ratings) **(A)** (N/A if no task difficulty- rate 9) **Questions. Therapist questions or reflection of observations guides client in reflecting on activity challenges or experiences (P)** ____ yes ____ no Below is sample criteria (C) *Guided Questions or therapist observations help client to (check those that apply)* ____ Self-recognize performance errors ____ Identify easy and hard aspects, (parts that went smoothly vs tricky, challenging) ____ Evaluate performance b) *Probing questions or why/ how if appropriate, to investigate challenges?* ____ yes ____ no ____ no opportunity ____ Missed Opportunity **OR** c) **Structured self-assessment** *with answer templates or checklists are used:* ____ yes ____ no d) *If needed, questions are asked during the self-assessment process to guide client in self-recognizing errors?* ____ yes ____ no ____ no opportunity		

Toglia & Foster: The Multicontext Approach to Cognitive Rehabilitation.

6. Strategy Post-Discussion **Reflection On Strategies or Task Methods Used**	*6. Strategy Discussion about Task Methods or Strategies used – includes therapist reflection of strategy observations and guided questions (A)* **Therapist uses guided questions to help client reflect on the methods or strategies used (P)__** *eg. Tell me how you went about doing this activity. What methods did you use? What was your plan?* Sample Criteria b) *Probing questions used, (general to specific) if strategies are vague or incomplete:* ____ yes ____ no c) *Positive feedback provided regarding strategy use or generation:* ____ yes ____ no ____ no opportunity (no task difficulty) d) *Observations of methods/ strategies used are shared by therapist for validation, if the person has difficulty identifying them?* ____ yes ____ no e) *Questions on generating alternate strategies are asked if strategies were lacking or ineffective* (e.g. would you do anything differently? ____ yes ____ no ____ no opportunity (no task difficulty) f) <u>If the client has difficulty generating alternate task methods or strategies</u> -*Therapist (check all that apply)* ____ Gently guides the client to strategies through questions (validation?) ____ Reminds the client of previous strategies ____ Provides choice of strategies or strategy suggestion (as last option) g) *Asks client to summarize successful task methods or strategies or identify what has been learned.*		
	Post Activity Discussion	A (1-2; 9)	P (0-3; 9)
7. Strategy Application	**7. Application of strategies or principles to past or future activities or situations are stated or discussed (A)** ____ yes ____ no **Therapist guides the person in identifying application of strategies, task methods, or principles to other activities or situations (P)** Therapist explicitly helps client connect activity experiences or relate strategies /task methods to past or future activities/situations: ____ yes ____ no Probes with (how, tell me) questions, if answers are incomplete. If client is unable to identify other activities/ situations. provides suggestions as *last option* if client cannot make connections. Helps the client reflect on what was learned from the session and how it applies it to other past or future activities or situations: ____ yes ____ no		
	**II. Therapeutic Support:** *General Observations Throughout Session (proficiency only; 0-3)*
1. Supports client in figuring out problems and fosters self-efficacy.		▓	
2. Questions are asked in a nonthreatening and supportive manner (neutral tone).		▓	
3. The focus is on what the person can do to enhance performance, rather than on deficits.		▓	
4. Therapist promotes a sense of supportive presence and makes excellent use of encouragement, praise, positive reinforcement, and validation.		▓	
5. Therapist reflects on observations of strategies or effective task methods; or reframes/rephrases or interprets client statements or observations.		▓	
	**III. Treatment Activities** *(Adherence only rating 1-2)*
1. Treatment Activities are **functionally relevant** (includes functionally relevant materials such as schedules, menus, bills, medications, food items, household or work-related tasks).			▓
2. Treatment Activities are different from previous session (same activity is not used or graded up in difficulty) (N/A if it is the first activity)			▓
3. Therapist uses activities that are structured horizontally or have similar cognitive demands to previous treatment activity. (N/A if it is the first activity)			▓
4. Activities are at optimal level of challenge (not too easy and not too hard) Optional: Circle one: *Not challenging, Mildly challenging, Moderately challenging, or Very challenging* See definitions at the end of Appendix C.13.2.			▓

Toglia & Foster: The Multicontext Approach to Cognitive Rehabilitation.

Appendix C.13.2. Multicontext Fidelity Tool Rating Criteria and Clarifications

Note: Refer corresponding MC fidelity rating score sheet for Adherence and Proficiency Ratings,

Fidelity Adherence Rating: *Clarifications on absence (1) or presence (2) or of treatment components.*

Orientation – The therapist describes activities and explains directions, <u>before</u> asking anticipation questions.

Anticipation – Discussion before task that relates to or potential task challenges or task difficulty, or things that need to be watched out for. This can include *ratings or predictions of difficulty level* or discussion of previous challenges or cognitive symptoms with similar tasks in the past. This component is absent if the person is presented with instructions and there is no discussion about task characteristics or potential task challenges (and it is not the first treatment session).

Strategy Generation – Discussion before the task, that relates to task methods (how the person plans to go about the task), strategies, or tricks. If client is instructed to use a particular strategy, *and No* questions or probes are asked, this component is absent. If strategy is provided by therapist but then therapist questions client about strategies or task methods, this component is present. If client initiates stating a strategy on their own, this component is considered present but an "a" is marked after it (2a to indicate the person stated the strategy themselves). Competency rating looks at probing of strategies, if appropriate.

Mediation – Discussion during the task that helps the person stop and reflect on task methods, generate strategies or check work. If therapist stops activity and reflects on observations ("it seems like it is getting challenging to keep track of everything"), this component is present. If therapist directly points out task errors or provides direct feedback <u>without any attempt to ask questions or reflect on observations</u>, this component is absent. If client asks for clarification of directions, or therapist asks client to review directions; this is not mediation. Repeating directions or asking the client what step they are at, is also not mediation. This component may be appropriately missing if the client self-recognizes errors or is able to progress through the activity without assistance.

Self-Assessment – Structured self-assessment (self-checking answers), self-ratings, or discussion that helps the person reflect on or evaluate their performance. Reflections on observations of the process of self-monitoring (e.g., I noticed that you checked yourself) as well as task challenges (e.g., it seemed like there was a lot of information all at once) are considered present. If errors are pointed out or the person is provided with direct feedback ***before a*ny questions are asked** or there are **no attempts** to describe observations of self-monitoring or task challenges or help the person reflect on performance or self-check their own work, this component is absent.

Strategy Post Discussion – Discussion after the task that relates to task methods, tricks or strategies or how the person went about doing the task including observations of strategy use. If therapist reflects on the process and methods or strategies observed, this component is present. <u>If there is no discussion of strategies, task methods, or reflection on strategies used, this component is absent.</u> If client spontaneously mentions strategies or task methods used during self-assessment and therapist reflects on observations, comments or discusses further, this component is considered present. If there is no discussion about strategies or task methods used, this component is absent.

Strategy Application – Discussion or mention of how the strategies used within the activity relate to past or future activities. If there is <u>no discussion or mention</u> about connection or application of the strategies or self-monitoring methods to other activities or situations (past or present), this component is absent. If therapist states how the strategies are linked to previous activities or future activities, this component is present.

Toglia & Foster: The Multicontext Approach to Cognitive Rehabilitation.

Fidelity Proficiency Rating Criteria: Score = 0 (missing or no evidence) to 3 (Proficient). If treatment component is absent, a 0 is assigned for proficiency. 9 = No opportunity. See Appendix C.13.1.

Item	Little Evidence (1)	Emerging/Adequate (2)	Proficient (3)
Anticipation	Therapist identifies challenges for the client almost immediately **after asking** initial question. Discusses challenges in similar or past activities without connections to current activity. Only has client rate difficulty level or predict performance with no discussion.	Makes a clear attempt to have client identify possible difficulties, challenges, or things to watch out for. Type of questions, wording and/or probing needs to be improved. May not follow up on incomplete responses.	Guided Questioning used before the task is performed. Questions are directed toward facilitating task analysis or assessing task demands and challenges. Additional questions are asked when responses are vague or incomplete. For example, why will that be challenging? What about __? Wording (neutral) and type of question (open) is good and progresses from general to specific if needed. If client confidently perceives the task as very easy, it is acceptable not to use additional probes.
Strategy Generation (this component is missing if strategies are provided without any questions)	Therapist provides strategy almost immediately **after asking initial question** or without giving the patient a chance to generate any strategies/ alternate strategies on their own. Or therapist states observations of strategies used and then asks strategy questions about strategy use, without questions related to alternate strategies.	Makes a clear attempt to have client identify strategies used and/or generate alternate strategies, although questions asked, wording, and use of probes may not be optimal (e.g. may include yes/no questions). Questions may be overly specific too quickly (does not go from general to more specific questions). Therapist could provide more probing or questioning, if client reports a strategy. (note: if strategy stated is specific, efficient, or appropriate, further probes are not needed and rating is 3). May provide strategy after other attempts fail.	Guided questions with good probes for strategy use and/or generation of alternate strategies are asked the majority of the time. Uses good follow up or probing questions. Probes vague or incomplete responses. Progresses from general to specific. If needed, highlights task challenges – e.g., what will you do to help manage all of the information on the page. Generally avoids yes/no questions and direct cues. May suggest strategy after other attempts fail. If client self-initiates a strategy, therapist asks client to describe strategy, if it is vague, partial or incomplete such as "I will plan first, or "Tell me more about how you would go about planning."
Mediation	Stops activity and provides feedback, reflects on observations about task methods without questions or probes or points out errors <u>quickly after asking initial question</u> or provides direct cues such as telling or pointing where to look, telling person what to do next, the majority of time. Jumps in as soon as errors are observed, without providing the client the opportunity to figure out what is wrong on their own.	Makes a clear attempt to help the person figure out what is wrong during the task but does not jump in too soon. Questions need improvement (e.g., may ask yes/no questions or Question may be too focused on task or task specific. If client indicates no challenges – this component is minimal.	Helps the person assess task methods, recognize errors or generate strategies. Guided questions with good probes are asked the majority of the time. Questions are open-ended or they progress from general to more specific questions. Self-discovery of errors or self-generation of alternate strategies represents successful mediation.
Self-Assessment	Asks client to rate task difficulty without discussion or structured self-assessment. Identifies challenges for the client **almost immediately after asking initial questions** or reflects upon observations regarding task challenges, before providing the client with an opportunity to self-reflect. Provides a structured self-assessment method but points out errors.	Makes a clear attempt to help the person self-check work or reflect on task difficulty level or challenges. May need to structure the process or provide the person with a method to help the person self-check (e.g., use piece of paper). Uses probes when needed although questions asked, wording, and use of probes may not be optimal (e.g., overly specific too quickly, yes/ no). Might be overly direct too quickly.	Facilitates self-checking and guides person in self-discovering errors. Guided questions with good follow-up probes or questions when needed are asked the majority of the time (questions are general and open-ended in nature and may progress to more specific questions). If client is aware, tries to have client identify task characteristics that were more challenging, if appropriate. Reframes task-specific responses to broader challenges. *If there are **no errors**,* this component is minimal. Reflections regarding why task was easy/ easier, what was different -should be used, if appropriate.

Toglia & Foster: The Multicontext Approach to Cognitive Rehabilitation.

Item	Little Evidence (1)	Emerging/Adequate (2)	Proficient (3)
Post strategy Discussion	Therapist identifies what strategies were observed without questions. Does not ask what methods were used or identifies methods observed almost **immediately after asking the question.**	Asks about task methods or strategies used during the task and/or asks about alternate/future strategies; however, questions are not optimal (overly specific too quickly, wording could be improved, focused on a specific task, yes/ no). Makes a clear attempt to help the person identify the task methods or strategies used to be successful (or could be successful), although questions asked and use of probes may not be optimal.	Guided questions with good follow up probes or questions when needed are asked the majority of the time. Questions are general and open-ended in nature and may progress to more specific questions after using more general quest). e.g., What methods did you use? Why do you think using your finger helped? What other methods could be used?" If strategies were observed but client doesn't mention them after questions, therapist shares observations and probes. e.g., "I noticed you were using your finger as you were reading– tell me more about that." Note – if no errors, strategies may not be needed so this component may be minimal.
Strategy Application	Therapist states the activities that the strategy could be applied to or relates strategy to previous activities for the client. If questions are asked, the therapist does not give the client a chance to respond and immediately provides examples.	Makes a clear attempt to help the person identify how strategies could be applied to future activities or how they are related to past activities. Or how present activity is related to other activities… Probing, questions or wording could be improved - at times too direct or asks yes/no questions)	Guided questions with good follow up probes or questions when needed are asked the majority of the time. Questions are initially general and open-ended in nature and may progress to more specific questions.

Note: For the category of proficient, questions should initially focus on the process (general method, self-checking) and not on the task or task outcome, with yes/ no questions avoided. Specific questions and direct suggestions follow the protocol, only after attempts at facilitating responses with other, more general questions have failed.

Therapeutic Support 0 (missing or no evidence) to 3 (Adequate).

Item	Little Evidence (1)	Emerging (2)	Adequate (3)
Focus on Figuring out Problems: Treatment supports client in figuring out performance problems and fosters Self Efficacy. (this component may be missing if there are no errors and the task was easy for the person)	Provides direct feedback, instruction or cues. Identifies problems or tells client what to do or provides strategies/ solutions. Or tells client what they observed with little opportunity for client to figure out on own.	Encourages client to figure out performance problems or identify things that might help prevent/ control cognitive symptoms some of the time; however, questions are not optimal. Question may be too task-specific or too close-ended at times.	Questions are guiding rather than direct. Yes/no questions are avoided. Questions focus on general process rather than the specific task. May progress from general to specific. Conveys confidence in client's ability to successfully address problems and achieve successful performance.
Supportive Tone Questions asked in a nonthreatening tone supportive manner.	Rushed, non-supportive tone. Tone may indirectly suggest the person is having difficulty.	Tone is neutral and supportive but Direct language is used that could be possibly threatening (Is this too difficult?, too hard?).	Tone is even, positive, calm, neutral. Allows time for client to respond. Avoids negative language.
Focus on Methods to Enhance Success Focus is on what the person can do to enhance performance, rather than on deficits, and what is wrong (this component may be missing if there are no errors and the task was easy for the person)	Direct negative/critiques client's performance feedback. Frequently points out problems or errors directly. Focuses on problems, errors. Uses negative language the majority of time (deficits, problems) and does not discuss *methods* that can promote success. May provide, direct, task specific advice.	May use some negative words (words that imply a deficit/weakness) used such as difficulty, problems, errors, but also asks client about things they can do to control errors or promote success. If needed, provides some suggestions for methods that promote success during discussion. Generally supports client in taking responsibility for managing their cognitive symptoms.	Asks clients about things they can do to control cognitive symptoms or promote success. Empowers client to take responsibility for managing their cognitive symptoms and identifying methods that optimize performance. Generally avoids negative language Avoids directly pointing out things that could be done differently. Helps to promote awareness of methods used for success- without directly stating them (regardless of whether there are errors)

Toglia & Foster: The Multicontext Approach to Cognitive Rehabilitation.

Item	Little Evidence (1)	Emerging (2)	Adequate (3)
Positive, supportive atmosphere: excellent use of encouragement, praise, positive reinforcement, or validation **Positive, supportive atmosphere, continued**	Provides minimal encouragement or positive reinforcement although opportunities are present.	Positive encouragement is provided some of the time (there are missed opportunities) or Feedback is overly general "great job" or focused more on task outcome rather than the process. (task methods, self-monitoring).	Provides positive feedback the majority of time with a focus on praising the process and methods used (if appropriate). Provides positive feedback that is specific or explains why methods or performance was good. Uses the sandwich method when appropriate (always starts with positive before providing constructive suggestions).
Reflection of Observations Reflects on past/present observations of strategies or effective task methods; or reframes/ rephrases or interprets client statements or observations. (This component may be missing if there are no errors and the task was easy for the person.)	No reflection, reframing is used, although opportunity is clearly present and could have facilitated strategy discussion or awareness.	Reflects on observations before allowing client to self-reflect on the process or task methods used themselves; may not always check if client accepts reflection made. I noticed that you…. It seems that….	Positively reframes, interprets or shares observations on positive task methods used by client. Reflects on observations appropriately, e.g. when client is stuck, or unable to identify strategies they used. Client has been asked questions or provided with some opportunity to self-reflect on the process or methods used before observations or interpretations are shared. Checks if client accepts re-framing, interpretations or observations made.

Treatment Activities: Only adherence is rated: (1= absent; 2 = yes, implemented).

1. Treatment Activities are functionally relevant (includes functionally relevant materials such as schedules, menus, bills, medications, food items, household or work-related tasks). Bean bags, puzzles, pegboard or worksheets with random shapes, letters, numbers, symbols or objects are not considered functionally relevant.

2. Treatment Activities are different from previous session – The activity should look different than the previous activity. The activity can have the same directions, with different materials and it can be a near transfer task (alternate version of a previous activity) but it should not be exactly the same. For example, if the same exact activity or exercise is presented but increased in difficulty, this is not considered sufficiently different from the previous sessions.

3. Activities are structured horizontally or have similar cognitive demands to the previous treatment activity. Activities share similarities with previous activities as outlined in treatment manual.

4. Activities are at optimal level of challenge – Activities that are mildly or moderately challenging may be at an optimal level of difficulty and scored a 2. See definitions below. If an activity is not challenging or very challenging, this treatment component is scored a 1.

Treatment activities level of challenge scale: In addition to rating, the therapist may want to indicate the level of challenge of the activity by circling one of the choices indicated on the form and defined below.

___ Not Challenging (no errors or self-corrections are needed, performed efficiently and quickly with no effort).

___ Mildly Challenging (optimal). Requires effort; slow but accurate or able to self-correct errors on own, may be inefficient or uses trial and error, occasionally stuck but eventually figures out solution on own; may make 1-2 errors that are not recognized, does not need prompts or mediation within the activity).

___ Moderately Challenging (Optimal). Requires effort, client makes several errors, loses track several times or becomes stuck at 1-2 points, may need prompts/ mediation at 1 or 2 points within the activity, may self-correct errors with questions or prompts.

___ Very Challenging. Client unable to progress within the activity, or makes multiple different errors and needs continual support or frequent cues, support or mediation throughout the entire task. Client may stop doing the task due to high level of challenge.

Toglia & Foster: The Multicontext Approach to Cognitive Rehabilitation.

Appendix C.14. Structured Journal Formats for Client

Sample 1

Activity	More Practice? 1 2 3 4 No Yes	What did I learn?	What will I do differently next time?

Sample 2

Activity	Challenges Anticipated	Result	What I learned

Toglia & Foster: The Multicontext Approach to Cognitive Rehabilitation.

Appendix C.15. Client Strategy Worksheet

Identify a strategy (or strategies) reviewed today that you felt was most helpful.

Identify specific activities and situations that you could practice this strategy over the next week	When? (Date)	Result and Self-Assessment
		How useful was the strategy? (circle one) 1 = Not useful 2 = A little 3 = Somewhat 4 = A Lot **How did it help? or Why didn't it help? What would you do differently next time?**
		How useful was the strategy? (circle one) 1 = Not useful 2 = A little 3 = Somewhat 4 = A Lot **How did it help? or Why didn't it help? What would you do differently next time?**
		How useful was the strategy? (circle one) 1 = Not useful 2 = A little 3 = Somewhat 4 = A Lot **How did it help? or Why didn't it help? What would you do differently next time?**

Additional Comments:

Toglia & Foster: The Multicontext Approach to Cognitive Rehabilitation.

Appendix C.16. Cognitive Strategy Action Plan

Cognitive Strategy Action Plan

PROBLEM When is it most likely to occur?	
GOAL AND PLAN *What strategy or methods will I try? How? Where?*	To help (above) _____, I will do the following: **Steps:** Situations or tasks that the strategies or above plan will be used with: What things could interfere with carrying out the plan? What could be done to manage obstacles or unexpected interference?
DO **Execute the Plan**	When or how often? _____ I will carry out the above plan by _____ (date).
REVIEW AND ASSESS *How did it go? What worked? What didn't? What changes or adjustments can be made so that it works better?* *What might I do differently next time?*	I will review and assess on: _____ What worked well? What parts went smoothly? What was most challenging in carrying out the plan? What parts need more practice? Identify any barriers or obstacles to carrying out the plan as intended What changes or adjustments should be made for next time?

Toglia & Foster: The Multicontext Approach to Cognitive Rehabilitation.

Appendix C.17. My Action Plan for Keeping Track

I seem to have the most challenges keeping track of things when…..	
Strategies to help me keep track of information	What can you do to help make sure you are keeping track of everything you need to?
Managing situations Next time I lose track of things in the middle of an activity, I will...	
Review and Assess Are revisions needed?	I will check my plan on _____ (date) How well did the plan help me keep track of information? What changes or adjustments should be made for next time? What should I do differently?

Toglia & Foster: The Multicontext Approach to Cognitive Rehabilitation.

Appendix C.18. Emotional Regulation Action Plan

	Emotional Regulation Action Plan
Problem When is it most likely to occur?	Problem: Context: When is it most likely to occur? Triggers?
Warning Signs	Earliest Signs: Signals/Alarms (How do you know that you have a problem?): *If others notice…what can they do to help?*
Strategies	What can you do to help yourself _____ Are there self-cues, phrases, mental alarms, or "mental images" that you can use to help yourself in this type of situation?
Review and Assess *What worked? What didn't? What changes or adjustments to the plan are needed?*	Review on _____ (date)

Toglia & Foster: The Multicontext Approach to Cognitive Rehabilitation.

Appendix C.19. Cognitive Log (Turn Sideways)

Log of Cognitive Lapses Name _____ Date _____

Date/Time of Event	Problem: What Happened? Describe troublesome cognitive experience or cognitive lapse or functional problem	When? Describe the context: Where were you? Were other people involved? What occurred immediately before, how did you feel at the time? (e.g., tired, relaxed, angry, etc.)	Why do you think this may have occurred?	Potential Solutions for Future? Adaptations? Strategies?

Toglia & Foster: The Multicontext Approach to Cognitive Rehabilitation.

Appendix C.20. Generic Self Evaluation

Did I....	Yes	Needs Improvement	Comments
review the directions carefully?			
take enough time to make a plan before beginning?			
stick to my original plan?			
complete everything I set out to do?			
keep track of the time?			
stay focused?			
follow all directions accurately?			
use strategies?			
complete everything efficiently?			
approach the task in an organized way?			
pay attention to all of the details?			
keep track of everything I needed?			
leave myself enough time to complete everything?			
run into any unexpected difficulties?			
double-check myself?			

Toglia & Foster: The Multicontext Approach to Cognitive Rehabilitation.

Appendix C.21. Simplified SELF RATINGS

1. This activity _____

    Needs improvement   **Does not need improvement**

2. *I am satisfied with how I went about doing this activity.*

    Not Satisfied   **Yes, Satisfied**

3. I used efficient methods to complete this task.   No   Yes

4. I was able to manage challenges during this activity.   No   Yes

5. I was able to successfully complete this activity.   No   Yes

6. I was able to stay focused during this activity.   No   Yes

7. I was able to keep track of everything I needed to do.   No   Yes

8. I was able to stay organized during this activity.   No   Yes

9. I was able to pace my speed (not too fast and not too slow).   No   Yes

Toglia & Foster: The Multicontext Approach to Cognitive Rehabilitation.

Appendix C.22. Simplified Self-Monitoring Ratings

My Timing was

| Too slow | Just Right | Too fast |

My Mental Energy is

High

Med

Low

Very Low

Self-Ratings – 4-point scale

1. *This activity*

| **1** | **2** | **3** | **4** |
| Needs improvement | | | Does not need improvement |

2. *I am satisfied with how I went about doing this activity*

| **1** | **2** | **3** | **4** |
| Not Satisfied | | | Yes, Satisfied |

3. *During this activity it was…*

| **1** | **2** | **3** | **4** |
| Very Hard to pay attention | | | Easy to pay attention |

Toglia & Foster: The Multicontext Approach to Cognitive Rehabilitation.

Appendix C.23. Strategy Self-Rating Scale

During the activity, I .....

Consistently used strategies to help keep track of information or items	4
Used a strategy to help keep track the majority of the time (50-90%)	3
Occasionally used a strategy to help keep track (<50%)	2
Did not use a strategy (e.g., verbal rehearsal or self-talk) to help keep track during the activity.	1

Self-Ratings – 10-point Scales of Targeted Cognitive Symptoms

During this activity it was…

1	2	3	4	5	6	7	8	9	10
Very Hard to stay focused									Very Easy to focus on task

1	2	3	4	5	6	7	8	9	10
Very Hard to get started									Easy to get started

1	2	3	4	5	6	7	8	9	10
Very Hard to keep track of everything									Easy to keep track of everything

1	2	3	4	5	6	7	8	9	10
Very Hard to pay attention to all the details.									Easy to keep pay attention to all the details.

Toglia & Foster: The Multicontext Approach to Cognitive Rehabilitation.

Appendix C.24. Pre-Made Goal Examples for Clients

I would like to be able to...
IADL

- Make a pasta and salad for dinner.
- Order from a meal delivery service online.
- Go shopping to the local mall by myself to purchase a birthday gift for a relative.
- Go to the local grocery store or drugstore to buy a list of 3-5 items.
- Pay my bills online.
- Take my pills on time at the right dosage during the day.
- Complete a list of daily errands.
- Find a new recipe/Make a new recipe.
- Plan meals for the next week.
- Keep track of time when I am involved in activities during the day.
- Organize my closets once a week so I can find things more easily.

Learning Technology: Learn or relearn how to use a device, App or software

- Use my phone to reply to a text message from my dad.
- Learn to use Instagram to view my grandsons __.
- Learn how to edit photos or videos of __.
- Learn to use an iPad to send e-mails to my granddaughter once a week.
- Use Skype or Facetime with my daughter
- Attach a photo to an e-mail I send to my daughter.
- Learn how to send an online greeting card to ____.
- Investigate an app to help me remember my medication.

Reading

- Read from a book at least 30 minutes a day and remember what I read.
- Read the newspaper for 15 minutes each day and have conversations with others about current events.
- Keep track of the thread of a story when reading a novel, so that I don't have to re-read sections.

Toglia & Foster: The Multicontext Approach to Cognitive Rehabilitation.

Remembering

- Know what I did yesterday without asking my wife.
- Know the upcoming events without asking my wife.
- Remember to put things I need to do in my phone calendar every day.
- Remember my grandchildren's names within the next 2 weeks.
- Follow a conversation in a group of 3-5 people.
- Remember to take important items (e.g., glasses, wallet, mobile phone) whenever I leave the house.
- Keep track of where I have placed my things (keys, phone, eyeglasses, wallet).
- Remember to check my online banking account 2 times a week.

Social/ Leisure

- Exercise 3 times a week or go to the gym 2 times a week.
- Enroll in a weekly class at the local community center in order to socialize with new people.
- Call a friend or a relative once a week.
- Answer e-mails from friends.
- Invite a friend over for lunch.
- Plan a social get together with friends within the next 2 weeks.

Toglia & Foster: The Multicontext Approach to Cognitive Rehabilitation.

Appendix C.25. Sample Goal Book

My Activities

My Interests: Activities that I like	Activities I need to do

My Strengths: Activities that I am good at	Activities I want to get better at

My Goals:	Methods I can use to help me meet my goals

Toglia & Foster: The Multicontext Approach to Cognitive Rehabilitation.

Appendix C.26. Subgoaling Worksheet

Areas of Concern (Sub-Goals)	Strengths within skill area	Subskills that need to be strengthened and sample strategies	Simulated tasks agreed upon by client and/or family member

Toglia & Foster: The Multicontext Approach to Cognitive Rehabilitation.

Appendix C.27. Goal Plan

Goal: _____

What do I need to do to prepare: _____
_____

Parts of this task I can do easily	Areas for Improvement	Strategies

Things I need to watch out for	
Other Activities that this Same Plan and/or Strategies might be useful with	

If my goal is met, I will be able to _____

Toglia & Foster: The Multicontext Approach to Cognitive Rehabilitation.

Appendix C.28. Goal Setting and Tracking

Date	Goal	Revised	Removed	Added

Toglia & Foster: The Multicontext Approach to Cognitive Rehabilitation.

Appendix C.29. Goal Rating Form

Functional Goal:

Levels of performance	Achievement	Rating
	Goal is met	5
	Almost met	4
	Partially met	3
	Lots of room for improvement	2
	0% or baseline	1

Specific Strategy Goal:

Levels of performance	Achievement	Rating
	Goal is met	5
	Almost met	4
	Partially met	3
	Lots of room for improvement	2
	0% or baseline	1

General Self-Monitoring Goal:

Levels of performance	Achievement	Rating
	Goal is met	5
	Almost met	4
	Partially met	3
	Lots of room for improvement	2
	0% or baseline	1

Toglia & Foster: The Multicontext Approach to Cognitive Rehabilitation.

APPENDIX D: Supplementary Material

APPENDIX D.1	Strategies for Specific Cognitive Domains or Performance Errors (Chapter 7)
APPENDIX D.2	Sample Activity Themes and Activities: Cognitive Demands that Remain Consistent Across a Series of Treatment Sessions (Chapter 8)
APPENDIX D.3	Sample of Everyday Treatment Materials for Cognitive Rehabilitation (Chapter 8)
APPENDIX D.4	Overview of Multicontext Activity Modules (Chapter 8)
APPENDIX D.5	Inpatient Activities: Simple Level 1 or 2 Structured Activities using Pre-made Multicontext Activity Modules (Chapter 8)
APPENDIX D.6	Sample Higher Level Activity Sequence from Multicontext Activity Modules (Chapter 8)
APPENDIX D.7	The Metacognitive Framework: Problems Encountered and How to Manage Them (Chapter 10)
APPENDIX D.8	Things to Remember During Mediated Learning (Chapter 10)
APPENDIX D.9	Examples of Multicontext Treatment Analysis and Fidelity Ratings (Chapter 11)
APPENDIX D.10	The Multicontext Approach Presented within the Rehabilitation Treatment Specification System (RTSS) (Chapter 11)
APPENDIX D.11	Levels of Awareness and Multicontext Treatment Implications (Chapter 14)
APPENDIX D.12	Completed Sample of Multicontext Treatment Planning Worksheet (Chapter 15; Blank form C.2)
APPENDIX D.13	SUB-GOALING Example (Chapter 12; Blank form C.25)
APPENDIX D.14	SUB-GOALING: Example 2 related to Work as a Claims Analyst (Chapter 12)
APPENDIX D.15	Example of a Completed Goal Plan (Chapter 12; Blank form, C.26)
APPENDIX D.16	Examples of Functional Goals Consistent with the Multicontext Approach (for therapist) (Chapter 12)
APPENDIX D.17	Example of Goal Rating (Chapter 12; Blank form C.28)

> **Appendix D.1. Strategies for Specific Cognitive Domains or Performance Errors**

Initiation

- Use verbal action cues to "get going."
- Use self-coaching cues for encouragement or to persist (e.g., "Just do it," "Keep going").
- Use images that prompt action and persistence.
- Place external cues in the environment that are linked with or prompt an action.
- Recollect (visualize) past experience with an activity that is similar or the same as the one the person is about to perform.
- Use broad, general categories before specifics for idea generation.
- Hum or play a rhythm, song, or music to pace activity (certain points in a song can become associated with completion of task components).
- Set visual, auditory, or tactile timers.
- Set external reminders (voice messages, alarm signals, etc.) themselves to prompt later actions.
- Use a checklist to prompt each step.

Disinhibition

Impulsivity

- Count to 10 (or tap foot 10x) before responding.
- Hum or play a rhythm, song, or music to pace actions or activity.
- Create personalized mental or visual images, metaphors, or external cues such as pictures or symbols to cue self to slow down and regulate timing (e.g., stop sign, a slow turtle crossing the road).
- Use verbal rehearsal to "slow down" during activity.
- Use mental rehearsal or visualization of "just right timing" or good timing (versus going too fast with an X over the too fast image) prior to an activity.
- Repeat instructions before beginning to prevent tendency to jump into tasks too soon.
- Point to each item before choosing.
- Cross or check each item/step off a list.
- Self-rate each response as "good timing" or "too fast" and keep a tally.
- Talk aloud or whisper steps or actions to pace actions.

Resisting Distractions

- Identify, select, or verbalize key attributes and priorities before starting.
- Eliminate, cover, or remove items that are irrelevant or unnecessary before starting.
- Verbally rehearse or mentally imagine end goal or product before starting.
- Create or use an external cue such as a picture of the goal or general image (e.g., photo of train tracks as a reminder to stay on track), if person has difficulty using internal cues.
- Set time goal and timer to resist tendency to wander and get sidetracked.
- Use periodic alerts to assess and monitor progress toward goal.
- Select visual image (internal or external) for staying focused and use during tasks.
- Remove or cross out irrelevant information.

Toglia & Foster: The Multicontext Approach to Cognitive Rehabilitation.

- Mentally rehearse completing task without getting sidetracked versus with getting sidetracked.
- Anticipate and plan for methods to reduce or manage distractions (if-then action plan).

Keeping Track (Working Memory)
- Verbal Rehearsal – Repeat keywords, phrases, or instructions several times to self.
- Mental Rehearsal – Mentally rehearse or imagine performing the steps or task procedures of an activity before performing it.
- Picture and rehearse what was just read, heard or said.
- Use verbal mediation, self-talk, or talk aloud through a task to focus attention.
- Break information or tasks into smaller parts.
- Group or associate similar items together into smaller chunks.
- Re-arrange or re-organize items before starting task.
- Create a mental or written checklist or follow a list.
- Plan for interruptions; If interrupted (e.g., phone call), place key item down or write note as a cue to where you left off or hold onto object last used as a cue.

Attending to Details
- Highlight, circle or identify most important information before beginning.
- Stimuli reduction – block out or cover irrelevant parts of stimuli array.
- Use finger to point to relevant task stimuli or features to enhance attention.
- Use pacing strategies (take frequent cognitive rest breaks)
- Double-check work.

Flexibility: When Stuck
- Use imagery.
- Search for a Different Way to represent the situations or problem:
    - Change point of view, re-examine problem in a different way.
    - Choose new sensory code (e.g., use imagery).
    - Use external representations when possible, such as charts or matrices, for keeping track of information and drawings or diagrams to find relations in the problem.
    - Reorganize information: classify or group information differently.
    - Summarize the main issues.
- Restate goal; summarize problem or goal.
- Brainstorm and/or use a concept map.
- Use verbal scripts: "If I get stuck, it is time to 'change plays.'"
- Make action plans: "If it doesn't go as expected, I should…"
- Prepare multiple plans (Plan A and Plan B).
- Choose an image of "letting it go" or "switching moves."
- Write out each possible course of action. For each course of action, list possible outcomes, both positive and negative.
- Talk aloud through each step.

Toglia & Foster: The Multicontext Approach to Cognitive Rehabilitation.

Remembering

Reading Retention (Green, 2012)

- Use visual imagery during reading – translate words or sentences into mental images.
- Take notes of keywords while reading; use a keyword list at the end of each paragraph or page.
- Restate the material, paraphrase or summarize information at the end of each page, paragraph, etc.
- Identify the main idea of the paragraph (gist).
- Self-Questioning: "Am I keeping track of everything? Am I following the story? Does it all make sense?"
- Preview context by skimming paragraphs and subtitles to obtain information on the context or big ideas before reading for specifics.
- Test oneself. After reading, ask self questions about the content then re-read to check answers.
- See also Exhibit 7.4 for specific memory strategies.

Remembering To Do Things (Prospective Memory)

- Turn time into event- or activity-based tasks so the cue for action is more obvious.
- Strategic clock monitoring – check the clock regularly and more frequently as the target time approaches.
- *Mental rehearsal* – Imagine or visualize yourself doing the future act at the correct time or to the correct cue. Think of the context – where you will be and what you will be doing – before and immediately after the targeted action (e.g., taking meds). Think of what would happen if you forget. Thinking about the time that you will need the information (retrieval) during the time of encoding links encoding and retrieval together and enhances the probability of recall. Additional forms of mental rehearsal are listed below
    - *Imagery-based episodic future thinking (EFT).* EFT is an approach of vividly imagining experiencing future situations and during which complex mental scenes are created (Altgassen et al., 2015).
    - *Imagery focused on the cue:* Imagine as much about the future cue (What will you see? Where will you be?) as possible from your own personal perspective and describe it in as much detail as possible (Raskin et al., 2019).
- *Implementation intentions* – Refer to the link between a specific cue and an intended behavior or action. "If I encounter situation X, then I will initiate action Y." Implementation intentions are then often repeated to oneself and combined with mental rehearsal (Brom & Kliegel, 2014; Gollwitzer, 1999; Radomski et al., 2018).
- Verbal rehearsal of intentions (Ihle et al., 2018)
- Content-free periodic cues such as STOP: Stop, Think, Organize, Plan (Fish et al., 2007).
- Identify environmental triggers or cues and associate them with the intended action.
- Put reminders (e.g., lists, signs) in key salient locations.
- Use an appointment book, daily schedule.
- Medication list/timers/pill box organizers.
- Set reminders on phone or watch, timers/alarms, voice messages or text messages to prompt future actions.
- Create a "things to do" checklist or use a checklist app.

Remembering Experiences and Events (Episodic Memory)

- Visual journal – Take photos and videos of information to be remembered during the day using a smartphone and replay in evening and/or next morning. Use digital journal with photo/video capability.
- Use a memory log, journal, electronic or digital journal to record or dictate daily events, conversations, etc.
- Identify most important points – Use of one- or two-word key retrieval cues and summaries.
- Predict need to write things down and self-test or predict what notes say and self-test.

Toglia & Foster: The Multicontext Approach to Cognitive Rehabilitation.

Remembering Where Things Are

- Choose key, consistent locations for items (glasses, keys).
- Retrace steps backward.
- Self-questioning: Where was I? What do I usually do on a Tuesday?
- Think of the overall context first.
- Anticipation – When placing object down, imagine yourself finding it.

Remembering Faces and Names

- Keep a list of names with key features in day planner or electronic journal.
- Associate the name with something familiar or the person's physical features.
- Review the name list daily.
- SALT Method (Herrmann, 1991, Graham-Scott, 2007).
    - Study = Familiarize and study the face.
    - Ask = Get the name of the person and use it immediately at least three times.
    - i.e., Use it once when introduced, again in the conversation, and finally when parting.
    - Leave = Move away from the person or group and rehearse the name.
    - Test = Return to the person at some point and use the name.
- SAVE Method
    - Say name at least three times in conversation.
    - Ask question about name.
    - Visualize.
    - End with name.

Organization

- Task Simplification – break task into chunks or smaller, more manageable steps before starting.
- Remove or cover items not needed or decrease the amount of information that is in view at any one time.
- Plan ahead – draw or write out plan.
- Look for similarities, patterns, clusters, categories or associations before starting; color code or group related information, materials or steps.
- Gather or rearrange materials before starting task (e.g., place objects in order of use).
- Episodic Cueing – ask person to think of a specific time and place where they carried out a similar activity in the past to facilitate planning and organization. (Hewitt et al., 2006).
- Mentally practice or rehearse an activity in one's mind.
- Think back to a previous similar activity experience to guide in planning and organizing information in a new situation.
- Create a list to plan a task.
- If overwhelmed, use task reduction or task segmentation methods to decrease the amount of stimuli that is attended to at any one time.
- Identifies overall context or "whole picture" before attending to the pieces.

Toglia & Foster: The Multicontext Approach to Cognitive Rehabilitation.

> **Appendix D.2. Sample Activity Themes and Activities: Cognitive Demands that Remain Consistent Across a Series of Treatment Sessions**

Different types of lists as described below can be used to represent distinct activity themes as described in Chapter 7 and 8. An example of each activity theme is presented below. Although each uses lists, the skills required are different, as described in Chapter 7.

- *Search and locate* or gather items on a list (e.g., kitchen supplies, stationery supplies, toiletries).
- *Checking and comparison*: Identify discrepancies (e.g., check off all items on the list that are in the closet or that are missing; make a list of the items in the cabinets/closets that are not on the list).
- *List of same task*: e.g., address cards, invitations, series of phone calls.
- *To-Do lists*: e.g., all activities involve following a list of five things to do (obtain information, find locations, deliver messages) within busy environments.
- *Follow a list of steps/directions* to a task that is provided. This requires translation of written or auditory directions into action. If activities require a fixed order, the person needs to understand how each step is connected to the next.
- *Break down complex activities* or directions into a list (simplification).
- *Create a list* from a schedule or provided information (e.g., create a list from shopping items circled on a page).
- *Use a list to enter information* into a schedule, form, invoice or bill.
- *Create a checklist* prior to starting a multiple-step task.
- *Generate a list of ideas* or things (brainstorm ideas) that need to be included on a list (e.g., to plan a webpage, PowerPoint presentation, etc.).
- *Keeping track or immediate recall* of items on a list, after studying or reading the list and looking away.

<u>Examples of Activities within Activity Themes:</u>

Activity Theme: Keeping track of items that are on a list

- Recall the last three items from a list or that were just put away into a cabinet or *recall where the last three grocery items were placed*.
- Remember the first 3-4 items from a list of food items (or ingredients from a recipe) and then retrieve items from kitchen cabinets.
- Remember the first 3-4 items from a shopping list and then find the items on Amazon.com.
- Recall four different items on a list and determine if they are in a supply cabinet.
- Look at a list of appointments and place two appointments into a calendar (remembering appointment, date and time) without looking back.
- Remember a person's name and address from a list and without looking back, address an envelope.
- Remember the first three items on a list and look up information, using your phone or computer (find closest restaurant or hotel, weather for tomorrow, headline news).

Activity Theme: Search and locate items that meet specific criteria or rules.
All activities involve holding in mind 1-2 pieces of information while searching or looking for information and updating or keeping track of information that is changing.

- Using the classified section, identify the number of one-bedroom apartments within certain locations or price range.
- On a menu, identify the number of entrees that are under $20.00.
- In kitchen pantry, look at nutritional labels and identify the number of items that have 3% or less of sodium.
- Find the number of advertisements for cars, clothes, or electronics/computers in a newspaper or magazine.

Toglia & Foster: The Multicontext Approach to Cognitive Rehabilitation.

- Using the TV calendar, identify the number of comedy shows playing during the week.
- Find the number of art exhibits available over the next two weeks within the local area.
- Using the schedule of classes and activities, find out the number of exercise classes this week.
- Using the menu, identify all of the vegetarian options.

The below activities involve holding in mind 3-4 pieces of key information while searching or looking for information. The person can be asked to figure out a method for keeping track of the items that meet the criteria. Alternatively, the person can also be asked to mentally keep track of what has been found.

- Using menu(s) online or on a table: Identify at least five vegetarian sandwiches, no more than 600 calories, are less than $9.00, and do not have cheese.
- Identify all the movies that are rated PG, starting time between 1:00 and 1:30 p.m., and in the area of _____ (specify).
- Identify all the automobiles on sale that are within a certain price range and are made by specific manufacturers.
- Identify all the one-bedroom apartments with _____, between a certain price range, and within a certain vicinity.
- Identify two clothing stores online and find all the XL, long-sleeve pullover shirts for a man that come in a solid color _____ and are under $34.00.
- Find items (e.g., microwave oven, TV, computer, watch, dishwasher, oven, book, clothes) that match 3-5 specific features and price range in a pile of catalogs or online.
- Using the internet, find a flight that is less than $450.00 and is on a weekend that flies nonstop to ____ and is not more than two hours long.

Activity Theme: Activities that involve searching and using or shifting between two or three different responses

- Cross off items on the list that are in the kitchen and circle the missing items.
- Using the monthly schedule, place a star on all MD appointments, circle all hair appointments, and * all _____ appointments on the calendar.
- Given a list of events on a three-month calendar, place a star on sporting events and a dot on concerts.
- In a newspaper, find all the one-bedroom apartments between a certain price range, then switch to finding two-bedroom apartments only within a certain vicinity.

Activity Theme: Activities that involve using or shifting back and forth between two or three pieces of information or locations to find information (three different computer screens, three different pages, to obtain answers).

- Using business cards, name list, and information sheet, identify the people who are on the list, registered for a convention, are from manufacturing, and have paid (from the Multicontext Business Activity Module).
- Using the calendar of sightseeing activities and the information sheet (with prices and locations), identify activities within _____ price range that are available on _____ days.

Activity Theme: Following multiple step directions (easily printed off internet or YouTube videos).

- Follow three- or four-step directions to a magic trick, origami, game, arts and crafts, directions to a new app, or to program an alarm or electronic device, etc.
- Follow steps to make an online birthday card, online word search puzzle, or invitation.
- Follow directions to make three different sandwiches for a picnic/kid's lunch.
- Follow a list of errands to carry out on a hospital floor, within a room/house, on the computer or phone.
- Video directions: "How to" directions on YouTube or other web sites.

Toglia & Foster: The Multicontext Approach to Cognitive Rehabilitation.

- Follow directions to find offices/unfamiliar locations within the building, using a floor map.
- On the internet, follow directions to send an e-card, or e-invite, make a crossword puzzle, design a t-shirt, make a word search puzzle, find or design a printable bookmark, make a picture collage with photos.

Activity Theme: Copy or duplicate information from a model – requires attention to detail and spatial relationships.

- Copy a table or place setting for 8-10 people from a photo, diagram, or model.
- Decorate cookies using a model; arrange cheese and crackers according to a model.
- Copy a page layout, flyer, or sign on the computer.
- Copy a chart, graph, or table.
- Copy information from one calendar to another.
- Copy a list, schedule, or recipe.
- Copy a room layout.
- Copy directions or route to a specific location from Google Maps because your printer is broken and your cell phone battery is low and you don't want to depend on it.

Activity Theme: Compare/contrast information that is provided (Provide coupons, advertisements, flyers, or internet; make a table that shows comparisons.)

- Review ads, coupons, or flyers and identify the best deal for rug cleaning, dry cleaning, taxi, car service, or shuttle rates to the nearest airport.
- Compare cell phone plans, college tuition, or prices for specific items at different stores.
- Compare credit card deals or checking account fees or saving interest rates at 3-4 different banks.
- Compare price, including delivery charge for ordering a large pizza pie.
- Compare parking garage prices in the nearest city or in the area (for weekend or particular date/time).
- Identify and compare three beauty salon hours within 30 minutes and their rates.
- Compare UPS and Fed-Ex rates for mailing a 30 lb. package OR find the least expensive (or quickest) method for mailing a 30 lb. package.
- Compare 3-4 health club/gym membership rates within the local area.
- Vacations: plane tickets, hotel prices, apartments with specifications (internet).

Activity Theme: Investigate or find specific information.

- Find out lunch specials in the cafeteria and prices.
- Find out the local headline news, biggest international news stories, entertainment news (from a particular day).
- Find out location and hours of nearest post office.
- Obtain information on the weather for next day or week in local area or at a specific location.
- Find a particular movie listing and reviews, or star ratings.
- Find concerts of a certain artist, price range, location, or dates.
- Find sport games for a specific team, time range, date or location.
- Find sports scores of a particular team, statistics on specific players, or player facts.
- Find the list of top 50 songs and identify the song that is # _____.
- Find the quickest (or least expensive) method of public transportation to get to a specified location.
- Find a book published by a certain author or books or article on a specified topic on a shelf, in the library, or online.

Toglia & Foster: The Multicontext Approach to Cognitive Rehabilitation.

- Find out what exhibit is at the local museum.
- Investigate the cost of sending a plant/flowers to someone in the hospital from two different flower shops.
- Find three stores that deliver pizza or lunch in the area and identify delivery fees (or find local pharmacies, florists that deliver and investigate delivery fees).
- Find a movie (comedy or specify type or name) playing at a movie theater within __ minutes.
- Find sports statistics (e.g., basketball player facts, statistics).

Activity Theme: Identifying the most important or relevant information

- Identify relevant information in a travel advertisement or a bill with a yellow highlighter.
- Identify the main idea or key points in a paragraph, news, or magazine article.
- Watch or listen to a radio or TV news report, or interview, conversation, etc. and take notes, summarize, or identify the most important points.
- Identify or summarize key points from an event, interview, or therapy session.
- Identify keywords to convey a message for a telegram writing situations or tweet (limited # of words).
- Summarize key information presented in graphs, charts, or tables.
- Provide scenarios such as the following example, which purposely contains unnecessary information. The person is asked to identify the information that is most relevant to answering the question: "Pat just bought a new shirt that would look great with navy blue pants. She likes the colors blue, gray, and green. She does not have any blue pants. Pat likes to shop online but when it comes to buying pants, Pat likes to go to the store in person so she can try them on. Most of the shirts she has are gray, beige, or green. What color pants should Pat buy?"

Activity theme: Figuring out a way to consolidate a lot of information

- Create a checklist from multistep/complex directions.
- Create a table to consolidate information presented.
- Create a table for price comparison (e.g., three different bank offers on credit cards, health plans or gym, etc.).

Activity theme: Generating ideas (or at least 2-3 options)

- Determine possible things to make for breakfast, lunch, dinner, or snack based on items in the kitchen.
- Given a controversial issue, generate different perspectives or arguments.
- Given a problem, generate a variety of different solutions.
- How many different combinations of coins can make 65 cents?
- How many different number sequences can you make with these five numbers?
- What are the different lunches you can order from the menu if you have $7.00?
- How many different combinations of items can you buy for $25.00 (use catalog)?
- Free Associations to a given topic: e.g., things that people drink; name as many different animals as you can; think of as many uses of as you can for the following objects: paper, toothpick, cards, pencil; name as many different things you see on the street; think of all the things that you would find in the dairy section of a supermarket.
- Write down all the things you do when you get up in the morning until lunch.
- In two weeks, you are leaving for a trip to Europe. You will be away for one month. List everything you will need to do before you leave. You will be away for six months. Revise your list.
- You are planning a surprise birthday party for _____. List everything that you will need to do.

Toglia & Foster: The Multicontext Approach to Cognitive Rehabilitation.

Activity theme: Create or generate methods of organizing information *e.g., Different ways to sort or organize...*

- Magazines/catalogs (e.g., by dates, topic/interest).
- Coupons (e.g., expired vs unexpired dates vs. food category vs. greater than 75 cents)
- Business cards (e.g., by business, or location), restaurant cards.
- Mail (junk mail or advertisements, flyers of event, household bills, store bills, coupons).
- Computer files into folders or file folders in a file drawer.
- Stack of bills.
- Items in a supply closet (or create an inventory system for items in a supply closet).
- Items in a cluttered drawer or closet.
- A shopping list.
- Items on a bulletin board (e.g., menus, notices or memos, event flyers).

Activity theme: Unstructured activities involving identifying steps to do, investigating information, planning or organizing

- Investigate a specified topic on the internet.
- Investigate best price on an iPad.
- Find the best deal for a weekend getaway within 60 miles, etc.
- Design a PowerPoint presentation on a topic of choice.
- Create a digital story or narrative on one's experiences.
- Create a webpage or blog post.
- Investigate different apps for photo organization or reminder apps or timer apps.

Additional Examples of Unstructured activities:

Planning a day's events
Material: Magazine, newspaper, flyers or brochures, computer
You are planning a 5-hour outing/sightseeing experience for a visitor from out of town. You have $35.00 to spend. You can do more than 1 activity, but you cannot come with more than $15.00.

Shopping Online: You have $95.00 to spend. You have to buy the following presents: Birthday gift for a 5-year-old niece; wedding anniversary present for close friends; a birthday present for a female friend's 40th birthday party; a graduation present for your 17-year-old nephew. What gifts will you buy? Here are some catalogs for you to look through.

Sample Group Planning Activities:
As a group, identify all the things that need to be done (brainstorm – broad categories first and then specifics) and then put steps in order. For example, When, where, who will be involved? How? What supplies, shopping list, cost? Divide the workload.

- Plan a holiday party, trip, bake sale, fundraiser, group lunch, picnic/barbecue;
- Plan a project (e.g. woodworking, small garden/planting).
- Plan to interview someone (e.g., physician, administrator, etc.) for a newsletter;
- Plan a mock news broadcast with current event topic, create a newsletter, webpage, or brochure for the program or group.

Toglia & Foster: The Multicontext Approach to Cognitive Rehabilitation.

Increasing cognitive load: To add cognitive load or multitasking demands to any of the above activities, the following can be included.

- **Interruptions during Activities**: Introduce interruptions that the person has to manage multiple times within a session (phone calls, text messages, irrelevant questions, people coming in asking a question, suddenly turning on radio, etc.).
- **Time Monitoring and Prospective Memory Activities**: e.g., set time goals or time limits for each sub-task or task; predict the time that will be needed for a task, estimate the time that has passed during an activity and the time remaining or include prospective memory tasks as listed below.

Prospective Memory: Fixed/ Recurring

- Every _____ minutes, circle the step you or up to or write a note in your planner with the time, the event you are up to and any notes to yourself that you would like for future reference.
- Every _____ minutes, check your e-mail to see if you received an e-mail from me.

Time-Based Prospective Memory Sample Tasks-indicate times (e.g. 5 min, 10 min) or specify exact time.
During this activity, (specified times) you have to

Time: _____ Find a take-out restaurant in the area that delivers lunch.
Time: _____ Put a pot of water on the stove to make some tea.
Time: _____ Check the pot on the stove and turn off the gas when the water boils.
Time: _____ Call the pharmacy and find out what time they close today.
Time: _____ Write your name, time, and date on this index card (or back of the page).
Time: _____ Check your cell phone for a text message.
Time: _____ Write a note in your planner.
Time: _____ Water plants in the room.
Time: _____ Take (or ask about) your medication.
Time: _____ Give this envelope to the receptionist or leave in room XX.
Time: _____ Call and leave me a message on my cell phone asking about your next appointment.
Time: _____ Stop and look up a phone number for _____.
Time: _____ Check your phone voicemail and write down any messages.
Time: _____ Check the refrigerator to see if you need to buy milk or eggs.
Time: _____ Check the weather for the weekend.
Time: _____ Ask me about our next appointment.
Time: _____ Stop and feed dog/cat or state that dog needs to be fed.
Time: _____ Let me know when we only have 10 more minutes left in our appointment.

Cue or Event-Based Prospective Memory Sample Tasks

- Whenever someone walks in the room, give them one of the message envelopes.
- When the alarm/ timer rings _____ (any of the above)
- When the phone rings, remind me to check my cell phone.
- I am leaving my bag here. Whenever I leave the room, remind me to take this bag.
- Whenever I introduce a new activity, write the time on this sheet of paper.
- At the end of the session, ask about your next appointment or check the calendar for the next appointment.

Toglia & Foster: The Multicontext Approach to Cognitive Rehabilitation.

Appendix D.3. Sample of Everyday Treatment Materials for Cognitive Rehabilitation

The sample activities in Appendix D.2 require that everyday materials be readily organized and accessible. This may involve organizing files or kits within a clinic for easy access. Below are suggested materials. Some of these materials, along with directions are also provided within the structured Multicontext Activity Modules.

- Variety of lists: lists of different birthday dates, anniversaries, appointments, etc. to place in monthly or year calendar; lists of websites or apps to locate; inventory lists for office supplies, closet, books (variety of lists are included within activity modules)
- Variety of schedules: class schedule, TV shows, sightseeing, things to do, sports, film festival (all included in Schedule Module); concerts, movies, theater, children's activities, event schedules, airplane, train, bus schedules or timetables. Can be printed off internet.
- Calendars: Wall calendars, monthly, weekly calendars of different sizes (Schedule Module).
- Food circulars (paper or accessed online)
- Wide variety of menus (Menu Module)
- Kitchen items on shelves that have different prices (mock simulation of grocery store)
- Restaurant cards (Menu Module)
- Variety of simple recipes
- Household bills
- Coupons (paper or online) or flyers
- Wide variety of greeting cards or invitations
- Brochures: travel, vacation, AAA travel book, sightseeing brochures
- Catalogs
- Newspapers and magazines
- Diagrams, room, floor or building layout, diagram of table setting or place setting, layout for flyer
- Sample mail items (junk mail, bills, etc.)
- Access to internet using phone, tablet, computer to print materials, view how-to videos, compare and contrast information on different sites, follow multiple-step written or video directions (how-to videos)
- Applications: Credit card, membership application, jobs, passport, driver's license
- Forms or certificates to complete (Business Module)
- Business cards (Business Module)
- Address lists and letters (Business Module); envelopes
- Graphs, charts, tables (Business Module)
- Data to copy into an Excel file (Business Module)
- File folders (sorting, filing, assembling, collating) (Business Module)
- Medication bottles with different instructions (for organization or scheduling)
- Invoices and receipts (Business Module)
- Multiple-step directions to follow (all Activity Modules)

Also:

- Stickers to add prices to any object (or greeting cards)
- Different-colored highlighters,
- Magnetic or bulletin board, magnetic tape, colored magnets (to place menus, schedules, lists)

Toglia & Foster: The Multicontext Approach to Cognitive Rehabilitation.

Appendix D.4. Overview of Multicontext Activity Modules

Module	Materials	Description
Schedule Module	Schedule Activity Module Manual 12 laminated wipe-off schedules: 4 alternate schedule activities each with 3 levels of difficulty. Items in each schedule can be grouped into three categories. 260 activity cards, 98 direction cards USB card with additional materials • Lists of varying lengths that accompany schedules • Detailed information sheets	Includes four parallel schedule activities (Class and Activity, Sightseeing, TV, and Things To Do). Activities are organized into 9 activity themes that are numbered: (1) Search and locate – lists, (2) Search and locate – cards, (3) Shifting, (4) Sorting, (5) Entering into schedules, (6) Entering information, (7) Finding information, (8) Creating lists, and (9) Complex questions + Supplementary activities. Within each theme, there is a range of activities that includes using lists to locate information on schedules, find items on schedules that meet select criteria, enter information into schedules, create lists of options from schedules, or use a combination of sources to select information from schedules.
Menu Module	Menu Activity Manual 2 laminated dry-erase picture menus and 3 laminated written menus that differ in the number of items and detail 108 small-sized cards (food cards, restaurant cards), 30 large-size direction/question cards USB card with additional materials • A variety of menus • Information sheet • Food item lists	Includes 3 levels and the same 9 activity themes + Supplementary activities as the Schedule Module. Activities include locating food items on menus, comparing lists and menus for discrepancies, selecting items that meet certain criteria, creating lists of options based on food preferences or price range, or using a combination of materials to choose restaurants or plan meals.
Business Module	Business Card Activity Manual 54 Business cards, 40 question cards 31 Direction Cards USB card with additional materials • Name Lists • Registration lists • Receipts and Invoices • Certificates and Invitations • Travel expense forms • Address lists	Includes 3 levels and the same 9 activity themes + Supplementary activities as the Schedule module. Activities revolve around the theme of a business convention. Activities involve comparing name lists and name cards for discrepancies, identifying people who meet certain criteria, entering information into tables, completion of receipts and invoices, work simulation activities such as preparing a mail merge, compiling, and assembling information for a mailing, files, or folders.

From: www.multicontext.net

Toglia & Foster: The Multicontext Approach to Cognitive Rehabilitation.

Appendix D.5. Inpatient Activities: Simple Level 1 or 2 Structured Activities using Pre-made Multicontext Activity Modules

Activity Theme: Search and locate using lists. Directions can focus on searching and locating information while managing and keeping track of items on a list, immediate recall or holding several items in mind at once or shifting between different rules and responses (not shown). Each session is presented within a metacognitive framework explained in Chapter 10.

Session	Materials	Search and Locate items from a list	Keeping track — Recall items from a list	Arrangement of Materials
Session 1	Classes and Activities Schedule TV Schedule *Schedule module*	1.1 Find the items on this list that are also on the schedule or menu. *Optional:* write day and time or price of items found OR Identify the cards that have matching items on the schedule or menu or list (2.1-2.2) *Note: Not all items from the list are on the menu. Directions do not explicitly state this and are purposely vague.*	1.5 This activity involves identifying items on the list that are also on the schedule. Study the list and try to remember several items from the list at once. Then turn the list over or look back at the list as few times as possible. *This requires a rehearsal strategy* (1.4 or 1.6 directions could also be used).	Items are spread far apart to place increased demands on motor skills and ability to hold information in mind during a task (working memory). Can be done in standing with list and calendar on a magnet board or on a table, placed behind or to the far left or right and calendar to opposite side to increase standing tolerance and weight shifting
Session 2	Sightseeing *Schedule module* Picture Brunch Menu			
Session 3	Things to Do calendar *Schedule module* (1.D1) Café menu or Michelle's menu or Peter's *Menu module*			
Session 4	Hospital 3-day *Menu module Level 1* (5a, 5.1) Name list *Business module*	Highlight the items on the menu that are also on the list (5a, 5.1 or 5.2) Circle the names that are on both lists (1.1) or Compare both invitation lists and identify the duplicate names. *(1.2 can also be used)*	*Same as above* 1.5 Study the list and try to remember several items from the list at once. Then turn the list over or look back at the list as few times as possible.	One list can be presented on a computer or menu. The other can be on table or lists/menu can be copied back-to-back to place more demands on ability to keep track.
Session 5	Restaurant cards *Menu module* Kitchen Food list (S1.1) (requires kitchen) *Schedule module: Supplemental lists* *Choose two activities for each session*	Identify the restaurants on the list that also have restaurant cards. (Menu module) Find and retrieve items from the list that are also in the kitchen. (S1) *Schedule module* *Optional:* Person writes location of restaurant or business or makes a shopping list of items not in the kitchen	*Same as above* Study the list and try to remember as many as you can. Turn over the list and retrieve as many items as you can before you look at the list again. 1.4 (Business module) can also be used	Cards and list are spread apart. List can be on bulletin board or table. Selected cards can be picked up or required to stay in place. Requires ambulation (walking, standing while thinking) or mobility to different areas of kitchen. To reduce mobility demands, items with distractors can be placed in same cabinet, closet or counter.
Session 6	Kitchen Supplies (S1.2) *Schedule module* Business cards *Business module*	Same directions as Kitchen food list. Identify the business cards that also have matching names on this list (2.1) or identify names on the list with matching cards). *Optional:* write business and/or location next to the person's name on list.	*Same as above* Using kitchen supply list or business card list.	

Toglia & Foster: The Multicontext Approach to Cognitive Rehabilitation.

Session	Materials	Search and Locate items from a list	Keeping track Recall items from a list	Arrangement of Materials
Session 7	Food Cards *Menu module* *Schedule module* Supplementary lists Toiletries (S1.4) *(requires bathroom or toiletry closet)*	Identify or choose the picture cards that have matching items on the list (2.2) or menu (2.1) *or* Identify items from the list that also have a matching card. *Optional:* Person checks menu and writes down price of food items on the list. Identify and gather the toiletry items that are also on the list.	*Same as above*	Cards and list are spread apart. List can be on bulletin board or table to increase demands on the ability to keep track. Alternatively, the client can hold the list as they are searching for and gathering items.
Session 8	*Schedule module* Supplemental lists: Packing list (s1.5) *(person's bedroom)*, Office supply list (S1.6), or Grocery store list (S1.3)	Identify and gather the items that are also on the packing list (or office supply list, grocery store list, etc.). *(requires real-life contexts or kitchen or food or office supply circular)*	*Same as above* Study the list and try to remember several items from the list at once. Then turn the list over or look back at the list as few times as possible.	

Note: The order of the activities within the treatment sessions above are not fixed (they can be interchanged) and are used for purposes of illustration only. Numbers correspond to # activities within the Multicontext Activity Modules (www.multicontext.net)

Appendix D.6. Sample Higher Level Activity Sequence from Multicontext Activity Modules

All below activities are Level 3 (#9 Complex Questions and Supplemental activities) and require similar cognitive demands:

- Use of detailed information (information sheets, directions, registration list).
- Selecting information and creating a list of options while following criteria.
- Shifting between two or more sources (information sheet and list, website and list, recipe and list).

Session	Materials	Directions
Session 1 Schedule Module	3.A9: Class and Activities Schedule and Information Question #10.	You and two coworkers would like to sign up for classes. Two of you are off of work Monday, Wednesday, and Friday; the third person is only available from 10:00 a.m.–2:00 p.m. on those days. Each person's budget is $50 for the month and the preference is for the Harrison Center and Main Street Community Center because they are handicapped accessible. Make a list of all possible classes and details that fit the budget and ensure availability for everyone.
Session 2 Schedule Module	3.E9: Sports Schedule and Information Sheet, Question # 9.	You are traveling alone to the East Coast in November. You would love to attend either a Surfs or Whales away game during that time. Your budget for the ticket is $50 and you can only attend weekend or Tuesday games. Put together a summary of possible games including all pertinent information.
Session 3 Schedule Module 3 Options	3.B9: Sightseeing Schedule and Information Sheet, Question #9.	You are on vacation in a city that you have never been to before. You are arriving on Monday at 11:00 a.m. and leaving on Saturday at 12:00 noon. You want to go on as many tours as possible paying cash only. Make a list of all of the possible tours that you could go on. Include all relevant information.
	3.C9: TV Schedule and Information Sheet, Question #1.	You prefer to watch Entertainment shows but you have to take care of your neighbor's dog every day after work this week so you are only able to watch shows from 8:00 p.m. to 10:00 p.m. Make a list of all the shows you can watch and include all details needed to watch them. Also, indicate which Entertainment show is the most popular and least popular.
	3.D9: Things to Do Schedule and Information Sheet Question #10.	Your neighbor wants to exercise more but has recently enrolled in college and does not have any extra money to spend. She has asked if she can join you on some of your activities away from the house that you walk or bike to. She is available on Mondays, Tuesdays, and Wednesdays. Make a list of all things to do that she could accompany you on that are less than 2 hours long and are no charge. Include the time, date, and duration of each activity.
Session 4 Menu Module	9a: Selecting restaurants: restaurant cards, restaurant info sheet, Question #9 (or other questions).	You and your friend are trying to decide on a restaurant. Your friend enjoys seafood, and you enjoy Greek food. You both agree to go to dinner on a Monday night and want a place that either does not require reservations or only recommends them and has a star rating between 3.0 and 4.2. You also do not like fast food, quick service or a diner. What are your choices?
Session 5 Business Module 3 Options	9a Preparing receipts and invoices, Question # 13. Need Registration list #1, price list, optional: invoice form 1 or 2.	9.13: Prepare a list of people who have registered for the convention but have not yet paid and are from either the West region of the United States or from outside the United States.
		Optional: These people will need an invoice. Complete invoices for each person on your list.
	Level 2: Convention Schedule Activity. Need Registration list, name card, schedule.	Here is a list of sessions and meetings at the convention as well as the day each will be held. People from Corporations, Imports, Manufacturing, and Pharmaceutical companies need to attend all of the meetings listed below. Those from Pharmaceutical companies and Corporations also need to attend the seminars while those from Manufacturing also need to attend the workshops. People from Technologies only need to attend the workshops. Indicate the estimated number of people for each session.

Toglia & Foster: The Multicontext Approach to Cognitive Rehabilitation.

Session	Materials	Directions
Session 6 **Menu or Business Module**	Supplemental Activity: Online Shopping activity: (online searching for flights and hotel).	Requires finding items from a list that meet criteria on two or three different websites. **Menu:** S.2. Online Drugstore Shopping (version 1 or 2) S.4 Online Shopping for Household Supplies (#4) S5. Online airline ticket activity S.6 Online Meal Delivery Service **Business:** S5.2 Convention Supplies S5.3 Online shopping for Office Supplies S5.1 Travels costs to attend Convention
Session 7 **Menu Module**	9B Meal Planning Question #1 (can use 1 menu or multiple menus provided).	In this activity, you need to plan what you will order for dinner for Tuesday, Wednesday, Thursday, and Friday using the menu(s). You will also need to determine the cost for each meal. For Tuesday, you prefer a fish entrée with a cold side, ice cream dessert and a cold beverage. For Wednesday, you prefer to start with a salad, a pasta entrée, hot beverage and a chocolate dessert. On Thursday, you would like an appetizer, a beef entrée with a hot side and a cold beverage. On Friday, you prefer a meat entrée, but you do not want to order beef since you had it yesterday. You also plan to order a soup, a cold side, and a chocolate dessert. Make a schedule of what you plan to order, including all necessary information and costs OR ask the client to prepare two different options.
Session 8 **Schedule Module**	Supplemental Activity: S4.2. Create a Shopping List: Peach Cobbler Recipe. Requires use of provided recipes, directions, list of items already in kitchen or use a real kitchen.	You are planning to make 24 peanut butter cookies and peach cobbler for a book club of 15 people that will be held at your house. The recipes are on the next page, but you will need to <u>double</u> the amounts for the cobbler recipe. You will also be serving beverages, including coffee, hot tea, and hot chocolate and iced tea and apple juice. Review the list of food and drink items that are already in the kitchen (listed on page labeled Kitchen Items) and make a shopping list of things that you will need on a separate piece of paper.

Note: The order of the activities within the treatment sessions above are not fixed (they can be interchanged) and are used for purposes of illustration only. Numbers correspond to # activities within the Multicontext Activity Modules.

Appendix D.7. Metacognitive Framework: Problems Encountered and How to Manage Them

Problem	Method	Sample
Before Task		
No Perceived Challenges *Before Task*	Move to activity Prompt connection to previous similar activity Draw attention to challenging task components	Person may need to experience challenges themselves if 1st or 2nd session. How is this activity like other activities we have done? What some of the challenges that were encountered last time? It seems like there is a lot of information (to keep track of, to sift through, etc.). How might that present a challenge?
No Strategy Generation *Before Task*	Move to Activity Prompt previous Connection OR Identify challenge (if not previously mentioned) Increase specificity of question, using knowledge of the person's symptoms and strategies (use task-specific strategy as a last resort).	If the person believes there is no need to use a strategy, the therapist should not try to convince them otherwise but should proceed to the activity, as strategies may be generated from activity experiences. Let's think back to our last session. How is this similar? What were some things that worked well/ did not work well? There is a lot of information and details in front of you. What can you do to help manage all of this? What can you do to help *keep track* of everything that needs to be done or what can you do to stay organized as you do this? What *could you say/repeat to yourself* that might make it easier to keep track?
Identified strategies are not really strategies (e.g., concentrate, pay attention, repeats steps or directions)	Probe for specificity Suggest strategies	Tell me more about that. What can you do to help you concentrate? There are a lot of directions. What could you do to keep track? Suggest strategies or present a choice of 2-3 strategies as a last resort or if the client repeatedly is unable to generate strategies, even after probing, directed questions, and previous task experiences.
During Task		
No Self-Monitoring	Prompt self-checking	How can you be sure....? e.g., that everything is in the right order or that you have included all the right information?
No Error Recognition	Stop and Review	Let's stop, review, and check how things are going. How can you be sure...? (same as above) Tell me your plan and how you are going about this. Let's take a careful look at ….
Symptoms or difficulties are observed	Gently reflect on observations	Seems like you might be stuck. Seems like things are getting confusing… Seems like things are not going smoothly. Let's stop and figure out some things that could help.
Strategies observed are ineffective	Encourage re-assessment of strategy Encourage alternate methods	Tell me how you are going about this? How well is _____ working? How you are keeping track of what step you are up to? Can you think of a plan to help make it easier to keep track? What else can you do to …?
Person appears to be getting overwhelmed	Stop and help person to work through it	It seems like this is getting overwhelming. Let's figure out a way to make this less overwhelming (simplify things). What could be done to break this apart? What information can be removed or covered?

Toglia & Foster: The Multicontext Approach to Cognitive Rehabilitation.

Problem	Method	Sample
	*After Task*		
Not aware of strategies	Share observations of methods that were used during the task if needed, and ask the person to explain how the methods may have helped.	What did you do to help you notice/keep track of the details? I noticed that you were underlining, can you tell me more about that. How/why did that help? I noticed you did an excellent great job of organizing the materials before you started (positive reinforcement). Tell me more about that.
Client statements are overly specific to the task	Therapist re-frame or re-interprets at a broader level	*Client mentions specific task item and therapist says....* • So it sounds like keeping track of everything was a bit challenging...let's think of what you can do to… • It seems like picking out the keywords in the instructions before you start helps to keep things on track.
Does not perceive any challenges Does not perceive any challenges, continued	Do not disagree or point out errors. Use mediation during and not after task. Consider alternate methods (video review)	Were there any parts that were easier than other parts? Provide structured self-assessment method. Focus on methods/strategies that promote success. Provide extra positive feedback on use of strategies/efficient task methods. If person is generating or using strategies, eliminate questions related to challenges. Address physical goals while simultaneously combining cognitive functional activities. Structure activity experiences to allow person to recognize errors themselves. If resistant, hostile, another approach may be more suitable.

Toglia & Foster: The Multicontext Approach to Cognitive Rehabilitation.

Appendix D.8. Things to remember During Mediated Learning

What to Do	What to Say
Probe vague responses	Expand on that. Tell me more about that. Explain that. Describe that more.
Avoid negative language (e.g., problems, difficulty)	Use words or phrases such as: challenge, obstacles, things you might need to watch out for, parts of the task that might be tricky.
"Strategy" substitutes (word substitutes)	Task methods, tricks, tips, efficient methods, smooth performance, ways to optimize performance; use special methods to stay a step ahead.
Focus on empowering the person to self-monitor & generate strategies	What could you do to . . . (e.g., manage/control, monitor, remind you)? How can you be sure that . . . ? What can you do to . . . (make things more manageable, simplify things, keep track)? Can you think of a different way you could organize this? "Let's take a look at this and try to figure it out. How can you be sure that you have all of the information you need? What could you do to help you manage all of the information on this page?
Positive reinforcement of strategy use	I noticed that . . . It's great that . . . "I noticed that you went in order and grouped the items that were similar together. That was a great idea." "It is great that you decided to underline the keywords in the directions. Why did you decide to do that?"
Reflect on observations	**It seems like it is challenging to**…. ignore some of the distractions. **Seems like things are** ….not going as smoothly as you would like….
Help the person understand why methods/strategies contributed to task success	How did that make a difference? Why did that help? "I noticed you crossed off each item in the list after you completed it. How did that help?" "I noticed it seemed to help you keep track of exactly where you were and what you needed to do next so that everything was completed."
Supportive atmosphere	Tone is even, positive, calm, neutral. Allow time for client to respond. Provide positive feedback on efficiency, task methods, monitoring. Use the sandwich method when appropriate (always starts with positive before providing constructive suggestions).
Reframe task-specific client statements	It seems . . . It like sounds like . . . "Pulling out the keywords and re-writing them into a list seems to be helping you to keep track. That is a great idea."
Miscellaneous phrases	- Let's try to figure out what is happening here. - How are you going about this? - Let's try to think of a way to make this more manageable. - What can you do to _____ (e.g., help keep track, remember, stay focused) - How can you be sure _____ (e.g., all steps were followed, everything is included) - Let's stop and review - Things are getting a bit confusing - Seems like you are stuck - Seems like it is tough to get started or figure out what to do first.

Appendix D.9. Examples of Multicontext Treatment Fidelity Analysis and Ratings

Tx Element	Therapist Transcript Examples (c=client)	Analysis	Proficient or Alternate Example
Pre-activity Discussion Anticipation and strategy generation	"What type of problems do you think you could have in a task like this?" C: *Following the directions.* "What about following the directions is difficult?" C: *I tend to gloss over things.* "Thinking about that, what are some of the strategies you can use so you follow the directions accurately?" C: *I will use the highlighter.* "Is there anything else you could do?"	The use of "challenge" instead of "difficult" or "problem" is suggested in the treatment guidelines (avoid negative language). The therapist used what the client identified as a problem to facilitate strategy generation, which nicely follows treatment guidelines. However, the word "accurately" places a focus on the task outcome or getting everything right, rather than the process. The therapist could have further probed use of the highlighter and asked a *yes/no* question, which should be avoided. *Rating:* Treatment components of anticipation and strategy generation are present, but words used and probing could be improved. This generally follows the treatment guidelines. The client vaguely identified challenges and the therapist appropriately probed further, but wording could be improved. *Adherence = 2; Proficiency = 2 emerging*	What parts of this task might be the most challenging? Tell me more about that. What about following the directions might be challenging?" Why might it be challenging to follow the directions? Tell me more about that. How will a highlighter help? What are some of the methods you can use to make it easier (or more efficient) to follow all the directions?
Pre-activity Discussion Strategy generation	After orientation to the task, therapist says, "It might be helpful to start by making a list. You did that yesterday and it really seemed to help."	Therapist does not ask client to generate strategies. The therapist is providing a strategy that she observed the client use in a previous task, but she does not ask the client to identify it. *Rating:* The treatment component of strategy generation is absent because no questions were asked that would help the client self-generate strategies. *Adherence = 1; Proficiency = 0 (since this component is missing).*	Strategy generation questions are increasingly structured when needed. "Let's look at this activity. What are some methods that you can use to help you do this task? Find all of the information that is needed? Make sure that you find all of the items on the list?"
Post-activity Discussion Challenge identification	"What challenges did you experience as you were doing this activity?" Client states she missed the location of an event and missed the time of another event. "So what you are saying is that noticing and managing all the details can be a bit challenging." "What can you do next time to make sure you can notice all the important details when there is a lot of information presented?"	The client identifies task-specific challenge, but the therapist reframes this to a broader error pattern and uses this to facilitate strategy generation. *Rating:* Treatment component is present and is considered. *Proficiency = 3.*	This is also an opportunity to provide positive feedback and reinforcement of the self-checking process. "It is great that you double-checked and corrected that." (this would be rated under general therapeutic techniques).
Post-activity Discussion Strategy Discussion	"I think you did an excellent job." "I noticed that you took time to plan ahead and stopped and checked yourself in the middle. You also did a great job of organizing all of the materials before you started".	The therapist is providing good feedback on the process and addresses strategy use in the after-task discussion, but the therapist is identifying the strategies used for the client. The treatment guidelines indicate that the client should be asked to reflect on methods used and strategy use, before sharing observations and feedback. *Rating:* Treatment component is present but little evidence of strategy discussion because no questions probing strategy use are used. *Proficiency = 1.* Use of positive feedback and encouragement is rated within the use of general therapeutic techniques section.	"Tell me how you went about doing this activity. "What methods did you use? How or why do you think they might have helped?" "Why do you think this activity went so smoothly? (compared to the last activity)? What was different?"

Toglia et al. (2020) For Additional Transcript Sample, see below website https://journals.sagepub.com/doi/suppl/10.1177/0308022619898091/suppl_file/BJO898091_Supplemental_Material2.pdf

Appendix D.10. The MultiContext (MC) Approach Presented within the Rehabilitation Treatment Specification System (RTSS)

The MultiContext (MC) Approach Presented within the Rehabilitation Treatment Specification System (RTSS) *

MC Treatment Component	Description (Key Ingredient)	Mechanism of action **Theoretical Rationale	Target for Treatment	**Treatment Differentiation (usual treatment)
Metacognitive Framework *Pre-Discussion* a) Anticipation	Guided Questioning used before each task that is directed at assessing task demands and challenges or facilitating analysis of task demands. *Questions before every task - gradually faded across treatment sessions*	*Mechanism of Action:* Metacognitive mental habit formation (size up task, assess challenge and generate strategy) with repeated practice in appraisal of task challenges or demands. *Rationale:* Directs attention to key features of task and builds anticipatory neural network. Evokes anticipatory processes. Anticipation of task challenge may engage additional neural circuitry and enhance initiation of strategies (Cicerone, 2012; Haskins, Cicerone, & Trexler, 2012; Wolf et al., 2016).	*Group:* Skills and Habits Increased ability to appraise task challenges or accurately estimate task demands in relation to abilities across different tasks.	Task is presented with directions and goals may be discussed. Guided questions about task demands are not used.
Metacognitive Framework *Pre-Discussion* b) Strategy generation	Questions that guide the person in self-generating and selecting strategies through questions and prompts. *Questions before every task - gradually faded across treatment sessions*	*Mechanism of Action:* Mental habit formation with repeated practice in self-generating (identifying and selecting) strategies before tasks. *Rationale:* Strategies that are self-generated may be more likely to be remembered and used effectively (generation effect) than those provided (Goverover, Chiaravalloti, & DeLuca, 2010; Lengenfelder, Chiaravalloti, & DeLuca, 2007). The ability to select effective strategies maximizes use of limited cognitive resources (Toglia, 2018).	*Group:* Skills and Habits Increased ability to identify effective strategies across different cognitive functional activities (with similar cognitive demands)	Therapist-directed strategy instruction Instructs the person on a strategy to use or provides strategies.
Metacognitive Framework *During Task* c) Mediates during activity if needed	Activity performance may be interrupted with brief periods of mediation or "stop and review" periods if needed, to guide the person in figuring out what is wrong and how to proceed. Mediation is used during a task if a person is unaware of performance errors or is aware but is unable to adjust methods or strategy use.	*Mechanism of Action:* opportunities to practice error management during activities; Learning by doing. *Rationale:* Mediation is effective in stimulating self-monitoring skills and helps people recognize errors or discover alternate strategies or solutions on their own. This is hypothesized to be more effective than directly pointing out errors or telling the person what to do. Awareness of performance errors within a task can facilitate strategy use (Kennedy & Coelho, 2005; Toglia & Kirk, 2000)	*Group:* Skills and Habits Improved self-monitoring skills such as error detection and correction across different tasks. Increase in initiation, frequency, appropriate timing or efficiency of strategy execution across tasks Improved error detection, correction and strategy adjustment when needed across functional tasks that have similar cognitive demands.	*If errors are observed, the therapist* Adapts task for the person to make it easier. Provides direct feedback on performance or errors are pointed out. Cues are used that provide progressive assistance or that tell a person what to do.
Metacognitive Framework *Post-Task Discussion* d) Self-assessment	Structured methods of self-checking work (e.g., checklist) or structured questions (from general to specific) are provided. Structure is gradually faded. *After every task.*	*Mechanism of Action:* Formation of mental habit with repeated practice in self-checking and self-assessing work. Repeated experience with probing questions facilitates self-reflection and appraisal of performance. *Rationale:* Self-awareness is more likely to emerge if the person discovers errors themselves. A structured method of self-checking makes it easier for the person to self-identify performance errors. Awareness of performance within the context of activities promotes strategy use and transfer of strategies to other situations (Kennedy & Coelho, 2005; Toglia, 2018).	*Group:* Skills and habits. Increased spontaneous self-checking or self-assessment across tasks. Increased ability to self-assess one's own performance (e.g., identify challenges). Increased accuracy across tasks (with similar cognitive demands).	Reviews task accuracy. Discussion on outcome rather than process. -Provides direct feedback or points out errors that need to be corrected.

Toglia & Foster: The Multicontext Approach to Cognitive Rehabilitation.

APPENDIX D: Supplementary Material 381

MC Treatment Component	Description (Key Ingredient)	Mechanism of action **Theoretical Rationale	Target for Treatment	**Treatment Differentiation (usual treatment)
Metacognitive Framework Post-Task Discussion e) Discusses strategies used	Guided questions that ask the person to explain and reflect upon task methods used and assess effectiveness. *After every task*	*Mechanism of Action:* Repeated practice in appraisal of effectiveness of strategies or task methods used. (mental habit). *Rationale:* Questions promote self-reflection and awareness of the task methods that promote success. This can eventually result in changes in knowledge, attitudes or beliefs regarding task methods, strategies and performance. Questions that prompt reflection help the person recognize that by adjusting methods or strategies used, performance can change. This increases perceived sense of control over cognitive symptoms and performance (self-efficacy) (Toglia, 2018).	*Group:* Skills and Habits Increased ability to identify effective task methods or "awareness of performance". Increased understanding of strategies and why or how they can enhance performance.	Discusses task itself and outcomes rather than the process. The session ends without reflection on the activity experience.
Metacognitive Framework Pre and/or Post-Task Discussion f) Connections between activities and strategy application	Therapist asks questions about how activity is similar to previous activities or everyday activities and/or how similar strategies could apply. *After every task*	*Mechanism of Action:* Repeated questions about similarities between tasks and strategy application provide practice in identifying connections between activity experiences (mental habit). *Rationale:* A key component of transfer involves detecting and connecting similarities across situations. Guided questions help to facilitate transfer or the ability to perceive connections between past, current, and future activity experiences (Bottiroli, Cavallini, Dunlosky, Vecchi, & Hertzog, 2017; Umanath, Toglia, & McDaniel, 2016). Repeated "bridging" questions also utilize retrieval practice and the spacing effect. This may help a person remember activity experiences, strategies or common characteristics better so that transfer occurs more easily (Sumowski et al., 2010).	*Group:* Skills and Habits. Increased ability to verbally identify similarities between activity experiences. Increased ability to identify application of strategies to other activities.	May discuss strategies that are used for the task, but discussion does not focus on application across tasks.
2. Practice of Cognitive Strategies	There is a focus on using and practicing cognitive strategies within/during activities.	*Mechanism of Action:* Learning by doing. Repeated opportunities to practice cognitive strategies within functional activities. *Rationale:* Strategies promote good information processing and are an inherent part of learning and effective performance (Pressley & Harris, 2009). Use of effective strategies may maximize cognitive resources. There is evidence that strategy-based cognitive training may increase connectivity within the cingulo-opercular and frontoparietal networks in individuals with TBI (Han, Chapman, & Krawczyk, 2018).	*Group:* Skills and Habits Increase in effectiveness of strategies observed within cognitive functional activities (increase in frequency, appropriate timing and efficiency of strategies). Increase in performance accuracy and efficiency within functional activities.	Focus on discrete cognitive impairments.
3. Activities structured to promote strategy transfer and generalization Use of multiple activities and contexts guided by use of a horizontal transfer continuum	Treatment activities are structured *horizontally* along a transfer continuum from near to far. *Variability and Practice:* The person practices strategy use in cognitive functional activities with similar cognitive demands across treatment sessions. Physical similarity between activities is gradually decreased. *Sideways (horizontal) learning:* Activities are not graded in difficulty or complexity level until application of strategies across situations are observed.	*Mechanism of Action:* Learning by doing. Repeated opportunities to practice recognizing error patterns and managing errors using the same strategies across activities. *Rationale:* It is easier to "detect and connect" activity experiences when activities look similar. Detection of similarities across activities is required for transfer and generalization (Perkins & Salomon, 2012). Repeated practice with different activities that share similarities provides opportunities to apply similar strategies broadly across different activities, over time. Learning that is spaced over time leads to better recall than massed learning (spacing effect) (Goverover, et al., 2009). Activities that have similar cognitive demands, and elicit the same performance error patterns, provide opportunities to recognize that the same error pattern occurs across activities (Toglia, 2018).	*Group:* Skills and Habit Increased transfer and generalization of strategies or Application or initiation of strategies observed *across* functional activities or situations, (resulting in increased accuracy). Increase in effectiveness of strategies observed across activities. Increased ability to self-detect or correct errors *across* tasks. Increased accuracy *across* different functional tasks (with similar cognitive demands).	Same tasks or cognitive exercises practiced until independence or mastery is achieved or... same task or cognitive exercise is gradually increased in difficulty (vertically).

Toglia & Foster: The Multicontext Approach to Cognitive Rehabilitation.

PART IV Tools, Resources, and Supplementary Material

MC Treatment Component	Description (Key Ingredient)	Mechanism of action **Theoretical Rationale	Target for Treatment	**Treatment Differentiation (usual treatment)
4. Therapeutic support focused on enhancing self-efficacy	Encourages client to figure out performance problems or identify things that might help prevent/ control cognitive symptoms. Focus is on the process or task methods used, rather that the outcome. Creates a positive and supportive atmosphere that avoids directly focusing on deficits or pointing out errors (non-confrontational). Restate/ rephrase and reframes statements; encouragement, positive feedback provided on the process (methods or strategies used, self-monitoring skills) There is an emphasis on staying a step ahead, or on what the person can do, and controlling cognitive symptoms.	*Mechanism of Action:* Attitudes, motivation/effort, Affective processing. *Rationale:* self-efficacy influences initiation of behaviors, choices about participation in activities and persistence in problematic situations. Beliefs, assumptions, and expectations about one's own cognitive functioning have a significant influence on functional performance (Rath, Hradil, Litke, & Diller, 2011). Beliefs can influence the top-down processing of information associated with successful strategy use and error correction. Helping a person anticipate and figure out successful task methods or strategies on their own can change beliefs and confidence in their ability to manage cognitive symptoms. This can also lead to changes in the functional activations and structural connectivity of the brain (Cicerone, 2012). Self-efficacy is determinant of functional performance and rehabilitation outcomes (Cicerone et al., 2008; Man, Soong, Tam, & Hui-Chan, 2006). Specifically, self-efficacy for management of cognitive symptoms has been shown to relate to life satisfaction, and community functioning in persons with TBI (Cicerone & Azulay, 2007).	*Group:* Representation. Increased cognitive self-efficacy (for strategy use and management of cognitive symptoms) Persistence and active engagement in treatment.	Identifies problems or obstacles for person and provides solutions Positive feedback on task outcome or problems (errors), rather than on the process and ability to monitor or control cognitive symptoms.
5. Cognitive activities are functionally relevant	Cognitively demanding activities include everyday functional materials so that the person readily perceives relevance.	*Mechanism of Action:* Affective processing and acquisition of self-knowledge regarding functional abilities and application of strategies. *Rationale:* Treatment activities that provide a closer resemblance to materials and activities that people use in daily life increase the likelihood of transfer of strategies to real-world functioning (Toglia, Johnston, Goverover, & Dain, 2010). Familiarity of activities also provides a benchmark from which to compare prior performance, thus facilitating the emergence of self-awareness (Toglia & Kirk, 2000). Activities that more relevant are likely to influence motivation, engagement and self-awareness (Fleming, Lucas, & Lightbody, 2006).	*Group:* Representation. Increased probability of transfer and generalization of strategies to everyday activities. Increased engagement and motivation within treatment. Increased ability to recognize connections between treatment activities, strategies used and daily life activities Increased understanding of functional abilities	Graded computerized games, exercises, or worksheets to address specific cognitive skills
6. Activities are at optimal level of cognitive challenge	Activities are not too easy and not too hard but are at an optimal challenge point.	*Mechanism of Action:* Affective processing; motivation. *Rationale:* Activities need to be at the optimal level of challenge to provide mastery experiences; that is, they allow individuals to experience and respond to actual challenges. This increases self-efficacy and engagement in treatment (Cicerone, 2012; Toglia & Kirk, 2000). The optimal level of challenge provides opportunities to practice strategies. If a task is too easy, strategies are not needed. If a task is too difficult, strategies are quickly abandoned because they are ineffective (Toglia, et al,2012).	*Group:* Representation. Increased cognitive self-efficacy Participation and engagement in treatment.	Not unique

Toglia & Foster: The Multicontext Approach to Cognitive Rehabilitation.

* Hart T, Whyte J, Dijkers M, Packel A, Turkstra L, Zanca J, Ferraro M, Chen C, Van Stan J: Manual of Rehabilitation Treatment Specification [https://mrri.org/innovations/manual-for-rehabilitation-treatment-specification/], accessed April, 2019.

** Theoretical rationale and treatment differentiation are not part of the RTSS framework and represent additional information included to clarify this approach.

Appendix D.11. Levels of Awareness and Multicontext Treatment Implications

Unawareness or Low Self-Awareness

Description: The person does not acknowledge cognitive concerns in an interview or vaguely acknowledges difficulties. Within the context of an activity, the person does not anticipate challenges or recognize the need to use special methods or strategies. The task is typically rated as easy. Performance difficulties are not recognized during or after activities at the start of treatment. The person is perplexed, surprised or neutral when errors are recognized.

	Treatment Considerations
Activities	• Use two shorter structured MC activities within 1 session, when feasible to provide the opportunity for same errors to emerge and same strategy to be practiced. Activities often simultaneously address physical goals because the person may be unaware of cognitive limitations. • Use activities along the MC transfer continuum for at least a minimum of first 4 sessions (8 activities) and then gradually progress to choosing from an activity list and then self-identifying activities.
Strategies	• Consider single strategy-specific training methods at start of treatment. For example, the same strategy such as a list is used across situations. Other strategies needed to use the main strategy effectively (underlining, checking) are gradually added. This does not require anticipatory skills and can be successful with those who have low awareness. Situational strategies may be also used or introduced as treatment progresses. • Technology such as repeated periodic text messages or alarm signals can be used to prompt self-checking or stop and review periods or provide reminders to use strategies. • Positive feedback provided for any attempts at using strategies (regardless of effectiveness), or recognizing or self-correcting errors.
Metacognitive Framework	• Eliminate pre-activity questions in initial 1-2 sessions. • Therapist will likely need to identify challenges as a context and focus for strategy generation in sessions 2-3. For example, "It might be tricky to **keep track** of all the directions. What special methods can you use to help you **keep track** of all 4 of these steps?" If no strategy generation is observed after a few activities, the therapist should suggest strategies. • Use more symptom-specific (above) or task-specific questions (e.g., It might be tricky to keep track of **which bills were paid**) early in treatment during guided questioning and then gradually broaden question content. • Use structured self-evaluation checklists whenever possible. • If client shows limited awareness with post-activity questions, video review with guided questions or **stop and review** periods within the task should be considered to facilitate error recognition and strategy generation. Role reversal techniques can also be considered.

Partial/Vague Self-Awareness

Description: The person might vaguely acknowledge cognitive concerns but minimize importance in an interview or be unable to provide specific examples. Within the context of activities, the person often overestimates performance and often does not anticipate difficulties or recognize errors during activities. After the activity, however, the person typically recognizes that the activity was more difficult than anticipated but may be unable to state why or identify performance errors unless guided to do so. The person may attempt to generate strategies, but they are often too general or ineffective. Strategy use is often inconsistent, ineffective, or inefficient. The person often does not recognize how performance difficulties in one activity relates to other activities.

	Treatment Considerations
Activities	• Structured activities are recommended with the first 4-6 activities or a minimum of 2-3 sessions and progress to either activities chosen from an activity list or self-chosen. • Once strategy use increases across situations, activities are graded vertically in difficulty.
Strategies	• Situational strategies (applied under certain conditions) or generic strategies (applied across situations) can be used. Gradually, combinations of strategies are added.
Metacognitive Framework	• Structured self-evaluation checklists are used in the first few sessions. • Anticipation questions should be skipped the first session. The person may need structured questions that facilitate links between the current activity to previous activities. • Therapist may need to initially identify challenges as a context and focus for strategy generation. For example, "There are a lot of details to watch out for. What could you do to make sure that you pay attention to all of the details?" • If ineffective or vague strategies are generated before the task, the therapist may prompt for specificity (e.g., Tell me more about that, what would you do first?) but does not provide alternate strategies. A greater emphasis is initially placed on helping the person assess strategy effectiveness within or immediately after the task. As treatment progresses, the pre-discussion is expanded to build anticipation. • The post-activity questions focus on awareness of methods used, identifying alternate strategies, or strategy revisions. • Structured journaling that includes identifying other activities where the same strategies could be used or focused action plans (e.g., to help me keep track when..., I will...) is recommended. • Guided questions are content free and focus on the process.

Toglia & Foster: The Multicontext Approach to Cognitive Rehabilitation.

Good Self-Awareness

Description: The person readily self identifies cognitive concerns and anticipates challenges. Strategies are generated, although they may not always be efficient, effective, or consistently used during activities. Strategies may be quickly abandoned, and excessive use of strategies may be observed. Errors may be recognized during and after activities, but the person may not always have a full understanding of why performance errors occurred. The person recognizes similarities between activities or situations and may become easily overwhelmed and anxious with cognitively challenging activities.

	Treatment Considerations
Activities	• Level 3 structured complex activities may be used as a starting point for managing multiple cognitive demands and coping with cognitive challenges (optional). • Self-chosen activities based on goals may be used from the start of treatment. If the person can readily recognize connections between activities, the horizontal transfer continuum may not be needed (all far and very far transfer activities can be used). • Challenging cognitive activities that the person no longer participates in should be explored. Structured cognitively challenging activities can sometimes help a person gain confidence in coping with cognitive challenges.
Strategies	• Focus on flexible strategy use including recognizing when strategies may be needed and using multiple strategies used simultaneously. A combination of strategies that are specific to certain problems or situations and generic strategies are often used. • **Cognitive logs** are used to help a person assess cognitive lapses and the current use and effectiveness of strategies. Strategy worksheets are used. • **Action or Goal Plans** are used for a person to identify problem situations along with multiple strategies that could be used • Emotional regulation strategies should be considered.
Metacognitive Framework	• Anticipation questions if needed, focus on analyzing task demands, understanding why certain task conditions present challenges or identifying unexpected problems or obstacles that could occur. • Strategy generation questions if needed, focus on identifying alternate (back-up) task methods and plans and identifying when a strategy needs to be revised or adjusted. • Guided questions are content free and focus on the process. • Structured self-evaluation checklists may not be needed. • There is a focus on helping the person assess strategy effectiveness, and make adjustments if needed • There is an emphasis on "staying a step ahead" and enhancing cognitive self-efficacy to control over managing cognitive lapses. • There is a focus on identifying other activities where the same task methods could be useful.

Toglia & Foster: The Multicontext Approach to Cognitive Rehabilitation.

Appendix D.12. Example of Multicontext Treatment Planning Worksheet (Case 1)

Client Interests/Occupations:

Worked as an inventory control manager for an electronic company and lived in his own apartment in an urban setting. Previously he prepared meals, took care of finances, grocery shopping, ordered items online such as books, music, electronics or food. Fred enjoyed going out to restaurants. He used a tablet and computer and enjoyed digital photography.

Functional Cognitive Limitations or Concerns (Activity Limitations and/or Participation Restrictions)	Cognitive Performance, Errors or Symptoms that go Across Activities	Strengths
Safety concerns Mobility (rushing, unsafe) Supervision for IADL: use of a stove in cooking Unable to accurately place pills into an organizer or appointments into a calendar, or pay bills. Unable to return to independent living.	Impulsivity observed. Jumps into tasks without preplanning and rushes without following directions accurately or adhering to rules and criteria. Performance is disorganized. Misses or omits information. Easily sidetracked by irrelevant thoughts or extraneous information.	Motivated to work on physical deficits. Demonstrates learning and retention. Recalls information from day to day. Initiates activities and conversation. Responsive to guided questions after tasks and self-recognizes some task errors with structured self-assessment. Spontaneously initiates strategies.

1. **Client Goals**
   - Goals are related to physical deficits (standing, balance, walking, increasing strength, or RUE). Would like to return to work, driving, and independent living.

2. **Client Perspective, Self-Awareness, and Metacognitive Skills** (outside and inside the context of activities)
   - Lacks general self-awareness of safety and cognitive concerns. Does not acknowledge cognitive concerns or limitations and does not recognize safety issues.
   - Online Awareness: Does not anticipate or recognize errors within activities. Acknowledges some task errors with structured self-assessment or questions after tasks but does not recognize behaviors that contributed to errors.

3. **Intervention Plan:**

   3a. What will be the initial focus of treatment? What are the targets for change?

   Build awareness and self-monitoring skills across simple IADL:
   - Ability to identify task challenges prior to an activity
   - Error recognition and/or correction during an activity
   - Recognize that similar performance errors are occurring across activities
   - Recognizes need for a strategy to manage performance errors across activities

   3b. Considerations and Reasoning: What will be the initial emphasis? How will treatment proceed?
   - The initial emphasis of treatment should be on online awareness of performance or helping Fred recognize the need to use different task methods. Treatment needs to work on building Fred's awareness of his need to pace and regulate his speed of actions within activities as a prerequisite to effective strategy use.
   - Since his stroke was only 2 weeks ago, Fred has not had the opportunity to resume many of his daily activities. Although he recognizes task errors after they occur, he is not aware that his speed of actions and tendency to become sidetracked are contributing to these errors.
   - All activities should incorporate Fred's physical goals (building standing tolerance, RUE strength and ambulation). Fred's concerns are related to his physical limitations, so treatment activities need to address his physical concerns and goals while simultaneously providing the opportunity to engage in cognitive functional activities.

Toglia & Foster: The Multicontext Approach to Cognitive Rehabilitation.

- Treatment will begin with structured cognitive activities. Repeated opportunity to experience activities that result in similar error patterns will help Fred self-recognize errors as well as strategies that can control the errors across activities, using the transfer continuum.
- Goal rating techniques are deferred until the client has had the opportunity to experience more activities. As awareness emerges, it is expected that Fred will revise and add goals. Targeted simplified self-ratings of speed of response will be used to help Fred recognize error patterns and learn to monitor his speed of response.

4. **Building Awareness/Self-Monitoring or Regulation of Symptoms:** How and when will awareness and self-monitoring skills be addressed (Before, during, after activities)? Are structured self-assessments needed? Do other techniques need to be considered (video review, role reversal)?

   - Pre-activity questions and mediation will be skipped in the first 1-2 sessions.
   - Use structured self-assessments for Fred to self-check work.
   - Used guided questions during and after activities initially to build self-awareness.
   - Consider targeted self-rating of timing (too fast, just right), video review, or role reversal if awareness doesn't show changes in the first 2 sessions.

5. **Strategies:**

   5a. Type of Strategy Training: flexible use of strategies that can be used across situations.

   5b. Identify possible strategies that would help the Fred control or reduce errors <u>across</u> different activities.

   Identifying effective strategies beforehand can help the therapist structure the strategy generation process if needed.

Identify Possible Strategies Internal or external strategy or a combination of both	Sample Structured Guiding questions (if needed) for strategy generation
Internal Strategies • Self-selected visual images, metaphors, pictures or symbols to cue self to regulate actions (e.g., calm ocean, stop sign) • Use a self-cue with an image • Stop, Plan, Review • Verbalize a plan ahead of time/verbal self-talk during activity to help regulate action	*If Fred has difficulty initiating strategies:* What type of image or picture can you think of to help you use "just right timing" or to control that tendency to go too quickly? What can you say to yourself to help you remember to stop and plan ahead? To use good "timing" as you do this activity?
External strategies, devices or adaptations used by client • Create a Checklist and imagine using it before action. • Alarm reminders or automatic text reminders with "Stop-plan-review". • Alarm to interrupt activity then stop and check (Am I using good timing? Am I sticking with my plan?). • Learn to remove distractions before beginning a task.	What can you do to remind yourself to ___ (e.g., Stop, Plan, Review)? Can you think of ways that technology might be able to help remind you to use "just right timing?" How could a alarm reminder help? What can you do to make it easier to stay focused? Ignore distractions or the tendency to become sidetracked? What can you remove to make it easier to focus?

   5c. Identify potential obstacles to strategy use and plans to address them:

   Self-awareness and lack of anticipation or recognition of errors withing performance

6. **Training for Generalization:** Think of activities that would require repeated practice in controlling key task errors or symptoms. Consider the starting point and the activity or environment characteristics that increase the likelihood of errors. Activities should be at an optimal level of challenge – not too easy and not too hard. Consider Multicontext Activity Modules, if appropriate.

   6a. Brainstorm sample activities that can be used to help client recognize error patterns in performance or practice generating and using similar strategies. Consider goals, interests, experiences, roles, or responsibilities as well as any physical considerations.

   Activities that involve standing, walking, reaching, and involve the kitchen, taking inventory, computers, online shopping.

Toglia & Foster: The Multicontext Approach to Cognitive Rehabilitation.

6b. After brainstorming activities, arrange activities on a horizontal continuum

Activity Theme: What activity demands will remain consistent across activities?

- Activities will involve using a list to locate items and record specific information or details while standing, reaching, or walking.

Very Similar:	Somewhat Similar:	Different:
1. *Initial Activity:* List On Counter. Retrieve Ingredients And Write Calories On List.	1. List On Table, Menu On Bulletin Board. Find The Items On The Menu And Write The Price Next To It.	1. Use List To Find Items On The Unit Or Floor And Write Location Next To Each Item On The List.
2. Search For And Locate Kitchen Supplies From A List, And Write Location Of Items On List Or Take Inventory (# Of Plates, Coffee Cups Etc).	2. List On Table. Search For And Locate Items And Supplies From The List And Take Inventory. Place Number Of Items Available Next To Each Item On The List.	2. Find Items In Gift Shop From A List And Write Down Price.

7. *Optional:* **Will goal rating, subgoaling or focused goal planning be used?**
   - Goal rating will be deferred until awareness emerges.

8. **Identify techniques that will be used for "strategy bridging" and reinforcement**
   - Help Fred identify similarities and connections between activities through guided questions and structured journaling if time permits.

9. **How will you collaborate with others (care partners, other professionals) to support intervention methods or goals?**
   - Work with PT and nursing to carry over guided use of strategies to control timing and pace of actions. If feasible, include Fred's significant others in treatment sessions.

10. **Other intervention considerations:**
    - Technology to support performance – Consider possible use of automatic text strategy reminders (see Chapter 14)
    - Specific task or environment adaptations (context dependent) - Consider adaptations for medication management.

Toglia & Foster: The Multicontext Approach to Cognitive Rehabilitation.

Appendix D.13. SUBGOALING Example

Main Goals

1. Increase independence in daily activities (fewer verbal reminders and less reliance on his wife).
2. Increase participation in social and leisure activities.
3. Ability to resume volunteer job.

Areas of Concern (Sub-Goals)	Strengths within skill area	Subskills that need to be strengthened and sample strategies	Simulated tasks agreed upon by Client and/or Family member
Spontaneously initiate household tasks without reminders	Can do all household tasks	"Getting started" without reminders and recognizing things that need to be done • Follow written lists or auditory reminder cues	Practice looking around at different environments (kitchen, clinic, home living room) and initiate making written lists of things that need to be done.
* Initiate social conversations, and activities (letters, telephone calls, etc.)	Gets along well with people	• Ability to generate or initiate a variety of ideas or topics • Cue card of topics • Outlines with broad categories	Practice in tasks requiring generating ideas or different options for conversations, letters.
* Initiate previous interests. Ability to plan and organize open-ended activities	Wide range of previous interests (music, movies, poetry, sports, woodworking)	• Tendency to get "stuck" • Ability to shift attention and keep track of all parts. • Use strategies such as checklists and metal practice	• Practice in unstructured activities requiring generating alternatives, planning, and organizing. • Plan and organize a woodworking project, investigate concerts, and compare prices.
** Less reliance on others to keep track of things to do and recall events that have occurred	Can follow routine lists, remembers parts of things	Ability to keep track of information. • Use of an organized system (daily planner) • Initiate efficient use of strategies: key retrieval cues, mental rehearsal	• Practice initiating and using an organized book for retrieval. • Practice rehearsing and summarizing key points from conversations, readings, movies, events.
Following instructions and lists to completion without verbal assistance or reminders	Can follow routine lists	Sometimes gets stuck on pieces "gets thrown off" Misinterprets instruction due to failure to "shift" • Time monitoring strategies • Underline key steps • Self-checking and comparison to original instructions.	Practice in following tasks with multiple-step task instructions (following a list requiring Xeroxing and collating forms according to rules, follow directions for an unfamiliar electronic device, follow directions on a map).

** Identified as the area of greatest concern; Placed on Goal Attainment Scale

Toglia & Foster: The Multicontext Approach to Cognitive Rehabilitation.

Appendix D.14 SUBGOALING Example 2 related to Work as a Claims Analyst (Chapter 12)

Skills needed for work as an Claims Analyst	Strengths within skill area	Subskills that need to be strengthened	Simulated tasks agreed upon by Client and/or Family member
Accurately recall conversations and reports which have been read	Remembers who was spoken to and the general topic of conversation or of what was read.	Needs to work on remembering all parts of a conversation or story as well as the important details.	Practice role-playing conversations; reading paragraphs using strategies to increase retention.
Compare and contrast information from different reports and pick-up inconsistencies	Comprehension of paragraphs is good	Work on summarizing 2 or 3 different paragraphs on the same subject and recognizing discrepancies between information from different sources.	Practice detecting inconsistencies within stories, written reports.
Prioritize tasks that need to be done during the day	Can generate a list of tasks that need to be done and makes a list	Work on organizing lists – for example, grouping similar tasks and prioritizing.	Practice prioritizing various scenarios of things that need to be done in a day.
Interview customers: probe, investigate, ask many questions	Friendly Personable Follows structured interview	Probe responses and work on recognizing inconsistencies in the person's report.	Role reversal with Therapist. Therapist plays a difficult, demanding customer with many inconsistencies in her story and a passive, quiet customer who requires extensive probing.
Write a summary of Interview	Good sentence structure. Reports things that have been said.	Summarize rather than state what has been said.	Given notes from an interview, pick out main points and then write a summary.

Toglia & Foster: The Multicontext Approach to Cognitive Rehabilitation.

Appendix D.15. Example of a Completed Goal Plan

Goal: Will make pasta and a salad for dinner and set the table one time a week.

What do I need to do to prepare: Identify day and time, discuss with John. Make a list of everything I need. Check kitchen. Make a shopping list for John of needed items.

Parts of this task I can do easily	Areas for Improvement	Strategies
Filling pot with water and cooking pasta Heating sauce Getting all the items I need Preparing the salad Setting the table	Plan amounts and stay organized. Keep track of what I just did. Keep track of pasta on the stove. Coordinate the timing and do things in the right order. Stay "on task"	Clean the counter and make sure it is not cluttered before I start. Write down what I need to do in order and then cross it off after I complete it Take out everything I need and place in order before I start. Plan how much I need in advance. Use the timer on the stove for the pasta. Set the table before I start.
Things I need to watch out for: Phone calls, text messages or interruptions Getting sidetracked by something else I see.		Will keep my cell phone in my bedroom so it will not distract me. Will repeat keywords to help me keep track. Will keep picturing my end goal "dinner on the table" to help me stay focused.
Other Activities that this Same Plan and/or Strategies might be useful with		Invite a friend over for lunch. Pay my bills online

Toglia & Foster: The Multicontext Approach to Cognitive Rehabilitation.

Appendix D.16. Examples of Functional Goals Consistent with the Multicontext Approach (for therapist)

Short-Term Goals Related to Self-Care Skills *(time frame needs to be included)*

- Client will use strategies to consistently choose relevant objects for safe and independent performance of grooming tasks (e.g., shaving, brushing teeth).
- Client will demonstrate reduced safety risk as demonstrated by accuracy in predicting need for assistance prior to transferring from wheelchair to bed 80% of the time.
- Client will sustain attention on a task for 5 minutes, as a prerequisite for safe performance during eating.
- Client will increase attention to environment as demonstrated by ability to identify four out of five potentially hazardous situations (obstacles, untied shoelace, unlocked brakes on wheelchair).
- Client will initiate left-sided visual scanning four out of five times to reduce safety risks and increase ability to attend to potentially hazardous obstacles present on the left side of the environment the majority of the time.
- Client will complete grooming with pre-selected items and a decreased level of verbal assistance (2-3 general cues rather than 2-3 directive cues).
- Client will refer to cue signs 50% of the time during dressing, as an initial step in decreasing need for continuous verbal assistance.
- Client will sustain attention towards a goal, using self-monitoring strategies, as demonstrated by independent completion of a 4- to 5-step simple meal preparation activity.
- Client will demonstrate use of talk aloud strategies 80% of the time to reduce speed of response and increase safety during self-care activities and decrease the need for verbal assistance to 20%.
- Client will remember to lock the wheelchair brakes prior to standing five out of six times.
- Caregiver will demonstrate ability to use appropriate cues and structure to enhance attention and decrease need for physical assistance during self-feeding.
- Family members will demonstrate proper cueing and task structuring and to elicit optimal participation (supervision only) in routine self-care activities.

Short-Term Goals Related to IADL and Productive Activities *(time frame needs to be included)*

Based on EFPT type of Baseline rating: (rating of underlying EF components)

- Client will be able to complete a bill-paying task with only 1-2 general cues for organization and sequencing.
- Client will be able to use a list to enter 10 appointments into a schedule (*baseline WCPA – 3 missing appointments*).
- Client will be able to accurately enter 8/10 items into a schedule (*baseline WCPA – 6/10*).
- Client will be able to make a hot lunch with an Executive Function Performance (EFPT) rating of 3-4 (EFPT baseline for oatmeal = 5-6; *higher scores indicate more assistance*).

Based on Kettle Task Rating or # of task steps/components completed independently

- Client will be able to complete five out of seven steps in a bill-paying task (or other task such as calling for information, making lunch) independently (baseline = 3/7 steps).

Based on types of errors (also includes counting of accurate steps)

- Client will demonstrate the ability to restrain impulsive responses and pre-plan prior to multiple-step activities as demonstrated by ability to accurately complete 5/8 errands from a list (independently).

Toglia & Foster: The Multicontext Approach to Cognitive Rehabilitation.

General Goals *(Therapist should add time frame, relate to client work or IADL activities)*

- Client will reduce safety risks through spontaneous self-checking and error monitoring as evidenced by ability to
  - Accurately enter eight pills into a medication organizer, according to directions from one medication bottle.
  - Adhere to budget and dietary restrictions items when ordering from a menu.
  - Accurately place doctor appointment or medication schedule into a calendar.
- Client will be able to consistently refer to a written list as a means of independently completing 5/8 steps to make a hot lunch *(baseline – refers to list 25% of time)*.
- Client will use goal management strategies to stay on task (without becoming sidetracked) 4 out of 5 times during _____ (e.g., meal preparation tasks, writing an e-mail, online shopping).
- Client will keep track of steps that have been completed through successful use of strategies, as demonstrated by ability to enter at least nine out of ten appointments into a daily calendar.
- Client will effectively use verbal rehearsal strategies to recall and carry out 2- to 3-step directions without reminders 90% of the time.
- Client will be able to remember 2-3 words that were just read as evidenced by ability to successfully gather 2-3 correct ingredients from a kitchen cabinet (as a prerequisite to meal preparation).
- Client will independently monitor and self-recognize 80% of errors in a 6- to 8-step activity (as a prerequisite for effective completion of multistep activities (e.g. making lunch).
- Client will anticipate the need to use a list with guided questions, as a prerequisite to initiating effective strategy use and successfully completing a 5- to 7-step simple cooking activity.
- Client will create and use a list 80% of the time as a means of effectively completing 6-8 multiple-step IADL activities (e.g., making a phone call to obtain information; ordering take-out food online, setting alarm reminders for daily errands).
- Client will complete four key daily tasks with alarm reminders 80% of the time.
- Client will set alarm reminders independently 70% of the time as a prerequisite to effectively managing appointments (or taking medications at scheduled time).
- Client will self-generate one effective strategy for accurate completion of 4- to 6-step tasks.
- Client will use cognitive strategies to select relevant information and attend to details as demonstrated by accurately copying information from a 10-item list into a weekly schedule.
- Client will follow an established schedule (or list of errands) 85% of the time as a prerequisite to return to work.
- Client will consistently follow a 6-step list, when performing a multistep task within a distracting environment, as a prerequisite to return to work.
- Client will initiate asking for medications using a checklist and alarm 75% of the time as a prerequisite to independence in medication management.
- Client will use strategies to keep track of steps (e.g., list, verbal rehearsal) as a means of safely preparing a 6-step hot lunch or dinner 90% of the time.
- Client will demonstrate increased visual scanning skills as demonstrated by ability to identify all important signs in a crowded environment and safely cross the street.
- Client will demonstrate increased awareness of limitations as evidenced by recognition of performance errors in 4- to 6-step activities, 80% of the time as a prerequisite to independent use of compensatory strategies.
- Client will increase accuracy and attention to detail in complex visual tasks (reading train schedule, map, scanning a grocery store shelf) to 85% as a prerequisite to returning to independent functioning within the community.

Toglia & Foster: The Multicontext Approach to Cognitive Rehabilitation.

- Client will demonstrate frequent self-monitoring or self-checking strategies to reduce omission errors and promote attention to 85% of relevant details within bill paying tasks. (medication management tasks).
- Client will effectively use electronic cognitive supports to independently carry out three selected daily tasks 90% of the time.
- Client will use effective strategies to identify relevant details in written instructions, 80% of the time as a prerequisite for work-related tasks.
- Client will use effective strategies to follow a 10-item list without errors (for example, searches and locates all items from a list within the kitchen).
- Client will demonstrate initiation of self-monitoring strategies 80% of the time to reduce errors on work-related tasks (or bill paying, copying lists, interpreting charts and graphs, etc.)
- Client will demonstrate talk aloud strategies to increase ability to shift attention in problem-solving tasks 80 % of the time (e.g., figuring out directions, bill paying) as a prerequisite to return to work.
- Client will initiate use of organizational strategies in unstructured tasks 85% of the time (shopping, investigating information, finding a new destination) as a prerequisite to return to independence in the community.

Long-Term Goals

- Increase efficiency of cognitive perceptual skills and strategies for independence in self-care activities.
- Increase efficient use of cognitive-perceptual strategies for independent functioning within the community.
- Increase awareness of deficits so that client can successfully use compensation strategies for independence in self-care (community).
- Increase ability of caregiver to select appropriate cues and use adaptations so that client can be managed at home.
- Maximize use of residual skills and strengths so that client can engage in productive activities such as part-time volunteer work.

Toglia & Foster: The Multicontext Approach to Cognitive Rehabilitation.

Appendix D.17 Example of Goal Ratings

Functional Goal: Manage my schedule without difficulty for one week.

Levels of performance	Achievement	Rating
Independently manages schedule without difficulty (100%)	Goal is met	5
Manages schedule without difficulty the majority of the week (75%)	Almost met	4
Manages schedule without difficulty about half the time (50%)	Partially met	3
Manages schedule occasionally without difficulty (25%)	Lots of room for improvement	2
Does not manage schedule without difficulty (daily errors of missing appointments, meetings, or errands, forgetting to enter appointments or events, double booking appointments) (0%)	0% or baseline	1

Specific Strategy Goal: Pre-plan in IADL tasks with > 5 steps.

Levels of performance	Achievement	Rating
Pre-plans all the time when needed (100%)	Goal is met	5
Pre-plans the majority of the time, when needed (75%)	Almost met	4
Stops and pre-plans the half of the time (50%)	Partially met	3
Stops and pre-plans some of the time (25%)	Lots of room for improvement	2
Jumps into task without pre-planning (e.g., does not review directions, outline what needs to be done or gather needed items) (0%)	0% or baseline	1

General Self-Monitoring Goal: Review and check work.

Levels of performance	Achievement	Rating
Reviews and checks work consistently (100%)	Goal is met	5
Reviews and checks work the majority of the time (75%)	Almost met	4
Reviews and checks work about half of the time (50%)	Partially met	3
Reviews and checks work occasionally (25%)	Lots of room for improvement	2
Does not stop to review or double-check work (0%)	0% or baseline	1

Toglia & Foster: The Multicontext Approach to Cognitive Rehabilitation.